Medicinal Chemistry and Pharmacology

Medicinal Chemistry and Pharmacology

Edited by Avianna Stokes

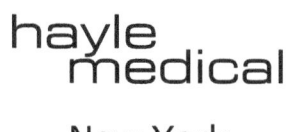

hayle
medical

New York

Hayle Medical,
750 Third Avenue, 9th Floor,
New York, NY 10017, USA

Visit us on the World Wide Web at:
www.haylemedical.com

ISBN: 978-1-63241-535-6

Cataloging-in-Publication Data

Medicinal chemistry and pharmacology / edited by Avianna Stokes.
   p. cm.
Includes bibliographical references and index.
ISBN 978-1-63241-535-6
1. Pharmaceutical chemistry. 2. Pharmacology. 3. Drug development. I. Stokes, Avianna.
RS403 .M44 2019
615.19--dc23

Table of Contents

Preface

Over the recent decade, advancements and applications have progressed exponentially. This has led to the increased interest in this field and projects are being conducted to enhance knowledge. The main objective of this book is to present some of the critical challenges and provide insights into possible solutions. This book will answer the varied questions that arise in the field and also provide an increased scope for furthering studies.

Medicinal chemistry and pharmacology are closely associated fields. They are concerned with the design and synthesis of drugs for the pharmaceutical industry. These drugs are generally organic compounds and can be divided into classes of biologics and small organic compounds. Medicinal chemistry is focused on the production of small organic molecules such as atorvastatin, fluticasone, clopidogrel, etc. The principles of synthetic organic chemistry, computational chemistry, enzymology, structural biology and chemical biology are integrated in medicinal chemistry. The study of drugs and their effects on the living body are explored in pharmacology. It involves the research, discovery and characterization of the chemicals that exhibit a biological effect. All therapies that are designed to target diseases, defects and pathogens and also advance preventive care, diagnostics and personalized medicine are a result of tremendous research in pharmacology. This book is a compilation of chapters that discuss the most vital concepts and emerging trends in the fields of medicinal chemistry and pharmacology. The various advancements in these fields are glanced at and their applications as well as ramifications are looked at in detail. This book is a vital tool for all researching and studying pharmaceutical science and medicinal chemistry.

I hope that this book, with its visionary approach, will be a valuable addition and will promote interest among readers. Each of the authors has provided their extraordinary competence in their specific fields by providing different perspectives as they come from diverse nations and regions. I thank them for their contributions.

Editor

Acute Co-Administration of the Cannabinoid Receptor Agonist WIN 55- 212,2 does not Influence 3,4-Methylenedioxymetamphetamine (MDMA)-Induced Effects on Effort-Based Decision Making, Locomotion, Food Intake and Body Temperature

Schulz S [1*], Gundelach J[1], Hayn L[1], Koch M[1] and Svärd HK[2]

[1]Brain Research Institute, Department of Neuropharmacology, University of Bremen, 28359 Bremen, Germany
[2]University of Oulu, Department of Biology, FIN-90140 University of Oulu, Finland

Abstract

Acute behavioural effects of co-administration of the illegal drug 3,4-methylenedioxymethamphetamine (MDMA, 7.5.mg/kg, s.c.) and the synthetic cannabinoid receptor agonist WIN55212-2 (WIN, 1.2mg/kg, i.p.) in rats were investigated. MDMA impaired performance on a T-maze effort-based decision making task. MDMA and MDMA+WIN treatment increased body temperature to a similar extent, whereas WIN increased temperature at an earlier time point. Locomotion, exploratory behaviour and food intake was comparable in MDMA and MDMA+WIN-treated animals. MDMA-induced decreased exploration anxiety in the open field was diminished by WIN. In summary, acute co-administration of the cannabinoid receptor agonist did not substantially modulate the MDMA-induced behavioural effects.

Keywords: MDMA; WIN 55212-2; Co-administration; Acute effects; Effort-based decision making; Body temperature; Locomotion; Food intake.

Introduction

Polydrug use has become a challenging issue in research involving human drug users [1]. For example, most 3,4-methylenedioxymetamphetamine (MDMA) users are polydrug users [2]. Cannabis is the most frequently taken illegal co-drug: 98% of a representative sample of MDMA users concomitantly use cannabis [3,4]. Combined effects on physiological, behavioural and cognitive measures are difficult to disentangle and may depend on frequency, duration, and amount of co-consumption. Furthermore, many human studies involve chronic and/or heavy polydrug users, thus causal relationships between single drugs and their effects are hard to discern. Many MDMA users report smoking cannabis concomitantly to enhance positive sensations (for example, euphoria, empathy, prosocial behaviour, energy) or sometime after MDMA consumption to alleviate adverse effects (anxiety, depression, anhedonia and agitation) of the "come-down" [5-7].

Acute MDMA administration leads to a transient, dose-dependent release and reuptake inhibition of the neurotransmitters serotonin (5-hydroxytryptamine, 5-HT) and dopamine (DA) and to a lesser extent noradrenaline (NA) and acetylcholine (ACh) [8], particularly in the medial prefrontal cortex (mPFC), striatum and hippocampus [7,9]. Increased 5-HT transmission contributes to the behavioural effects of MDMA in a complex way which additionally seems to depend on the interaction with DA transmission (10). In accordance with reported effects in human users, acute effects of MDMA-administration in animals include hyperthermia [8,11], hyper-locomotion [12], anxiety (Cole and Sumnall), and hypophagia [13,14]. Few studies have tested the acute effects on more complex behaviour. A decrease in impulsivity in humans as well as a dose-dependent increase of lever pressings for reinforcement in animals' byVollenweider et al [15] was shown after MDMA administration.

In contrast, the main psychoactive compound of cannabis, delta9-tetrahydrocannabinol (delta9-THC) acts as an inhibitory transmitter on presynaptic cannabinoid (CB) type 1 (CB1) and type 2 (CB2) receptors within the endo cannabinoid system. Activation of CB1 seems to modulate neurotransmission [16]. In the CNS, a high abundance of CB1 receptors has been found in basal ganglia, cerebellum, olfactory bulb and hippocampus, moderate density appears in cortical areas [17]. Results from acute studies in animals employing delta9-THC, or one of the more potent synthetic CB1 receptor agonists (e.g., WIN 55-212,2, CP 55,940) or antagonists (e.g., SR 171416) support reports obtained from human studies in that cannabinoids are implicated in the acute regulation of several physiological processes. For example, acute consumption of delta9-THC increases heart rate and postural instability, impulsive responding on certain tasks, decreases alertness and influences time- estimations in humans [18,19]. In animals, activation of CB receptors increases food intake and heart rate, dose-dependently affects locomotor behaviour and decreases body temperature [20-22].

Behavioural and neurobiological effects of sole administration of MDMA or cannabis are well documented (for review see [7,23,24]) and some studies examine the long-term cognitive consequences of co-consumption of these drugs [25-27]. Literature on the consequences of acute co-consumption is less thorough. One human study demonstrated mixed effects: co-administration of cannabis prolonged the onset and duration of MDMA-induced increases in temperature, but had no additive influence on deficits in memory. Delta9-THC-induced psychomotor impairments independent of MDMA [28].

Corresponding author: Sybille Schulz, Brain Research Institute Department of Neuropharmacology, University of Bremen, Hochschulring 18, Room 212028359 Bremen, Germany, E-mail: s.schulz@uni-bremen.de

Positive subjective ratings were increased for the combination of the drugs compared to each drug effects alone [29]. Some evidence from rodent studies shows regulatory effects of co-administration on locomotion, body temperature, and reinforcing effects. For example, prevention of MDMA-induced hyperthermia, anxiety, and a decrease of MDMA-induced hyperactivity due to delta9-THC was observed in rats [12]. Impairment of working memory upon co-administration of low and medium doses of MDMA plus delta9-THC was shown (Young et al., 2005). In terms of drug reinforcing properties, intra-cerebroventricular (i.c.v.) self-administration studies demonstrate a modulation of MDMA- induced reinforcing effects (self-administration or conditioned place preference (CPP)) by cannabinoid agents [30,31]. In mice, exposure to WIN in adolescence later facilitated MDMA-induced CPP [32] or potentiated the rewarding effects of MDMA [33]. In the latter study, the CB1 antagonist SR 171416 did not block the effects of WIN. Furthermore, in CB1-knock-out mice, pre-treatment with delta9-THC still prevented MDMA-induced acute responses [34] pointing towards a CB1-independent mechanism of interaction. The effects of acute co-administration on cognitive tasks, for example choice behaviour, have not been investigated.

This study aimed to further elucidate the interactive effects seen after acute co-administration of MDMA and Cannabis. The synthetic specific CB receptor agonist WIN 55212-2-2 (WIN) was used to investigate interactions of MDMA and CB receptor stimulation, aiming to narrow the range of effects of delta9-THC in the central nervous system. For the first time, the effect of acute MDMA administration as well as the combined administration of MDMA and a cannabinoid agonist on effort-based choice behaviour is investigated, in addition to locomotion, food intake and body temperature measures.

Material and Methods

Animals

In total, 39 adult naive male Wistar rats (Harlan, Borchen, Germany) weighing 230-300 grams were used in these experiments. Upon arrival, animals were allowed to habituate for 4-5 days in a vivarium under standardized conditions (4-6 animals per Makrolon type IV cage; tap water ad libitum; 12 hour light/dark circle, lights on at 7am; temperature 22+/- 2°C) and were handled regularly. During the habituation and handling period, standard lab chow was available ad libitum. Controlled feeding (12g/animal/day) started two days before the first training session. All animal experiments were conducted in accordance with the principles of animal care and the international laws on animal experiments (Directive 2010/63/EU) and were approved by the local authorities.

Drugs

All drugs were prepared freshly before administration and were injected in a volume of 1ml/kg. WIN 55212-2-2 (SIGMA-Aldrich, Steinheim, Germany) was dissolved in 2% Tween®80 (Serva, Heidelberg, Germany) and 98% NaCl solution (0.9% NaCl, Fresenius Kabi GmbH, Bad Homburg, Germany) and injected at a dose of 1.2mg/kg, intraperitoneally (i.p.). MDMA hydrochloride (synthesized in the Institute of Inorganic Chemistry, Prof. Nagel, University of Tübingen. Identity and chemical purity was verified) was dissolved in phosphate buffered saline (PBS), stabilizing a well-tolerated pH-value of the solution, and injected at a dose of 7.5mg/kg, subcutaneously (s.c.). PBS injection served as vehicle control. Single doses which have been shown to be behaviourally relevant (Drews et al., 2005; Young et al., 2005) were chosen in order to minimize the number of animals used in this study.

Behavioural tests

Behavioural testing was conducted in a between subjects design. Each treatment group consisted of n=10 rats, except the combination (MDMA+WIN) group (n=9). Each animal underwent the same training and testing procedures. However, the sequence of tests was altered in order to minimize the influence of repeated substance administration and previous behavioural tasks. All animals started with training and subsequent testing in the effort-based decision making task. Half of each treatment group were tested in an open field one week later, followed by a food preference test another week later. The second half of the group underwent the food preference task first, followed by the open field tests. After each tests, a wash-out period of seven days was allowed for all animals. Contrary to other reports [35], there were no observable adverse effects upon first, or subsequent, exposure to the cannabinoid agonist. MDMA was administered 30mins and WIN 10mins prior to testing to allow examination of behaviour during the peak time of effect. The combined treatment was timed in such a way that the peak time of the effects accumulated at the time of testing. Half (n=5) of the control (vehicle) group was injected 10mins prior to testing, the other half (n=5) 30mins before.

Effort-based decision making

The effects of MDMA, WIN, and the combination of both drugs on effort-based decision making were tested in a T-maze paradigm. This task allows monitoring of cost-benefit choice behaviour, i.e., how much effort the animal is willing to exert to obtain a (larger) reward. At the end of the reward arms of the T-maze (measurements of each arm: 60 cm x 15 cm x 30 cm (L x W x H)) either two or four pellets (Bio-Serv©, UK Dustless Precision Pellets©, 45mg) were placed in a metal food well. While the arm containing two pellets (low reward arm, LR) was freely accessible for the rats, a 30 cm barrier made of wire mesh was placed in the arm containing four pellets (high reward arm, HR). The HR was the right side T-maze arm for half of the animals, and left side for the other half. All animals were habituated to the apparatus as well as increasing heights of the barrier and pre-trained until as a group they reached baseline level of ≥ 80% choice of HR for three consecutive days. Intertrial interval (ITI) was 1 min. Habituation and pre-training sessions took place once a day for an average of 16 days (for further detail on apparatus and training method see [36], adapted from the original study by Salamone (1994)). For the test the animals received drugs or vehicle as described above and performed two forced choice runs (one to each arm, in pseudo-randomized order), prior to ten free choice runs. The percentage of choices for the HR arm was calculated for each treatment group.

Body temperature

Temperature was measured with an in-ear thermometer (Thermoscan, IRT3020 CO, Braun, Switzerland) at three different time points: A baseline measurement one day before the first testing in the effort-based task was done in order to rule out effects of the injection procedure. A second measurement was done before the animals were tested (i.e., at the respective peak times of effects of the substances, T1), and a third time 1 hour after the test (T2). At each time point, temperature was measured three consecutive times, and the mean of these three measures was considered the temperature value for that time point.

Locomotor activity

Animals were placed in infrared beam-controlled acrylic glass chambers (ActiMot-system; TSE, Bad Homburg, size: 44.7 cm x

Acute Co-Administration of the Cannabinoid Receptor Agonist WIN 55-212,2 does not Influence...

3

44.7 cm x 44 cm) measuring horizontal and vertical locomotion. Locomotion and exploratory behaviour was automatically recorded by a PC (ActiMot Software; TSE, Bad Homburg) for 35 minutes and stored as aggregated data in seven intervals. Parameters analysed were number of rearings, total activity (%), and time spent in centre (%) per 5-minute interval.

Food preference test

Animals were placed in a standard Makrolon type II cage with two glass food wells each containing pellets (Bio-Serv©, UK Dustless Precision Pellets©, 45mg) or breeding chow (Altromin, Lage, Germany). Breeding chow and pellets only differed in palatability, not in protein (22.5%, 18.7%, respectively) or fat (5%, 5.6%, respectivley) content. Animals were allowed to free-feed for 10mins. Animals had not eaten for 20+/-2 hours when testing was conducted. Mass of eaten food was weighed for each animal.

Data analysis

For statistical analysis, analyses of variance (ANOVAs) were conducted with SigmaStat2.03 for Windows (SPSS Inc., Chicago, IL, USA), followed by post hoc Tukey tests for pairwise multiple comparisons. For all measurements, $p < 0.05$ was considered a significant difference.

Results

Effort-based decision making

One animal from the MDMA+WIN group was unable to complete the task and therefore was excluded, thus yielding n=10 for MDMA, WIN and vehicle groups, and n=8 for the MDMA+WIN group for the statistical analysis. MDMA- and MDMA+WIN-treated animals chose the high reward (HR) arm less often compared to the WIN and vehicle groups (51% and 57% vs. 82% and 95%, respectively, Figure 1). A one-way ANOVA yielded a significant difference of HR choices between treatment groups [$F(3,34)= 3.50, p=0.026$]. The post-hoc test revealed a significant difference between the vehicle and MDMA group (mean HR choice= 95%, 51%, respectively, p= 0.034). While the combined treatment (MDMA+WIN) reduced choices for the HR, this effect failed to reach significance (Mean: 57%, p=0.117). (Figure 1)

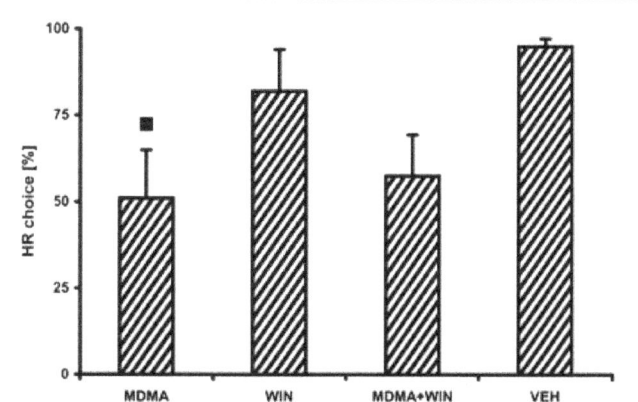

Figure 1: Effects of acute MDMA (n=10), WIN (n=10), MDMA+WIN (n=8) and vehicle (n=10) administration on effort-based decision making. Bars depict the percentage means (+SEM) of HR choices (large reward obtained by climbing the 30cm barrier) during the behavioral test sessions. Closed square denotes p<0.05 compared to vehicle.

Body temperature

One hour after behavioural testing (T2), body temperature was increased in rats treated with MDMA (mean: 37.4°C) and MDMA+WIN (mean: 37.5°C) compared to baseline (BL) and to measurements 30 minutes after administration (T1). WIN-treated animals showed an increase in temperature 10 minutes after administration (37.3°C, BL: 36.6.°C; (Figure 2). A two-way ANOVA yielded a significant effect of time point of measurement [$F(2,44)=15.41, p<0.001$] as well as a significant interaction of time point x substance ($F(6,44)= 3.40, p=0.008$). Post-hoc test revealed significant differences comparing treatment groups MDMA+WIN vs. WIN measured before the first run (T1) (p=0.007). Furthermore, significant differences were found within MDMA and MDMA+WIN groups between measurements taken one hour after behavioural testing (T2) and BL (p=0.001 and p<0.001) as well as between T1 and T2 (p=0.017 and p<0.001). Within the WIN group, the difference between T1 and BL was significant (p<0.001).

Locomotor activity and exploratory behaviour

MDMA and MDMA+WIN-treated animals showed an increase in activity (mean: 63% and 61%, respectively) as well as in number of rearings (mean: 53 and 43, respectively), compared to the WIN (20% and 12) or vehicle (20% and 18) group (Figure 3). In addition, MDMA-treated rats spent more time in the centre of the open field than the remaining three treatment groups (mean: 15% vs. 8% (MDMA+WIN), 4% (WIN) and 6% (vehicle)). For locomotor activity, a two-way ANOVA yielded significant effects of treatment group [$F(3,244)= 310.74, p<0.001$], time interval [$F(6,244)= 27.46, p<0.001$], and interaction of substance x time interval [$F(18,244)= 2.18, p=0.004$]. Post-hoc test revealed significant differences between MDMA and MDMA+WIN groups compared to WIN- and vehicle-treated groups (p<0.001) over all 35 minutes, as well as within each 5-minute time interval (p<0.001). WIN- and vehicle-treated animals significantly reduced their activity between the first and all subsequent intervals (p<0.001), as well as between the second and the second last (WIN, p=0.05) or the third last (vehicle, p=0.011) intervals.

A two-way ANOVA comparing the number of rearings yielded significant effects for substance [$F(3,244)= 73.56, p<0.001$] and time interval [$F(6,244)= 3.24, p=0.004$]. Post-hoc test revealed significantly increased number of rearings for the MDMA group compared to the other three treatment groups (p<0.001 (WIN and vehicle), p=0.021 (MDMA+WIN)), as well as for the MDMA+WIN group compared to the WIN and vehicle groups (p<0.001).

In terms of differences within time intervals, MDMA-treated animals reared significantly more often than WIN- and vehicle-treated groups in all but the very first time interval (p<0.001 to p=0.006). MDMA+WIN-treated animals reared significantly more often than both WIN- and vehicle-treated animals in the last three intervals (p<0.001) and the third interval (p=0.029; p=0.044, respectively), as well as compared to WIN during the second and fourth interval (p=0.003 and p=0.042, respectively). Vehicle-treated animals showed a reduction in the number of measured rearings between the first and third to seventh time interval (p<0.001 to p=0.025) (For significant differences (p<0.001) within the time intervals, see Figure 3). A two-way ANOVA analysing the time spent in the centre of the open field yielded a significant effect for substance [$F(3,244)=17.88, p<0.001$]. Post-hoc test confirmed that MDMA-treated animals spent significantly more time in the centre compared to all three remaining treatment groups (p<0.001).

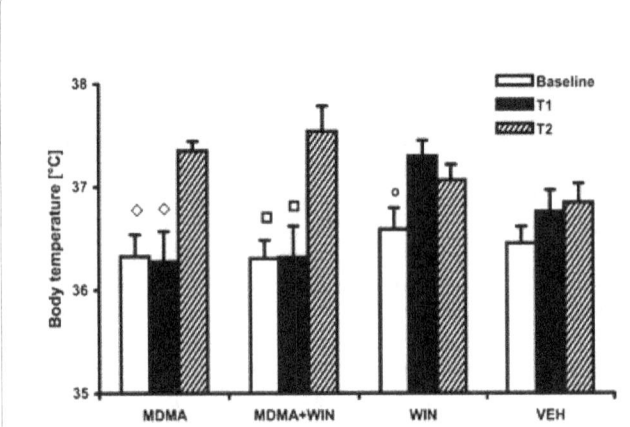

Figure 2: Effects of administration of MDMA (n=10), WIN (n=10), MDMA+WIN (n=9) and vehicle (n=10) on body temperature (°C). Data are means (+SEM) of three measurements for each animal at each time point. Closed triangle denotes significant difference (p<0.05) compared to WIN at T1; open symbols represent differences within the same treatment group compared to T2 (p<0.001).

Open triangles and open circles indicate differences between the first and the denoted time interval within vehicle and WIN groups, respectively. Closed triangles and squares denote differences between MDMA vs. WIN and vehicle groups, respectively. Closed circles and rhombuses indicate differences between MDMA+WIN and WIN and vehicle groups, respectively.

Food preference test

All animals consumed more pellets than breeding chow. When comparing the amount of pellets consumed, MDMA- and MDMA+WIN-treated animals are less than the vehicle and WIN-treated groups (mean: 4.5 and 2.8 grams vs. 6.0 and 6.8 grams, respectively) (Figure 4). A two-way ANOVA yielded significant effects for type of food [$F(1,70)=167.66$, p<0.001], substance [$F(3,70)=6.14$], p<0.001], and the interaction substance x type of food [$F(3,70)= 4.88$, p=0,004]. Post-hoc tests revealed that all animals preferred pellets over breeding chow (p<0.001). Rats from the vehicle group consumed significantly more pellets than the MDMA (p=0.017) and MDMA+WIN group (p<0.001). WIN-treated animals consumed significantly more pellets than the MDMA+WIN group (p<0.001). When comparing total amount of food intake, vehicle and WIN-treated groups ate significantly more than MDMA+WIN-treated animals (p=0.004 and p=0.002, respectively). MDMA+WIN-treated animals consumed less food than MDMA-treated animals (2.8grams vs. 4.7grams), however this difference was not statistically significant.

Discussion

Various studies suggest an interaction of MDMA influence on different neurotransmitters and the inhibitory effects of CB receptors on transmitter release in a range of brain regions. For example, the synthetic CB1 receptor antagonist SR141617A increased serotonergic and dopaminergic neurotransmission, especially in the mPFC [37], whereas delta9-THC decreases 5-HT neurotransmission in the nucleus accumbens [38,39]. Furthermore, CB1 receptors are expressed on 5-HT and DA neurons not only pre-synaptically, but also on dendrites, and may interfere with the serotonin transporter (SERT) and dopamine transporter (DAT) [40]. The abundant and overlapping distribution of CB1 receptors may cause an indirect inhibition on dopaminergic and serotonergic neurons by influencing GABAergic

inhibition of DA neurons [41]. An effect of WIN on glutamatergic [42] and cholinergic [43] synapses has been shown as well, offering further sites for interaction. Therefore, the DA and 5-HT release and reuptake inhibition properties of MDMA would hereby interact with the inhibitory effects of WIN via the CB1 receptor and result in opposing, additive or regulative effects in motivation and effort, as well as temperature regulation and locomotor behaviour.

Effort- based decision making

MDMA impaired choice behaviour based on effort irrespective of co-administration of WIN. As far as to current knowledge, no previous study has investigated the effect of acute MDMA administration on effort-based choice behaviour. Exact mechanisms on how MDMA-induced alterations in 5-HT and DA release could influence the fronto-striatal circuitry [44] or DA release in the nucleus accumbens [45] responsible for regulating effort-based choice remain speculative. The impact of central 5-HT release on general aspects of behaviour, e.g. motivation, may be important here. Furthermore, acute MDMA administration did not impair locomotion, but decreased food intake (see below). Therefore, increased 5-HT release might have decreased appetite and thus, motivation for climbing the barrier to obtain the high reward. Whatever the underlying causes, our data indicates that acute MDMA effects do not only include physiological responses like hyperthermia or increased activity, but may also immediately impair cognitive functions like decision making.

Although only MDMA-alone significantly differed from the control group, responses of the combined treatment group closely paralleled those of MDMA-treated animals. The lack of a significant effect is probably due to side effects observed in the MDMA+WIN-treated animals such as increased head waving, defecation, salivation and overall slow responses and movements. One MDMA+WIN-treated animal was excluded from the analysis due to inability to move further than the decision point of the T-maze. These impairments may have been adverse effects upon the first acute simultaneous administration of MDMA and WIN, as this behavioural pattern was not, or to a lesser extent, observed in subsequent experiments. Young et al. (2005) reported similar behavioural impairments upon combined administration of delta9-THC (1mg/kg) and MDMA (5mg/kg) in a within subjects design. As in our study, no major adverse effects of administration of either MDMA or the cannabinoid agonist alone were evident, thus observed impairments seem to be due to the combination, not the single doses, of the substances. Overall, and especially taking into account the observed side effects of co-administration, it is not possible to draw firm conclusions about the influence of the combined consumption on effort-based decision making based on these results. However, MDMA-administration seems to have an effect on effort-based choice behaviour with or without WIN co-administration.

Our results show no effect of WIN (1.2mg/kg) on effort-based decision making in rats. This contrasts with an earlier study employing operant chambers showing that acute treatment with 1.2 mg/kg or 1.8 mg/kg WIN significantly reduced the number of lever presses for pellets ("break point") in a progressive-ratio task compared to a lower dose of WIN (0.6mg/kg) or vehicle treatment. Moreover, a significant decrease in the total number of lever presses was detected, indicating a complex role of cannabinoids in the control of reward-related behaviour [46]. However, although both paradigms aim at investigating the influence of CB1 activation on effort-based reward obtainment, there are of course differences between T-maze- and instrumental tasks, which preclude a direct comparison. However, our data indicate no influence of CB1 receptor activation on this behavioural paradigm.

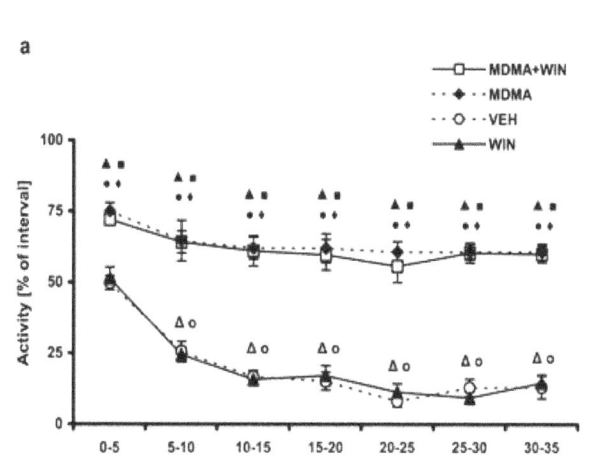

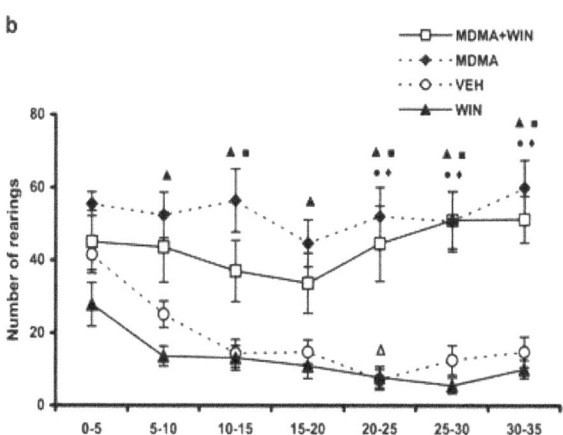

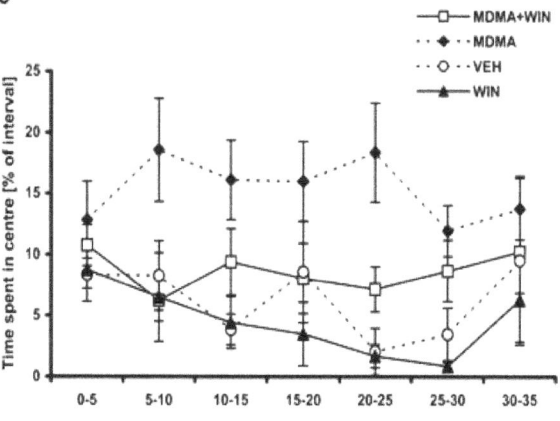

Figure 3: Effects of MDMA, WIN, MDMA+WIN and vehicle (n=10;10;9;10, respectively) on locomotion (a), exploratory (b) and anxiety-like (c) behaviour. (a) and (c) are depicted as % time of 5-minute intervals for a total of 35 minutes, (b) as absolute number of rearings per interval. Significant differences of p<0.001 are depicted only. Open triangles and open circles indicate differences between the first and the denoted time interval within vehicle and WIN groups, respectively. Closed triangles and squares denote differences between MDMA vs. WIN and vehicle groups, respectively. Closed circles and rhombuses indicate differences between MDMA+WIN and WIN and vehicle groups, respectively.

Body temperature

Our results support previous studies demonstrating an increase in body temperature upon consumption of MDMA in humans [47,48] and rats [7]. The peak temperature measured 1hr after behavioural testing contrasts with previous findings showing significant increases compared to baseline levels at 20-30 minutes after administration of MDMA (12.5mg/kg, i.p.) [9]. However, depending on the route of administration (s.c. versus i.p. injection) hyperthermic effects can vary in time due to different absorption and metabolizing rates. Furthermore, according to Green at al. (2003) peak temperatures are observed 40-60 minutes after i.p. administration.

Co-administration of WIN did not influence MDMA-induced hyperthermia. Significantly higher temperature compared to both baseline and pre-test was measured 1hr after behavioural testing for the MDMA+WIN group. In fact, temperature changes were akin to those seen in the MDMA group. These results are in contrast with a finding by Morley (2004), showing that delta9-THC and CP 55,940 prevent MDMA-induced hyperthermia in rats. However, these cannabinoid agents were administered according to a different injection scheme (4x 2.5 mg/kg). A study in humans demonstrated that delta9-THC co-administration does not prevent MDMA-induced temperature increase [28]. Our results do not support the modulatory role of acutely administered CB1/2 receptor ligands on MDMA-induced hyperthermia. Rather, a modulation of the WIN- induced rise in temperature by MDMA appears.

WIN (1.2mg/kg) led to a significant increase in body temperature 10 minutes after administration compared to baseline. Earlier studies on cannabinoid effects on body temperature found that low doses of delta9-THC (0.05 and 0.1 mg/kg) caused hyperthermia, while doses of 1.0, 2.0 and 5.0 mg/kg induced hypothermia [49]. In contrast to our study, cannabinoid receptor agonists WIN55,212-2 and CP55,940 led to hypothermia, which was reversed by the selective CB1 receptor antagonist SR 141716 [35]. On the other hand, it was recently shown that the endogenous cannabinoid anandamide increases temperature when administered intracerebroventricularly, an effect which is reduced by co-administration of a CB1 receptor antagonist [50]. Furthermore, low

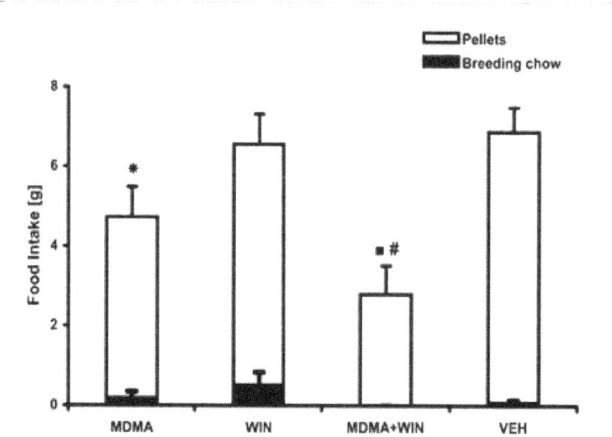

Figure 4: Effects of acute administration of MDMA, WIN, MDMA+WIN and vehicle (n=10;10;9;10, respectively) on food preference. Closed square shows significant difference (p<0.005) in total food intake compared to vehicle and WIN groups; hash symbol denotes difference (p<0.001) in amount of pellets consumed compared to vehicle and WIN groups; asterisk shows difference (p<0.05) in amount of pellets consumed compared to vehicle group.

doses of delta9-THC significantly reduce, but doses of 1.0, 2.0 and 5.0 mg/kg increase the levels of 5-HT metabolites in the whole brain [49]. The dose used in the current study may have had an indirect increasing effect on body temperature by elevating 5-HT levels.

Locomotor activity and exploratory behaviour

MDMA as well as MDMA+WIN treatment significantly increased locomotor activity compared to the WIN- as well as vehicle- group (Figure 3a). These effects were stable over the 35 minutes test duration and support other studies demonstrating hyperactivity upon acute MDMA-administration [7,51]. Rats treated with 1.2 mg/kg WIN showed activity levels akin to the vehicle group. Co-administration of WIN therefore does not have an attenuating effect on MDMA-induced increases in locomotor activity.

Compared to MDMA-treated animals, MDMA+WIN administration led to a significant overall reduction in exploratory behaviour (number of rearings) over the 35 minute measurement (Figure 3b). No habituation was observed over time. However, there was no difference when comparing any of the individual time intervals. Therefore, co-administration of WIN seems to have a small, if any, modulating effect on MDMA-induced exploratory behaviour. In contrast to these results, rodent studies administering delta9-THC and MDMA found that the cannabinoid had an attenuating effect on MDMA-induced hyperactivity in rats [12] and mice [34]. The discrepancy between the previously described and our results may be due to the different test paradigms, dose-dependent biphasic effects of cannabinoids [35], and a more unspecific effect of delta9-THC compared to WIN.

In terms of the time spent in the centre of the open field, a measure for exploration anxiety, MDMA+WIN-, WIN- and vehicle-treated animals spent significantly less time in the centre than MDMA-treated animals (see Figure 3c). MDMA seems to have an anxiolytic effect. In contrast, increased anxiety levels were found in MDMA-only treated rats [52] and mice [53] on various anxiety-related measures. However, this result is congruent with Morley et al. (2005) demonstrating a decreasing effect of delta9-THC on MDMA-induced anxiety measured in an emergence test. The attenuating effect of WIN on MDMA-induced decreased exploration anxiety is not due to differences in locomotion as the MDMA+WIN group displayed equal levels of hyperactivity as the MDMA group whilst not differing from vehicle group in the anxiety measure. Future studies seeking to elucidate the influence of CB1 agonism on (MDMA-induced) anxiety should employ a more direct measure as well as various CB agents.

Rats treated with 1.2 mg/kg WIN showed activity, vertical exploratory behaviour as well as exploration anxiety levels akin to the vehicle group. Furthermore, there were no differences in habituation, i.e. a reduction of activity over the measured intervals within the 35 minutes occurred in WIN- and vehicle-treated animals equally. As noted previously, CB1 agonists may have biphasic effects according to dose, inducing hyperactivity at low doses and severe motor deficits at larger doses [35]. In line with this, locomotor activity in the open field has been reported to be increased by 0.6 mg/kg, but not by higher doses of WIN [46]. A dose of 1 mg/kg does not affect either ambulation or the frequency of rearings, while higher doses (3 or 5.6mg/kg) reduce both measures [54]. Various reports point to involvement of CB1 antagonism (for example, by SR 141716), but not agonism, in anxiogenic effects [55-58]. In the current experiment, WIN-only treatment did not affect any of the measures.

Food preference

MDMA reduced intake of pellets, which is congruent with previous studies demonstrating that MDMA consumption reduces food intake and appetite in humans [59,60] and animals [13,61]. Co-administration of WIN does not seem to have an effect on MDMA-induced hypophagia, as MDMA+WIN treated animals consumed even less than the MDMA group (means of total food intake: 2.79 vs 4.55 grams), but this difference was not statistically significant. Although i.c.v. administration of WIN has been shown to decrease extracellular 5-HT and 5-HIAA in hypothalamic brain areas [62], this effect seems to be overruled by the strong MDMA-induced increase of 5-HT release and the associated reduction in food intake [63]. Food intake is a process mediated by stimulation of 5-HT receptors [62,63].

WIN-treated animals did not differ from the vehicle-treated group in terms of food consumption. This result was somewhat unexpected since previous studies demonstrated an increase in food intake after delta9-THC or WIN administration compared to vehicle groups [64]. For example, i.p. administration of WIN at doses of 0.5, 1 and 2 mg/kg caused a significant increase in food intake from 1h-6h after injection [62]. However, Merroun et al. (2009) did not find significant differences when comparing the non-cumulative amounts of food intake between vehicle- and WIN- (1 or 2 mg/kg) treated animals. As with activity levels and body temperature, activsation of CB1/2 receptors tends to evoke dose-dependent biphasic responses. WIN at doses of 1 and 2 mg/kg promoted hyperphagia, whereas administration of a higher dose (5 mg/kg) significantly inhibited food intake in partially satiated rats [62]. Drews et al. (2005) even found a significant reduction in the amount of pellets consumed by animals treated with 1.8 mg/kg WIN. If orexigenic effects of WIN appear subsequent to maximal blood concentration levels, hyperphagia may have been evoked only partially in the current study as testing took place 10 minutes after administration.

Conclusion

MDMA led to decreased choices of the HR option in an effort-based decision making task. Furthermore, previously well-documented increases in activity and body temperature as well as decreased food intake were replicated. Overall, our behavioural tests do not support a modulatory role of WIN regarding MDMA-induced acute effects. Apart from an augmenting effect on body temperature, WIN administration alone did not yield effects distinct from vehicle treatment. Although there was a wash-out period of seven days between each test, additive or habituation effects cannot be completely ruled out. Future studies could vary the administration schedule and doses. In the current study, we used doses which in other animal studies have been shown to be behaviourally relevant (e.g., [44,65]. However, since the dosage used in these experiments was relatively high, a lower dose of MDMA could reveal a putative potentiating effect of WIN. Many MDMA users consume cannabis concomitantly to enhance positive sensations or sometime after MDMA consumption to alleviate adverse effects of the "come-down" [66,67]. The neurobiological mechanisms underlying behavioural effects of MDMA, as well as co-consumption of cannabis, remain somewhat unclear as a complex interplay between 5-HT and DA release as well as activation of different 5-HT subtypes must be considered. Administration of specific CB1 agonists and manipulation of certain 5-HT receptors, and/or verification of DA and 5-HT-transmitter levels in brain areas known to be involved in behavioural responses, could further elucidate underlying pharmacological mechanisms. From these experimental tests in rats, we conclude that acute co-administration of a CB agonist does not substantially attenuate the MDMA-induced behavioural effects.

Disclosures and Acknowledgements

This manuscript has not been published elsewhere and has not been submitted simultaneously for publication elsewhere. H.K.S. was supported by an Erasmus Placement Grant from the EU. All authors contributed in a significant way to the manuscript and have read and approved the final manuscript. There are no real or potential conflicts of interest.

We thank Prof. Nagel, laboratory of inorganic chemistry University of Tübingen, for kindly providing MDMA. Dr. Andreas von Ameln-Mayerhofer (University of Tübingen) is gratefully acknowledged for helpful discussions on MDMA. We also thank MSc. Sven Büttner for conducting preliminary studies.

References

1. Editorial team (2010) The EMCDDA annual report 2010: the state of the drugs problem in Europe. Euro Surveill 15.

2. Danielsson AK, Wennberg P, Hibell B, Romelsjö A (2012) Alcohol use, heavy episodic drinking and subsequent problems among adolescents in 23 European countries: does the prevention paradox apply? Addiction 107: 71-80.

3. Wu LT, Parrott AC, Ringwalt CL, Yang C, Blazer DG (2009) The variety of ecstasy/MDMA users: results from the National Epidemiologic Survey on alcohol and related conditions. Am J Addict 18: 452-461.

4. Parrott AC, Milani RM, Gouzoulis-Mayfrank E, Daumann J (2007) Cannabis and Ecstasy/MDMA (3,4-methylenedioxymethamphetamine): an analysis of their neuropsychobiological interactions in recreational users. J Neural Transm 114: 959-968.

5. Parrott AC, Gouzoulis-Meyfrank E, Rodgers J, Solowij N (2004) Ecstasy/MDMA and cannabis: the complexities of their interactive neuropsychobiological effects. J Psychopharmacol 18: 572-575.

6. Boys A, Marsden J, Strang J (2001) Understanding reasons for drug use amongst young people: a functional perspective. Health Educ Res 16: 457-469.

7. Green AR, Mechan AO, Elliott JM, O'Shea E, Colado MI (2003) The pharmacology and clinical pharmacology of 3,4-methylenedioxymethamphetamine (MDMA, "ecstasy"). Pharmacol Rev 55: 463-508.

8. Cole JC, Sumnall HR (2003) The pre-clinical behavioural pharmacology of 3,4-methylenedioxymethamphetamine (MDMA). Neurosci Biobehav Rev 27: 199-217.

9. Mechan AO, Esteban B, O'Shea E, Elliott JM, Colado MI, et al. (2002) The pharmacology of the acute hyperthermic response that follows administration of 3,4-methylenedioxymethamphetamine (MDMA, 'ecstasy') to rats. Br J Pharmacol 135: 170-180.

10. Bankson MG, Cunningham KA (2001) 3,4-Methylenedioxymethamphetamine (MDMA) as a unique model of serotonin receptor function and serotonin-dopamine interactions. J Pharmacol Exp Ther 297: 846-852.

11. Docherty JR, Green AR (2010) The role of monoamines in the changes in body temperature induced by 3,4-methylenedioxymethamphetamine (MDMA, ecstasy) and its derivatives. Br J Pharmacol 160: 1029-1044.

12. Morley KC, Li KM, Hunt GE, Mallet PE, McGregor IS (2004) Cannabinoids prevent the acute hyperthermia and partially protect against the 5-HT depleting effects of MDMA ("Ecstasy") in rats. Neuropharmacology 46: 954-965.

13. Frith CH, Chang LW, Lattin DL, Walls RC, Hamm J, et al. (1987) Toxicity of methylenedioxymethamphetamine (MDMA) in the dog and the rat. Fundam Appl Toxicol 9: 110-119.

14. De Souza I, Kelly JP, Harkin AJ, Leonard BE (1997) An appraisal of the pharmacological and toxicological effects of a single oral administration of 3,4-methylenedioxymethamphetamine (MDMA) in the rat. Pharmacol Toxicol 80: 207-210.

15. Byrne T, Baker LE, Poling A (2000) MDMA and learning: effects of acute and neurotoxic exposure in the rat. Pharmacol Biochem Behav 66: 501-508.

16. Wilson RI, Nicoll RA (2002) Endocannabinoid signaling in the brain. Science 296: 678-682.

17. Herkenham M, Lynn AB, Johnson MR, Melvin LS, de Costa BR, et al. (1991) Characterization and localization of cannabinoid receptors in rat brain: a quantitative in vitro autoradiographic study. J Neurosci 11: 563-583.

18. McDonald J, Schleifer L, Richards JB, de Wit H (2003) Effects of THC on behavioral measures of impulsivity in humans. Neuropsychopharmacology 28: 1356-1365.

19. Zuurman L, Ippel AE, Moin E, van Gerven JM (2009) Biomarkers for the effects of cannabis and THC in healthy volunteers. Br J Clin Pharmacol 67: 5-21.

20. Ameri A (1999) The effects of cannabinoids on the brain. Prog Neurobiol 58: 315-348.

21. Elphick MR, Egertová M (2001) The neurobiology and evolution of cannabinoid signalling. Philos Trans R Soc Lond B Biol Sci 356: 381-408.

22. Iversen L (2003) Cannabis and the brain. Brain 126: 1252-1270.

23. Morton J (2005) Ecstasy: pharmacology and neurotoxicity. Curr Opin Pharmacol 5: 79-86.

24. Howlett AC, Breivogel CS, Childers SR, Deadwyler SA, Hampson RE, et al. (2004) Cannabinoid physiology and pharmacology: 30 years of progress. Neuropharmacology 47 Suppl 1: 345-358.

25. Daumann J, Hensen G, Thimm B, Rezk M, Till B, et al. (2004) Self-reported psychopathological symptoms in recreational ecstasy (MDMA) users are mainly associated with regular cannabis use: further evidence from a combined cross-sectional/longitudinal investigation. Psychopharmacology (Berl) 173: 398-404.

26. Croft RJ, Mackay AJ, Mills AT, Gruzelier JG (2001) The relative contributions of ecstasy and cannabis to cognitive impairment. Psychopharmacology (Berl) 153: 373-379.

27. Rodgers J, Buchanan T, Scholey AB, Heffernan TM, Ling J, et al. (2001) Differential effects of Ecstasy and cannabis on self-reports of memory ability: a web-based study. Hum Psychopharmacol 16: 619-625.

28. Dumont GJ, Kramers C, Sweep FC, Touw DJ, van Hasselt JG, et al. (2009) Cannabis coadministration potentiates the effects of "ecstasy" on heart rate and temperature in humans. Clin Pharmacol Ther 86: 160-166.

29. Dumont GJ, van Hasselt JG, de Kam M, van Gerven JM, Touw DJ, et al. (2011) Acute psychomotor, memory and subjective effects of MDMA and THC co-administration over time in healthy volunteers. J Psychopharmacol 25: 478-489.

30. Sala M, Braida D (2005) Endocannabinoids and 3,4-methylenedioxymethamphetamine (MDMA) interaction. Pharmacol Biochem Behav 81: 407-416.

31. Braida D, Sala M (2002) Role of the endocannabinoid system in MDMA intracerebral self-administration in rats. Br J Pharmacol 136: 1089-1092.

32. Rodríguez-Arias M, Manzanedo C, Roger-Sánchez C, Do Couto BR, Aguilar MA, et al. (2010) Effect of adolescent exposure to WIN 55212-2 on the acquisition and reinstatement of MDMA-induced conditioned place preference. Prog Neuropsychopharmacol Biol Psychiatry 34: 166-171.

33. Manzanedo C, Rodríguez-Arias M, Daza-Losada M, Maldonado C, Aguilar MA, et al. (2010) Effect of the CB1 cannabinoid agonist WIN 55212-2 on the acquisition and reinstatement of MDMA-induced conditioned place preference in mice. Behav Brain Funct 6: 19.

34. Touriño C, Ledent C, Maldonado R, Valverde O (2008) CB1 cannabinoid receptor modulates 3,4-methylenedioxymethamphetamine acute responses and reinforcement. Biol Psychiatry 63: 1030-1038.

35. Chaperon F, Thiébot MH (1999) Behavioral effects of cannabinoid agents in animals. Crit Rev Neurobiol 13: 243-281.

36. Walton ME, Bannerman DM, Rushworth MF (2002) The role of rat medial frontal cortex in effort-based decision making. J Neurosci 22: 10996-11003.

37. Darmani NA, Janoyan JJ, Kumar N, Crim JL (2003) Behaviorally active doses of the CB1 receptor antagonist SR 141716A increase brain serotonin and dopamine levels and turnover. Pharmacol Biochem Behav 75: 777-787.

38. Sano K, Mishima K, Koushi E, Orito K, Egashira N, et al. (2008) Delta 9-tetrahydrocannabinol-induced catalepsy-like immobilization is mediated by decreased 5-HT neurotransmission in the nucleus accumbens due to the action of glutamate-containing neurons. Neuroscience 151: 320-328.

39. López-Moreno JA, González-Cuevas G, Moreno G, Navarro M (2008) The

pharmacology of the endocannabinoid system: functional and structural interactions with other neurotransmitter systems and their repercussions in behavioral addiction. Addict Biol 13: 160-187.

40. Lau T, Schloss P (2008) The cannabinoid CB1 receptor is expressed on serotonergic and dopaminergic neurons. Eur J Pharmacol 578: 137-141.

41. Pistis M, Porcu G, Melis M, Diana M, Gessa GL (2001) Effects of cannabinoids on prefrontal neuronal responses to ventral tegmental area stimulation. Eur J Neurosci 14: 96-102.

42. Shen M, Piser TM, Seybold VS, Thayer SA (1996) Cannabinoid receptor agonists inhibit glutamatergic synaptic transmission in rat hippocampal cultures. J Neurosci 16: 4322-4334.

43. Gessa GL, Casu MA, Carta G, Mascia MS (1998) Cannabinoids decrease acetylcholine release in the medial-prefrontal cortex and hippocampus, reversal by SR 141716A. Eur J Pharmacol 355: 119-124.

44. Floresco SB, St Onge JR, Ghods-Sharifi S, Winstanley CA (2008) Cortico-limbic-striatal circuits subserving different forms of cost-benefit decision making. Cogn Affect Behav Neurosci 8: 375-389.

45. Assadi SM, Yücel M, Pantelis C (2009) Dopamine modulates neural networks involved in effort-based decision-making. Neurosci Biobehav Rev 33: 383-393.

46. Drews E, Schneider M, Koch M (2005) Effects of the cannabinoid receptor agonist WIN 55,212-2 on operant behavior and locomotor activity in rats. Pharmacol Biochem Behav 80: 145-150.

47. Freedman RR, Johanson CE, Tancer ME (2005) Thermoregulatory effects of 3,4-methylenedioxymethamphetamine (MDMA) in humans. Psychopharmacology (Berl) 183: 248-256.

48. Mohamed WM, Ben Hamida S, Cassel JC, de Vasconcelos AP, Jones BC (2011) MDMA: interactions with other psychoactive drugs. Pharmacol Biochem Behav 99: 759-774.

49. Taylor DA, Fennessy MR (1977) Biphasic nature of the effects of delta9-tetrahydrocannabinol on body temperature and brain amines of the rat. Eur J Pharmacol 46: 93-99.

50. Fraga D, Zanoni CI, Rae GA, Parada CA, Souza GE (2009) Endogenous cannabinoids induce fever through the activation of CB1 receptors. Br J Pharmacol 157: 1494-1501.

51. Spanos LJ, Yamamoto BK (1989) Acute and subchronic effects of methylenedioxymethamphetamine [(+/-)MDMA] on locomotion and serotonin syndrome behavior in the rat. Pharmacol Biochem Behav 32: 835-840.

52. Morley KC, McGregor IS (2000) (+/-)-3,4-methylenedioxymethamphetamine (MDMA, 'Ecstasy') increases social interaction in rats. Eur J Pharmacol 408: 41-49.

53. Ferraz-de-Paula V, Stankevicius D, Ribeiro A, Pinheiro ML, Rodrigues-Costa EC, et al. (2011) Differential behavioral outcomes of 3,4-methylenedioxymethamphetamine (MDMA-ecstasy) in anxiety-like responses in mice. Braz J Med Biol Res 44: 428-437.

54. Järbe TU, Ross T, DiPatrizio NV, Pandarinathan L, Makriyannis A (2006) Effects of the CB1R agonist WIN-55,212-2 and the CB1R antagonists SR-141716 and AM-1387: open-field examination in rats. Pharmacol Biochem Behav 85: 243-252.

55. Moreira FA, Grieb M, Lutz B (2009) Central side-effects of therapies based on CB1 cannabinoid receptor agonists and antagonists: focus on anxiety and depression. Best Pract Res Clin Endocrinol Metab 23: 133-144.

56. Rodgers RJ, Evans PM, Murphy A (2005) Anxiogenic profile of AM-251, a selective cannabinoid CB1 receptor antagonist, in plus-maze-naïve and plus-maze-experienced mice. Behav Pharmacol 16: 405-413.

57. Patel S, Cravatt BF, Hillard CJ (2005) Synergistic interactions between cannabinoids and environmental stress in the activation of the central amygdala. Neuropsychopharmacology 30: 497-507.

58. Haller J, Varga B, Ledent C, Freund TF (2004) CB1 cannabinoid receptors mediate anxiolytic effects: convergent genetic and pharmacological evidence with CB1-specific agents. Behav Pharmacol 15: 299-304.

59. Vollenweider FX, Gamma A, Liechti M, Huber T (1998) Psychological and cardiovascular effects and short-term sequelae of MDMA ("ecstasy") in MDMA-naïve healthy volunteers. Neuropsychopharmacology 19: 241-251.

60. Kirkpatrick MG, Gunderson EW, Perez AY, Haney M, Foltin RW, et al. (2012) A direct comparison of the behavioral and physiological effects of methamphetamine and 3,4-methylenedioxymethamphetamine (MDMA) in humans. Psychopharmacology (Berl) 219: 109-122.

61. Jean A, Conductier G, Manrique C, Bouras C, Berta P, et al. (2007) Anorexia induced by activation of serotonin 5-HT4 receptors is mediated by increases in CART in the nucleus accumbens. Proc Natl Acad Sci U S A 104: 16335-16340.

62. Merroun I, Errami M, Hoddah H, Urbano G, Porres JM, et al. (2009) Influence of intracerebroventricular or intraperitoneal administration of cannabinoid receptor agonist (WIN 55,212-2) and inverse agonist (AM 251) on the regulation of food intake and hypothalamic serotonin levels. Br J Nutr 101: 1569-1578.

63. Lam DD, Garfield AS, Marston OJ, Shaw J, Heisler LK (2010) Brain serotonin system in the coordination of food intake and body weight. Pharmacol Biochem Behav 97: 84-91.

64. Kirkham TC (2005) Endocannabinoids in the regulation of appetite and body weight. Behav Pharmacol 16: 297-313.

65. Young JM, McGregor IS, Mallet PE (2005) Co-administration of THC and MDMA ('ecstasy') synergistically disrupts memory in rats. Neuropsychopharmacology 30: 1475-1482.

66. Winstock AR, Griffiths P, Stewart D (2001) Drugs and the dance music scene: a survey of current drug use patterns among a sample of dance music enthusiasts in the UK. Drug Alcohol Depend 64: 9-17.

67. Schulz S (2011) MDMA & cannabis: a mini-review of cognitive, behavioral, and neurobiological effects of co-consumption. Curr Drug Abuse Rev 4: 81-86.

Antimicrobial and Anti-Inflammatory Properties of *Anchomanes difformis* (Bl.) Engl. and *Colocasia esculenta* (L.) Schott.

Christian Agyare[1]*, Yaw Duah Boakye[1], John Antwi Apenteng[2], Susana Oteng Dapaah[1], Theresa Appiah[1] and Adobea Adow[1]
[1]*Department of Pharmaceutics, Kwame Nkrumah University of Science and Technology, Kumasi, Ghana*
[2]*Department of Pharmaceutical Science, Central University College, Accra, Ghana*

Abstract

   Anchomanes difformis (Blume) Engl. and *Colocasia esculentus* (L.) Schott. of the family Araceae are plants widely distributed in Africa. The leaves and roots of these plants are traditionally used to treat various disease conditions including dysentery, cough, kidney pains and stomach disorders. This study aimed at investigating the antimicrobial, antioxidant and anti-inflammatory properties of methanol extracts of *A. difformis* leaves (ADL) and roots (ADR), and *C. esculentus* leaves (CEL). Antimicrobial activity was evaluated using micro-dilution methods against typed strains of *Escherichia coli, Staphylococcus aureus, Pseudomonas aeruginosa* and clinical stains of *Streptococcus pyogenes* and *Candida albicans*. The antioxidant activities of the extracts were determined using 1, 1-diphenyl-2-picryl-hydrazyl (DPPH) free radical scavenging, total antioxidant capacity and total phenol content methods. The anti-inflammatory activity of ADL, ADR and CEL were evaluated using the carrageenan-induced foot pad oedema in 7-day old chicks. ADL, ADR and CEL demonstrated broad spectrum antimicrobial activity with MIC ranging from 12.5 to 50 mg/mL. All the extracts exhibited antioxidant activity with CEL demonstrating the highest with IC_{50} value of 146.9 µg/mL. The methanol extracts further demonstrated a significant anti-inflammatory ($p < 0.001$) at the concentrations tested with 30 and 300 mg/kg body weight each extract showing better activity than the 100 mg/kg body weight. Phytochemical screening revealed the presence of saponins, phenols, tannins flavonoids, and triterpenoids in especially in ADR and CEL. The above findings may justify the medicinal uses of the plants.

Keywords: *Colocassia esculentus*; *Anchomanes difformis* ; Antimicrobial; Inflammation; Anti-inflammatory; Antioxidant

Introduction

The use of medicinal plants to treat various ailments inflicting man has been in existence since the onset of time. In Africa, about 80% of the populace relies on medicinal plants in managing various forms of infections which are endemic in the sub-region [1]. Over the years, medicinal plants have proven to be a remarkable source of newer and potent therapeutic agents and have therefore taken the central stage in most research centers in the world [2,3]. However, with the identification and development of newer and potent antimicrobial interventions to treat microbial infections, the number of resistant microorganisms being identified currently, increases exponentially. It has therefore become imperative that more medicinal plants be screened to identify and develop newer and cost-effective antimicrobial agents to treat infections caused by resistant microorganisms.

Anchomanes difformis (Blume) Engl. belongs to the family Araceae. *A. difformis* is a large herbaceous plant which grows in the tropical zones especially in various parts of Africa [4]. Traditionally *A. difformis* is used to manage a vast range of ailments in West and Central Africa. In Nigeria, a decoction of the root is used to treat cough, diabetes, dysentery and throat related problems [5]. The rhizomes are used topically as vesicants and rubefacient. Both roots and leaves are used to treat oedemas, kidney pains, jaundice and as a diuretic in treating urethral discharge [6]. Studies conducted have shown that the plant possesses insecticidal activity [7]. Methanol extract of the rhizome has also found to possess trypanocidal activity [8]. Bero et al. [9] have also shown that the plant exerts antiplasmodial activity.

Colocasia esculentus (L.) Schotts (Family Araceae) is an herbaceous perennial plant that is thought to be a native of India but is widely cultivated in the tropical Africa. Traditionally, a decoction of the leaves is drunk to promote menstruation and together with other parts of the plants, it is used to relieve stomach problems and to treat cysts. *C. esculenta* has been reported to possess hypoglycemic effect due to the presence of cyanoglucoside [10]. Hypolipidemic activity has also been revealed and attributed to the presence of arabinogalactan [11] and mono and digalactocyl diacylglycerols [12]. It has also been reported to possess antifungal activity due to presence of cystatin [13].

This study therefore seeks to determine pharmacological properties including antimicrobial, antioxidant and anti-inflammatory properties of the methanol extracts of *A. difformis* leaves (ADL) and roots (ADR) and *C. esculentus* leaves (CEL).

Materials and Methods

Chemicals and reagents

All chemicals and reagents were purchased from Sigma-Aldrich, St. Louis, AM, USA unless otherwise stated.

Preparation of plant materials

The leaves and roots of *A. difformis* and leaves of *C. esculentus* were collected in the month of October, 2014. The plants parts were authenticated by Dr. G.H. Sam and voucher specimens of each plant material have been deposited at the Herbarium of Department of Pharmacogncosy, Faculty of Pharmacy and Pharmaceutical Sciences,

---

*Corresponding author: Dr. Agyare Christian, Department of Pharmaceutics, Kwame Nkrumah University of Science and Technology, Kumasi, Ghana, E-mail: cagyare.pharm@knust.edu. gh; chrisagyare@yahoo.com

Kwame Nkrumah University of Science and Technology, Kumasi, Ghana. The plants parts were washed under tap water to remove debris. The leaves samples were dried in a hot air oven at 40°C for 48 h whiles the roots of *A. difformis* were cut into smaller pieces and oven-dried under similar conditions. The dried plant samples were then pulverized into coarse powder using a laboratory mill machine (Christy and Norris, London, UK).

Extraction of plant materials

A quantity of 500 g of the powdered leaves of *A. difformis* was soaked overnight in 2.5 L 70% v/v methanol and homogenized using ultra-turrax T-50 (Janke & Kunkel KG, Hamburg, Germany) for 3 min under ice cooling. The suspension obtained was then filtered using filter paper (Whatmann No. 10) with the aid of a vacuum pump. The residue was homogenized with more solvent and filtered to ensure maximum extraction of plant material. The filtrates obtained were then concentrated using a rotary evaporator (Buchi, Konstanz, Germany) at 40°C and the concentrates lyophilized. The dry extracts obtained were then kept in a refrigerator at 4°C until needed. The above extraction procedure was repeated for 500 g of powdered leaves of *C. esculentus* and 400 g of powdered root of *A. difformis* using 3 L and 2.5 L of 70% v/v methanol, respectively.

Phytochemical screening

Preliminary phytochemical screening was performed on all the extracts for the presence tannins, saponins, flavonoids, steroids and alkaloids [14,15].

Test organisms

The test organisms used for the antimicrobial determination included: *Escherichia coli* ATCC 25922, *Staphylococcus aureus* ATCC 25923, *Pseudomonas aeruginosa* ATCC 25922 and clinical strains of *Streptococcus pyogenes* and *Candida albicans*. The inoculum size of 1.0×10^6 (CFU)/mL of the test organisms was used in all the antimicrobial determinations.

Determination of antimicrobial activity

Determination of minimum inhibitory concentrations (MIC): The MICs of the extracts were determined using the micro-dilution method [3,16]. Ciprofloxacin and ketoconazole were used as standard antibacterial and antifungal agents, respectively. Stock solutions of extracts and standards were prepared. The microtitre plates were initially filled with 100 μL double strength nutrient broth (Oxoid, London, UK) and 20 μL of 24 h organisms culture suspension. Calculated volumes of the stock solutions (plant extracts, ciprofloxacin and ketoconazole) were filled into labelled wells to obtain a final volume of 200 μL with varying sample concentrations. The plates were then incubated at 37°C for 24 h. The MIC was determined as the lowest concentration of test sample that inhibited microbial growth which was indicated by the absence of purple colouration upon the addition of 30 μL of 125 mg/mL of 3-(4,5-dimethylthiazol -2-yl)-2,5-diphenyltetrazolium bromide) (MTT) solution [3]. The experiment was independently carried out in triplicates.

Determination of antioxidant activity

DPPH free radical scavenging activity: Antioxidant activities of the extracts were determined according to the method described by Chizzola et al. [17] using the free radical 1,1-diphenyl-2-picryl-hydrazyl (DPPH). Solutions of concentrations within the range of 7.8125 to 1000 μg/mL of the extracts and reference antioxidant (α-tocopherol) were prepared in methanol. The solutions were placed in a 96-well micro-titer plate. A concentration of 0.10 mM DPPH solution was also prepared in methanol. A volume of 10 μL of the DPPH solution was added to 100 μL of the various extracts and α-tocopherol solutions in the 96-well microtiter plates. The tubes were kept in the dark for 30 min after which absorbance of excess DPPH was measured at 517 nm using a MTP reader (MTX Lab Systems, Inc., Virginia, USA). The percentage inhibition of radical scavenging was then calculated using the following equation; Inhibition $(\%) = [(A_0 - A_1) / A_0] \times 100$, where (A_0) is the absorbance of a blank solution containing equal volume of methanol and DPPH, (A_1) is the absorbance of the samples at 517 nm. Inhibitory Concentration, IC_{50} was determined as the concentration of sample that scavenged 50% of DPPH free radical in solution.

Determination of total phenolic content

The total phenolic content of the extracts was determined by the Folin-Ciocalteu method [18,19]. Hundred microliters (0.1 mL) of 0.5 N Folin-Ciocalteu reagent was added to 0.5 mL sample solutions of concentrations 1000 to 5000 μg/mL and incubated at room temperature for 15 min. Two (2) mL of 2% sodium carbonate was added to each test tube containing the extract and Folin-Ciocalteu mixture. Tannic acid of concentrations 15.6 to 125 μg/mL was used as reference substance. Absorbance was read at 760 nm with a plate reader. The experiment was independently performed in triplicates.

Determination of total antioxidant capacity

Extract concentrations ranging from 2.0 to 5.0 mg/mL were prepared. To a volume of 1 mL of the extract solutions, 3 mL of mixed reagents (28 mM disodium Phosphate, 4 mM ammonium Molybdate and 0.6 M H_2SO_4) solution was added and incubated at 95°C for 90 min. Absorbance was then read at 695 nm after incubation [19].

Determination of anti-inflammatory activity

Ethical clearance: The *in vivo* anti-inflammatory studies were approved by the Faculty of Pharmacy Animal Ethical Committee (FPPS-AEC/CA01/13), Faculty of Pharmacy of Pharmacy and Pharmaceutical Sciences, Kwame Nkrumah University of Science and Technology, Kumasi, Ghana and also in compliance with internationally accepted principles for laboratory animal use and care (EEC Directive of 1986: 86/609 EEC). The procedure was performed in accordance with the guide for care and use of laboratory animals.

Carrageenan-induced foot oedema: Carrageenan induced inflammation of the footpad of chicks was employed to assess the anti-inflammatory property [20] of ADL, ADR and CEL. The chicks were randomly divided into eleven (11) groups with each group consisting of five (5) chicks. The chicks were weighed and their foot volumes measured using electronic calipers.

Chicks in the groups 1 to 3 were orally administered with 30, 100 and 300 mg/kg body weight of ADL, respectively. Group 4 to 6 received 30, 100 and 300 mg/kg of ADR orally, respectively. Groups 7 to 9 were orally administered with doses of 30, 100 and 300 mg/kg body weight of CEL, respectively whiles Groups 10 and 11 were administered orally with aspirin (positive control) (100 mg/kg) orally and vehicle (distilled water). Inflammation or oedema was induced by a sub-plantar injection of carrageenan (0.10 mL of a 2% w/v solution in normal saline) into the right footpad of the chicks 1 h post treatment. The foot pad volumes were determined immediately before the experiment (time zero) and every hour until 6 h post-carrageenan injection. Drug effects were evaluated by comparison of the pre-treated chicks with the control groups. Percentage inhibition of oedema was also calculated for each dose from the AUC using the equation below:

$$\% \text{ Inhibition} = \frac{AUC\ Control - AUC\ Treatment}{AUC\ Control} x100\%$$

Statistical analysis

All results were plotted and analysed with GraphPad Prism 5.0 for windows (GraphPad software, San Diego, CA, USA) and analysed by two-way ANOVA followed by Bonferroni post-test analysis which recognises $*p < 0.05$, $**p < 0.01$, $***p < 0.001$ as statistically significant.

Results

Phytochemical screening

Phytochemical screening of the extracts revealed the presence of saponins, phenols, tannins flavonoids and triterpenoids in ADR and CEL. Majority of the secondary metabolites tested were found absent in ADL. Alkaloids were found to be absent in all the extracts (Table 1).

Minimum inhibitory concentration (MIC)

The extracts demonstrated broad spectrum antibacterial and antifungal activity against the test microorganisms. ADL and ADR showed MIC values within the ranges of 12.5 to 50 mg/mL whiles CEL was within ranges of 25 to 50 mg/mL (Table 2).

Antioxidant activity

The extracts demonstrated very good antioxidant activity at the concentrations tested. CEL, demonstrated the highest antioxidant activity amongst the extracts with the lowest IC_{50} value. (Table 3 and Figure 1). Total antioxidant capacity and total phenolic content revealed an increase in these parameters with increase in extract concentration (Figures 2 and 3).

Anti-inflammatory activity

ADR, ADL and CEL demonstrated anti-inflammatory activities at the doses used. All the doses of extracts (ADL, ADR and CEL) tested at 30 and 300 mg/kg body weight exhibited significant ($p < 0.001$) activity over the course of duration of the experiment than the dose of 100 mg/kg (Figure 4).

Discussion

Studies conducted on the roots and leaves of *A. difformis* and leaves of *C. esculenta* showed that these plants possess some pharmacological or biological properties [5,21]. The preliminary phytochemical screening of the roots and leaves of *A. difformis* revealed the presence of saponins, tannins, flavonoids and phenols in the roots of the plant while these secondary metabolites were absent in the leaves. The leaves were found to have triterpenoids and sterols present. Alkaloids were not observed in all the extracts. These findings confirm earlier research conducted on these plant parts [5,21]. The leaves of *C. esculenta* revealed the presence of phenols, tannins, glycosides, flavonoids, triterpenoids and sterols.

All the plant extracts demonstrated antimicrobial activity against both Gram-negative and Gram-positive bacteria as well as the fungus (*C. albicans*). ADR exerted better antimicrobial activity than ADL as reported by Abah et al. [21] and Oyetayo [5]. The antimicrobial activity can be attributed to the secondary metabolites present in the extracts [22] which were present in ADR and CEL.

Constituents	ADR	ADL	CEL
Saponins	+	-	+
Phenols	+	-	+
Tannins	+	-	+
Glycosides	-	-	+
Alkaloids	-	-	-
Flavonoids	+	-	+
Triterpenoids	+	+	+
Sterols	-	+	+

ADL: *A. difformis* Leaf Extract; ADR: *A. difformis* Root Extract; CEL: *C. esculentus* Leaf Extract; +: Present; -: Absent of Secondary Metabolite

Table 1: Phytochemical screening of extracts.

Organism	Minimum Inhibitory Concentration				
	CEL	ADL	ADR	Ciprofloxacin	Ketoconazole
	mg/mL			µg/mL	mg/mL
E. coli	25.00	12.5	12.5	5.0	NA
S. aureus	50.0	50.0	50.0	10.0	NA
P. aeruginosa	50.0	50.0	25.0	5.0	NA
S. pyogenes	50.0	50.0	25.0	5.0	NA
C. albicans	50.0	50.0	25.0	NA	10.0

ADL: *A. difformis* Leaf Extract; ADR: *A. difformis* Root Extract; CEL: *C. esculentus* Leaf Extract; NA: No Activity

Table 2: Minimum inhibitory concentration (MIC) of extracts (ADR, ADL and CEL) and reference antibiotics.

Extract / Compound	IC_{50} (µg/mL)
α- tocopherol	4.176
ADR	627.3
ADL	669.9
CEL	146.9

ADL: *A. difformis* Leaf Extract; ADR: *A. difformis* Root Extract; CEL: *C. esculentus* Leaf Extract

Table 3: Antioxidant activity of α- tocopherol and extracts (ADR, ADL and CEL).

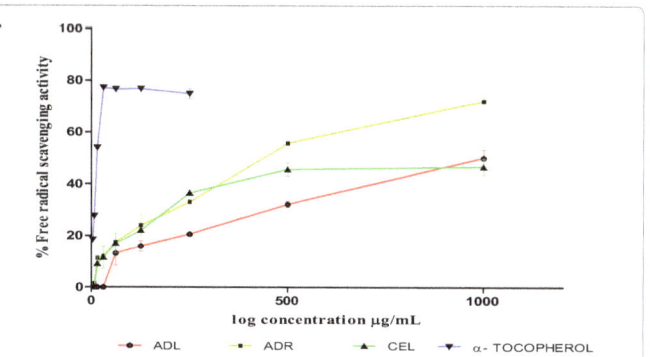

Figure 1: Free radical scavenging activity of ADL, ADR and CEL. N=3; Values are means ± SEM; ADL: *A. difformis* Leaf Extract; ADR: *A. difformis* Root Extract; CEL: *C. esculentus* Leaf Extract

The DPPH free radical scavenging, total antioxidant activity and total phenolic content methods were used in assessing the antioxidant activity of the extracts due to high speed and sensitivity and because it is imperative to use more than one method to evaluate antioxidant nature or capacity of plant materials due to the complex nature of the phytochemicals present in them [23]. The IC_{50} value indicates the extent of antioxidant activity with lower values indicating potent antioxidant activity. CEL had the highest radical scavenging activity as compared to the other two extracts with ADL lowest antioxidant property (Table 3). Antioxidant activity has been attributed to the presence of phenolic compounds in plants which were present in ADR and CEL [3,24,25]. The results from the total phenolic content revealed increasing phenolic content with increase in extract concentration. This was also similar with the total antioxidant capacity. Antioxidant activity can therefore be said to increase with increase in phenolic content which supports our findings.

The anti-inflammatory studies revealed that ADR, ADL and CEL possess significant anti-inflammatory activity. The time course curve shows a reduction in oedema in ADR, ADL and CEL-treated rats when compared to the control. This implies that the extracts possess significant inhibitory effects on preformed mediators such as histamine and serotonin which are involved in the initial phase of the acute inflammatory process. The inhibitory effect of the extracts extended

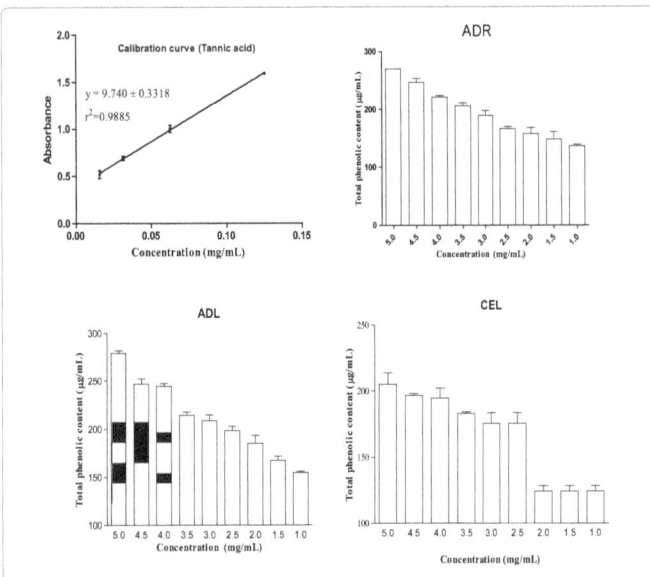

ADL: *A. difformis* Leaf Extract; ADR: *A. difformis* Root Extract; CEL: *C. esculentus* Leaf Extract, N=3; Values are means ± SEM

Figure 2: Calibration curve of tannic acid and total phenolic content of ADL, ADR and CEL.

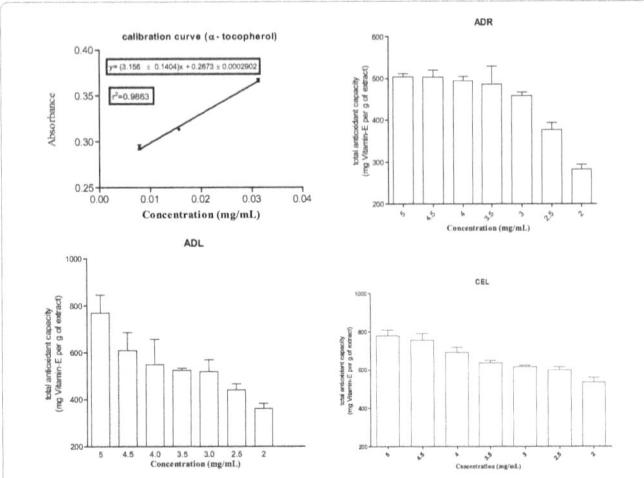

Figure 3: Calibration curve of α-tocopherol and total antioxidant capacity of ADL, ADR and CEL. ADL: *A. difformis* Leaf Extract; ADR: *A. difformis* Root Extract; CEL: *C. esculentus* Leaf Extract; N=3; Values are means ± SEM.

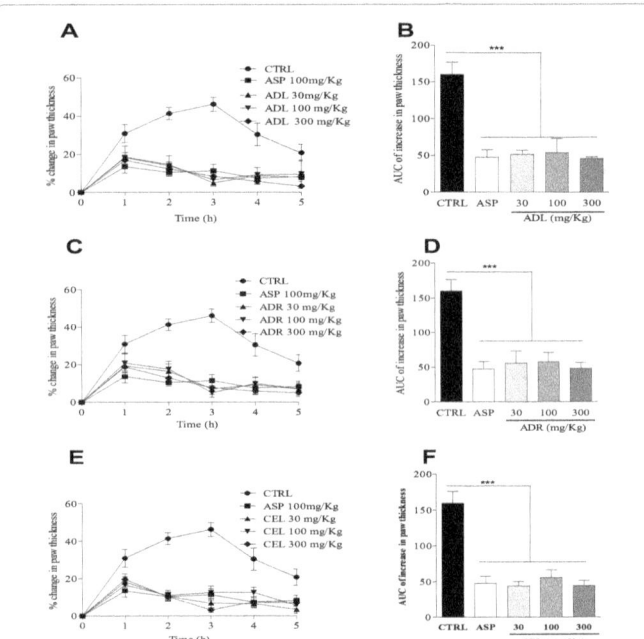

Figure 4: Influence of aspirin and extracts (ADR, ADL and CEL) on carrageenan-induced inflammation in chicks. **A**: Effect of *A. difformis* leaf extract on time-course curve; **B**: Effect of *A. difformis* leaf extract on auc of carrageenan induced oedema; **C**: Effect of *A. difformis* root extract on time-course curve; **D**: Effect of *A. difformis* root extract on auc of carrageenan induced oedema; **E**: Effect of *C. esculentus* leaf extract on time-course curve; **F**: Effect of *C. esculentus* leaf extract on auc of carrageenan induced oedema; ADL: *A. difformis* Leaf Extract; ADR: *A. difformis* Root Extract; CEL: *C. esculentus* Leaf Extract; *$p < 0.05$, ***$p < 0.001$ Compared to Vehicle-Treated Group (Two-way ANOVA followed by Bonferroni's *post hoc* test); $N = 5$, Values are means ± SEM.

to the later phase implicating the role of arachidonic acid metabolites as well as polymorphonuclear cells in the inflammatory process [26]. *A. difformis* and *C. esculentus* therefore exhibit prophylactic efficacy against inflammation in chicks. The anti-inflammatory activity could be due to the presence of steroids in the extracts. Steroids are known to reduce inflammation by preventing phospholipase A2 from hydrolysing arachidonic acid from phospholipids in the cell membrane. This eventually results in a reduction in prostaglandins and thromboxanes which are important for inflammatory effects Aspirin which was used as a control is a non-steriodal anti-inflammatory drug (NSAID) which inhibits cyclooxygenase enzyme (COX-2) hence inhibiting prostaglandin and thromboxane [27]. The phytochemical screening revealed the presence of steroids in the extracts which could have been responsible for the anti-inflammatory activity. ADR, ADL and CEL at the doses tested demonstrated better anti-inflammatory activity than aspirin. The mechanism of action could be due to the inhibition of the arachidonic pathway. There is need to isolate the bioactive agents responsible for the above observed biological activities. These findings could therefore justify the folkloric use of *A. difformis* and *C. esculenta*.

Conclusion

Methanol extracts of *A. difformis* and *C. esculenta* possess broad spectrum antimicrobial and antioxidant activity. Extracts (ADR, ADL and CEL) exhibited significant anti-inflammatory activity.

Acknowledgement

Authors acknowledge the technical support of Mr. Francis Amankwah, Department of Pharmaceutics (Microbiology Section) and Mr. Thomas Ansah in the

Department of Pharmacology, Faculty of Pharmacy and Pharmaceutical Sciences, Kwame Nkrumah University of Science and Technology, Kumasi, Ghana.

References

1. Agyare C, Asase A, Lechtenberg M, Niehues M, Deters A, et al. (2009) An ethnopharmacological survey and in vitro confirmation of ethnopharmacological use of medicinal plants used for wound healing in Bosomtwi-Atwima-Kwanwoma area, Ghana. J Ethnopharmacol 125: 393-403.

2. Iwu M W, Duncan A R, Okunji C O (1999) New antimicrobials of plant origin. In: Janick J (Eds), Perspectives on new crops and new uses, ASHS Press, Alexandria, VA 457-462.

3. Agyare C, Dwobeng AS, Agyepong N, Boakye YD, Mensah KB, et al. (2013) Antimicrobial, Antioxidant, and Wound Healing Properties of Kigelia africana (Lam.) Beneth. and Strophanthus hispidus DC. Adv Pharmacol Sci 2013: 692613.

4. Tchiakpe L, Balansard G, Bernard P, Dalziel JM (1979) The useful plants of west tropical Africa. Planta Med 39: 257.

5. Oyetayo VO (2007) Comparative Studies of the phytochemical and antimicrobial properties of the leaf, stem and tuber of Anchomanes difformis. J Pharm Toxicol 2: 407-410.

6. Burkill HM (2000) The useful plants of west tropical Africa. Royal Botanic Gardens, Kew, UK.

7. Akinkuolere R O (2007) Assessment of the insecticidal properties of Anchomanes difformis (P. Beauv.) powder on five beetles of stored produce. J Entomol 4: 51-55.

8. Atawodi SE, Bulus T, Ibrahim S, Ameh DA, Nok AJ, et al. (2003) In vitro typanocidal effects of methanolic extract of some Nigerian savannah plants. Afr J Biotechnol 2: 317-321.

9. Bero J, Hannaert V, Chataigné G, Hérent M, Quetin-Leclercq J (2011) In vitro antitrypanoasomal and antileishmanial activity of plants used in Benin in traditional medicine and bio-guided fractionating of the most active extract. J Ethnopharmacol 137: 998-1002.

10. Phillip BA, Grindleya OF, Asemotaa HN, Errol Y, Morrisona A (2002) Carbohydrate digestion and intestinal Atpases in streptozotocin-induced diabetic rats fed extract of yam (Dioscorea cayenensis) or dasheen (Colocasia esculenta). Nutr Res 22: 333-341.

11. Boban PT, Nambisan B, Sudhakaran PR (2006) Hypolipidaemic effect of chemically different mucilages in rats: a comparative study. Br J Nutr 96: 1021-1029.

12. Tanaka R, Sakano Y, Nagatsu A, Shibuya M, Ebizuka Y, et al. (2005) Synthesis of digalactosyl diacylglycerols and their structure-inhibitory activity on human lanosterol synthase. Bioorg Med Chem Lett 15: 159-162.

13. Yang AH, Yeh KW (2005) Molecular cloning, recombinant gene expression, and antifungal activity of cystatin from taro (Colocasia esculenta cv. Kaosiung no. 1). Planta 221: 493-501.

14. Evans WC (2008) Trease and Evans' Pharmacognosy, 15th (Edn), WB Saunders, UK.

15. Sofowora AE (1993) Medicinal plants and traditional medicine in Africa, 2nd (Edn), Spectrum Books Ltd., Ibadan, Nigeria 289.

16. Eloff JN (1998) A sensitive and quick microplate method to determine the minimal inhibitory concentration of plant extracts for bacteria. Planta Med 64: 711-713.

17. Chizzola R, Michitsch H, Franz C (2008) Antioxidative properties of Thymus vulgaris leaves: comparison of different extracts and essential oil chemotypes. J Agric Food Chem 56: 6897-6904.

18. Wolfe K, Wu X, Liu RH (2003) Antioxidant activity of apple peels. J Agric Food Chem 51: 609-614.

19. Chanda S, Dave R (2009) In vitro models for antioxidant activity evaluation and some medicinal plants possessing antioxidant properties: An overview. Afr J Microbiol Res 3: 981-996.

20. Roach JT, Sufka KJ (2003) Characterization of the chick carrageenan response. Brain Res 994: 216-225.

21. Aliyu AB, Ibrahim MA, Musa AM, Musa AO, Kiplimo JJ, et al. (2013) Free radical scavenging and total antioxidant capacity of root extracts of Anchomanes difformis Engl. (Araceae). Acta Pol Pharm 70: 115-121.

22. Abah SE, Egwari LO, Mosaku TO (2011) In vitro antimicrobial screening on Anchomanes difformis (Blume) Engl. leaves and rhizomes against selected pathogens of public health importance. Adv Biol Res 5: 221-225.

23. Salazar R, Pozos ME, Cordero P, Perez J, Salinas MC, et al. (2008) Determination of the antioxidant activity of plants from northeast Mexico. Pharm Biol 46: 166-170.

24. Ayoola GA, Folawewo AD, Adesegun SA, Abioro OO, Adepoju-Bello AA, et al. (2008) Phytochemical and antioxidant screening of some plants of Apocynaceae from south eastern Nigeria. Afr J Plant Sci 2: 124-128.

25. Dudonné S, Vitrac X, Coutière P, Woillez M, Mérillon JM (2009) Comparative study of antioxidant properties and total phenolic content of 30 plant extracts of industrial interest using DPPH, ABTS, FRAP, SOD, and ORAC Assays. J Agric Food Chem 57: 1768-1774.

26. Gupta M, Mazumder UK, Gomathi P, Selvan VT (2006) Antiinflammatory evaluation of leaves of Plumeria acuminata. BMC Complement Altern Med 6: 36.

27. Cashman JN (1996) The mechanisms of action of NSAIDs in analgesia. Drugs 52 Suppl 5: 13-23.

3

Can Pharmacological Targeting of Advanced Glycation End Products Provide Protection against Experimentally Induced Liver Fibrosis?

Baraka AM* and Guemei A

Department of Clinical Pharmacology, Faculty of Medicine, Alexandria University, Egypt

Abstract

Aim: The aim of the current study was to assess the possible protective effects of advanced glycation end product (AGE) inhibitors against liver fibrosis and the possible underlying mechanisms.

Material and Methods: The present study was conducted on 48 male Wistar albino rats that were grouped into six groups of 8 rats each. Groups I-III; normal groups that were injected intraperitoneally (I.P.) with normal physiological saline, and either received no treatment (Group I), or received aminoguanidine (group II) or lisinopril (group III) daily for 4 weeks by I.P. injection. Group IV included untreated liver fibrosis group in which liver fibrosis was induced by thioacetamide. Groups V and VI included treated liver fibrosis group in which aminoguandine and lisinopril were injected I.P., daily for 4 weeks, concomitantly with thioacetamide. At the end of the treatment period (4 weeks), serum was collected to measure aminotransferases (AST and ALT) activities. Hepatic levels of AGEs, transforming growth factor-B1 (TGF-β1), tissue inhibitor of matrix metalloproteinase (TIMP), malondialdehyde (MDA), reduced glutathione (GSH) and hydroxyproline levels were assessed. Histopathological examination of liver was also carried out.

Results: TAA administration resulted in hepatic fibrosis evidenced histologically and by a significant increase in hepatic hydroxyproline level. TAA also resulted in a significant increase in serum AST, ALT activities as well as hepatic AGEs, TGF-β1, MDA and TIMP concentrations, together with a significant decrease in hepatic GSH. Administration of either aminoguanidine or lisinopril resulted in significant amelioration of above mentioned parameters.

Conclusion: Targeting AGEs could represent a therapeutic option for patients at risk for developing liver fibrosis.

Keywords: Advanced glycation end products; Lisinopril; Aminoguanidine; Thioacetamide; Fibrosis

Introduction

Liver cirrhosis is a serious irreversible disease and is the tenth leading cause of death in developed countries. If treated properly at fibrosis stage, cirrhosis could be prevented. Several experimental ameliorative strategies have been tested. However, there is still a remarkable lack of definitive evidence supporting specific therapies in these settings that can either cure or at least halt the progress of liver injury to liver fibrosis. Therefore, better strategies and /or drugs are desperately needed that would reduce the risk of liver fibrosis.

Although the pathophysiology of liver cirrhosis is not completely understood, some key events leading to tissue injury and thereby to liver fibrosis have been identified [1]. Much attention has been paid in the recent years to the nonenzymatic glycation and advanced glycation end products (AGEs) hypothesis. This hypothesis has been issued based on the fact that diabetes is featured by hyperglycemia, which facilitates the formation of AGEs and diabetes is commonly accompanied by non-alcoholic steatohepatitis, which could cause hepatic fibrosis. Indeed, Elevated levels of serum AGEs were observed in patients with non-alcoholic steatohepatitis [2].

Non-enzymatic glycation involves the reaction of the carbonyl group of sugar aldehydes with the N-terminus of free amino groups of proteins, resulting in the formation of Schiff's base that is subsequently rearranged to amadori products in a reaction called Maillard reaction. These amadori products or glycated proteins may then react with other proteins, lipids or DNA resulting in irreversible crosslinking and the formation of AGEs (post-amadori or glycotoxins) [3]. Although AGEs formation happens as a result of normal aging, it occurs at an accelerated rate in diseases as diabetes mellitus [4], renal failure [5], diabetic nephropathy [6], inflammatory conditions [7] and liver cirrhosis [8]. Recently, AGEs have been reported to significantly increase in hepatic fibrosis and to play a critical role in stimulating extracellular matrix (ECM) synthesis [9].

Several possible mechanisms could account for the ability of AGEs to stimulate liver fibrosis. AGEs can increase oxidative stress; induce production of pro-inflammatory cytokines as tumor necrosis factor-α (TNF-α), and transforming growth factor-β (TGF-β) [3]. Effects of AGEs are mediated by their receptor system, which could be generally divided into two categories. Receptor for AGEs (RAGE) facilitates oxidative stress (OS), cell growth and inflammation [10] and AGE receptors (AGE-Rs), eg. AGE-R1 (also called OST-48), is responsible for detoxification and clearance of AGEs [11].

Inhibition of AGEs formation, blockade of AGEs-RAGE interaction, suppression of RAGE expression, interruption of its signaling and induction of AGE-R1 expression are, thus, novel therapeutic strategies for targeting AGE-mediated diseases [12,13].

AGE inhibitors, as aminoguanidine, carnosine, acarbose and pyridoxamine, vary widely in structure, but they have common mechanism of action, which is the trapping of reactive carbonyl groups

*Corresponding author: Baraka AM, Department of Clinical Pharmacology, Faculty of Medicine, Alexandria University, Egypt, E-mail: azza.baraka@alexmed.edu.eg

for intermediates in the glycation synthetic pathway. Some of them may also exhibit free radical scavenging properties as aminoguanidine and pyridoxamine [14].

Another recent finding is that angiotensin-converting enzyme inhibitors (ACEi) are potent inhibitors of the formation of AGE. It has been postulated that ACE inhibition reduces the accumulation of AGEs in diabetes partly by increasing the production and secretion of AGE-Rs into plasma. This increase in sRAGE could act as a mechanism to divert AGE from binding to the full-length RAGE receptor, acting as a "decoy" because this truncated form of the receptor has no downstream signaling capacity [15].

The aim of this study was to examine the contribution of AGEs in thioacetamide-induced liver fibrosis in rats and to assess the possible protective effect of AGE inhibitors, namely aminoguanidine as well as the angiotensin converting enzyme inhibitor; lisinopril.

Material and Methods

Animals

Male Wistar albino rats (150-200 g) were obtained from the Animal House, Faculty of Medicine, Alexandria University. The animals were kept in a room under standard conditions of light, feeding and temperature. Animals used in this study were handled and treated in accordance with the strict guiding principles of the guide for care and use of laboratory animals of the Faculty of Medicine at Alexandria University. The experimental design and procedures were approved by the Ethical Committee of Faculty of Medicine -Alexandria University.

Experimental protocol

The animals were randomly divided into six groups, each of 8 animals as follows:

Group I (Normal control group): received physiological saline intraperitoneal (i.p) twice a week for 4 weeks.

Group II (Aminoguanidine control group): received aminoguanidine (Sigma-St. Louis, MO) in a dose of 100mg/ kg/d, i.p. [16] daily for 4 weeks starting from the first day of physiological saline administration.

Group III (Lisinopril control group): received Lisinopril (Zestril-AstraZeneca Pharmaceuticals LP) in a dose of 10mg/ kg, i.p. [17] daily for 4 weeks starting from the first day of physiological saline administration.

Group IV (Thioacetamide (TAA) group): hepatic fibrosis was induced by i.p. injection of TAA (Sigma-St. Louis, MO) in a dose of 200 mg / kg twice a week for 4 weeks [18].

Group V (TAA-Aminoguanidine-treated group): received i.p. aminoguanidine (Sigma-St. Louis, MO) in a dose of 100mg/ kg, daily for 4 weeks starting from the first day of TAA administration.

Group VI (TAA- Lisinopril-treated group): received i.p. Lisinopril (Zestril-AstraZeneca Pharmaceuticals LP) in a dose of 10mg/ kg, daily for 4 weeks starting from the first day of TAA administration.

Collection of samples

At the end of the experimental period (4 weeks), rats were anaesthetized using thiopental sodium (40 mg/kg), blood samples were collected and serum separated for determination of AST and ALT activities [19].

Preparation of liver homogenate: Liver tissue was washed by cold normal saline solution, then it was homogenized in a homogenization buffer (0.05 M Tris-HCl pH 7.9, 25% glycerol, 0.1 mM EDTA, and 0.32 M $(NH_4)2SO_4$) containing a protease inhibitor tablet (Roche, Germany). The resulting solution was sonicated in an ice bath for 10 seconds followed by centrifugation at 13000 rpm, 4°C for 5 minutes. The supernatant was aliquoted and stored at -80°C and assayed for protein concentration using BCA kit (Pierce, Rockford, USA) using bovine serum albumin diluted in the lysis buffer as standard. The homogenate was used for the determination of:

Malondialdehyde(MDA) concentration: As a marker for oxidative stress, the amount of hepatic TBARS was measured by the thiobarbituric acid assay (TBA) as previously described by Buege and Aust [20]. MDA concentrations were calculated by the use of 1,3,3,3 tetra-ethoxypropane as a standard. The results were expressed as nmol/g wet tissue weight.

Reduced glutathione (GSH) concentration: Reduced glutathione was determined as previously described by Owens and Belcher [21] based on the reaction of 5, 5- dithiobis-(2-nitrobenzoic acid) (DTNB) with the GSH present. The results were expressed as μmol / g wet tissue weight.

Transforming growth factor-beta1 (TGF-β) concentration: Hepatic level of TGF-β was determined using an enzyme-linked immunosorbent assay (ELISA technique) [22].

Tissue inhibitor of matrix metalloproteinase (TIMP-1) concentration: TIMP-1 protein concentration in liver homogenate was determined with a TIMP-1 sandwich ELISA kit from Rand D Systems (Mannheim, Germany) [23].

Advanced glycation end products (AGE) concentration: AGE concentration in liver homogenate was determined with AGE ELISA kit, Roche Diagnostics (Mannheim, Germany) [24].

Hydroxyproline (HPO) concentration: Collagen concentration in liver homogenate was determined with HPO ELISA kit, Biosource [25].

Histological evaluation

Portions of the livers were processed for light microscopy. This processing consisted of fixing the specimens in a 5% neutral formol solution, embedding the specimens in paraffin, making 5μm thick sections, and staining the sections with hematoxylin and eosin and Masson's Trichome staining.. The tissue slices were scanned and scored blindly. Pathological alterations consistent with fibrosis, enlargement, inflammatory infiltration, and breaking up of the hepatocellular limiting plates were observed in the portal tracts [26]. Liver sections were processed together for routine hematoxylin-eosin (HE) stain. Pathological diagnosis of each liver specimen was graded from 0 to VI according to the criteria described by Wang et al [27] (Table 1).

Statistical analysis: The results were expressed as mean values ± S.E.M. The data were analyzed by one-way analysis of variance (ANOVA) followed by Tukey-Kramer multiple comparisons test as *post hoc* test. $P < 0.05$ was considered statistically significant.

Results

Biochemical results

TAA administration resulted in a significant increase in serum AST and ALT activities as well as hepatic AGEs, MDA, TGF-β1, TIMP and HPO concentrations together with a significant reduction in GSH concentration in TAA group as compared to normal. Treatment with either aminoguanidine or lisinopril resulted in a significant decrease in serum AST, ALT activities and in hepatic AGEs, MDA, TGF-β1, TIMP and HPO concentrations as well as a significant increase in GSH concentration as compared to non-treated TAA group. No significant difference was found between untreated normal group and aminoguanidine-treated as well as lisinopril-treated control groups (Table 1).

Histopathological results

Administration of TAA progressively induced several histological markers of cell death and liver fibrosis. In this regard, the tissue sections of untreated TAA animals showed numerous signs of portal and periportal hepatitis. Centrilobular degeneration of hepatocytes, in which hepatocytes appeared swollen with faint staining cytoplasm and some hepatocytes appeared unnucleated. Sinusoids in between appeared obliterated. Both aminoguanidine and lisinopril administration significantly reduced the histological signs of cell damage (Figure 1).

Histopathological stages of the normal control as well as aminoguanidine and lisinopril control groups were all determined to be stage 0. TAA administration resulted in hyperplasia of connective tissues, but most of the histopathological stages were not above III. Aminoguanidine as well as Lisinopril-treated TAA rats resulted in obvious regression of fibrosis score (Table 2).

Degree of fibrosis	Score
No fibrosis	0
Slight fibrosis expanding to some portal areas and central veins	1
Marked fibrosis expansion, but without portal to portal bridging	2
Fibrosis expanding to most portal areas with occasional portal to portal bridging	3
Pseudolobules formed and partly replacing the normal architecture of the liver lobules	4
Occasional pseudolobules formed (incomplete cirrhosis)	5
Congested with pseudolobules, and between pseudolobules wide hyperplastic collagen fiber existed (complete cirrhosis)	6

Table 1: Scoring system assessing the degree of fibrosis.

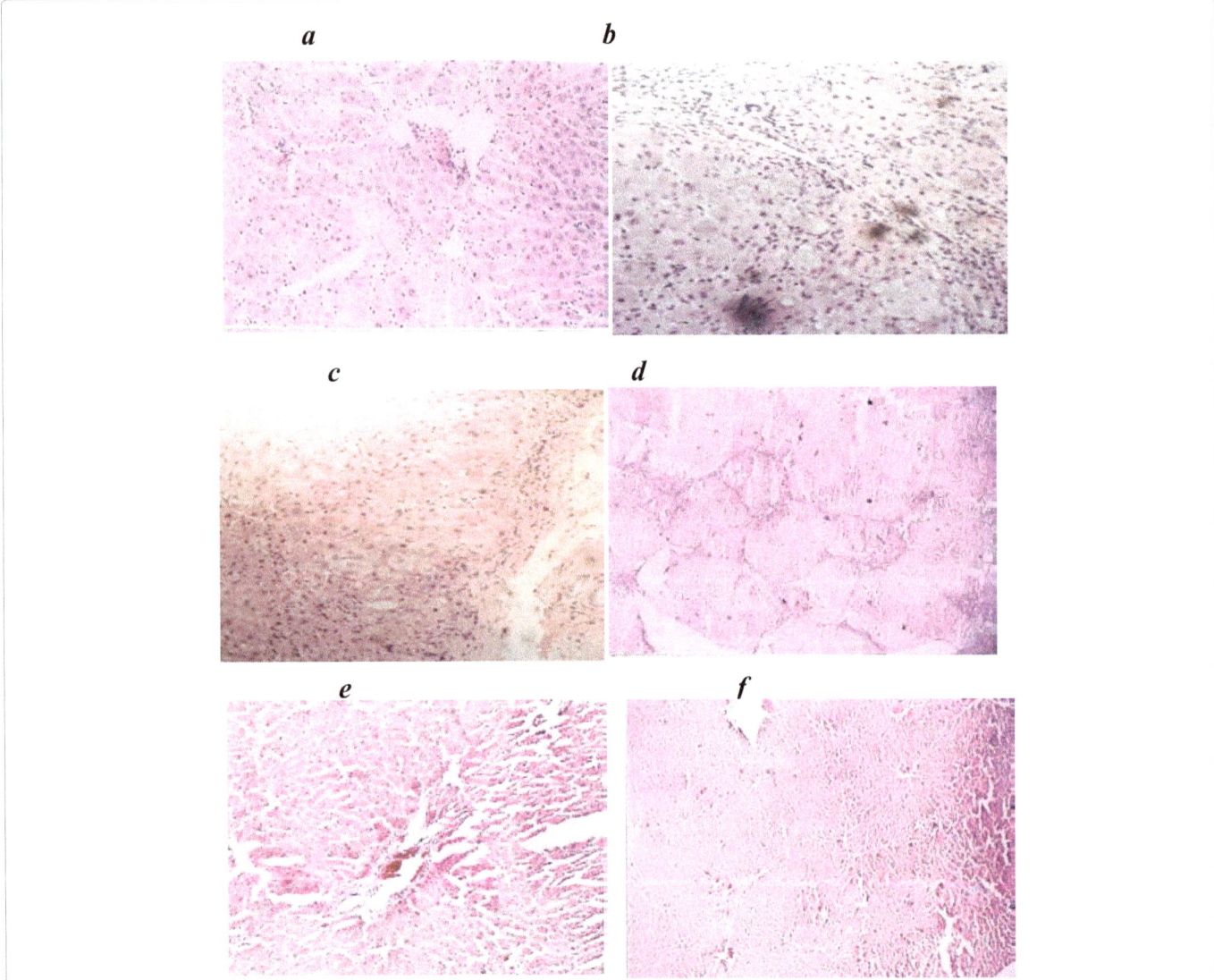

Figure 1: Light photomicrograph of H&E stained sections: (a) Control group (b) Aminoguanidine Control group (c) Lisinopril Control group (d) Thioacetamide group (e) Thioacetamide group treated with aminoguanidine (f) Thioacetamide group treated with lisinopril (X400).

Group	Hepatic fibrosis score	Serum ALT (U/L)	Serum AST (U/L)	Hepatic AGE (U/µg protein)	Hepatic MDA (nmol/g wet tissue)	Hepatic TGF-β1 (ng/ml)	Hepatic GSH (mg/g/g wet tissue)	Hepatic TIMP (ng/g wet liver)	Hepatic HPO (µg/g wet liver)
Normal control	0 ± 0	48 ± 15	85 ± 17	0.07 ± 0.02	18.31 ± 4.66	367.2 ± 14.6	124.2 ± 10.39	10.46 ± 2.6	42.4 6 ± 14.1
Aminoguanidine control	0 ± 0	51 ± 13	90 ± 12	0.09 ± 0.06	18.84 ± 5.10	389.7 ± 12.8	126.3 ± 15.12	10.79 ± 1.0	39.95 ± 10.21
Lisinopril control	0 ± 0	53 ± 11	89 ± 16	0.08 ± 0.04	19.09 ± 4.09	360 ± 14.7	127.7 ± 19.34	11.15 ± 2.7	41.76 ± 11.32
TAA	3.5 ± 0.2	137 ± 40*	312 ± 76*	0.30 ± 0.07*	96.25 ± 9.63*	1000 ± 28.4*	73.9 ± 9.62*	20.76 ± 5.7*	288.46 ± 76.5*
TAA-Aminoguanidine	1.5 ± 0.1	69 ± 10&	103 ± 5 7&	0.17 ± 0.05&	28.29 ± 5.15&	629 ± 18.3&	111.5 ± 22.13&	14.71 ± 3.9&	79.96 ± 10.13&
TAA-Lisinopril	1.4 ± 0.1	75 ± 16&	110 ± 37&	0.15 ± 0.06&	25.85 ± 6.20&	585 ± 21.4&	113.2 ± 19.5&	13.53 ± 4.5&	89.31 ± 9.15&
F value	78.83	66.95	57.96	39.16	42.73	82.52	43.28	52.76	75.92
P	<0.001	<0.001	<0.001	<0.001	<0.001	<0.001	<0.001	<0.001	<0.001

n: Number of rats in each group
*Significant compared to normal control group
&Significant compared to TAA group

Table 2: Hepatic fibrosis score, serum aspartate aminotransferase (AST) and alanine aminotransferase (ALT) activities and hepatic advanced glycation end products (AGEs), malondialdehyde (MDA), transforming growth factor beta-1 (TGFβ1), reduced glutathione (GSH), tissue inhibitor of matrix metalloproteinase (TIMP) and hydroxyproline (HPO) concentrations (Mean ± S.E.M.) of the studied groups, four weeks after thioacetamide administration in rats.

Discussion

In the present study, a significant increase in AGEs could be detected in TAA-induced liver fibrosis supporting the notion that these products might play a role in the pathogenesis of HSC activation and fibrosis.

AGEs are a heterogeneous group of molecules, formed in vivo both by non-oxidative and oxidative reactions of sugars and their adducts to proteins and lipids. It is now well established that formation and accumulation of AGEs progress during normal aging, and at an extremely accelerated rate under certain disease conditions, thus being implicated in various types of AGEs-related disorders such as diabetic vascular complications, neurodegenerative diseases ,cancers and fibrosis [28]. There is a growing body of evidence that activation of RAGE (receptor for AGEs) system is also implicated in these devastating disorders. Indeed, the engagement of RAGE with AGEs is shown to elicit oxidative stress generation and subsequently evoke inflammatory responses in various types of cells [29].

Liver is not only a target organ, but also an important site for clearance and catabolism of circulating AGEs. Although there are several studies to suggest the involvement of AGEs-RAGE system in various types of liver diseases such as non-alcoholic steatohepatitis, liver cirrhosis and cancers [30], as far as we know, there are no studies that have tested the effect of AGE inhibitors in liver fibrosis. Therefore, in this study, we investigated the pathological role of AGEs and the possible protective role of AGE inhibitors in TAA-induced liver fibrosis.

Enhanced RAGE expression in hepatic fibrogenesis has been previously shown in rats with cirrhosis induced by BDL and TAA treatment [31]. Our results are also in line with prior findings in CCl4-induced hepatic fibrosis where RAGE transcript and protein levels were upregulated until 6 weeks after the completion of CCl4 treatment [32]. Furthermore, it has been shown that α-SMA-positive HSC/myofibroblasts of the septal or portal interface, representing the prominent fibrogenic effectors, expressed RAGE in both fibrosis models.

AGEs have been reported to induce HSC proliferation by inducing cell proliferation and expression of genes relevant to HSC activation [33].

HSCs have been recently shown to express five advanced glycation end product receptors: Galectin-3, CD36, SR-AI, SR-BI and RAGE. All receptors, except SR-BI, showed up-regulation during HSC activation [34].

Indeed, a recent study conducted by Cai et al [35] demonstrated that specific targeting of RAGE using siRNA may inhibit RAGE gene expression effectively in the rat hepatic fibrosis model and attenuate the progression of established hepatic fibrosis. This therapeutic effect may be mediated via inhibition of the expression of NF-κB. These findings suggest that RAGE may be a new target to prevent hepatic fibrosis.

Another recent study investigated the effect of specific siRNAs targeting RAGE on the development of hepatic fibrosis (HF), using primary rat HSCs, which were isolated and cultured in vitro. The expression levels of RAGE together with IL-6, TNF-α, TGF-β1, connective tissue growth factor, laminin, hyaluronic acid and N-terminal procollagen III in the treated primary HSCs were significantly downregulated compared with those in the untreated. Thus, it can be deduced that RAGE-specific siRNAs inhibited the expression of RAGE in primary rat HSCs and inhibited the development of HF [36].

The current study demonstrated an increase in hepatic MDA concentration in TAA-induced liver fibrosis and this might be a possible mechanism whereby AGEs induce liver fibrosis. Our results support the findings of Guimarães et al [34] who demonstrated that AGEs induce reactive oxygen species generation in HSCs and they concluded that this unveils a potential new route through which AGEs induce liver fibrosis in the metabolic syndrome.

Our results also demonstrated the possible mechanistic role by which AGE inhibitors may provide protection against liver fibrosis. This is possibly achieved by acting upon many possible sites in the proposed pathway; first by preventing oxidative stress, second by inhibiting the synthesis of proinflammatory cytokines (TGF-b) and thirdly by combating extracellular matrix accumulation via upregulating TIMPs. Previous results have reported the ability of AGEs to induce oxidative stress as well as proinflammatory cytokines [34] and the ability of aminoguanidine to inhibit oxidative stress [35] and to decrease lung fibrosis [36].

It is possible that the high TIMP-1 activity in the liver microenvironment prevents apoptosis of HSC and thus contributes to the fibrogenic progress on liver injury. Alternatively, it has been shown that TIMP can act as a transcription factor [37].

Our study also confirmed a growing evidence of cross-talk between the renin angiotensin system (RAS) and AGEs pathways [38], where the current study demonstrated that lisinopril suppressed the level of AGEs and resulted in a significant decrease in TGF-b, MDA and hydroxyproline levels as well as a significant increase in hepatic GSH and TIMPs. These results are in accordance with other results reporting an inhibitory effect of drugs targeting RAS on AGEs [39].

The mechanism(s) by which AGEs activate RAS might be through the RAGE-PI3-K/Akt-dependent pathway [40]. Conversely, angiotensin II can stimulate AGEs and upregulate RAGE expression [41]. Indeed, other studies reported the ability of the angiotensin receptor blocker; telmisartan, to inhibit AGEs production [42-46].

Our study opens new areas of therapy and provides new modalities for the management of liver injury. Targeting AGEs could represent a therapeutic option for patients at risk of developing liver fibrosis. Patients with hepatitis B or C infections, patients with autoimmune hepatitis, patients with nonalcoholic steatohepatitis due to obesity or type 2 diabetes, and perhaps elective transplant recipients might be candidates.

References

1. Ginès P, Cárdenas A, Arroyo V, Rodés J (2004) Management of cirrhosis and ascites. N Engl J Med 350: 1646-1654.

2. Hyogo H, Yamagishi S, Iwamoto K, Arihiro K, Takeuchi M, et al. (2007) Elevated levels of serum advanced glycation end products in patients with non-alcoholic steatohepatitis. J Gastroenterol Hepatol 22: 1112-1119.

3. Vlassara H, Palace MR (2002) Diabetes and advanced glycation endproducts. J Intern Med 251: 87-101.

4. Singh R, Barden A, Mori T, Beilin L (2001) Advanced glycation end-products: a review. Diabetologia 44: 129-146.

5. Heidland A, Sebekova K, Schinzel R (2001) Advanced glycation end products and the progressive course of renal disease. Am J Kidney Dis 38: S100-106.

6. Zhou G, Li C, Cai L (2004) Advanced glycation end-products induce connective tissue growth factor-mediated renal fibrosis predominantly through transforming growth factor beta-independent pathway. Am J Pathol 165: 2033-2043.

7. Miyata T, Ishiguro N, Yasuda Y, Ito T, Nangaku M, et al. (1998) Increased pentosidine, an advanced glycation end product, in plasma and synovial fluid from patients with rheumatoid arthritis and its relation with inflammatory markers. Biochem Biophys Res Commun 244: 45-49.

8. Ahmed N, Lüthen R, Häussinger D, Sebeková K, Schinzel R, et al. (2005) Increased protein glycation in cirrhosis and therapeutic strategies to prevent it. Ann N Y Acad Sci 1043: 718-724.

9. Goodwin M, Herath C, Jia Z, Leung C, Coughlan MT, et al. (2013) Advanced glycation end products augment experimental hepatic fibrosis. J Gastroenterol Hepatol 28: 369-376.

10. Schmidt AM, Yan SD, Yan SF, Stern DM (2000) The biology of the receptor for advanced glycation end products and its ligands. Biochim Biophys Acta 1498: 99-111.

11. Lu C, He JC, Cai W, Liu H, Zhu L, et al. (2004) Advanced glycation endproduct (AGE) receptor 1 is a negative regulator of the inflammatory response to AGE in mesangial cells. Proc Natl Acad Sci U S A 101: 11767-11772.

12. Sourris KC, Forbes JM (2009) Interactions between advanced glycation end-products (AGE) and their receptors in the development and progression of diabetic nephropathy-are these receptors valid therapeutic targets. Curr Drug Targets 10: 42-50.

13. Yamagishi S, Nakamura K, Matsui T, Ueda S, Fukami K, et al. (2008) Agents that block advanced glycation end product (AGE)-RAGE (receptor for AGEs)-oxidative stress system: a novel therapeutic strategy for diabetic vascular complications. Expert Opin Investig Drugs 17: 983-996.

14. Price DL, Rhett PM, Thorpe SR, Baynes JW (2001) Chelating activity of advanced glycation end product inhibitors. J Biol Chem 276: 48967-48972.

15. Forbes JM, Thorpe SR, Thallas-Bonke V, Pete J, Thomas MC, et al. (2005) Modulation of soluble receptor for advanced glycation end products by angiotensin-converting enzyme-1 inhibition in diabetic nephropathy. J Am Soc Nephrol 16: 2363-2372.

16. Tsuji M, Higuchi Y, Shiraishi K, Kume T, Akaike A, et al. (2000) Protective effect of aminoguanidine on hypoxic-ischemic brain damage and temporal profile of brain nitric oxide in neonatal rat. Pediatr Res 47: 79-83.

17. Lakshmia KS, Sharma S (2010) Lisinopril fails to protect rat lens against sodium selenite-induced experimental cataractogenesis. Pharmacologyonline 2: 559-567.

18. Müller D, Sommer M, Kretzschmar M, Zimmermann T, Buko VU, et al. (1991) Lipid peroxidation in thioacetamide-induced macronodular rat liver cirrhosis. Arch Toxicol 65: 199-203.

19. Reitman S, Frankel S (1957) A colorimetric method for the determination of serum glutamic oxalacetic and glutamic pyruvic transaminases. Am J Clin Pathol 28: 56-63.

20. Buege JA, Aust SD (1978) Microsomal lipid peroxidation. Methods Enzymol 52: 302-310.

21. Owens CW, Belcher RV (1965) A Colorimetric Micro-Method for the Determination of Glutathione. Biochem J 94: 705-711.

22. Charan S, Palmer K, Chester P, Mire-Sluis AR, Meager A, et al. (1997) Transforming growth factor-beta induced by live or ultraviolet-inactivated equid herpes virus type-1 mediates immunosuppression in the horse. Immunology 90: 586-591.

23. Oggionni T, Morbini P, Inghilleri S, Palladini G, Tozzi R, et al. (2006) Time course of matrix metalloproteases and tissue inhibitors in bleomycin-induced pulmonary fibrosis. Eur J Histochem 50: 317-325.

24. Münch G, Keis R, Wessels A, Riederer P, Bahner U, et al. (1997) Determination of advanced glycation end products in serum by fluorescence spectroscopy and competitive ELISA. Eur J Clin Chem Clin Biochem 35: 669-677.

25. Woessner JF (1961) The determination of hydroxyproline in tissue and protein samples containing small portions of this imino acid. Arch Biochem Biophys 93: 440-447.

26. Gan BH, Ng GL, Bay BH, Chang CF (2005) Altered CD38 expression in thioacetamide-induced rat model of liver cirrhosis. Liver Int 25: 1233-1242.

27. Wang BE, Wang ZF, Ying WY, Huang SF, Li JJ. The study on animal model of experimental liver fibrosis. Zhonghua Yixue.

28. Wang BE (1989) [Animals with liver fibrosis induced by albumin immunization]. Zhonghua Yi Xue Za Zhi 69: 503-505, 36.

29. Singh VP, Bali A, Singh N, Jaggi AS (2014) Advanced glycation end products and diabetic complications. Korean J Physiol Pharmacol 18: 1-14.

30. Franko B, Brault J, Jouve T, Beaumel S, Benhamou PY, et al. (2014) Differential impact of glucose levels and advanced glycation end-products on tubular cell viability and pro-inflammatory/profibrotic functions. Biochem Biophys Res Commun 451: 627-631.

31. Hyogo H, Yamagishi S (2008) Advanced glycation end products (AGEs) and their involvement in liver disease. Curr Pharm Des 14: 969-972.

32. Lohwasser C, Neureiter D, Popov Y, Bauer M, Schuppan D (2009) Role of the receptor for advanced glycation end products in hepatic fibrosis. World J Gastroenterol 15: 5789-5798.

33. Xia JR, Liu NF, Zhu NX (2008) Specific siRNA targeting the Receptor for Advanced Glycation End Products Inhibits Experimental Hepatic Fibrosis in Rats. Int J Mol Sci 9: 638-661.

34. Lin J, Tang Y, Kang Q, Chen A (2012) Curcumin eliminates the inhibitory effect of advanced glycation end-products (AGEs) on gene expression of AGE receptor-1 in hepatic stellate cells in vitro. Lab Invest 92: 827-841.

35. Guimarães EL, Empsen C, Geerts A, van Grunsven LA (2010) Advanced glycation end products induce production of reactive oxygen species via the activation of NADPH oxidase in murine hepatic stellate cells. J Hepatol 52: 389-397.

36. Cai XG, Xia JR, Li WD, Lu FL, Liu J et al. (2014) Anti-fibrotic effects of specific-siRNA targeting of the receptor for advanced glycation end products in a rat model of experimental hepatic fibrosis. Mol Med Rep 10: 306-314.

37. Xia JR, Chen TT, Li WD, Lu FL, Liu J et al. (2015) Inhibitory effect of receptor for advanced glycation end product specific small interfering RNAs on the development of hepatic fibrosis in primary rat hepatic stellate cells. Mol Med Rep.

38. Torreggiani M, Liu H, Wu J, Zheng F, Cai W, et al. (2009) Advanced glycation end product receptor-1 transgenic mice are resistant to inflammation, oxidative stress, and post-injury intimal hyperplasia. Am J Pathol 175: 1722-1732.

39. Giardino I, Fard AK, Hatchell DL, Brownlee M (1998) Aminoguanidine inhibits reactive oxygen species formation, lipid peroxidation, and oxidant-induced apoptosis. Diabetes 47: 1114-1120.

40. Yildirim Z, Turkoz Y, Kotuk M, Armutcu F, Gurel A, et al. (2004) Effects of aminoguanidine and antioxidant erdosteine on bleomycin induced lung fibrosis in rats. Nitric Oxide 11: 156-165.

41. Yoshiji H, Kuriyama S, Yoshii J, Ikenaka Y, Noguchi R, et al. (2002) Tissue inhibitor of metalloproteinases-1 attenuates spontaneous liver fibrosis resolution in the transgenic mouse. Hepatology 36: 850-860.

42. Miller AG, Zhu T, Wilkinson-Berka JL (2013) The renin-angiotensin system and advanced glycation end-products in diabetic retinopathy: impacts and synergies. Curr Clin Pharmacol 8: 285-296.

43. Ono Y, Mizuno K, Takahashi M, Miura Y, Watanabe T (2013) Suppression of advanced glycation and lipoxidation end products by angiotensin II type-1 receptor blocker candesartan in type 2 diabetic patients with essential hypertension. Fukushima J Med Sci 59: 69-75.

44. Cheng CL, Tang Y, Zheng Z, Liu X, Ye ZC, et al. (2012) Advanced glycation end-products activate the renin-angiotensin system through the RAGE/PI3-K signaling pathway in podocytes. Clin Invest Med 35: E282.

45. Rüster C, Bondeva T, Franke S, Tanaka N, Yamamoto H, et al. (2009) Angiotensin II upregulates RAGE expression on podocytes: role of AT2 receptors. Am J Nephrol 29: 538-550.

46. Fukui Y, Yamashita T, Kurata T, Sato K, Lukic V, et al. (2014) Protective effect of telmisartan against progressive oxidative brain damage and synuclein phosphorylation in stroke-resistant spontaneously hypertensive rats. J Stroke Cerebrovasc Dis 23: 1545-1553.

4

Effect of *Ficus benghalensis* L. Latex Extract (FBLE) on Cisplatin Induced Hypotension and Renal Impairment in Wistar Rats

Yogesh Chand Yadav*

Department of Pharmacology, Pharmacy College Saifai, Uttar Pradesh University of Medical Sciences, UP, India

Abstract

Background and objective: *Ficus benghalensis* is a remarkable tree that sends down its branches and great number of shoots. It is used for treatment of neuralgia, rheumatism, lumbago, bruises, nasitis, gonorrhoea, inflammations, cracks of the sole and skin diseases and in ayurveda for diarrhea, dysentery, and piles". To evaluate protective activity of *F. benghalensis* latex extract (FBLE) on cisplatin induced hypotension and renal impairment in wistar rats.

Materials and methods: Rats were divided five groups and duration study 16 days. 1st group administered 5 ml/kg normal saline; 2rd group FBLE treated group 400 mg/kg per day; 3rd group (cisplatin treated) with single dose of cisplatin (5 mg/kg, i.p.) on 1st day and keep animals up to 6 days; 4th Group and 5th Group FBLE treated (200 and 400 mg/kg, p.o.) of for 1st to 10th day and single dose of cisplatin (5 mg/kg, i.p.) on 11th day.

Results: Phytochemical screening of FBLE has revealed presence of glycoside, alkaloids, tannin, flavonoids and amino acids, IC_{50} values for DPPH, and phosphor-molybdenum were 28.63 µg/ml ± 0.16 µg/ml, and 31.84 µg/ml ± 0.12 µg/ml respectively. The cisplatin-treated 3rd group showed a significant (**$P < 0.01$) changes renal functions biochemical parameters, blood pressure and histopathology were significantly (**$P < 0.01$) monitored by 200 mg/kg and 400 mg/kg protective groups.

Conclusion: These findings demonstrated that the FBLE and their constituents have excellent nephroprotective and normalized blood pressure.

Keywords: *Ficus benghalensis;* latex; Cisplatin; Hypotension; Renal impairment

Introduction

Ficus benghalensis is a remarkable tree from India that sends down its branches and great number of shoots, which take root and become new trunks [1]. Its chemical constituent's flavonoids leucoanthrocyanidin, leucoanthocyanin, friedelin, β sitosterol, quercetin-3-glactoside and rutin. Earlier, glucoside, 20-tetratriaconthene-2-one, 6-heptatriacontene-10-one, pentatriacontan-5-one, beta sitosterol-alpha-D-glucose, and meso-inositol have been isolated from the bark of the *F. benghalensis* and it latex contains Caoytchoue (2.4%), Resin, Albumin, Cerin, sugar, and Malic acid [2] and used for treatment of neuralgia, rheumatism, lumbago, bruises, nasitis, gonorrhoea, inflammations, cracks of the sole and skin diseases [3] and in ayurveda for diarrhea, dysentery, and piles [4]. The extract of *F. benghalensis* was reported to inhibit insulinase activity from the liver and kidney and it was also found to inhibit the lipid peroxidation. *F. benghalensis* was traditionally used for the treatment of mehavikar or urinary disorders [5] but no scientific studies have been undertaken to verify these claims. Thus, the purpose of current study was to investigate whether oral administration of *F. benghalensis* latex extract has possible protective effect against cisplatin induced hypotension and renal impairment in wistar rats.

Materials and Methods

Phytochemical standardization

Phytochemical identification and standardization of FBLE performed by TLC Method and HPTLC (CAMAG Switzerland, Linomet 5, and Scanner 3, Win Cat Software) Mobile phase: Butanol: Formic acid: Water (7.5 ml: 1.5 ml: 1.0 ml). HPTLC analysis performed by use of various standard amino acid markers like glutamine, glycine, cysteine, methione, lysine, arginine etc., and extract in which one compound was identified on the extract track and their RF value 0.56 was similar to standard methionine marker. The methionine content of FBLE standardized that was found 0.842 ± 0.0364 % of standard methionine.

Determination of total phenolic and flavonoid contents in FBLE

The total Phenolic and Flavonoid content of latex extract determined by method [6,7] respectively.

In vitro antioxidant activity

In vitro antioxidant studies of FBLE evaluated by Method DPPH [8] ferric chloride [9] phosphor-molybdenum [10] free radical scavenging.

Animals

Adult male Wistar rats (180-210 g) have an access to water and food ad libitum, and maintained under constant (25 ± 1°CAS), humidity (65 ± 10%) and a 12 h light/dark cycle. The experiment was carried out in accordance to the guidelines mentioned in the CPCSEA, and IAEC approved the experiment protocols (SVU/PH/IAEC/26.03.2010/02).

Acute toxicity study

Each group of Wistar rats fasted overnight prior to the experiment. Each group of rats fed FBLE dissolved in normal saline with increasing

*Corresponding author: Yogesh Chand Yadav, Department of Pharmacology, Pharmacy College Saifai, Uttar Pradesh University of Medical Sciences, Saifai-206130, Etawah, UP, India, E-mail: drycy31@gmail.com

dose like 5, 50, 100, 200, 400, 1000 2000 mg/kg body weight. The animals observed continuously for 2 h and then every 2 h up to 24 and 72 h for gross behavior changes. So LD_{50} cut off of the extract was 2000 mg/kg body weight. FBLE dose regimen prepared like $1/10^{th}$ and $1/5^{th}$ of the respective LD_{50} cut off values.

Cisplatin-induced renal injury

Five groups of rats (n=6) used, in which 1st group administered 5 ml/kg normal saline throughout the experiment for 16 days; 2rd control group received FBLE 400 mg/kg per day for 16 days; 3nd group (cisplatin treated) with single dose of cisplatin (5 mg/kg, i.p.) on 1st day and keep animals up to 6 days; 4th Group and 5th Group (Protective) FBLE (200 and 400 mg/kg, p.o. for 1st to 10th day and single dose of cisplatin (5 mg/kg, i.p.) on 11th day and keep animals up to 16 days [11].

On the 6th day in cisplatin control and 16th day in control, protective were measured blood pressure by help of student physiograph (instruments & chemicals PVT. LTD, Ambala, India) after then blood withdrawn from retro-orbital sinus of rats for biochemical estimation for serum urea and creatinine levels using diagnostic kit from Span Diagnostic, "Kolkata on chemical analyzer (Microlab 3000) and also dissected out the kidneys for estimation of *in vivo* antioxidant enzymes and histopathological works [12]."

In vivo Antioxidant activity

Rat kidneys homogenized and centrifuged at 10,000 rpm at 0°C for 20 min. The supernatant used for estimation of antioxidant enzymes level by calorimetric method using spectrophotometer (Merck thermo spectronic, Model NO. UV-1, double beam), Glutathione reductase (GSH) estimated by method [13] Lipid peroxidation by thiobarbuturic acid-reactive substances (TBARS) methods [14] Superoxide dismutase (SOD) by method [15] Catalase (CAT) by colorimetric assay [16] and the sediment of the centrifuge used for estimation of the $Na^{+}K^{+}ATPase$ by method [17] $Ca^{2+}ATPase$ [18] $Mg^{2+}ATPase$ [19].

Statistical analysis

Result were expressed as mean ± SEM, Statistical Analysis were performed with one way analysis of variance (ANOVA) followed by Dunnett's test. P value less than <0.05 was considered significant.

Results

FBLE has revealed presence of glycoside; alkaloids, tannin (Phenolic compound), Flavonoids, and methionine amino acid (Figures 1 and 2). Total Phenolic and flavonoids content had obtained 2.76 ± 0.84 mg GAE/g and 1.84 ± 0.5 mg QE/g extract respectively.

In vitro antioxidant potential of FBLE was evaluated by scavenging effect of DPPH, ferric chloride, and phosphor-molybdenum. IC_{50} values for DPPH, and phosphor-molybdenum were 28.63 ± 0.16 µg/ml, and 31.84 ± 0.12 µg/ml respectively (Figures 3 and 4).

Blood pressure of cisplatin-treated was decreased to 70 mmHg which is significantly increased 100 mmHg in protective groups.

The cisplatin-treated showed a significant increase urine volume, serum urea and creatinine levels, lipid peroxidation and decrease body wt. (Figure 2), GSH, SOD, CAT, Na^{+}/K^{+} ATPase, Ca^{++} ATPase, $Mg^{++}ATPase$ of kidney (Tables 1-3), on the 6th day as compared to the group I. They were significantly (p<0.01) recovered in protective regimen with treated dose at 200 and 400 mg/kg of FBLE.

Histopathological sections of the kidneys showed marked vasoconstriction, hyaline droplets, proinflammatory and tubular necrosis were observed cisplatin treated group III (Figure 5; Plates 1A-1C) and in the protective regimen extract (200 and 400 mg/kg body wt., p.o.) reduced hyaline droplets, tubular dilation and recovery of tubular necrosis in which 400 mg/kg more effective reduction than 200 mg/kg (Figure 5; Plate 1D and 1E) respectively.

Discussion

In the present study, cisplatin-induced renal impairment was evidenced by an increase in serum urea and creatinine and acute tubular necrosis. These changes observed on 6th day after administration of a single dose 5 mg/kg cisplatin. FBLE normalized, raised serum urea, creatinine levels, lipid peroxidation and decreased blood pressure, GSH, SOD, CAT, Na^{+}/K^{+} ATPase, Ca^{++} ATPase, $Mg^{++}ATPase$ of kidney. The histopathological report supported the biochemical findings.

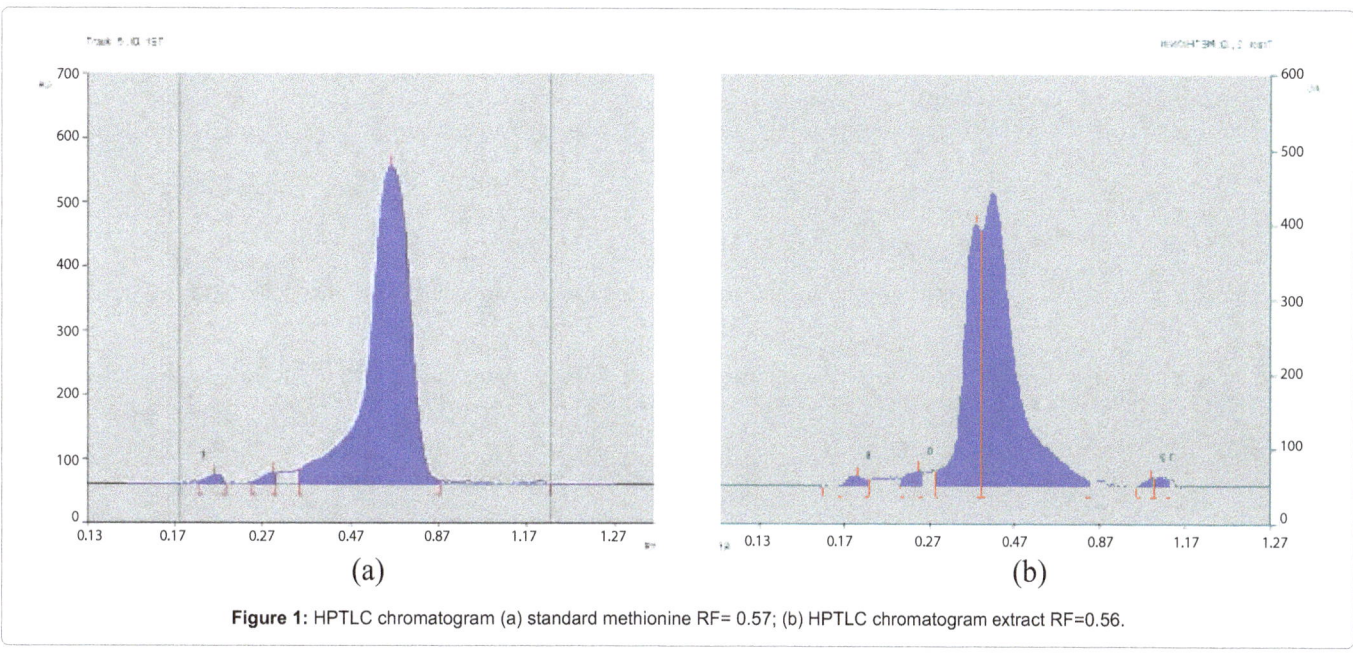

Figure 1: HPTLC chromatogram (a) standard methionine RF= 0.57; (b) HPTLC chromatogram extract RF=0.56.

Groups	Urine volume (ml/24 h)	Urea level in serum (mg/dl)	Creatinine level in blood serum (mg/dl)
Control	5.33 ± 0.33	24.16 ± 1.04	0.94 ± 0.05
Extract FBL	6.66 ± 0.66[b*]	25.18 ± 1.85[b*]	0.96 ± 0.03[b*]
Cisplatin treated	14.66 ± 0.88[a]	76.66 ± 2.24[a]	2.32 ± 0.10[a]
Protective (200 mg/kg)	8.66 ± 0.36[b*]	50.66 ± 2.82[b']	1.53 ± 0.01[b*]
Protective (400 mg/kg)	10.66 ± 0.42[b**]	61.66 ± 1.05[b**]	1.85 ± 0.08[b**]

[a]: P<0.01 as compared to the control; [b]: **P<0.01 as compared to the cisplatin treated group; [b]: *P<0.05 as compared to cisplatin treated group.

Table 1: Effects of methanol extract of *Ficus benghalensis* latex L. on the Urinary volume, Urea and Creatinine level in serum on 6th day after cisplatin administration.

Groups	μmol GSH/g	n Mol MDA/g. Ml	Unit SOD/g	CAT (μ mole of H_2O_2/g
Control	69.50 ± 1.54	14.00 ± 0.57	21.83 ± 0.94	323.33 ± 1.75
Extract FBL	68.34 ± 2.28[b]	14.98 ± 0.36[b*]	20.43 ± 0.59[b*]	319.53 ± 5.24[b*]
Cisplatin treated	45.33 ± 1.66[a]	24.50 ± 0.61[a]	07.16 ± 0.60[a]	201.67 ± 3.33[a]
Protective (200 mg/kg)	58.66 ± 2.82[b*]	15.00 ± 2.39[b*]	15.83 ± 0.60[b]	285.83 ± 8.00[b*]
Protective (400 mg/kg)	59.51 ± 2.44[b**]	18.16 ± 0.74[b**]	12.66 ± 0.66[b**]	232.50 ± 4.42[b**]

[a]: P<0.01 as compared to the control; [b]: **P<0.01 as compared to the cisplatin treated group; [b]: *P<0.05 as compared to cisplatin treated group.

Table 2: Effect of methanol extract of *Ficus benghalensis* latex L. on the lipid peroxidation and antioxidant enzymes of kidney on 6th day after cisplatin administration.

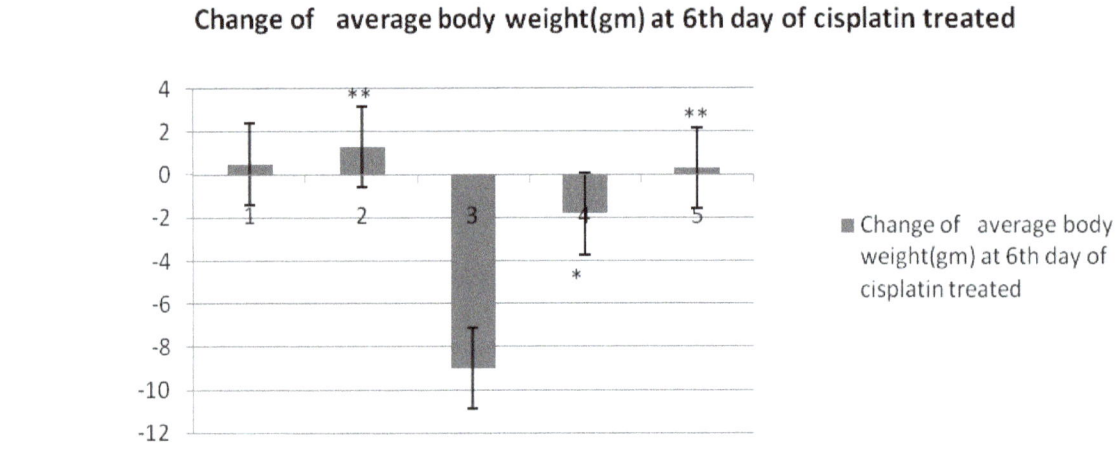

1: Control; 2: Extract FBL; 3: Cisplatin treated; 4: Protective 200 mg/kg; 5: Protective 400 mg/kg, dose of extract

Figure 2: Effect methanol *Ficus benghalensis* L. latex extract on average change body weight of various groups as compared to cisplatin treated group (3). Each group represents mean ± S.D. of six animals, **P<0.01,*P>0.05, **P>0.01, **P<0.01, **P>0.01 as compared to the cisplatin treated group.

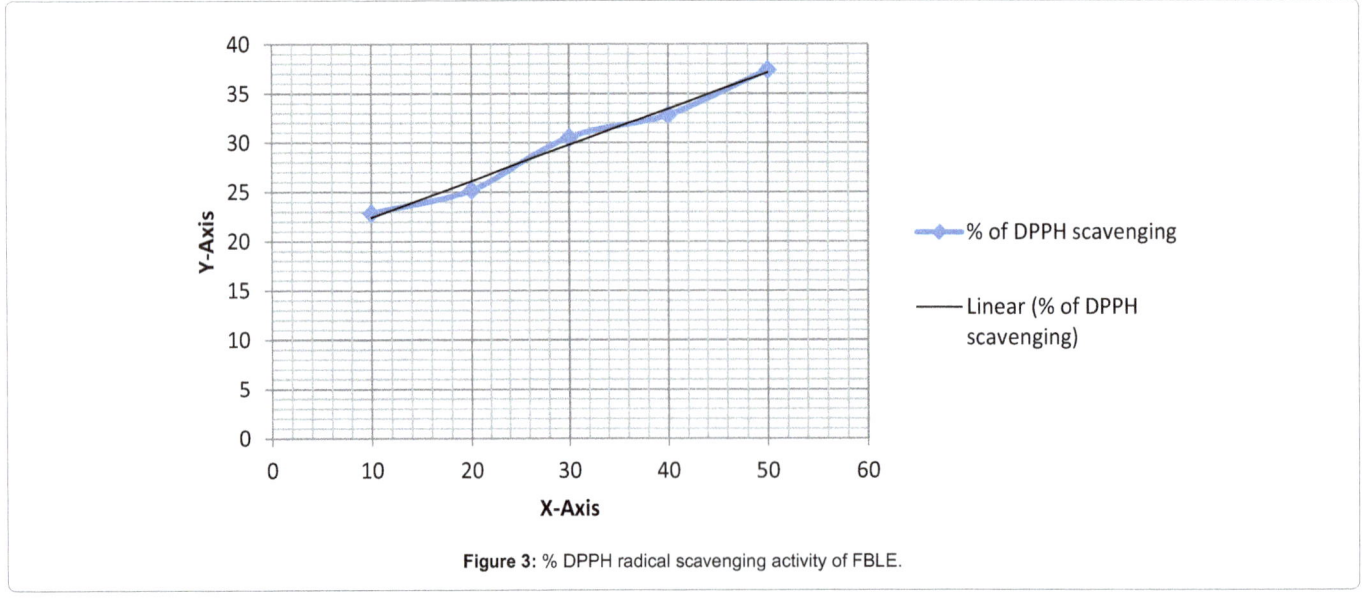

Figure 3: % DPPH radical scavenging activity of FBLE.

Groups	Na$^+$/K$^+$ ATPase (mM of phosphate librated/mg tissue)	Ca^{++} ATPase (mM of phosphate librated/mg tissue	Mg^{++} ATPase (mM of phosphate librated/mg tissue)
Control	210.83 ± 2.64	102.83 ± 2.31	152.67 ± 0.88
Extract FBL	210.34 ± 2.37[b*]	101.51 ± 2.31[b*]	154.66 ± 1.66[b*]
Cisplatin treated	135.17 ± 2.51[a]	64.33 ± 1.05[a]	81.66 ± 1.05[a]
Protective (200 mg/kg)	159.83 ± 2.06[b*]	71.53 ± 2.25[b']	98.00 ± 2.19[b*]
Protective (400 mg/kg)	186.56 ± 2.46[b**]	98.28 ± 2.16[b**]	116.16 ± 2.56[b**]

[a]: P<0.01 as compared to the control; [b]: **P<0.01 as compared to the cisplatin treated group; [b]: *P<0.05 as compared to cisplatin treated group.

Table 3: Effects of methanol extract of *Ficus benghalensis* L. latex on ATPase in kidney tissue of various groups on 6th day after cisplatin administration.

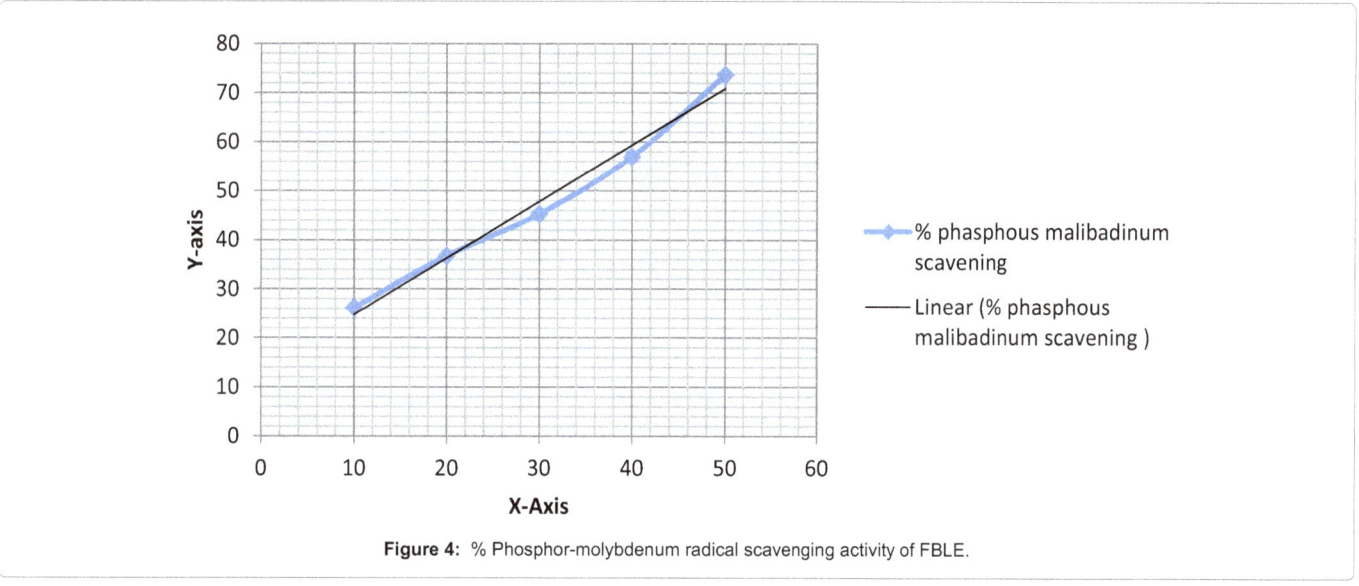

Figure 4: % Phosphor-molybdenum radical scavenging activity of FBLE.

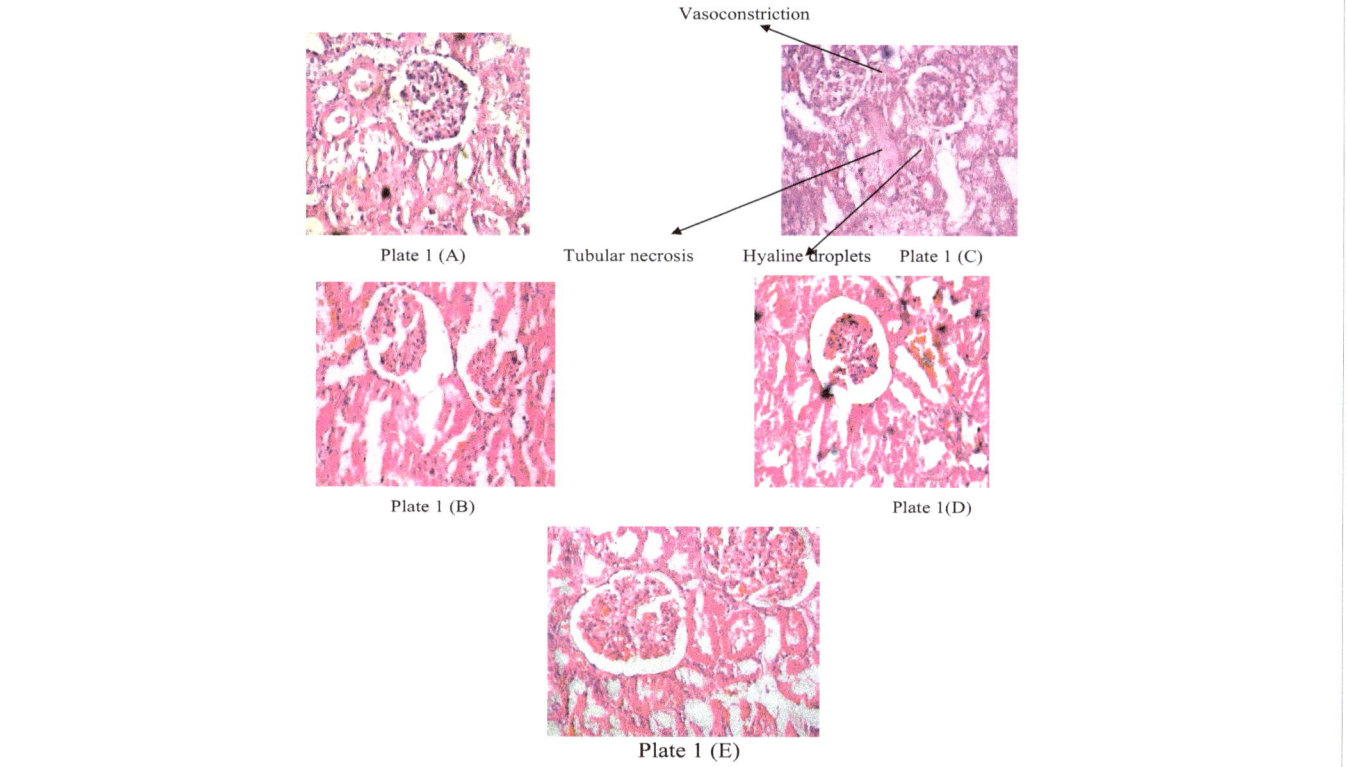

Figure 5: "Histopathology sections of kidney; Plate 1(A) Vehicle-treated, Plate 1 (B) FBLE treated, Plate 1 (C) Cisplatin-treated rats (5 mg/kg, 6 days), Plate 1 (D) Protective (200 mg/kg), and Plate 1 (E) Protective (400 mg/kg)".

The FBLE treated dose 400 mg/kg body weight was observed more significant than 200 mg/kg body wt.

According to previous findings, it was conformed that the single dose of cisplatin (5 mg/kg, i.p.) causes a significantly increase in two serum markers of the kidney function, viz. serum urea and creatinine [20]. Present study was revealed that significantly decrease the level of urea and creatinine in blood serum after treatment with FBLE that was indicate FBLE has nephroprotective activity. A relationship between oxidative stress and nephrotoxicity had well demonstrated in many experimental models Evidence point. The regulation up to normal blood pressure could be protective effect of renal impairment and activation sympathetic nerves system.

In vitro studies of FBLE evaluated for its good antioxidant potential revealed DPPH, ferric chloride, phosphor-molybdenum of free radical scavenging effect with lower IC_{50} values. FBLE has been found to be a rich source of Caoytchoue (2.4%), Cerin, and Malic acid and present phytochemical data have been revealed tannin, Flavonoids, methionine. Yadav [21] also reported hepatoprotective effect of *Ficus religiosa* latex on cisplatin induced liver injury in Wistar rats.

Deegan et al. [22], also reported that nephrotoxicity, cytotoxicity and renal handling of a cisplatin methionine complex in male wistar rats. The present phytochemical screening data has observed methionine which was antagonized cisplatin nephrotoxicity.

Conclusion

Finally, it is concluded that FBLE could be an ameliorated cisplatin hypotension and nephrotoxicity.

Acknowledgement

This investigation was supported by MJRP University Jaipur.

References

1. Subramanian PM, Misra GS (1978) Chemical constituents of Ficus bengalensis (part II). Pol J Pharmacol Pharm 30: 559-562.

2. Joy PP, Thomas J, Mathew S, Skaria BP (1999) The Wealth of India, Volume-(F-G). In: A Dictionary of Indian Raw Materials and industrial products. Vol. 4. New Delhi: Council of Scientific and Industrial Research pp: 24-30.

3. Warrier PK, Nambiar VPK, Ramankutty C (1995) Indian Medicinal Plants. Orient Longman Ltd., Madras pp: 1-5.

4. Mukherjee PK, Saha K, Murugesan T, Mandal SC, Pal M, et al. (1998) Screening of anti-diarrhoeal profile of some plant extracts of a specific region of West Bengal, India. J Ethnopharmacol 60: 85-89.

5. Vaidya BA (2005) Nighantu. Chaukhambha Prakashan p: 471.

6. Taga MS, Miller EE, Pratt DE (1984) Chia seeds as a source of natural lipid antioxidants. J Am Oil Chem Soc 61: 928-931.

7. Li Y, Guo C, Yang J, Wei J, Xu J, et al. (2006) Evaluation of antioxidant properties of pomegranate peel extract in comparison with pomegranate pulp extract. Food Chem 96: 254-260.

8. Blois MS (1958) Antioxidants determinations by the use of stable free radical. Nature 181: 1199-11100.

9. Benzie IF, Strain JJ (1996) The ferric reducing ability of plasma (FRAP) as a measure of "antioxidant power": the FRAP assay. Anal Biochem 239: 70-76.

10. Prieto P, Pineda M, Aguilar M (1999) Spectrophotometric quantization of antioxidant capacity through the formation of a phosphor-molybdenum complex: Specific application to the determination of vitamin E. Anal Biochem 269: 337-341.

11. Annie S, Rajagopal PL, Malini S (2005) Effect of Cassia auriculata Linn. Root of extract on cisplatin and gentamicin-induced renal injury. Phytomedicine 12: 555-560.

12. Sedlak M, Lindsay R (1968) Estimation of total, protein-bound and non-protein sulfhydryl groups in tissue with Ellman's reagent. Anal Biochem 25: 192-205.

13. Mihara M, Uchiyama M (1978) Determination of malonaldehyde precursor in tissues by thiobarbituric acid test. Anal Biochem 86: 271-278.

14. Misra HP, Fridovich I (1972) The role of superoxide anion in the autoxidation of epinephrine and a simple assay for superoxide dismutase. J Biol Chem 247: 3170-3175.

15. Sinha AK (1972) Colorimetric assay of catalase. Anal Biochem 47: 389-394.

16. Bonting SL (1970) Presence of enzyme system of mammalian tissue. Wiley Inter Sci 197: 257.

17. Hjerken S, Pan H (1982) Purification and characterization of two form of the low affinity calcium ion ATPase from erythrocyte membrane. Biochem Biophys Acta 728: 281-288.

18. Ohnishi T, Suzuki T, Suzuki Y, Ozawa K (1982) A comparative study of plasma membrane Mg2+ -ATPase activities in normal, regenerating and malignant cells. Biochim Biophys Acta 684: 67-74.

19. Chandrasekaran SK, Benson H, Urquhart J (1978) Methods to achieve controlled drug delivery: The biochemical engineering approach. In: Robinson JR (ed.) Sustained and Controlled Drug Delivery Systems. New: Marchel Dekker pp: 557-593.

20. Francescato HD, Costa RS, Rodrigues Camargo SM, Zanetti MA, Lavrador MA, et al. (2001) Effect of oral selenium administration on cisplatin-induced nephrotoxicity in rats. Pharmacol Res 43: 77-82.

21. Yadav YC (2015) Hepatoprotective effect of Ficus religiosa latex on cisplatin induced liver injury in Wistar rats. Rev Bras Famacogn 3: 278-283.

22. Deegan PM, Pratt IS, Ryan MP (1994) The nephrotoxicity, cytotoxicity and renal handling of a cisplatin-methionine complex in male Wistar rats. Toxicology 89: 1-14.

5

Effect of Vitamin C and Vitamin E on Mercuric Chloride-Induced Reproductive Toxicity in Male Rats

Muthu K[1] and Krishnamoorthy P[2]*

[1]Department of Zoology, Raja Serfoji College, Thanjavur-622 404, Tamil Nadu, India
[2]Department of Biotechnology, J.J.College of Arts and Science, Pudukottai-622 404, Tamil Nadu, India

Abstract

To evaluate the protective effects of Vitamin C and Vitamin E against Mercuric chloride -induced reproductive toxicity and to study the mechanisms underlying these effects. Male Wistar rats were orally administered mercuric chloride (10 mg/100 gm b.wt), (10 mg/100 gm b.wt) of mercuric chloride + (40 mg/100 gm b.wt) of Vitamin C and (10 mg/100 gm b.wt) of mercuric chloride + (20 mg/100 gm b.wt) of Vitamin E were administered orally to male albino rats for 30 days. Treatments with either Vitamin C or Vitamin E resulted in a significant protection of reproductive function. Both vitamins reduced the extent of mercuric chloride-induced reproductive toxicity, as evidenced by decrease in sperm abnormality and increase in sperm motility. Mercuric chloride-induced alterations in testis lipid peroxidation (MDA) were also markedly improved by test vitamins, and mercuric chloride -induced alterations in the testis antioxidation defense system were profoundly prevented by vitamins. In groups, where mercuric chloride was combined with either Vitamin C or Vitamin E, antioxidation enzymes like superoxide dismutase (SOD), reduced glutathione (GSH), and catalase (CAT) were significantly elevated compared to the mercuric chloride-treated group. The results provide further insight into the mechanisms of mercuric chloride-induced reproductive toxicity and confirm the antioxidant potential of both Vitamin C and Vitamin E.

Keywords: Mercuric chloride; Testicular toxicity; Protection; Male rats; Testis; Oxidative stress; Antioxidants; Vitamin C; Vitamin E

Introduction

Mercury is a naturally occurring metal, which can exist in several forms. Metallic mercury is a shiny, silver-white, odorless liquid, which forms a colorless, odorless gas if heated. Mercury combines with other elements such as chlorine, sulfur, or oxygen to form inorganic mercury compounds or salts, which are usually white solids. Mercury also combines with carbon to make organic mercury compounds, the most common of which is methyl mercury [1].

Historically, mercuric chloride ($HgCl_2$) pollution has posed a serious health hazard to humans. Mercuric chloride ($HgCl_2$) from industries surrounding the area was discharged directly into the bay, producing elevated levels in fish [1]. The extreme morbidity and mortality in humans who consumed these fish clearly demonstrated the relationship between $HgCl_2$ ingestion and human health. Adverse effects of $HgCl_2$ on fish-eating mammals have also been reported [2], suggesting a link between environmental $HgCl_2$ and wildlife health. Although strict regulations now limit the discharge of $HgCl_2$ directly into bodies of water, indirect contamination continues. Augmented output of airborne $HgCl_2$ from anthropogenic sources, such as coal-fired utilities and the burning of municipal wastes are likely to be responsible for observed increases in atmospheric levels [3]. Although controversial, reports have indicated that exposure to $HgCl_2$ might impair male reproductive health. For example, several reports have indicated that $HgCl_2$ ingestion can cause reduced spermatogenesis and steroidogenesis in rodents [4].

Inorganic mercury-induced testicular damage is a known fact in experimental animals [5]. In humans, mercury induces loss of libido [6], hypospermia, astheno-spermia and teratospermia [7]. Owing to the relative spermiotoxicity of $HgCl_2$, almost all patients under chemotherapy will show temporary or permanent azoospermia. The damage to both spermatogenesis and testicular endocrine function can be temporary or permanent base on the applied dose of $HgCl_2$ [8]. Testicular damage is also developed in various animal species [9,10].

Within days of $HgCl_2$ injection, animals develop severe testicular damage, which is characterized by spermatogenic damages, germ cell apoptosis, Leyding cell dysfunction and testicular steroidogenic disorder [10].

Many environmental contaminants have been reported to disturb the pro-oxidant or antioxidant balance of the cells thereby inducing oxidative stress [11]. Oxidative stress in biological systems originates as the result of an imbalance between the generation of oxidizing species and cellular antioxidant defences [11,12]. The radical chain reaction of lipid peroxidation appears to be a continuous physiological process. The process, if out of control, can alter essential cell functions to cell death [13]. Oxidative stress has been shown to mediate the $HgCl_2$ -induced reproductive toxicity [14].

A major contributor to non-enzymatic protection against lipid peroxidation (LP) is vitamin E and vitamin C, a known free radical scavenger [12]. Vitamin E as a lipid soluble, chain breaking antioxidant [13] plays a major role against oxidative stress, and prevents the production of lipid peroxides by scavenging free radicals in biological membranes [15]. Vitamin C, an endogenous water-soluble natural antioxidant, chain breaking antioxidant and is found in both intra cellularly and extra cellularly [16]. It prevent lipid peroxidation due to peroxy radicals, protects against DNA damage by hydrogen peroxide radical. Vitamin E and Vitamin C have been widely investigated due to

*****Corresponding author:** Krishnamoorthy P, Department of Biotechnology, J.J.College of Arts and Science, Pudukottai-622 404, Tamil Nadu, India, E-mail: sindhues.muthu15@gmail.com

its action against oxidative stress [17], its protective role on biological membranes [18].

The administration of antioxidants such as vitamin E [19], or vitamin C [14] has been reported to prevent different $HgCl_2$-associated side effects. On the other hand, the mechanism of $HgCl_2$-induced testicular toxicity is not quite understood yet and protective remedies against $HgCl_2$-induced testicular damage are scarce. This investigation was set to evaluate the protective effects of Vitamin C and Vitamin E against $HgCl_2$-induced testicular toxicity in male rats and to study the mechanisms underlying these effects.

Materials and Methods

Chemicals

Mercuric chloride, Vitamin C, Vitamin E, Thiobarbituric acid, reduced glutathione, 5,5-dithiobis (2- nitrobenzoic acid), Folin's reagent, epinephrine, SOD enzyme, H_2O_2 and bovine serum albumin were obtained from Sigma Chemical Co., Mumbai, India. All other chemicals were obtained from local commercial suppliers.

Experimental animals

Twelve - week-old adult Wister albino male rats weighing between 175 - 225g, along with supplies of their standard diet, were obtained from animal house centre of "Jawaharlal Nehru Institute of Post Graduate Medical Educations and Research" (JIPMER), Pondicherry. The study design was approved "Animal ethic committee" J. J. College of Arts and Science, Pudukottai, Tamil nadu, India.

Treatment regime

Animals were divided into six groups of six rats each for 30 days. Group I was received distilled water and served as the control. Group II was administered mercuric chloride (10 mg/100 gm. b.wt). Group III received mercuric chloride (10 mg/100 gm b.wt) and Vitamin C (40 mg/100 gm b.wt), Group IV was administered mercuric chloride (10 mg/100 gm. b.wt) and Vitamin E (30 mg/100 gm. b.wt), Group V was received (40 mg/100 gm b.wt) of Vitamin C and Group VI was administered (30 mg/100 gm. b.wt) of Vitamin E.

Sample preparation

Following diethyl ether anesthesia, blood was collected from the retro-orbital plexus [20]. Following sacrifice, testes and epididymis were removed and weighed. The organ weight/body weight ratio x 100 was calculated and expressed as a relative organ weight. For histopathological examination, one testis was immediately fixed in 10% buffered formalin. For biochemical determination, another testis was homogenized in ice-cold KCl_4 (150 mM). The ratio of tissue weight to homogenization buffer was 1:10. From the latter, suitable dilutions for determination of the levels of GSH, LP product MDA, total proteins, and activities of SOD and CAT were prepared in suitable different buffers. To obtain serum, blood was collected in centrifuge tubes and centrifuged in a refrigerated centrifuge (4°C) at 3000 r.p.m. for 20 minutes.

Sperm motility, sperm count and abnormality test

After removing each epididymis, it was immediately weighed, minced in 5ml of physiological saline and then incubated at 37°C for 30 minutes to allow sperms to swim from the epididymal tubules. After mixing, one drop was placed onto a warm microscope slide and cover slip was placed over the droplet. The percentage of motile sperm was recorded with a phase contrast microscope at 400X magnification. The cover slip was removed and sperms were allowed to air dry and then stained with 1% eosin and examined for morphology abnormalities. Three hundred sperm from different fields were examined with a phase contrast microscope. Total sperm number was determined by using a Neubauer hemocytometer by a method of Yokoi et al. [21]. The total number of sperm per gram of epididymis was then calculated.

Biochemical assays and histopathology

The GSH content of testis homogenate was determined using the method described by Van Dooran et al. [22]. The GSH determination method is based on the reaction of Ellman's reagent 5, 5-dithiobis (2-nitrobenzoic acid) (DTNB) with the thiol group of GSH at pH 8.0 to produce 5-thiol-2- nitrobenzoate, which is yellow. Malondialdehyde (MDA) is the most abundant individual aldehyde resulting from lipid peroxidation (LP) breakdown in biological systems and is used as an indirect index of LP [23]. Determination of MDA in biological materials, as described in Uchiyama and Mihara [24], is based on its reaction with thiobarbituric acid (TBA) to form a pink complex with absorption maximum at 535 nm. The activity of SOD enzyme in testis homogenate was determined according to the method described by Sun and Zigman [25]. This method is based on the ability of SOD to inhibit the auto-oxidation of epinephrine to adrenochrome and other derivatives at alkaline pH. These derivatives can easily be monitored in the near-UV region of the absorption spectrum. CAT activity was determined by measuring the exponential disappearance of H_2O_2 at 240 nm and expressed in units/mg of protein as described by Aebi [26]. The total protein content of testis was determined according to the Lowry method as modified by Peterson [27]. Absorbance was recorded using Shimadzu recording spectrophotometer (UV-160) in all measurements. For the histological examinations, pieces of testis were fixed in 10% neutral phosphate-buffered formalin and hydrated tissue sections, 5μm in thickness, were stained with Hematoxylin and Eosin. The sections were examined under a Nikon light microscope.

Testosterone levels

Serum was collected by allowing trunk blood to clot overnight at 4°C. Interstitial fluid was collected into a centrifuge tube by perforating the tunica albuginea at the distal pole of the testis several times with a needle and centrifuging at $54 \times g$ at 0°C for 15 min [28]. Samples were stored at −20°C. For each rat, testosterone levels in trunk blood and in the interstitial fluid of the testes were measured using fully automated chemiluminescence analyser at Vivek laboratories, Nagarkovil, Tamil nadu, India.

Statistical analysis

The results were expressed as Mean ± SD, and statistical analysis was performed using Student "t" test.

Results

Effects of $HgCl_2$ on the weights of reproductive organs

Administration of $HgCl_2$ individually treated rats showed significantly ($p<0.05$) decreased relative weights of the testes (Figure1a) and epididymis (Figure 1b). However, No significant changes were observed in the relative weights of testes and epididymis in animal groups treated with a combination of Vitamin C or Vitamin E and $HgCl_2$ treatment (Figure 1a and 1b).

Protective effect of Vitamin C and Vitamin E on sperm parameters

The number of sperm per gm of epididymis was significantly reduced (P<0.01) in the $HgCl_2$ a lonely treated rats (Figure 2a). A combination of $HgCl_2$ with Vitamin C had no effect on this parameter; similar results were obtained in $HgCl_2$ treatment with vitamin E. The effect of $HgCl_2$ on sperm motility and abnormality is shown in (Figure 2b). The results indicate that sperm motility was reduced (P<0.001) and sperm abnormality was increased (P<0.05) in $HgCl_2$ treated rats (Figure

2c). While the treatment with Vitamin C or Vitamin E was found to protect against the changes of $HgCl_2$ induced parameters.

Significantly declined (P<0.05) in testicular content of reduced GSH (Figure 3a), activities of CAT and SOD (Figure 4a and 4b) in $HgCl_2$ – treated rat, while significantly increased (P<0.05) in the level of MDA was recorded after $HgCl_2$ treatment (Figure 3b). These markers of oxidative stress did not differ significantly from control level, when Vitamin C or Vitamin E was administered with $HgCl_2$.

Testosterone level

Serum concentration of testosterone significantly (P < 0.01) decreased in the $HgCl_2$ treated rats than control groups (Figure 5). Similarly, testicular testosterone also significantly decreased (P < 0.01) in $HgCl_2$ treated animals as compared to control rats (Figure 5). However, did not evoke any significant changes in the concentration of serum testosterone and testicular testosterone in the combination of $HgCl_2$ vitamin C or vitamin E treated animals and same results were

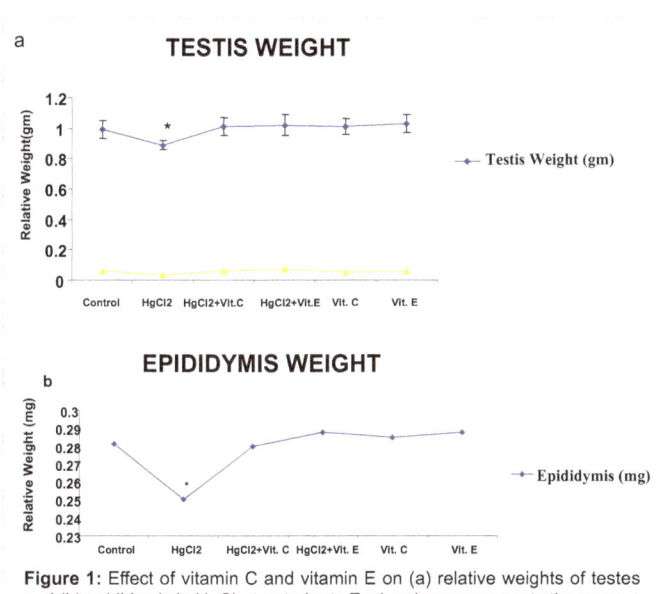

Figure 1: Effect of vitamin C and vitamin E on (a) relative weights of testes and (b) epididymis in $HgCl_2$- treated rats Each column represents the mean ± SE *P<0.05 vs control.

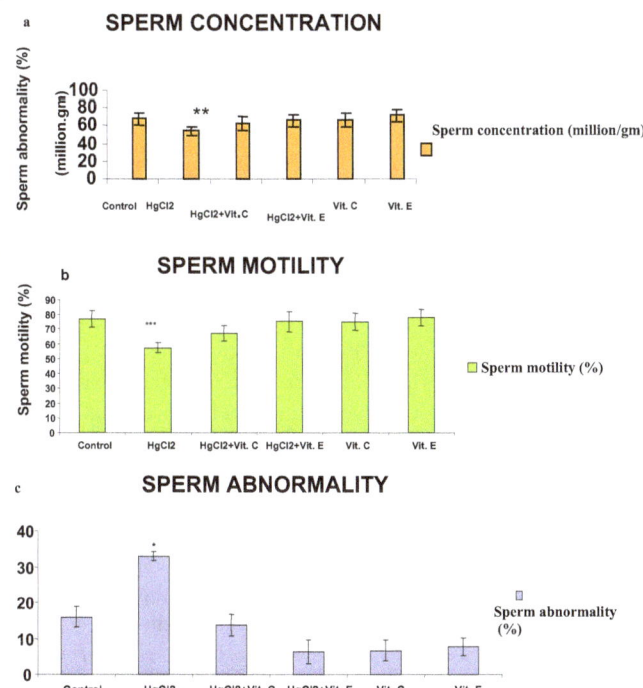

Figure 2: Effect of vitamin C and vitamin E on (a) epididymal sperm concentration and (b) sperm motility and abnormality (c) in - $HgCl_2$ treated rats. Each column represents the mean ± SE. * P < 0.05; **P<0.001;*** P<0.001.

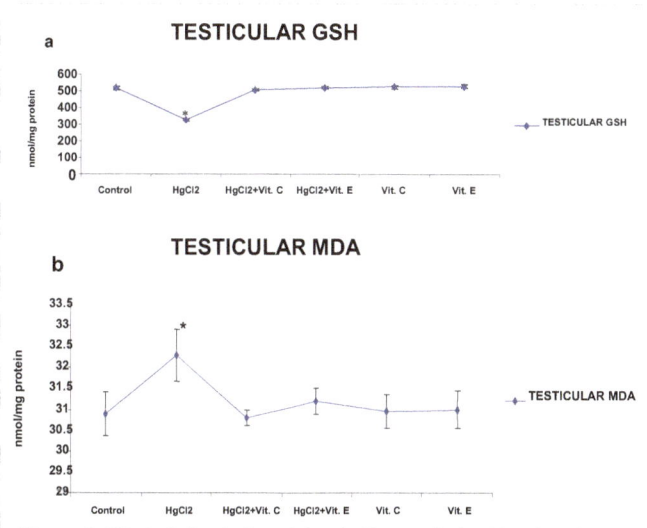

Figure 3: Effect of vitamin C and vitamin E on testicular (a) reduced glutathione content (GSH) and (b) malondialdehyde level (MDA) in $HgCl_2$-treated rats. Each column represents the mean ± SE. * P<0.05 vs control.

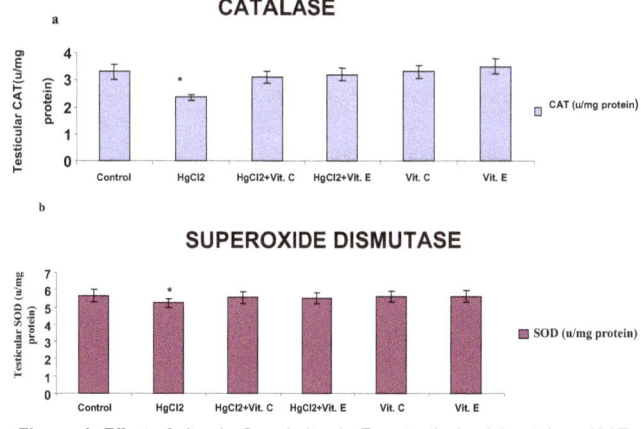

Figure 4: Effect of vitamin C and vitamin E on testicular (a) catalase (CAT and (b) superoxide dismutase (SOD) activities (u / mg protein) in control- and $HgCl_2$ - treated rats. Each column represents the mean ± SE. *P < 0.05 vs control.

measured in vitamin C or vitamin E individually treated rats for serum testosterone and testicular testosterone (Figure 5).

Histopathological effect of Vitamin C and Vitamin E

Severe degeneration of seminiferous tubules, depletions in germ cells and reduction in Leydig cells were clearly seen in the HgCl$_2$-treated group. Debris from the degeneration of cellular components was seen in the lumen. Congestion of blood vessels was also observed between tubules. Animals treated with Vitamin C or Vitamin E showed normal testicular morphology and spermatogenesis with slight degeneration of spermatids and spermatozoa (Figure 6).

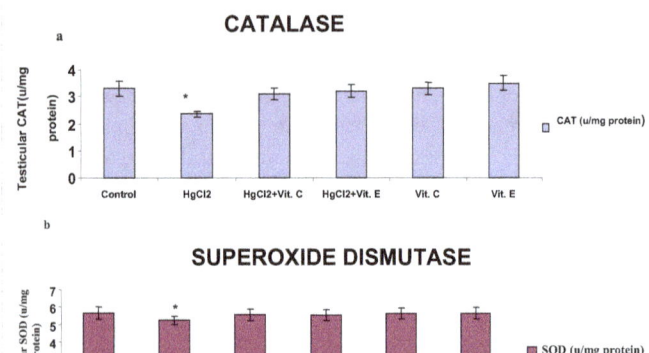

Figure 5: Effect of vitamin C and vitamin E on serum testosterone (ng/ml) and testicular testosterone (ng/gm of tissue) in control- and HgCl$_2$ - treated rats. Each column represents the mean ± SE. *P < 0.05 vs control.

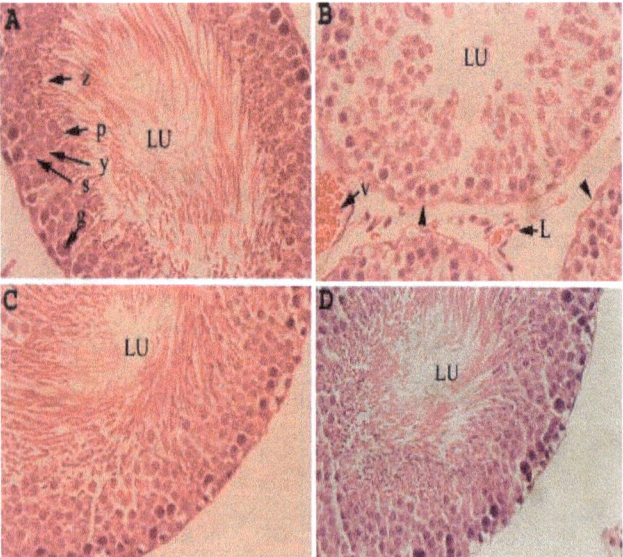

Figure 6: Photomicrograph of the seminiferous tubules of control (a) showing the normal arrangement of germ cells at different stages of spermatogenesis. The tubule contains spermatogonia (g), Sertoli cell (s), spermatocytes (y), spermatids (p) and spermatozoa (z) in the lumen (LU).Testis of HgCl$_2$- treated rats (b) showing extensive degeneration in some tubules (arrowheads) and depletion of germ cells. There are few Leydig cells (L) and congestion of blood vessel (v) between the tubules. Group of rats treated with Vitamin C (c) or Vitamin E (d) with HgCl$_2$ treatment showing normal testicular morphology and spermatogenesis with slight degenerations in spermatids and spermatozoa (H&E, X 400).

Discussion

The protective effect of vitamin C and vitamin E on testicular toxicity of HgCl$_2$, were investigated in male albino rats. To our knowledge, the present study planned to evaluates the protective effect of vitamin C and vitamin E against testicular damage induced by HgCl$_2$ toxicity in experimental animals. In this report, a single dose of HgCl$_2$ (10 mg/100 gm b wt) induced severe reproductive toxicity in adult male rats. Treatment with HgCl$_2$ has been shown to cause testicular damage in various animal species and in humans [9,10]. The HgCl$_2$-induced testicular damage in animals is commonly associated with spermatogenic damage, germ cell apoptosis, Leydig cell dysfunction and testicular steroidogenic disorder [29].

B. The present result showed a significant reduction in the relative weight of testes and epididymis as well as a decreased in the quality of epididymal sperm (sperm count, motility and morphology) after treatment with HgCl$_2$ [30]. The results of this study suggest that a diet containing low levels of HgCl$_2$ can lead to elevated concentrations of HgCl$_2$ in the testes, decreased levels of testosterone in serum and testicular interstitial fluid, a decreased in cauda epididymal sperm storage [1]. This HgCl$_2$-induced testicular damage was also confirmed by histopathological lesions [31]. Many investigators have reported a correlation between MDA and HgCl$_2$-induced complications [14,32]. In this study, HgCl$_2$-treated animals showed an elevation in testicular MDA level versus the control group. A possible explanation for the increased MDA concentration might be the decreased formation of antioxidants in HgCl$_2$-induced tissues, which in view of the augmented activity of reactive oxygen species (ROS) in HgCl$_2$ treated tissues, potentially explains the resulting increase in MDA production. GSH concentration and activities of CAT and SOD in the testes were also lower in the HgCl$_2$-treated animals relative to control animals. It has been suggested that HgCl$_2$ generates free radicals by interacting with DNA [33], which interferes with antioxidant defense system and results in the tissue injury. Therefore, over production of free radicals and hence oxidative stress may account, at least in part, for testicular injury associated with HgCl$_2$ treatment. Recently, much attention has been focused on the protective effects of antioxidants and naturally-occurring substances against HgCl$_2$-induced nephrotoxicity [14,32].

However, little is known about vitamin C and vitamin E act as protective agents against HgCl$_2$-induced testicular toxicity. Administration of vitamin C or vitamin E with HgCl$_2$ treatment clearly restored the testicular damage and quality of sperm, in addition to retaining the control values of oxidative stress markers. Accumulating evidence suggests that the protective effect of vitamins against oxidative damage could be attributed to its anti-oxidative properties [34]. This prevention of the HgCl$_2$-induced oxidative stress damage in rat with vitamin C and vitamin E supports the hypothesis that part of the mechanism of testis damage is attributed to the overproduction of free radicals. (Figure 6): Photomicrograph of the seminiferous tubules of control (a) showing the normal arrangement of germ cells at different stages of spermatogenesis. The tubule contains spermatogonia (g), Sertoli cell (s), spermatocytes (y), spermatids (p) and spermatozoa (z) in the lumen (LU). Testis of HgCl$_2$- treated rats (b) showing extensive degeneration in some tubules (arrowheads) and depletion of germ cells. There are few Leydig cells (L) and congestion of blood vessel (v) between the tubules. Group of rat treated with vitamin C (c) or vitamin E (d) and HgCl$_2$ showing normal testicular morphology and spermatogenesis with slight degenerations in spermatids and spermatozoa (H&E, X 400).

Administration of vitamin C or vitamin E with $HgCl_2$ treatment also attenuated testicular damage induced by $HgCl_2$ treatment as shown by the normal sperm count, normal sperm morphology and low histopathological changes in comparison to the $HgCl_2$-treated animals. The protective effect of vitamin C or vitamin E is accompanied by normalization of antioxidant activity in testis and associated decrease of MDA. Vitamin C, which would neutralize H2O2 and would protect the plasma membrane from lipid peroxidation [14,35], Vitamin E has been shown to lower lipid peroxidation and increased glutathione content in blood of rats [36]. Indeed, the protective effect of Vitamin E against $HgCl_2$ toxicity might be mediated not only by its potent antioxidant properties but through its androgenic activities as well. This activity was reflected by the increase of testis weight and serum testosterone levels [37].

In conclusion, we showed that oxidative stress contributes to the testicular toxicity induced by $HgCl_2$ in male rats. Either vitamin C or vitamins E were shown to have a potent protective effect on $HgCl_2$-induced testicular damage and oxidative stress in rats. The protective effect of vitamin C or vitamin E may be due to their antioxidant properties.

Acknowledgements

Authors are wishing to thank the Management of J. J. College of Arts and Science, Pudukottai, Tamil nadu, India for providing the facilities.

References

1. Aebi H (1984) Catalase in vitro. Methods Enzymol 105: 121-126.

2. Ahmed RS, Seth V, Banerjee BD (2000) Influence of dietary ginger (Zingiber officinales Rosc) on antioxidant defense system in rat: comparison with ascorbic acid. Ind J Exp Biol 38: 604-606.

3. Appenroth D, Fröb S, Kersten L, Splinter FK, Winnefeld K (1997) Protective effects of vitamin E and C on cisplatin nephrotoxicity in developing rats. Arch Toxicol 71: 677-683.

4. Aulerich RJ, Ringer RK, Iwamoto S (1974) Effects of dietary mercury on mink. Arch Environ Contam Toxicol 2: 43-51.

5. Gangadharan B, Murugan MA, Mathur PP (2001) Effect of methoxychlor on antioxidant system of goat epididymal sperm in vitro. Asian J Androl 3: 285-288.

6. Burton GV, Meikle AW (1980) Acute and chronic methyl mercury poisoning impairs rat adrenal and testicular function. J Toxicol Environ Health 6: 597-606.

7. Chance B, Sies H, Boveris A (1979) Hydroperoxide metabolism in mammalian organs. Physiol Rev 59: 527-605.

8. Chowdhury AR, Arora U (1982) Toxic effect of mercury on testes in different animal species. Indian J Physiol Pharmacol 26: 246-249.

9. Colpi GM, Contalbi GF, Nerva F, Sagone P, Piediferro G (2004) Testicular function following chemo-radiotherapy. Eur J Obstet Gynecol Reprod Biol 113 Suppl 1: S2-6.

10. Devi Priya S, Shyamala Devi CS (1999) Protective effect of Quercetin in cisplatin-induced cell injury in the rat kidney. Ind J Pharmacol 31: 422-426.

11. Draper HH, Hadley M (1990) Malondialdehyde determination as index of lipid peroxidation. Methods Enzymol 186: 421-431.

12. Antunes LM, Darin JD, Bianchi Nde L (2001) Effects of the antioxidants curcumin or selenium on cisplatin-induced nephrotoxicity and lipid peroxidation in rats. Pharmacol Res 43: 145-150.

13. Halliwell B, Gutteridge JM (1986) Oxygen free radicals and iron in relation to biology and medicine: some problems and concepts. Arch Biochem Biophys 246: 501-514.

14. Heath JC, Banna KM, Reed MN, Pesek EF, Cole N, et al. (2010) Dietary selenium protects against selected signs of aging and methylmercury exposure. Neurotoxicology 31: 169-179.

15. Jayanthi R, Subash P (2010) Antioxidant effect of caffeic Acid on oxytetracycline induced lipid peroxidation in albino rats. Indian J Clin Biochem 25: 371-375.

16. De AK, Darad R (1988) Physiological antioxidants and antioxidative enzymes in vitamin E-deficient rats. Toxicol Lett 44: 47-54.

17. Lee IP, Dixon RL (1975) Effects of mercury on spermatogenesis studied by velocity sedimentation cell separation and serial mating. J Pharmacol Exp Ther 194: 171-181.

18. Malarvizhi D, Mathur PP (1996) Effects of cisplatin on testicular functions in rats. Indian J Exp Biol 34: 995-998.

19. Masuda H, Tanaka T, Takahama U (1994) Cisplatin generates superoxide anion by interaction with DNA in a cell-free system. Biochem Biophys Res Commun 203: 1175-1180.

20. McFarland RB, Reigel H (1978) Chronic mercury poisoning from a single brief exposure. J Occup Med 20: 532-534.

21. Noguchi T, Cantor AH, Scott ML (1973) Mode of action of selenium and vitamin E in prevention of exudative diathesis in chicks. J Nutr 103: 1502-1511.

22. Peterson GL (1977) A simplification of the protein assay method of Lowry et al. which is more generally applicable. Anal Biochem 83: 346-356.

23. Popescu HI (1978) Poisoning with alkylmercury compounds. Br Med J 1: 1347.

24. Chowdhury AR, Arora U (1982) Toxic effect of mercury on testes in different animal species. Indian J Physiol Pharmacol 26: 246-249.

25. Chowdhury AR, Vachhrajani KD, Chatterjee BB (1985) Inhibition of 3 beta-hydroxy-delta 5-steroid dehydrogenase in rat testicular tissue by mercuric chloride. Toxicol Lett 27: 45-49.

26. Saalu LC, Oluyemi KA, Omotuyi IO (2007) a-Tocopherol (vitamin E) attenuates the testicular toxicity associated with experimental cryptorchidism in rats. African Journal of Biotechnology 6: 1373-1377.

27. Slemr F, Langer E (1992) Increase in global atmospheric concentrations of mercury inferred from measurements over the Atlantic Ocean. Nature 355: 434-437.

28. Suga T, Watanabe T, Matsumoto Y, Horie S (1984) Effects of long-term vitamin E deficiency and restoration on rat hepatic peroxisomes. Biochim Biophys Acta 794: 218-224.

29. Sun M, Zigman S (1978) An improved spectrophotometric assay for superoxide dismutase based on epinephrine autoxidation. Anal Biochem 90: 81-89.

30. Turner TT, Jones CE, Howards SS, Ewing LL, Zegeye B, et al. (1984) On the androgen microenvironment of maturing spermatozoa. Endocrinology 115: 1925 1932.

31. Mihara M, Uchiyama M (1978) Determination of malonaldehyde precursor in tissues by thiobarbituric acid test. Anal Biochem 86: 271-278.

32. van Doorn R, Leijdekkers CM, Henderson PT (1978) Synergistic effects of phorone on the hepatotoxicity of bromobenzene and paracetamol in mice. Toxicology 11: 225-233.

33. Wang CJ, Wang JM, Lin WL, Chu CY, Chou FP, et al. (2000) Protective effect of Hibiscus anthocyanins against tert-butyl hydroperoxide-induced hepatic toxicity in rats. Food Chem Toxicol 38: 411-416.

34. Wang X, Falcone T, Attaran M, Goldberg JM, Agarwal A, et al. (2002) Vitamin C and vitamin E supplementation reduce oxidative stress-induced embryo toxicity and improve the blastocyst development rate. Fertil Steril 78: 1272-1277.

35. Yousef MI, Awad TI, Elhag FA, Khaled FA (2007) Study of the protective effect of ascorbic acid against the toxicity of stannous chloride on oxidative damage, antioxidant enzymes and biochemical parameters in rabbits. Toxicology 235: 194-202.

36. World Health Organization (1990) WHO Environmental Health Criteria 101, Methylmercury.

37. Yokoi K, Uthus EO, Nielsen FH (2003) Nickel deficiency diminishes sperm quantity and movement in rats. Biol Trace Elem Res 93: 141-154.

6

Effects of N-Butanol Fraction of *Gongronema Latifolium* Leave Extract on Some Liver Function and Histological Parameters in Ccl$_4$-Induced Oxidative Damage in Wistar Albino Rats

Okpala JC[1]*, Igwe JC[2] and Ifedilichukwu HN[3]

[1]*Department of Biochemistry, Ahmadu Bello University, Zaria, Kaduna State, Nigeria*
[2]*Department of Pharmaceutical Microbiology, Ahmadu Bello University, Zaria, Kaduna State, Nigeria*
[3]*Department of Medical Biotechnology, National Biotechnology Development Agency, Abuja, Nigeria*

Abstract

Effects of n-butanol fraction of *Gongronema latifolium* leave extract on some liver function and histological parameters in CCl$_4$-induced oxidative damage in Wistar albino rats were assessed. Fifty-four (54) Wistar albino rats were divided into treatment group and LD$_{50}$ groups. Group A (normal control) was given feed and water, Group B (vehicle control) was injected with olive oil intraperitoneally, while the rest groups (C, D, E, F and G) were injected intraperitoneally with a single dose of CCl$_4$ (148 mg/kg) as a 1:1 (v/v) solution in olive oil and all the animals were fasted for 36 hours. This was repeated once every week for a period of four (4) weeks. At the end of 28 days of treatment, liver marker enzymes studies showed that there was significant ($p < 0.05$) increase in the serum activities of ALT, AST, ALP and bilirubin concentrations in CCl$_4$-induced control group when compared with the normal control and induced treated groups but there was no significant ($p > 0.05$) difference of these liver marker enzymes and bilirubin levels between the normal control and induced treated groups. Antioxidant assay on the liver homogenate showed that there was significant ($p < 0.05$) decrease in SOD, CAT, GPx and a significant increase ($p < 0.05$) in MDA of CCl$_4$-induced control rats when compared to the normal control rats but there was no significant ($p > 0.05$) difference between the normal control and induced treated groups. These findings suggested that n-butanol fraction of methanolic leave extract of *G. latifolium* may have anti-hepatotoxic and antioxidative effects against CCl$_4$-induced liver damage in rats.

Keywords: *Gongronema latifolium*; Antioxidant; n-butanol; CCl$_4$; Histology

Introduction

Gongronema latifolium (Asclepiadaceae), is a perennial climber forest leafy vegetable with woody hollow glaborous stems below and characterized by greenish yellow flowers [1]. It is widespread in tropical Africa such as Senegal, Chad and DR Congo as well as grows in the forest of south eastern and western Nigeria where it is widely used for medicinal and nutritional purposes [2]. *G. latifolium* occurs in rainforest, deciduous and secondary forests, and also in mangrove and disturbed roadside forest, from sea-level up to 900 m altitude. In Nigeria, information available from the indigenous traditional healers claimed that a decoction of the chopped [3] leaves of *G. latifolium* has been used in the production of several herbal products which are taken orally [1] for the treatment of stomach upsets and pains, dysentery, malaria, typhoid fever, worm and cough [4]. Asthma patients chew fresh leaves to relieve wheezing [1] and a decoction of the roots, combined with other plant species, is taken to treat sickle cell anaemia. A maceration of the leaves in alcohol is taken to treat bilharzia, viral hepatitis and as a general antimicrobial agent [5]. It is also taken as a tonic to treat loss of appetite [4]. Previous studies have revealed that other plants with polyphenols exhibit clear anti-hepatotoxic properties [1], and that flavonoids could protect the liver against oxidative injury induced by CCl$_4$ in vivo [4]. Although many other plants have been reported to possess anti-hepatotoxic properties, the scientific authentication of most of them such as *G. latifolium* which is used traditionally to treat several diseases is unavailable [3]. The qualitative phytochemicals screening of the methanolic leave extract of *G. latifolium* revealed the presence of glycosides, alkaloids, saponin, flavonoids, tannins, and the absence of free anthraquinone. The quantitative analysis of phytochemical constituents of *G. latifolium* leaves is presented in Table 1. The crude extract showed high tannin content followed by glycosides, alkaloids and saponin. The results in Table 2 also showed

that the n-butanol fraction has higher flavonoids, polyphenols and ascorbic acid content than the ethylacetate fraction. The aim of this work is to provide some scientific support for the health benefit of G. latifolium. To achieve this, studies were carried out to investigate the phytochemical constituents of *G. latifolium* and to evaluate the anti-hepatotoxic activities of n-butanol fraction of methanolic leave extract of *G. latifolium* against oxidative damage induced by CCl$_4$ in Wistar albino rats.

Materials and Methods

Chemicals/reagents

All assays kits were from Randox Laboratories Ltd. Ardmore, Co. Antrm UK. Chemicals and reagents used were purchased from Sigma Chemical Company St. Louis U.S.A. and chemicals used were of analytical grade. Folin ciocalteu phenol reagent, gallic acid, carbon tetrachloride (Sigma-Aldrich), distilled water, normal saline.

Plant material and extraction

Fresh leaves (blend) of *G. latifolium* were obtained from a

*Corresponding author: Okpala JC, Department of Biochemistry, Ahmadu Bello University, Zaria, Kaduna State, Nigeria, E-mail: judeokpch@yahoo.co.uk

Leave	Alkaloids (mg/g)	Saponins (mg/g)	Glycosides (mg/g)	Tannins (mg/g)
Crude	1.26	0.82	2.57	10.60

Table 1: Quantitative Analysis of the Phytochemical Constituents (mg/g) of G. latifolium

Fractions	Polyphenols (mg/g)	Flavonoids (mg/g)	Ascorbic acid (mg/g)
n- Butanol	4.53	5.15	2.24
Ethylacetate	2.39	4.51	0.62

Table 2: Quantitative Analysis of the Phytochemical Constituents (mg/g) of fractions ofG. latifolium

homestead garden at Isuofia, Aguata L.G.A., Anambra State, Nigeria in the month of February 2013 and authenticated at the herbarium unit by Gallah U.J. in the Department of Biological Sciences, Ahmadu Bello University, Zaria, Kaduna State, Nigeria where a voucher specimen with voucher number 1274 was deposited. The collected plants were rinsed in clean water and air dried at room temperature for two weeks. The dried leaves were pulverized into powder using Thomas-Wiley laboratory mill (model 4) manufactured by Arthur H. Thomas Company, Philadelphia, PA., U.S.A. before being extracted. A portion of five hundred grams (500 g) of the pulverized plant leaves was suspended in 2.5 L of methanol for 48 hours in large amber bottles with intermittent shaking. At the end of the extraction, the crude methanol extract was filtered using Whatmann No. 1 filter paper (1mm mesh size) and then concentrated in a water bath maintained at 45°C until greenish black residues were obtained. Certain gram of the crude extract was then subjected to phytochemical analysis using standard procedures [6]. Also, 51 g of the crude extract was reconstituted with 250 ml of methanol for further fractionation and the fractions were kept in sealed containers and refrigerated at 2-4°C for further use. The percentage yield of both the crude methanol leaves extract and fractions were determined as a percentage of the weight (g) of the extract to the original weight (g) of the dried sample used.

Fractionation of crude extract

The crude extract of G. latifolium was subjected to liquid- liquid partition separation to separate the extract into different fractions. 250 ml of the reconstituted extract was placed in a separator funnel and 250 ml of n-hexane, ethylacetate and n-butanol solvents were added sequentially as a 1:1 (v/v) solution and rocked vigorously [7]. The sample was left standing for 30 minutes for each solvent on the separator funnel until a fine separation line appear clearly indicating the supernatant from the sediment before it was eluted sequentially. The process was repeated thrice in order to get adequate quantity for each fraction. The n-hexane, ethylacetate, n-butanol as well as the aqueous residue fractions were evaporated to dryness in a water bath to afford four fractions in (grams) respectively.

Preliminary phytochemical screening

Test for Glycosides was carried out according to the method of Trease and Evans, 1983 [8].

Test for Anthraquinones derivatives was carried out according to the method of Trease and Evans, 1983 [8].

Test for Saponins was carried out according to the method of Trease and Evans, 1983 [8].

Test for Flavonoids was carried out according to the method of Trease and Evans, 1983 [8].

Test for Tannins was carried out according to the method of Trease

and Evans, 1983 [8].

Test for Alkaloids was carried out according to the method of Sofowora, 1982 [9].

Quantitative analysis of phytochemicals

Determination of saponin was carried out according to the gravimetric method of AOAC, 1984 [10].

Determination of total flavonoids was done using the method of Boham and Kocipal-Abyazan [11].

Determination of tannin was done using the standard method described by AOAC [12].

Determination of Glycosides was done using the standard method described by AOAC [10].

Determination of total phenolic contents (TPC) using the Folin-Ciocalteu method adopted by Amin et al. [13] was used.

Ascorbic Acid Contents was determined using the method described by Barros et al. [14].

Determination of Alkaloids was carried out using the procedure described by Harbone (1973) with slight modification by Edeoga et al. [15].

Animals

A total of 54 apparently healthy Wistar albino rats of both sexes weighing between 100-150 g were obtained from the animal house, Department of Pharmacology, Ahmadu Bello University, Zaria, Kaduna State. The animals were separated into male and female in well aerated laboratory cages in the animal house, Department of Pharmacology, Ahmadu Bello University, Zaria, Kaduna State and were allowed to acclimatize to the laboratory environment for a period of two weeks before the commencement of the experiment. They were fed daily with grower mash from Vital Feeds Company and water ad libitum during the stabilization period.

Acute toxicity study

The median lethal dose (LD_{50}) of n-butanol fraction was conducted in order to select a suitable dose for the evaluation of the effects of n-butanol fraction. This was done using the method described by Lorke (1983) [16]. In the initial phase, rats were divided into 3 groups of 3 rats each and were treated with 10 mg, 100 mg and 1000 mg of n-butanol fraction per kg body weight orally. They were observed for 24 hours for signs of toxicity, including death. In the final phase, 3 rats were divided into 3 groups of one rat each, and were treated with n-butanol fraction based on the findings in the first phase. The LD_{50} was calculated from the results of the final phase as the square root of the product of the lowest lethal dose and the highest non-lethal dose, i.e., the geometric mean of the consecutive doses with 0 and 100% survival rates were recorded.

Animal grouping

A total of 54 Wistar albino rats were used. The rats were divided into carbon tetrachloride induced liver damage group of 6 rats each and LD_{50} group.

Carbon tetrachloride induced group

Group A: Normal control Rats were given feed and water only. This served as the normal control group (NC).

Group B: Rats were treated with olive oil and served as vehicle control group (VC).

Group C: Rats were treated with 148 mg/kg b.wt. carbon tetrachloride (CCl₄) in olive oil. This serves as the CCl₄-induced liver damage group (IC).

Group D: Rats were treated with 148 mg/kg b.wt. CCl₄ in olive oil+100 mg/kg b.wt. Silymarin as standard drug (CCl₄+Std).

Group E: Rats were treated with 148 mg/kg b.wt. CCl₄ in olive oil+100 mg/kg b.wt. n-butanol fraction (CCl₄+BF).

Group F: Rats were treated with 148 mg/kg b.wt. CCl₄ in olive oil + 150 mg/kg b.wt. n-butanol fraction (CCl₄+BF).

Group G: Rats were treated with 148 mg/kg b.wt. CCl₄ in olive oil + 200 mg/kg b.wt. n-butanol fraction (CCl₄+BF).

Induction of liver damage

The liver damage was induced by the administration of carbon tetrachloride (CCl₄). Rats were injected intraperitoneally with a single dose of CCl₄ (148 mg/kg body weight) as a 1:1 (v/v) solution in olive oil and were fasted for 36 hours before the administration of n- butanol fraction [17]. This was done once a week for a period of four weeks. The administration of n- butanol fraction was done daily by oral intubation for the period of 28 days.

Collection and preparation of sera samples

At the end of 28 days of treatment, the animals were sacrificed by decapitation using chloroform anaesthesia and blood samples were collected from the head wound in plain bottles (for biochemical parameters). The Blood samples collected in plain tubes were allowed to clot and the serum separated by centrifugation using Labofuge 300 centrifuge (Heraeus) at 3000 rpm for 10 minutes and the supernatant (serum) collected was subjected to biochemical screening.

Collection of liver

Immediately after the blood was collected, the liver was quickly excised, trimmed of connective tissues, rinsed with saline to eliminate blood contamination, dried by blotting with filter paper and weighed (so as to calculate the relative weight) and kept on ice. Certain gram of the liver was crushed in 50 mM potassium phosphate buffer (pH 7.4) using mortar and pestle (homogenization) while the rest of the organs were placed in freshly prepared 10% formalin for histopathological studies. It was then centrifuged at 4000 rpm (2700xg) for 15 minutes. Then the supernatant was collected using Pasteur pipette. The percentage change in organ weight of each of the animals was calculated as follows;

$$\% \text{ change in weight} = \frac{organ\ weight}{animal\ weight} \times 100$$

Heamatological assay

Determination of Packed Cell Volume (PCV): The PCV is the volume of red blood cells (RBC) expressed as a fraction of the total volume of the blood. The microhaematocrit method was used.

Biochemical Studies

Assessment of Aspartate Aminotransferase (AST) activity: AST activity was determined by the method described by Amador and Wacker [18].

Assessment of Alanine Aminotransferase (ALT) activity: ALT activity was determined by method described by Amador and Wacker [18].

Assessment of Alkaline Phosphatase (ALP) activity: Serum activity of alkaline phosphatase (ALP) was determined by the method described by Haussament [19].

Determination of Serum Bilirubin Concentration: The serum total and direct bilirubin levels were determined by the method Jendrassik and Gróf [20].

Determination of Total Protein Level: Total protein was determined colorimetrically according to the method described by Fine [21].

Determination of Albumin Level: The serum albumin was determined by the method of Doumas et al. [22].

Estimation of Superoxide Dismutase (SOD) Activity : Superoxide dismutase activity was measured using the method described by Martin et al. [23].

Estimation of Catalase Activity: Catalase activity was determined using the method described by Aebi and Bergmeyer [24].

Estimation of Glutathione Peroxidase: Glutathione peroxidase assay was determined using the method adapted by Paglia and Valentine [25].

Estimation of Thiobarbituric Acid Reactive Substance (TBARS): Thiobarbituric acid reactive substance (TBARS) in the tissues was estimated in the form of MDA using the method described by Fraga et al. [26].

Histopathological studies

A portion of the liver of the animals was cut into two to three pieces and fixed in 10% formalin. The paraffin sections were prepared and stained with haematoxylin and eosin. The thin sections of livers were made into permanent slides and examined under high (X250) resolution microscope with photographic facility and photomicrographs were taken.

Statistical analysis

The data were analyzed by the analysis of variance (ANOVA) using SPSS program (version 17.0 SPSS Inc., Chicago, IL, USA). The differences between the various animal groups were compared using the Duncan Multiple Range Test. The results were expressed as mean ± standard error of mean (SEM). P value less than 0.05 was considered as significant ($P<0.05$).

Results

The Percentage Yield of Methanolic Leave Extract and Fractions of G. latifolium

The percentage yield (w/w) of the crude extract is (10.24%) and the various fractions have aqueous residue as the highest yield (45.80%), followed by n-butanol fraction (25.14%), ethylacetate fraction (10.70%) and n-hexane fraction has the lowest yield (6.66%).

Lethal Dosage (LD_{50}) determination for n-butanol fraction of *G. latifolium*

No death was recorded after the oral administration up to a dose of 5000 mg per kg body weight.

Effects of n-butanol fraction of *G. latifolium* on Packed Cell Volume

The effect of sub-chronic oral administration of n-butanol fraction of *G. latifolium* methanolic leaves extract and silymarin (Standard drug) at 100 mg/kg b.wt, 150 mg/kg b.wt and 200 mg/kg b.wt. on packed cell volume in CCl_4-induced liver damage in albino rats for 28 days is shown in Figure 1. The result showed that the packed cell volume (PCV) level of induced control group was significantly *(P<0.05)* lowered than the PCV level of normal control group, but there was no significant *(P>0.05)* difference between the PCV level of the normal control animals and all the induced treated animals.

Effects of n-Butanol fraction of *G. latifolium* on body and organ weight change

Changes in body weight of rats induced liver damage treated with n-butanol fraction of *G. latifolium* methanolic leaves extract and silymarin (Standard drug) for a period of 28 days is represented in Figure 2. The results showed no significant *(P>0.05)* difference in the body weight change of all the induced treated groups compared with the normal control group. However, the CCl_4 induced liver damage control group shows a significant *(P<0.05)* decrease in body weight compared with the induced treated and normal control groups.

Changes in organ weight of rats induced liver damage treated with n-butanol fraction of *G. latifolium* methanolic leaves extract and silymarin (Standard drug) for a period of 28 days is represented in Table 3. The result showed that there was no significant *(P>0.05)* difference between the percentage change in liver weights of the entire induced treated group compared with the normal control rats. However, the induced control rats presents a significant *(P<0.05)* higher percentage change in liver weights compared with the normal control rats.

Biochemical studies

Assessment of liver function indices: Liver function indices of alanine aminotransferases (ALT), aspartate amino transferases (AST), alkaline phosphatases (ALP), total protein (TP), albumin (ALB) and bilirubin (DB and IB) concentrations in the serum of CCl_4-induced liver and kidney damage rats after the daily oral administration of n-butanol fraction of *G. latifolium* and silymarin for 28 days is represented in Tables 4 and 5. There was significant *(P<0.05)* increase in activities of all these liver marker enzymes (ALT, AST and ALP) in the CCl_4-induced liver damage control group when compared with the normal control. The activities of ALT, AST and ALP in the induced treated groups were however significantly *(P<0.05)* reduced when compared with induced not treated group. The n-butanol fraction and silymarin significantly *(P<0.05)* increase the serum total protein levels of the induced treated groups compared with the induced not treated group but there was no significant *(P>0.05)* difference between the serum total protein levels of all the induced treated groups and the normal control group. Also serum albumin concentrations of the induced not treated group was significantly *(P<0.05)* lower than the normal control and the induced treated groups, but there was no significant *(P>0.05)* difference between the serum albumin levels of all the induced treated groups and the normal control group. Also, the levels of bilirubin in the

induced treated groups were however significantly *(P<0.05)* reduced when compared with induced not treated group, but there was no significant *(P>0.05)* difference between the bilirubin levels of all the induced treated groups and the normal control group.

In vivo antioxidant studies

Effects of n-butanol fraction of *G. latifolium* on some endogenous antioxidant enzymes in the liver of CCl_4-induced liver damage albino rats: The effects of daily oral administration of n-butanol fraction of *G. latifolium* and Silymarin for 28 days on the level of malondialdehyde (MDA) and some endogenous antioxidant enzymes (catalase, glutathione peroxidase and superoxide dismutase) of the liver of CCl_4 induced liver damage rats is represented in Table 6. There was

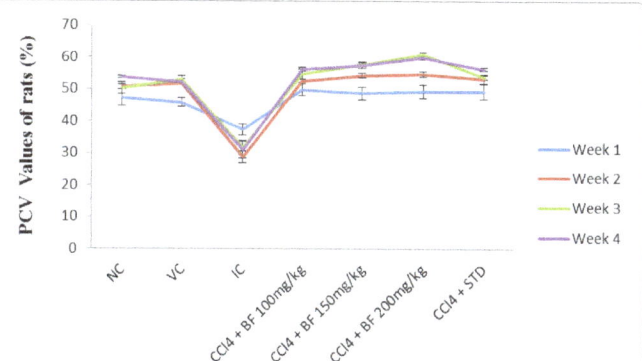

Figure 1: Mean changes in PCV values of CCl_4-induced Liver damage rats treated daily with oral administration of n-butanol fraction of G. latifolium and silymarin (STD).

Values are presented as mean with six replicates for each group.

NC: Normal Control rat, VC: Vehicle control rats, CCl_4: Carbon tetrachloride, IC: CCl_4 Induced liver damage control rats, CCl_4 + BF: CCl_4 Induced liver damage rats+100mg/kg b.wt. of n-butanol fraction, CCl_4 + BF: CCl_4 Induced liver damage rats+150 mg/kg b.wt. of n-butanol fraction, CCl_4 + BF: CCl_4 Induced liver damage rats+200 mg/kg b.wt. of n-butanol fraction, CCl_4 + Std: CCl_4 Induced liver damage rats+100 mg/kg b.wt. of Standard Drug (Silymarin).

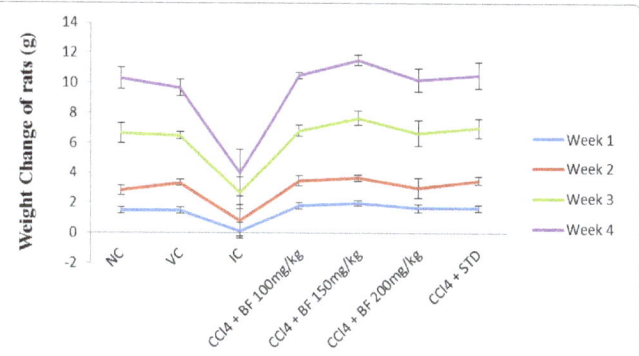

Figure 2: Mean Changes in body weights of CCl_4-induced Liver damage rats treated daily with oral administration of n-butanol fraction of G. latifolium and silymarin (STD).

Values are presented as mean with six replicates for each group.

NC: Normal Control rat, VC: Vehicle control rats, CCl_4: Carbon tetrachloride, IC: CCl_4 Induced liver damage control rats, CCl_4 + BF: CCl_4 Induced liver damage rats+100 mg/kg b.wt. of n-butanol fraction, CCl_4 + BF: CCl_4 Induced liver damage rats+150 mg/kg b.wt. of n-butanol fraction, CCl_4 + BF: CCl_4 Induced liver damage rats+200 mg/kg b.wt. of n-butanol fraction, CCl_4 + Std: CCl_4 Induced liver damage rats+100 mg/kg b.wt of Standard Drug (Silymarin).

a significant *(P<0.05)* increase in the level of malondialdehyde (MDA) and a significant *(P<0.05)* decrease in the level of catalase (CAT), glutathione peroxidase (GPx) and superoxide dismutase (SOD) of the CCl_4 induced liver damage control rats compared with the normal control. There was no significant *(P>0.05)* difference in the levels of MDA and endogenous antioxidant enzymes of all the induced treated groups when compared with the normal control group.

Histopathological studies

Effects of n-butanol fraction of *G. latifolium* on liver: The histological section of the liver of CCl_4-induced oxidative damage rats treated with n-butanol fraction of *G. latifolium* methanolic leave extract and silymarin for 28 days is shown in Plate 1. The histopathological examinations of liver section of normal control group showed normal cellular architecture with distinct hepatic cells. CCl_4-induced control group liver showed an intense hepatic necrosis with vascular congestion, vacoulation, lymphocyte hyperplasia and degeneration of normal hepatic cells. The induced treated groups showed almost normalization of the hepatic cells. On daily oral administration of n-butanol fraction of *G. latifolium* methanolic leave extract and silymarin brought the liver back to moderate hepatic necrosis.

Discussion

The preliminary phytochemical studies revealed the presence of glycosides, saponins, tannins, alkaloids, and flavonoids in the crude methanolic leave extracts of G. latifolium. The presence of these

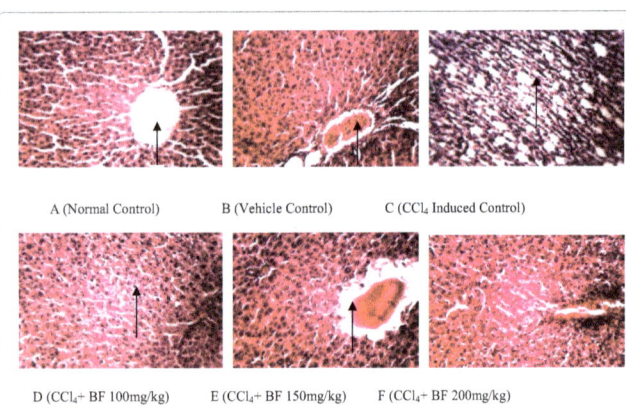

A (Normal Control)   B (Vehicle Control)   C (CCl_4 Induced Control)

D (CCl_4+ BF 100mg/kg)   E (CCl_4+ BF 150mg/kg)   F (CCl_4+ BF 200mg/kg)

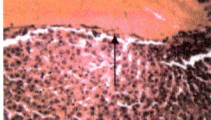

G (CCl_4 + STD 100mg/kg)

A: Normal hepatocytes

B: Slight vascular congestion

C: Intense vascular congestion, vacoulation, lymphocyte hyperplasia and hepatic necrosis

D: Moderate hepatic necrosis with vacoulation

E: Slight vascular congestion and vacoulation

F: Slight vascular congestion

G: Moderate vascular congestion with slight vacoulation

Plate 1: The Representative Liver Region of CCl4-Induced Liver damage rats treated with n-butanol fraction of G. latifolium and silymarin (H&E STAIN X250).

Groups (n=6)	% Change in Liver Weight (g)
NC	4.31±0.14a
VC	4.58±0.32a
IC	6.94±0.38b
CCl_4+ BF	4.70±0.17a
CCl_4+ BF	4.21±0.53a
CCl_4+ BF	4.40±0.14a
CCl_4+ Std	4.64±0.14a

Table 3: Mean Changes in Organ Weights of CCl_4-Induced Liver Damage Rats Treated Daily with Oral Administration of Silymarin and n-Butanol Fraction of G. latifolium

Values are Means ± SEM. Values with different superscript down the columns are significantly different (P<0.05)

NC: Normal Control rat, VC: Vehicle control rats, CCl_4: Carbon tetrachloride, IC: CCl_4 Induced liver damage control rats, CCl_4 + BF: CCl_4 Induced liver damage rats+100mg/kg b.wt. of n-butanol fraction, CCl_4 + BF: CCl_4 Induced liver damage rats+150mg/kg b.wt. of n-butanol fraction, CCl_4 + BF: CCl_4 Induced liver damage rats+200mg/kg b.wt. of n-butanol fraction, CCl_4 + Std: CCl_4 Induced liver damage rats+100mg/kg b.wt. of Standard Drug (Silymarin).

Group (n=6)	ALT (IU/L)	ALT (IU/L)	ALP (IU/L)
NC	45.8±2.85a	42.5±1.63ab	60.2±2.18a
VC	44.5±3.24a	41.3±1.89a	59.5±1.77a
IC	60.3±3.02b	56.8±2.18c	76.0±3.44b
CCl_4 + BF	48.0±2.15a	47.3±1.54b	64.7±2.33a
CCl_4 + BF	47.3±1.63a	43.8±1.74ab	62.2±1.11a
CCl_4 + BF	45.5±1.73a	44.5±1.71ab	61.8±1.78a
CCl_4 + Std	48.3±2.03a	46.7±1.71ab	64.0±1.81a

Values are Means ± SEM. Values with different superscript down the columns are significantly different (P<0.05)

NC: Normal Control rat, VC: Vehicle control rats, CCl_4: Carbon tetrachloride, IC: CCl_4 Induced liver damage control rats, CCl_4 + BF: CCl_4 Induced liver damage rats+100mg/kg b.wt. of n-butanol fraction, CCl_4 + BF: CCl_4 Induced liver damage rats+150mg/kg b.wt. of n-butanol fraction, CCl_4 + BF: CCl_4 Induced liver damage rats+200mg/kg b.wt. of n-butanol fraction, CCl_4 + Std: CCl_4 Induced liver damage rats+100mg/kg b.wt. of Standard Drug (Silymarin).

ALT: Alanine aminotransferase, AST: Aspartate aminotransferase, ALP: Alkaline phosphatase.

Table 4: Effects of Daily Doses of n-butanol fraction of G. latifolium on Serum Liver Function Parameters (ALT, AST and ALP) of CCl_4-Induced Liver Damage Albino Rats

Group (n=6)	TP (g/dl)	ALB (g/dl)	DB (mg/dl)	IB (mg/dl)
NC	61.2±1.82cd	37.2±2.09c	6.68±0.41a	5.30±0.69a
VC	60.3±1.94bcd	33.5±1.52bc	7.13±0.68a	5.10±0.23a
IC	44.8±2.21a	24.8±1.74a	10.5±0.57b	6.82±0.24b
CCl_4 + BF	55.2±2.02bc	32.2±1.30bc	7.70±0.89a	5.78±0.25ab
CCl_4 + BF	59.5±1.48bcd	29.5±2.49ab	7.62±0.95a	4.72±0.24a
CCl_4 + BF	63.3±2.06d	33.3±1.71bc	6.83±0.78a	5.55±0.33a
CCl_4 + Std	54.5±2.45b	33.0±1.93bc	8.23±0.62a	4.83±0.51a

Values are Means ± SEM. Values with different superscript down the columns are significantly different (P<0.05)

NC: Normal Control rat, VC: Vehicle control rats, CCl_4: Carbon tetrachloride, IC: CCl_4 Induced liver damage control rats, CCl_4 + BF: CCl_4 Induced liver damage rats+100mg/kg b.wt. of n-butanol fraction, CCl_4 + BF: CCl_4 Induced liver damage rats+150mg/kg b.wt. of n-butanol fraction, CCl_4 + BF: CCl_4 Induced liver damage rats+200mg/kg b.wt. of n-butanol fraction, CCl_4 + Std: CCl_4 Induced liver damage rats+100mg/kg b.wt. of Standard Drug (Silymarin).

TP: Total protein, ALB:Albumin, DB: Direct bilirubin, IB: Indirect bilirubin.

Table 5: Effects of Daily Doses of n-butanol fraction of G. latifolium on Serum Total Protein, Albumin, Direct and Indirect Bilirubin of CCl_4 Induced Liver Damage Albino Rats

Group (n=6)	MDA (µM/ml)	SOD(U/ml)	CAT (U/ml)	GPx(mU/ml)
NC	1.32±0.06a	2.45±0.08b	50.0±2.93b	50.8±1.17b
VC	1.52±0.07a	2.25±0.08b	51.2±2.06b	49.5±1.89b
IC	2.53±0.09b	1.43±0.09a	40.3±1.17a	37.7±1.67a
CCl$_4$ + BF	1.53±0.11a	2.23±0.10b	52.0±1.27b	47.2±1.64b
CCl$_4$ + BF	1.52±0.11a	2.45±0.09b	53.0±1.32b	49.8±1.30b
CCl$_4$ + BF	1.48±0.13a	2.43±0.09b	54.5±1.18b	51.0±1.53b
CCl$_4$ + Std	1.58±0.10a	2.35±0.11b	52.5±1.34b	49.83±2.34b

Values are Means ± SEM. Values with different superscript down the columns are significantly different (P<0.05)

NC: Normal Control rat, VC: Vehicle control rats, CCl$_4$: Carbon tetrachloride, IC: CCl$_4$ Induced liver damage control rats, CCl$_4$ + BF: CCl$_4$ Induced liver damage rats+100mg/kg b.wt. of n-butanol fraction, CCl$_4$ + BF: CCl$_4$ Induced liver damage rats+150mg/kg b.wt. of n-butanol fraction, CCl$_4$ + BF: CCl$_4$ Induced liver damage rats+200mg/kg b.wt. of n-butanol fraction, CCl$_4$ + Std: CCl$_4$ Induced liver damage rats+100mg/kg b.wt. of Standard Drug (Silymarin).

MDA: Malondialdehyde, SOD: Superoxide dismutase, CAT: Catalase, GPx: Glutathione peroxidase

Table 6: Effects of Daily Doses of n-butanol fraction of G. latifolium on Some Endogenous Antioxidant Enzymes in the Liver of CCl$_4$-Induced Liver Damage Albino Rats

phytochemicals in the plant, accounts for its usefulness as medicinal plant [27]. The quantitative phytochemical analysis showed that tannins had the highest concentration in the crude extract (Table 1) whereas the n-butanol fraction had the highest concentration of flavonoids, ascorbic acid and polyphenols [28,29] when compared to the ethylacetate fraction (Table 2). Plant phenolics, flavonoids and ascorbic acid constitute major groups of phytochemicals acting as primary *in vitro* antioxidants or free radical terminators [30]. Therefore, it was reasonable to determine their concentration in the n-butanol and ethylacetate plant fractions with the aim of utilising the fraction with the highest concentration of *in vitro* antioxidant [31,32]. Polyphenols, flavonoids and ascorbic acid scavenging potentials and metal chelating ability is [33] dependent upon their unique structure, the number and position of the hydroxyl groups [34-36]. The potential health benefits associated with these phytochemicals has generated great interest among scientists for the development of natural *in vitro* antioxidant compounds from plants [37,38].

Haematological investigation provides information on the general pathophysiology of the blood and reticuloendothelial system [39,40]. Fairbarks [41] showed that xenobiotics causes low PCV level which may be associated with the oxidization of sulphydryl groups of the erythrocyte membrane thus, inflicting injury to the erythrocytes membrane. This is in agreement with the present study as packed cells volume (PCV) values in rats exposed to CCl$_4$ gave low levels of PCV. The n-butanol fraction appeared to boost blood cells as the values of PCV approached the normal control (Figure 1). This finding suggests that the administration of the n-butanol fraction of the methanolic leave extract of G. *latifolium* to patient with remarkable low PCV level may increase their packed cell volume. It implies that the n-butanol fraction may possess constituents that would trigger the production of more blood cells [42,43].

Changes in the body weight after CCl$_4$ dosing have been used as a valuable index of CCl$_4$-related organ damage by [44,45] and thus, will be applicable in this study in order to justify the effects of CCl$_4$ on the body and organ weights of these animals. The decrease in changes in body weight (Figure 2) and consequent increase in liver weights seen in CCl$_4$-induced control group was considered to be as a result of direct toxicity of CCl$_4$ and/or indirect toxicity that lead to liver damage (Table

3). This indicates that CCl$_4$ may have induced hypertrophy of the cells of these organs as well as elicit remarkable tissue damage [46] which may have led to the observed effects on the body and organ weights of these animals. However, all the induced treated groups experienced a significant increase in body weight changes as well as reduced change in organ weights, suggesting the possible curative effects of the n-butanol fraction of G. *latifolium* against liver injury after CCl$_4$ induction.

Assessment of liver can be made by estimating the activities of serum ALT, AST and ALP which are enzymes originally present at higher concentration in cytoplasm [47]. When there is hepatopathy, these enzymes leak into the blood stream in conformity with the extent of liver damage [48,49]. Administration of CCl$_4$ caused a significant ($P<0.05$) elevation of these liver marker enzyme levels and a consequent decrease in the level of serum proteins when compared to normal control group (Tables 4 and 5). The elevated level of these marker enzymes with a corresponding decrease in serum proteins level observed in the CCl$_4$-induced not treated group corresponded to the extensive liver damage induced by CCl$_4$ which may lead to an impaired protein turnover. These results are in agreement with previous finding that the activity levels of serum ALT, ALP and AST were significantly elevated as well as a significant decrease in serum protein levels in rats after CC14 administration [50-53].

Also, the significant ($P<0.05$) elevation of bilirubin levels in the CCl$_4$-induced not treated group when compared to the normal control and the induced treated groups may be as a result of haemolytic anaemia that may be associated with oxidative damage to red blood cells thus, leading to elevated bilirubin level since bilirubin is an intermediate product in haemoglobin breakdown in the liver [47]. Again, this elevated bilirubin level may also be associated with reduced hepatocyte uptake of bilirubin, impaired conjugation of bilirubin and reduced hepatocyte secretion of bilirubin [48,49]. However, since there are significant elevation of direct (conjugated) and indirect (unconjugated) bilirubin levels in the blood serum of CCl$_4$-induced not treated group, this may be attributed to the inability of the hepatocyte to secrete conjugated bilirubin as envisioned in elevated direct bilirubin level as a result of liver necrosis or may be due to inability of the liver to conjugate bilirubin in the case of elevated indirect bilirubin which can be attributed to the inability of the necrotic liver to conjugate bilirubin or the inability of the hepatocytes to take up bilirubin [50-52]. Also, elevated bilirubin may also be due to obstruction in the flow of bile within the liver or in the bile duct as a result of severe liver damage [43].

There was significant ($P<0.05$) restoration of these liver marker enzymes activities as well as bilirubin and serum proteins levels on administration of the n-butanol fraction and silymarin for 28 days at a dose of 100 mg/kg b.wt., 150 mg/kg b.wt. and 200 mg/kg b.wt. The reversal of these serum liver marker enzymes in CCl$_4$-induced treated groups towards a near normalcy by the n-butanol fraction observed in this study may be due to the prevention of the leakage of these intracellular enzymes as a result of the presence of polyphenols, flavonoids and ascorbic acid in the n-butanol fraction as well as their membrane stabilizing activity which may be attributed to their ability to mop up free radicals that attack cell membranes. Also, the repeated contact of these *in vitro* antioxidants with hepatocytes may lead to increased stability of the cell membrane [54]. Again, the ability of the n-butanol fraction to reduce the bilirubin level to near normalcy may be as a result of its ability to assist in the regeneration of the hepatocytes by reducing oxidative damage to red blood cells which may lead to reduction in haemoglobin breakdown by the liver. This is in agreement with the commonly accepted view that serum levels of transaminases, bilirubin and serum proteins returns to normalcy with the healing of hepatic parenchyma cells as well as the regeneration of hepatocytes [14]. It is therefore, a clear manifestation of the hepatocurative effects of the n-butanol fraction of G. latifolium. Following the administration of the n-butanol fraction of *G. latifolium* and silymarin, the hepatocytes showed close to normal cellular architecture which may be as a result of regeneration and repair of liver cells [43,53].

Antioxidant activity or scavenging activity of the generated free radicals is important in the curative effect of CCl_4-induced hepatotoxicity. The body has an effective defence mechanism to prevent and neutralize free radicals-induced damage. This is accomplished by a set of endogeneous antioxidant enzymes such as superoxide dismutase, glutathione peroxidase and catalase. Decrease in enzyme activity of superoxide dismutase (SOD) is a sensitive index in hepatocellular damage and is the most sensitive enzymatic index in liver injury [55,56]. The increased level of malondialdehyde (MDA) in the liver tissue of the rats administered CCl_4 (Table 6) may be as a result of the enhanced membrane lipid peroxidation by free radicals generated and failure of antioxidant defence mechanisms to prevent formation of excessive free radicals [50,57,58]. Also, the decreased activity of SOD, GPx and CAT in the liver tissues of CCl_4-induced rats may be due to high concentration of these free radicals generated by CCl_4 which may lead to decreased level or inactivation of these endogenous antioxidant enzymes [59]. Treatment with n-butanol fraction of *G. latifolium* significantly ($P<0.05$) increased the levels of SOD, GPx and CAT activities and a consequent significant ($P<0.05$) reduction in MDA. The effects of the n-butanol fraction were comparable to the standard drug (Silymarin). Thus, this result suggests that n-butanol fraction of *G. latifolium* contains free radical scavenging activity due to the presence of *in vitro* antioxidants, which could exert beneficial action against pathophysiological alterations caused by the presence of superoxide and hydroxide free radicals as well as hydrogen peroxide indicating the regeneration of damaged liver cells [2,53].

The histopathological studies of the liver in the CCl_4-induced control group showed that CCl_4 caused an intense vascular congestion, vacoulation, lymphocyte hyperplasia and necrosis (Plate 1) indicating its hepatotoxicity. This result is in agreement with [60]. Following the administration of the n-butanol fraction of *G. latifolium* and silymarin, the hepatocytes showed close to normal cellular architecture which may be as a result of regeneration and repair of liver cells [43,53]. In line with these findings, it's obvious that histopathological examinations are in agreement with observed biochemical analysis. This result is in agreement with the report [2,53,61-68].

Conclusions

The result of this study has scientifically justified the traditional use of *G. latifolium* in the management of human diseases. The result showed that the n-butanol fraction of methanolic leave extract of *G. latifolium* possess *in vitro* antioxidants which may have contributed to its significant anti-hepatotoxic properties. The histological examination showed that the n-butanol fraction of *G. latifolium* has curative effect on the liver in CCl_4-induced liver damage rats. The n-butanol fraction of *G. latifolium* is comparable to the standard drug (silymarin). This work provides the phytotherapeutic potential of n-butanol fraction of *G. latifolium* that may be useful to scientists and researchers in the nutraceutical industry.

Recommendations

1. There is need to carry out a bioactivity-guided fractionation, isolation and identification of the bioactive constituents of the n-butanol

fraction which is responsible for the observed pharmacological activities.

2. There is need to carry out chronic toxicity studies of the n-butanol fraction of the plant so as to ascertain the safety of long term usage on animals.

References

1. Ugwu GC, Eze EI (2010) In vivo evaluation of the effects of ethanolic leaf extract of *Gongronema latifolium* on AST and bilirubin secretions in albino rats. J Med Appl Biosci 2: 1-2.

2. Ugochukwu NH, BabadyNE, Cobourne M, Gaset SR (2003) The effect of *Gongronema latifolium* extracts on serum lipid profile and oxidative stress in renal and hepatocytes of diabetic rats. J Biosci 28: 1-5.

3. Ajibola AO, Satake M (1992) Contributions to the phytochemistry of medicinal plants growing in Nigeria as report in the 1979- 1990 literature- A review. Afr J Pharm Sci 22: 172-201.

4. Akpan PA (2004) Food from Nigeria Forest African farming September/ October. 23.

5. Okigbo RN, Anuaga CL, Amadi JE (2009) Advances in selected medicinal and aromatic plants indigenous to Africa. J Med Plants Res 3: 086-095.

6. Sofowora A (1993) Spectrum Books Limited, Medicinal Plants and Traditional Medicine in Africa. (2nd Edn) Ibadan, Nigeria1-153.

7. Abbot D, Andrews RS (1970) An Introduction to chromatography 2nd ed. Longman press, London 72-78.

8. Trease GE, Evans WC (1983) Pharmacognosy. (12th Edn), Bailliere and Tindale, London 774-775.

9. Sofowora EA (1982) Traditional Medicine Methods and Techniques. John Wiley and Son Ltd., New York, Pp. 2626-2253.

10. AOAC (1984) Official Methods of Analysis of the Association of Official Analytical Chemists. (14th edn), Arlington, Virginia 114-119.

11. Boham BA, Kocipal-Abyazan R (1974) Flavonoids and condensed tanins from the leaves of Hawaiian Vaccinium vaticulatum and V. calycinium. Pacific Science 48: 458-463.

12. AOAC (1980) Official Method of Analysis Association of official analytical Chemists. (13th edn), Washington D.C. 376-384.

13. Amin I, Zamaliah MM, Chin WF (2004) Total antioxidant activity and phenolic content in selected vegetables. Food Chemistry 87: 581- 586.

14. Barros L, Joao Ferreira M, Queiros B, Ferreira IC, Baptista P (2007) Total phenol, ascorbic acid, β-carotene and lycopene in Portuguese wild edible mushroom and their antioxidant acitivities. Food Chemistry 103: 413-419.

15. Edeoga HO, Okwu DE, Mbacble BO (2005) Phytochemical constituents of some Nigerian medicinal plants. African Journal of Biotechnology 4: 685-688.

16. Lorke D (1983) A New Approach to Practical Acute Toxicity Testing. Arch Toxicol 53: 275-289.

17. Manoj B, Aqued K (2003) Protective effect of Law sonalba L. against CCl_4-induced hepatic damage in albino rats. Indian Journal expo on Biology 4: 85-87.

18. Amador E, Wacker W (1962) Analytical methods for quantitative determination of liver marker enzymes. Clinical Chemistry 8: 343.

19. Haussament TU (1977) Quantitative determination of serum alkaline phosphatase. Clinica Chimica Acta 35: 271-273.

20. Jendrassik L, Grof (1938). In-vitro determination of total and direct bilirubin in serum. Journal of Biochemistry. 299:81-88.

21. Fine J (1935) Quantitative determination of serum proteins by colorimetric method. Biochemistry Journal 29: 799.

22. Doumas BT, Watson WA, Biggs HG (1971) Albumin standards and the measurement of serum albumin with bromcresol green. Clin Chim Acta 31: 87-96.

23. Martin JP, DaileyM, Sugarman E (1987) Negative and Positive Assays of Superoxide Dismutase based on Heamatoxylin Autoxidation. Arch Biochemistry Biophysiology 255: 329-336.

24. Aebi HE, Bergmeyer HU (1983) Methods in enzymatic analysis. New York Academic press Inc. 3: 276-286.

25. Paglia DE, Valentine WN (1967) Studies on the quantitative and qualitative characterization of erythrocyte glutathione peroxidise. J Lab Clin Med 70: 158-169.

26. Fraga CG, Leibovitz BE, Tappel AL (1988) Lipid peroxidation measured as thiobarbituric acid-reactive substances in tissue slices: Characterization and comparison with homogenates and microsomes. Free Radic Biol Med 4: 155-161.

27. Jayathilakan K, Sharma GK, Radhakrishna K, Bawa AS (2007) Antioxidant potential of synthetic and natural antioxidants and its effect on warmed over-flavour in different species of meat. Food Chemistry 105: 908-916.

28. Venkatalakshmi P, Eazhisaivallabi D, Ambika R (2012) Preliminary Phytochemical Analysis and Antimicrobial Screening of Hygrophilla spinosa. Int J Pharm Technol Res. 4: 466-468.

29. Omonkhelin JO, Eric KIO, Osahon O (2007) Antifungal and antibacterial activities of the ethanolic and aqueous extract of Kigelia africana (Bignoniaceae) stem bark. African Journal of Biotechnology 6: 1671-1680.

30. El-Sayed S Abdel-Hameed, Salih A Bazaid, Mohamed M Shohayeb (2012) Total Phenolics and Antioxidant Activity of Defatted Fresh Taif Rose, Saudi Arabia. British Journal of Pharmaceutical Research 2: 129-140.

31. Kumbhare MR, Guleha V, Sivakumar T (2012) Estimation of total phenolic content, cytotoxicity and in-vitro antioxidant activity of stem bark of Moringa oleifera. Asian Pacific Journal of Tropical Disease 2:144-150.

32. Makepeace W, Dobson AT, Scott D (1985) Interference phenomena due to mouse ear and king devil hawkweed. New Zealand Journal of Botany 23: 79-90.

33. Wang H, Gao XD, Zhou GC, Cai L, Yao WB (2008) In vitro and in vivo antioxidant activity of aqueous extract from Choerospondias axillaris fruit. Food Chem 106: 888-895.

34. Pazos M, Gallardo JM, Torres JL, Medina I (2005) Activity of grape polyphenols as inhibitors of the oxidation of fish lipids and fish muscle. Food Chemistry 92: 547-557.

35. Smith IF, Eyzaguine PB (2007) African leafy vegetables: Their role in the World Health Organization's Global Fruit and Vegetable Initiative. African Journal of Food Agriculture and Nutrition Development 7: 1-17.

36. Kumar A, Lavarasan RI, Jayachandran T, Decaraman M, Aravindhan P, et al. (2009) phytochemical investigation on a tropical plant, Syzygium cumini from Kattuppalayam, Erode District, Tamil Nadu, chupandia South India. Pak J Nutr 8: 83-85.

37. Rohman A, Riyanto S, Yuniarti N, Saputra WR, Utami R (2010) Antioxidant activity, total phenolic, and total flavaonoid of extracts and fractions of red fruit (Pandanus conoideus Lam). International Food Research Journal 17: 97-106.

38. Masoumeh M, Parastoo Z, Moghaddam, Hooman B, Mohammed RZ, et al. (2011) Iranian Journal of Plant Physiology 1: 169-176.

39. Baker FJ, Silverton RF (1985) Introduction to medical laboratory technology, Butterworth and co publishers. 316-334.

40. Mishra AK, Mishra A, Kehri HK, Sharma B, Pandey AK (2009) Inhibitory activity of Indian spice plant Cinnamomum zeylanicum extracts against Alternaria solani and Curvularia lunata pathogenic dematiaceous moulds. Annals for Clinical Microbiology and Antimicrobial 8: 1-7.

41. Fairbarks VF (1967) Mechanism of haemolytic drug action. Lancet 1: 512-520.

42. Patrick – Iwuanyanwu KC, Wegwu MO, Ayalogu EO (2007) The Protective Nature of Garlic, Ginger and Vitamin E on CCl4-Induced Hepatotoxicity in Rats. Asian Journal of Biochemistry 2: 409-414.

43. Emeka EJI, Obioa O (2009) Effect of a long term consumption of a diet supplemented with leaves of Gongronema latifolium Benth on some biochemical and histological parameters in male albino rats. Journal of Biological Sciences 9: 859-865.

44. Bruckner JV, MacKenzie WF, Muralidhara S, Luthra R, Kyle GM, et al. (1986) Oral Toxicity of Carbon Tetrachloride: Acute, Subacute and Subchronic Studies in Rats. Fundam Appl Toxicol 6: 16-34.

45. Pradeep K, Mohan CV, Anand KG, Karthikeyan S (2005) Effect of Pretreatment of Cassia fistula Linn. Leaf Extract against Subacute CCl4-Induced Hepatotoxicity in Rats. Indian J Exp Biol 43: 526-530.

46. Li W, Zhang M, Zheng YN, Li J, Wang YP, et al. (2011) Snailase Preparation of Ginsenoside M1 from Protopanaxadiol-Type Ginsenoside and Their Protective Effects against CCl4-Induced Chronic Hepatotoxicity in Mice. Molecules 16: 10093-10103.

47. Reham AM, Reham SR, Lamiaa AA (2009) Effect of Substituting Pumpkin Seed Protein Isolate for Caseinon Serum Liver Enzymes, Lipid Profile and Antioxidant Enzymes in CCl4-intoxicated Rats. Advances in Biological Research 3: 9-15.

48. Nkosi CZ, Opoku AR, Terblanche SE (2005) Effect of Pumpkin Seed (Cucurbita Pepo) Protein Isolate on the Activity Levels of Certain Plasma Enzymes in CCl4-Induced Liver Injury in Low Protein Fed Rats. Phytotherapy Research 19: 341-345.

49. Dominic Amalraj A, Parkavi C, Murugaiah K, Dhanaraj TS (2012) Hypolipidemic Activity of Cyperous rotundus on CCl4-Induced Dyslipidemia in Rats. Asian J Pharm Tech 2: 51-53.

50. Khan MR, Siddique F (2012) Antioxidant effects of Citharexylum spinosum in CCl4-induced nephrotoxicity in rat. Exp Toxicol Pathol 64: 349-355.

51. Battu GR, Rao YV, Dasari VSP (2012) Antihepatotoxic effect of Elephantopus scaber L. on carbon tetrachloride-induced hepatotoxicity in rats. Recent Research in Science and Technology 4: 21-24.

52. Shahid SM, Shamim S, Mahboob T (2012) Protective effect of green tea on CCl4-induced hepatoxicity in experimental rats. African Journal of Pharmacy and Pharmacology 6: 1958-1963.

53. Etim O, Akpan E, Usoh I (2008) Hepatotoxicity of carbon tetrachloride: protective effect of Gongronema latifolium. Pak J Pharm Sci 21: 269-274.

54. Chavan Sandeep D, Patil Sandeep B, Naikwade NS (2012) Biochemical and Histopathological Studies of Butea Monosperma (Lam) Taub Leaves on Paracetamol-Induced Hepatotoxicity In Albino Rats. Journal of Pharmacy Research 5: 4006-4008.

55. Mohajeri D, Amouoghli Tabrizi B, Yousef D, Nazeri M (2011) Protective Effect of Turnip Root (Brassica Rapa. L) Ethanolic Extract on Early Hepatic Injury in Alloxanized Diabetic Rats. Journal of Applied Sciences Research 5: 748-756.

56. Tamilarasi R., Sivanesan D, Kanimozhi P (2012) Hepatoprotective and antioxidant efficacy of Anethum graveolens linn in carbon tetrachloride-induced hepatotoxicity in albino rats. Journal of Chemical and Pharmaceutical Research. 4: 1885-1888.

57. Liu J, Tan H, Sun Y, Zhou S, Cao J, et al. (2009) The preventive effects of heparin-superoxide dismutase on carbon tetrachloride-induced acute liver failure and hepatic fibrosis in mice. Mol Cell Biochem 327: 219-228.

58. Kim HY, Kim JK, Choi JH, Jung JY, Oh WY, et al. (2010) Hepatoprotective effect of pinoresinol on carbon tetrachloride-induced hepatic damage in mice. J Pharmacol Sci 112: 105-112.

59. Showkat AG, Ehtishamul H, Akbar M, Mohmmad AZ (2010) Amelioration of carbon tetrachloride-induced oxidative stress in kidney and lung tissues by ethanolic rhizome extract of Podophyllum hexandrum in Wistar rats. Journal of Medicinal Plant Research 4: 1673-1677.

60. Venkatanarayana G, Sudhakara G, Sivajyothi P, Indira P (2012) Protective Effects of Curcumin and Vitamin E on Carbon Tetrachloride-Induced Nephrotoxicity in Rats. Experimental and clinical Journal 11: 641-650.

61. Khan MR, Ahmed D (2009) Protective effects of Digera muricata (L.) Mart. on testis against oxidative stress of carbon tetrachloride in rat. Food Chem Toxicol 47: 1393-1399.

62. Khan MR, Zehra H (2011) Amelioration of CCl4-induced nephrotoxicity by oxalis corniculata in rat. Exp Toxicol Pathol 65: 327-334.

63. Cheesbrough M (2000) District laboratory practice in tropical countries (2ndedn) Cambridge University Press. Pp. 297-298.

64. Harborne JB (1973) Plant phenolics. In: BELL EA, CHARLWOOD BV (eds). Encyclopedia of Plant Physiology, Volume 8 Secondary Plant Products, Springer-Verlag, Berlin Heidelberg New York 329-395.

65. Khan RA, Khan MR, Ahmed M, Sahreen S, Shah NA (2012) Antioxidant and hepatoprotective effects of oxalis corniculata against carbon tetrachloride (CCl4) induced injuries in rats. African Journal of Pharmacy and Pharmacology 6: 2255-2267.

66. Khan MR, Rizvi W, Khan GN, Khan RA, Shaheen S (2009) Carbon tetrachloride-induced nephrotoxicity in rat: protective role of Digera muricata. J Ethnopharmacol 122: 91-99.

67. Lillie RD (1965) Nuclei, nucleic acid, general oversight stains. In: Histopathology Technique and Practical Histochemistry. (3rd edn), McGraw Hill Book Company, Pp: 142-179.

68. Palanivel MG, Rajkapoor B, Senthil Kumar R, Einstein JW, Prem Kumar E (2008) Hepatoprotective and Antioxidant Effects of Pisonia Aculeata L. against CCl$_4$- Induced Hepatic Damage in Rats. Scientia Pharmaceutica 76: 203-215.

7

Effects of Passive Immunization against Peptide Tyrosine Tyrosine on the Activity of Digestive Enzymes in Rats

Fan Zhiyong1,2*, Zhang Guanglei1, Zhou Dinggang3, Liang Zhe3, Wu Xin4 and Wang Fenglai2

¹Engineering Research Center for Feed Safety and Efficient Utilization of Ministry of Education, Institute of Animal Nutrition, Hunan Agricultural University, Hunan, 410128, China
²State Key Laboratory of Animal Nutrition, Beijing 100081, China
³College of Animal Science and Technology, Sichuan Agricultural University, Yaan, 625014, China
⁴Hunan Provincial Engineering Research Center of Healthy Livestock, Key Laboratory of Agro-ecological Processes in Subtropical Region, Institute of Subtropical Agriculture, Chinese Academy of Sciences, Changsha, Hunan 410125, China

Abstract

The object of this study was to investigate the effect of serum antibody of peptide tyrosine tyrosine on activities of digestive enzymes in rats. A total of sixty sprague-dawley (SD) rats weighing 87.77 ± 1.61 g were randomly allocated to 1 of 4 dose treatment:0 (control), 50 µL, 100 µL, or 200 µL peptide tyrosine tyrosine antiserum during the 21-d experimental period. The activity of amylases and lipases in the pancreas and duodenum as well as gastric pepsin was measured at the end of the study. The results showed that the activity of lipases in the pancreas and duodenum increased with increasing peptide tyrosine tyrosine antiserum level, but obvious tendency of pancreatic lipases activity between all treatments was not observed($P > 0.05$). The lipase activity in the duodenum showed a significant increase ($P < 0.05$) in the groups treated with 100 µL or 200 µL of peptide tyrosine tyrosine antiserum compared with the control group. The amylase activity in the pancreas and duodenum increased with the increasing peptide tyrosine tyrosine antiserum dose, and the group treated with 200 µL of peptide tyrosine tyrosine antiserum was significantly higher ($P < 0.05$) than the other groups. The amylase activity in the duodenum showed no significant difference ($P > 0.05$) among groups, but the group treated with 200 µL of PYY antiserum showed the highest activity. In conclusion, the injection of peptide tyrosine tyrosine antiserum improved nutrition utilization rate and activity of digestive enzymes in a dose dependent manner in rats.

Keywords: Peptide tyrosine; Tyrosine; Antiserum; Digestive enzymes; Rat

Introduction

The gut hormone peptide tyrosine tyrosine (PYY) is a 36-amino acid peptide and two main endogenous forms PYY1–36 and PYY3–36, have been identified, with PYY3–36 being the predominant circulating form [1-3]. Peptide tyrosine tyrosine is released from specialized enteroendocrine cells called L-cells, which are found predominantly within the distal GI tract [4,5]. PYY may be secreted by the stomach and pancreatic endocrine cells, while it is also found in the central nervous system (hypothalamus, brain stem, medulla, pons and spinal cord) and the peripheral nervous system neurons [6,7]. Peptide tyrosine tyrosine is secreted alongside hormone glucagon-like peptide 1, and it is released after eating, circulates in the blood and functions by binding to receptors in the brain. The binding of these receptors then causes a decreased appetite and makes people feel full after eating. Moreover, peptide tyrosine tyrosine had important effects on the function of the stomach and intestine to slow down the movement of food through the digestive tract.

Peptide tyrosine tyrosine exerts its action through neuropeptide Y (NPY) receptors to inhibit gastric motility and increase water and electrolyte absorption in the colon [8]. Expression of Y2 receptor is the most abundant PYY receptor on pancreatic cancer cell. This indicated that peptide tyrosine tyrosine may also affect pancreatic secretion [9]. In the pancreatic, PYY occurs in islet cells of the mouse pancreas, most of which are glucagon cells, and that PYY inhibits stimulated insulin and glucagon secretion in vivo in the mouse.[10]. This indicated that it played an important role in the proliferation and differentiation during the development of the pancreatic [7]. Peptide tyrosine tyrosine can regulate the function of digestive system by slowing the gastric emptying; hence, it increases efficiency of digestion and nutrient absorption after a meal. Peptide tyrosine tyrosine also

plays a very important role in energy homeostasis by regulating food intake via the neuroendocrine system (brain-gut axis). Previous study indicated that PYY may affect directly the hypothalamic arcuate nucleus of its neurons after secreted by the intestinal endocrine cells by G protein-coupled way and have an ingibitory effect on the ingestion of animals; Or else PYY may affect the feed intake of animal in the way of negative feedback. That means the negative feedback of PYY can block the ventrolateral thalamic nucleus under the excitement and express of NPY caused by ingestion [1]. PYY-knockout rats, on the other hand, are resistant to obesity, but have higher fat mass and lower glucose tolerance when fed a high-fat diet, compared to control rats. High PYY concentrations cause a decrease in appetite and food intake. Moreover, high PYY concentrations are associated with diseases where there is dramatic weight loss, such as anorexia nervosa, coeliac disease, inflammatory bowel disease (Crohn's disease and ulcerative colitis) and some cancers. Low PYY concentrations are associated with an increase in appetite and food intake. There has been some research into using PYY as a medication for obesity, aiming to decrease the appetite of people who are overweight.

*Corresponding author: Fan Zhiyong, Engineering Research Center for Feed Safety and Efficient Utilization of Ministry of Education, Institute of Animal Nutrition, Hunan Agricultural University, Hunan, 410128, China, E-mail: fzyong04@163.com

PYY is the satiety factor physiologically inhibiting food intake in animals, and it regulates a variety of gastrointestinal hormones [11]. As shown by both in vitro and in vivo studies, PYY inhibits the secretion of insulin. PYY can also reduce gastric acid secretion and slow down gastric emptying. In addition, a relationship between PYY and regulating factors associated with feeding has been observed in animals. However, future investigation is needed. Moreover, active immunization against PYY decreases its level in serum, but the resulting effects on the hormones and enzymes related to feeding in animals still remain largely unexplored. Therefore, the objective of this study was to investigate effects of passive immunization against PYY on activities of digestive enzymes in rats.

Methods and Materials

Animal management

PYY antiserum was derived from rabbits and prepared before the experiment. Sprague–Dawley (SD) rats were obtained from the Laboratory Animal Center of the Chinese Academy of Sciences (Hunan, China). The rats were housed in a pathogen-free house and had free access to food and drinking water. Feed intake was recorded.

Study design

Sixty SD rats weighing about 70 g were randomly assigned to three active treated groups and one control group, with five replicates in each group and three rats for each replicate. The rats were injected with 50 (group 1), 100 (group 2), 200 (group 3) μL of PYY antiserum or 0.9% physiological saline (control) respectively. The rats were treated once a week for three weeks and the experiment lasted for 21 days.

Digestion experiment

The digestion experiment began on the day of 21. The digestion trial consisted of a 3-day adaptation period followed by a 7-day feces collection period. During the digestion trial, the rats had free access to food. The feces were collected twice daily (8 AM and 8 PM) and stored at -20°C. The feces were thawed, mixed well, dried in a 60-70°C oven, and ground to pass a 40 mesh screen for analysis of dry matter, crude protein, and gross energy.

Sample collection

At the end of the trial, one rat from each replicate was sacrificed, and the stomach, duodenum, pancreas were removed and weighed immediately. The samples were snap frozen in liquid nitrogen and stored at -20°C until further analysis.

Measurement of digestibility of nutrients

Measurement of original moisture: The original sample was dried in a 65°C oven for 8-12 hours, and the weight was taken after leaving the sample at room temperature for resurgence for 24 hours. After weighing the sample, it was dried in a 65°C oven for 2 hours and left at room temperature for resurgence for 24 hours before achieving the weight again. The procedure was repeated till the difference between two weights was less than 0.5 g, and the lowest value of the weights was used for the calculation of original moisture.

Original moisture = (initial weight-dried weight) / initial weight × 100%

Measurement of dry matter: The air-dried sample was dried in a 105 ± 2°C oven till the stable weight was achieved. The bound moisture was measured and the dry matter was calculated by the following formula. Determination of dry matter content of the drying method, reference GB/T 6433-2006 [12].

Water = (W1-W2) / (W1-W0) ×100%

`W1 (g) is the total weight of the sample and the container before the sample was dried in a 105±2°C oven; W2 (g) is the total weight of the sample and the container after the sample was dried in a 105±2☒ oven; W0 (g) is the weight of container.

Total water =[A+(1—A)×B]×100%

`A is the measured original moisture (%); B is the bound moisture of dried sample (%).

Measurement of crude protein: Crude protein were measured using FOSS Kjeltec 2300 (Foss, Denmark). Determination Kjeldahl method crude protein content, reference GB/T 6432-1994 [13].

Energy measurement: The Energy was measured by using HXR-6000 precision automatic calorimeter.

Measurement of enzyme activity: The tissue of stomach, pancreas, or duodenum was homogenized in chilled 0.9% physiological saline to obtain a 10% (for pepsin and amylase) or 20% (for lipase) homogenate (w/v) which was then centrifuged at 2500 rpm for 10 min. The resulting supernatant was used for analysis of stomach pepsin activity with an ELISA assay kit (Nanjing Jiancheng Bioengineering Institute) according to the manufacturer's instructions.

The lipase activity in the pancreas and duodenum was analyzed according to the Kaumas brilliant blue method using a lipase kit (Nanjing Jiancheng Bioengineering Institute) according to the manufacturer's instructions

The amylase activity in the pancreas and duodenum was determined using an amylase assay kit (Nanjing Jiancheng Bioengineering Institute) according to the manufacturer's instructions. The protein content in the tissue was also measured with an assay kit (Nanjing Jiancheng Bioengineering Institute) using Coomassie brilliant blue method.

Statistical analysis

Data were processed using Excel and analyzed by SPSS 11.5. Tukey test was used for multiple comparisons. The significance level was set at 0.05. The results were expressed as mean ± standard deviation (X ± SD).

Results

Effects of PYY antiserum on nutrition utilization rate

As shown in Figure 1, the difference of utilization ratio of dry matter among groups was not significant (P>0.05), with the highest in the control group and the lowest in the group 2. Utilization ratio of crude protein was improved by 76.65 % (P<0.05) in group 3 and numerically increased (P>0.05) by 24.4% in group 1 and 38.13 % in group 2 when compared with the control. Utilization ratio of energy was enhanced (P<0.05) by 161.11% in group 3 and numerically increased (P>0.05) by 46.88% in group 1 and 19.90 % in group 2 relative to the control.

Effects of PYY antiserum on activity of digestive enzymes

The activity of pancreatic lipases increased numerically with the increasing dose of PYY antiserum, but the difference among groups was not significant (P>0.05). Compared with the control group, pancreatic lipases activity increased by 7.80%, 27.96% and 38.58% in groups 1, 2, and 3, respectively. The activity of lipases in the duodenum increased with the increasing dose of PYY antiserum, and group 3 had a significant (P<0.05) increase compared with the control and group 1. Lipase activity in the duodenum of group 3 increased by 14.31%, 10.21% and 2.37% compared to the control, group 1 and group 2, respectively. Group 2 had an 11.67% increase (P<0.05) of lipase activity in the duodenum compared with the control group (Figure 2).

As shown in Figure 3 the activity of amylases in the pancreas and duodenum increased as the dose of PYY antiserum increased. The activity of pancreatic amylases of group 3 increased (P<0.05) by 52.94%, 44.44% and 36.84% compared with the control, group 1 and group 2, respectively. The activity of amylases in the duodenum did not show a significant difference among groups (P>0.05), but group 3 had the highest activity, with an increase of 96.24%, 75.69% and 24.24% compared with the control, group 1 and group 2, respectively (Figure 3).

As shown in table 1, the activity of gastric pepsin increased as the dose of PYY antiserum increased, but the difference among groups was not significant (P>0.05). After the injection of PYY antiserum, the protein content in the pancreatic and gastric tissues was not significantly different among groups (P>0.05), and the group 3 has the lowest protein content in the pancreatic tissue. The difference of

the protein content in the duodenum was significant among groups, with the control, groups 1 and 2 being 16.13%, 11.29% and 8.06%, respectively, lower (P<0.05) than group 3 (Figure 4).

Discussion

Effects of PYY antiserum on nutrition utilization rate

PYY is released from the gut into the circulation in a nutrient-dependent manner. PYY levels are low in the fasting state, rapidly increase in response to food intake, reach a peak at 1–2 h after a meal and then remain elevated for several hours [14]. PYY3–36 has additional metabolic beneficial effects on energy expenditure and fuel partitioning. PYY regulates body weight by reducing food intake and increasing energy expenditure [15]. Several studies suggested a role of endogenous PYY in satiety regulation in humans [5,16]. And some benefits were observed in experimental subjects in reducing hunger and promoting weight loss [2]. This would help explain the weight-loss experienced with high-protein diet. Blockade of endogenous PYY by administration of PYY antiserum resulted in increased food intake in rats that had undergone jejuno-intestinal bypass [17-18].

The effects of the injection of PYY antiserum on the growth and endocrine in rats have been proved to some degree, but the effect of

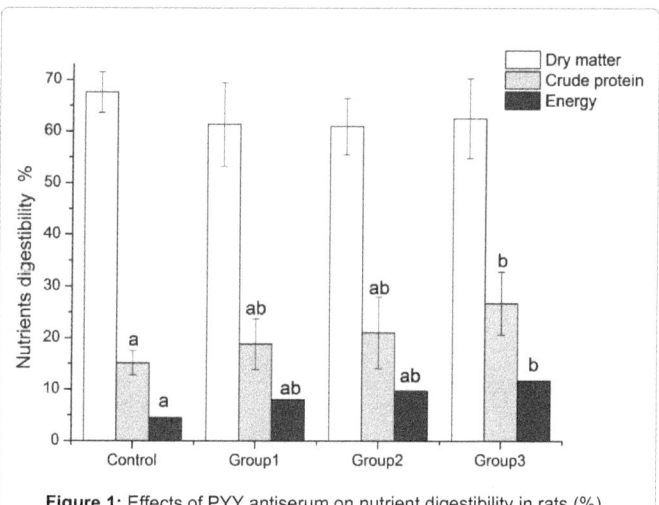

Figure 1: Effects of PYY antiserum on nutrient digestibility in rats (%).

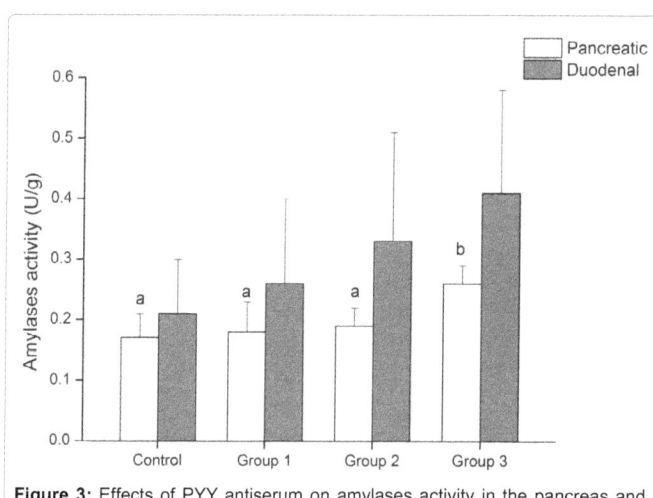

Figure 3: Effects of PYY antiserum on amylases activity in the pancreas and duodenum.

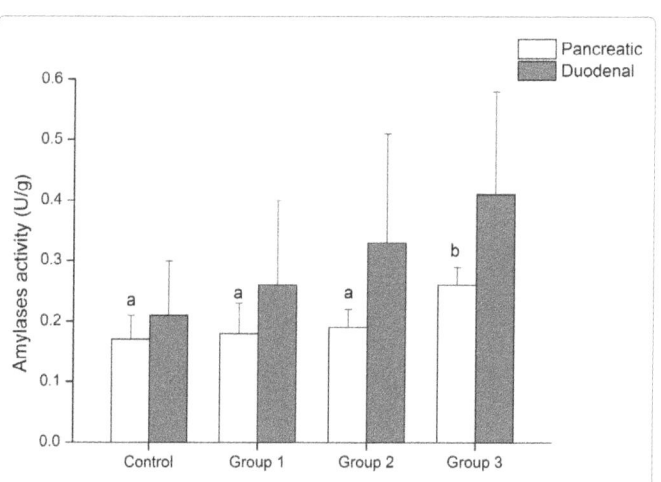

Figure 2: Effects of PYY antiserum on the lipases activity in the pancreas and duodenum.

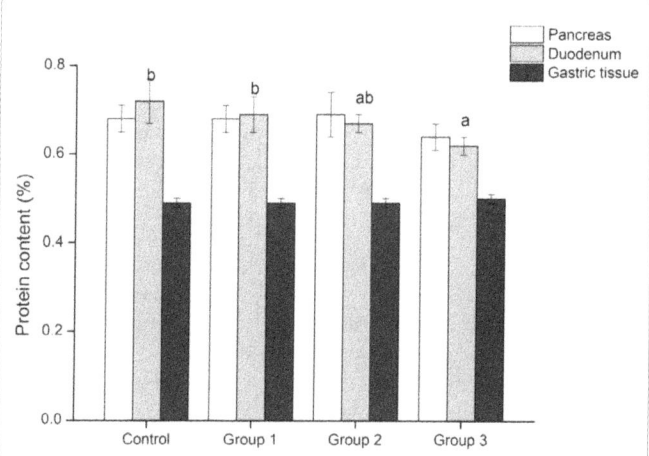

Figure 4: Effects PYY antiserum on protein content of the pancreatic, duodenal and gastric tissue.

PYY antiserum on the nutrient absorptivity in rats are not well studied [19]. Our study showed that dry matter digestibility was not affected by PYY in a dose dependent manner, and the difference among groups was not significant. Digestibility of crude protein increased with the increasing dose of PYY antiserum, and the difference between the treated groups and the control group was significant. Digestibility of energy also increased with the increasing dose of PYY antiserum in rats, which indicates that the injection of PYY antiserum affected the metabolic rate, facilitated the metabolism of food, and improved the growth of animals.

Effects of passive immunization against PYY on the digestive enzymes

Exocrine pancreas (mainly pancreatic juice) plays an important role in digestion and absorption of food. Irregular secretion of pancreatic juice leads to abnormal digestion and absorption, affects the growth of animals, and harms the production [20]. Pancreatic juice is maintained at a normal level under the neuronal and homeostatic regulation. It is the colorless and odorless alkaline solution, mainly including water, inorganic and organic chemicals [21]. The organic chemicals are mostly composed of multiple digestive enzymes, including pancreatic amylases, lipases, proteases and intestinal kinases. PYY regulates growth, digestion and absorption in the gut and pancreas, and its physiological function in the immunization and nutrient absorption are through decreasing cell factors and releasing amylases. Although the mechanism is still unclear, the glandular level of PYY is believed to be associated with many cell transcription factors. PYY stimulates the secretion of pancreatin, CCK and insulin, and inhibits the secretion of glucagon, somatostatin and pancreatic polypeptide [22]. PYY inhibits endocrine and exocrine secretion of the pancreas, reduces the pancreatic blood flow, suppresses the growth of the pancreas stimulated by pancreatin, and inhibits the basal pancreatic secretion and the secretion of pancreatic juice stimulated by vagus nerve [23]. As shown in Figures 2 and 3, the activity of pancreatic lipases, pancreatic amylases and duodenal amylases increased with the increasing dose of PYY antiserum, which is consistent with previous studies.

Pepsin hydrolyzes the protein in the food, and its primary role is to hydrolyze protein and peptide containing phenylalanine or tyrosine, and the decomposed products are mainly peptone, with polypeptide or amino acids as minor products. Pepsin only functions in the acidic environment, and the optimistic pH is 2. The activity of protease decreases as the pH increases, and the protease is irreversibly denatured if the pH rises to more than 6. Therefore, stomach proteases and stomach acid are closely related. Previous research has shown that intravenous injection of 50 pmol/kg/h of GLP-1 or PYY in dogs suppressed the secretion of stomach acid, and completely inhibited secretion of stomach acid if injected with both drugs. Studies also showed that taking 10 pmol/kg of PYY and 0.05 CU/kg of secretin hourly inhibited the secretion of stomach acid stimulated by pentagastrin in human [24-25].

PYY suppresses the secretion of stomach acid through the regulation of central nervous system. Research showed that PYY regulates the secretion of stomach acid via vagus nerve, and most of them are through vagus nerve at the pyloric part of stomach [26]. PYY and Y2 receptor agonists regulate the secretion of stomach acid via dorsal motor nucleus of vagus nerve in the in vitro and in vivo experiments [27,28].

As shown in Table 1 the activity of pepsin decreased with the increased dose of PYY antiserum. A possible mechanism could be that the effects of inhibiting the secretion of stomach acid by PYY reduced with the passive immunization of PYY, which caused the raising of pH in the stomach, and thus decreased the activity of pepsin. However, further investigation is still needed.

	Pepsin
Control group	52.25 ± 14.02
Group 1	58.12 ± 10.47
Group 2	63.27 ± 10.64
Group 3	65.26 ± 5.71

Table 1: Effects of PYY antiserum on pepsin activity (U/g).

Conclusion

The injection of PYY antiserum affected digestibility of crude protein and energy, which increased with the increasing dose of PYY antiserum. However, PYY antiserum had no obvious effect on the digestion of dry matter. Injection of PYY antiserum improved the activity of pancreatic lipases, pancreatic amylases, duodenal lipases and duodenal amylases in a dose-response manner. But the activity of gastric pepsin decreased with the increasing dose of PYY antiserum. The injection of PYY antiserum had no effects on protein content in pancreas and gastric tissue, and the injection of high dose of PYY antiserum (200 μl/rat) decreased the protein content in duodenum.

Immunizing rats with the PYY antiserum could improve the nutrient utilization rate and digestive enzyme activity, and the effects increased with the increasing dose of PYY antiserum. The possible mechanism of this effect is that PYY antiserum specifically neutralizes the endogenous PYY thus decreases its biological effects in rats.

Acknowledgment

This research was jointly supported by grants from the State Key Laboratory of Animal Nutrition (2004DA125184F1305), National Key Technology Research and Development Program of the Ministry of Science and Technology of China (2012BAD39B00).

References

1. Batterham RL, Cowley MA, Small CJ, Herzog H, Cohen MA, et al. (2002) Gut hormone PYY(3-36) physiologically inhibits food intake. Nature 418: 650-654.
2. Batterham RL, Heffron H, Kapoor S, Chivers JE, Chandarana K, et al. (2006) Critical role for peptide YY in protein-mediated satiation and body-weight regulation. Cell Metab 4: 223-233.
3. Korner J, Inabnet W, Conwell IM, Taveras C, Daud A, et al. (2006) Differential effects of gastric bypass and banding on circulating gut hormone and leptin levels. Obesity (Silver Spring) 14: 1553-1561.
4. Lundberg JM, Tatemoto K, Terenius L, Hellström PM, Mutt V, et al. (1982) Localization of peptide YY (PYY) in gastrointestinal endocrine cells and effects on intestinal blood flow and motility. Proc Natl Acad Sci U S A 79: 4471-4475.
5. Challis BG, Pinnock SB, Coll AP, Carter RN, Dickson SL, et al. (2003) Acute effects of PYY3-36 on food intake and hypothalamic neuropeptide expression in the mouse. Biochem Biophys Res Commun 311: 915-919.
6. Pieribone VA, Brodin L, Friberg K, Dahlstrand J, Söderberg C, et al. (1992) Differential expression of mRNAs for neuropeptide Y-related peptides in rat nervous tissues: possible evolutionary conservation. J Neurosci 12: 3361-3371.
7. Ekblad E, Sundler F (2002) Distribution of pancreatic polypeptide and peptide YY. Peptides 23: 251-261.
8. Liu CD, Aloia T, Adrian TE, Newton TR, Bilchik AJ, et al. (1996) Peptide YY: A potential pro-absorptive hormone for the treatment of mal-absorptive disorders. Am Surg 62: 232-236.
9. Li H, Wang Z, Dong L, Jiang J, Xu X, et al. (2014) Peptide tyrosine-tyrosine combined with its receptors exhibits an anti-cancer potential in pancreatic cancer MiaPaCa-2 cell. Chin Med J (Engl) 127: 4235-4242.
10. Böttcher G, Ahrén B, Lundquist I, Sundler F (1989) Peptide YY: Intra-pancreatic

localization and effects on insulin and glucagon secretion in the mouse. Pancreas 4: 282-288.

11. Adams SH, Won WB, Schonhoff SE, Leiter AB, Paterniti JR Jr (2004) Effects of peptide YY [3-36] on short-term food intake in mice are not affected by prevailing plasma ghrelin levels. Endocrinology 145: 4967-4975.

12. National Feed Industry Standardization Technical Committee. (2006) GB / T 6433-2006 Determination of crude fat diet [S]. Beijing: China Standard Press.

13. National Feed Industry Standardization Technical Committee. (2006) GB / T 6432-1994 Determination of crude protein [S]. Beijing: China Standard Press.

14. Adrian TE, Savage AP, Sagor GR, Allen JM, Bacarese-Hamilton AJ, et al. (1985) Effect of peptide YY on gastric, pancreatic, and biliary function in humans. Gastroenterology 89: 494-499.

15. Pfluger PT, Kampe J, Castaneda TR, Vahl T, D'Alessio DA, et al. (2007) Effect of human body weight changes on circulating levels of peptide YY and peptide YY3-36. J Clin Endocrinol Metab 92: 583-588.

16. Roth CL, Enriori PJ, Harz K, Woelfle J, Cowley MA, et al. (2005) Peptide YY is a regulator of energy homeostasis in obese children before and after weight loss. J Clin Endocrinol Metab 90: 6386-6391.

17. le Roux CW, Aylwin SJ, Batterham RL, Borg CM, Coyle F, et al. (2006) Gut hormone profiles following bariatric surgery favor an anorectic state, facilitate weight loss, and improve metabolic parameters. Ann Surg 243: 108-114.

18. le Roux CW, Batterham RL, Aylwin SJ, Patterson M, Borg CM, et al. (2006) Attenuated peptide YY release in obese subjects is associated with reduced satiety. Endocrinology 147: 3-8.

19. Ding GZ, Liang Z, Fan ZY, Liu GH, Zhou P, et al. (2013) Effects of passive immunization against peptide tyrosine tyrosine on the growth performance and endocrine hormone levels in blood serum of rats [A]. Advance Journal of Food Science and Technology 5: 99-105.

20. Fung LC, Chisholm C, Greenberg GR (1998) Glucagon-like peptide-1-(7-36) amide and peptide YY mediate intraduodenal fat-induced inhibition of acid secretion in dogs. Endocrinology 139: 189-194.

21. Guan D, Rivard N, Morisset J, Greeley GH Jr (1993) Effects of peptide YY on the growth of the pancreas and intestine. Endocrinology 132: 219-223.

22. Vona-Davis L, McFadden DW (2007) PYY and the pancreas: Inhibition of tumor growth and inflammation. Peptides 28: 334-338.

23. Stanley S, Wynne K, Bloom S (2004) Gastrointestinal satiety signals III. Glucagon-like peptide 1, oxyntomodulin, peptide YY, and pancreatic polypeptide. Am J Physiol Gastrointest Liver Physiol 286: G693-697.

24. En ÃFY, ImeryÃN, Akin L, TuroÄŸlu T, Dede F, et al. (2001) Inhibition of gastric emptying by acarbose is correlated with GLP-1 response and accompanied by CCK release. Am J Physiol Gastrointest Liver Physiol 281: G752-763.

25. Morínigo R, Moizé V, Musri M, Lacy AM, Navarro S, et al. (2006) Glucagon-like peptide-1, peptide YY, hunger, and satiety after gastric bypass surgery in morbidly obese subjects. J Clin Endocrinol Metab 91: 1735-1740.

26. Yang H, Kawakubo K, Wong H, Ohning G, Walsh J, et al. (2000) Peripheral PYY inhibits intracisternal TRH-induced gastric acid secretion by acting in the brain. Am J Physiol Gastrointest Liver Physiol 279: G575-581.

27. Singh G, Singh L, Raufman JP (1992) Y2 receptors for peptide YY and neuropeptide Y on dispersed chief cells from guinea pig stomach. Am J Physiol 262: G756-762.

28. Janssen P, Verschueren S, Rotondo A, Tack J (2012) Role of Y(2) receptors in the regulation of gastric tone in rats. Am J Physiol Gastrointest Liver Physiol 302: G732-739.

Hepatoprotective and Antioxidative Effects of *Terminalia Arjuna* against Cadmium Provoked Toxicity in Albino Rats (*Ratus Norvigicus*)

Muhammad Tahir Haidry* and Arif Malik

Institute of Molecular Biology and Biotechnology, The University of Lahore-Pakistan, Pakistan

Abstract

The extract of bark of *Terminalia arjuna* was investigated for its hepatoprotective and antioxidative effects on cadmium provoked toxicity. It was found that cadmium (Cd) significantly ($P<0.05$) elevated the serum levels of following biomarkers alanine amino transferase (ALT), aspartate amino transferase (AST), alkaline phosphatase ALP, and malondialdehyde (MDA) simultaneously, it lowered the protein and depleted the antioxidant enzymes superoxide dismutase (SOD), catalase (CAT), and glutathione (GSH) upon administration of cadmium chloride (5 mg/kg) to albino rats. Study results indicated that the treatment of these rats with extracts of *Terminalia arjuna* (200 mg/kg) significantly reversed the effects of cadmium and proved that it has hepatoprotective, and antioxidative potential. The results also suggested that the phytochemicals present in the extract of bark of T. *arjuna* have potential therapeutic value.

Keywords: Cadmium chloride; Stress; Toxicity; *Terminalia arjuna*; Hepatoprotective; Antioxidative

Introduction

The liver performs an array of functions and the most important one is its role in metabolism so no other organ is more important for healthy metabolism than the liver. It is accountable for detoxifying the poison or any foreign substance by converting and excreting waste and toxin [1]. Other major functions of liver are the metabolism of carbohydrates, lipid, protein and secretion of bile. Thus the maintenance of healthy liver is vital for overall health [2]. It is considered as one of the most vital organs due to the handling the metabolism and excretion of drugs and other xenobiotics thus it provides protection against foreign substances by detoxifying and eliminating them [3]. It is frequently abused by the environmental toxins, heavy metals, poor eating habits, alcohol, prescription and the counter drug use thus it is damaged and weakened ultimately leads to the hepatitis, cirrhosis and alcoholic liver disease. Various toxicants, chemo-therapeutic agents, carbon tetrachloride (CCl_4), thioacetamide, lead, chromium, cadmium, chronic alcohol consumption and microbes are well studied for liver cell injury. Many synthetic drugs are used for the treatment of liver diseases also damage the liver [4].

Human health is under the serious threat of heavy metal pollution which is a gift of modern age of industrialization [5]. Cadmium is environmental pollutant and toxicant that can affect liver, kidney, lungs, bones, brain, testis and cardiovascular system [6]. It became commercial in 20th century due to its agricultural and industrial applications and then these actions cause the entry of cadmium into the soil and drinking water. Extremely soluble characters of compounds of cadmium make its entry into the plants and crops that are used to get food and feed [7]. Other sources of cadmium are smoking, occupational disclosure and house dirt [8]. Respiratory tract and gastrointestinal tract are two main ways of absorption of cadmium. It competes with iron during absorption so iron status of individual is more important thus iron deficiency increase its absorption [9]. Although there is no specific transporter for its absorption but divalent metal ion transporters are used to take up free cadmium ion from cadmium [10].

As cadmium enters the blood circulation taken up by the red blood cells or get attach with albumin in blood plasma. Within first six hours cadmium is taken into the hepatocytes and makes new complex with metallothionein [11], with other proteins or peptides and glutathione (GSH) [12]. From liver it is send to kidney for excretion. While passing through the proximal tubules, it is reabsorbed and stored in these cells [13].

Oxidative stress is the basic mechanism of cadmium toxicity but cadmium is incapable to induce the production of reactive oxygen species (ROS) directly because of being a non-fenton metal. Indirectly it provokes stress via dislodgment of metal ions e.g. Fe+2, reduction of ROS scavengers, denaturation of enzymes and rollout of ETC (electron transport chain) cause the production of ROS [14,15]. The important way of production of hydroxyl radical is fenton reaction [16]. Hydroxyl radical is most reactive and damaging to lipids proteins and DNA, it damages membranes by initiating lipid peroxidation (LPO) results in production of malondialdehyde (MDA) from the breakdown of polyunsaturated fatty acids [17].

Medicinal plants are the major source of drugs and have been proven for the presence of hepatoprotective potential. Extracts of such plants are widely used for the treatment of liver diseases like hepatitis, cirrhosis, and loss of appetite and the *Terminalia arjuna* is one of such plants that are used for liver diseases [18]. *Terminalia arjuna* is an ever green, 20-30m long, South Asian plant, generally known as 'Arjuna. Antibacterial and antioxidant nature of T. arjuna has been well explored *in vitro* [19]. T. *arjuna* has antioxidant properties due to presence flavonoids, tannins and oligomeric proanthocyanidins [20].

Aims and Objectives

The present work was aim to determine the hepatoprotective and antioxidative effects of *Terminalia arjuna* against the Cd-provoked hepatotoxicity and oxidative stress in albino rats.

*Corresponding author: Muhammad Tahir Haidry, Institute of molecular biology and biotechnology, The University of Lahore-Pakistan, Pakistan, E-mail: biochemistmth@gmail.com

Material and Methods

Animals

Fifteen albino rats were selected from the population of 50 rats and placed in animal house of institute of molecular biology and biochemistry (IMBB) the University of Lahore (UOL). They were placed in cages made up of stainless steel at constant $25 \pm 5°C$ temperature with alternating day and night cycles, and standard pellets and water were in free access (ad libitum). This project was approved by the ethic committee of IMBB the University of Lahore.

Chemicals

All chemicals and regents were of analytical grades. Cadmium chloride (CdCl2) was purchased from Merck Pharmaceutical Company Germany.

Experimental design

Out of 50 total rats only 15 male healthy rats were chosen and were separated in three groups each having 5 rats. Group I: Normal control kept on normal diet and tap water. Group II: Rats were given $CdCl_2$ @ 5 mg/kg B.Wt in drinking water till the end of research for six weeks [21]. Group III: Rats were given $CdCl_2$ @ 5 mg/kg B.Wt in drinking water for three weeks then they were given standardized extract of bark Terminalia arjuna @ 200 mg/kg B.Wt. for next three weeks.

Biochemical analysis

LFT (Liver functioning test include AST, ALT, ALP) was measured by using spectrophotometric method as described by Anonymous, 1996 [22]. Levels of total protein were estimated by Lowry Method [23]. SOD activity was measured by Kakkar method [24]. TBARS was measured by the method of Ohkawa et al. [25]. Catalase activity was measured by Aebi's method [26]. Glutathione was measured by method described by Moron et al. [27]

Statistical Analysis

The values were reported in mean ± SD (n=5). Experimental results were statistically analyzed by using analysis of variance (ANOVA) by Duncan's multiple range tests.

Results

Table1 showed that Cadmium had a significant effect on alanine aminotransferase (ALT), aspartate aminotransferase (AST), alkaline phosphatase (ALP) and total protein (TP) level in serum. The administration of Cadmium 5mg/kg in rats provokes significant (P<0.05) increase in ALT, AST, ALP levels as compared to group A denoting the presence of liver dysfunction. The treatment with Terminalia arjuna 200 mg/kg group C significantly (P<0.05) decreased the toxic effect of Cadmium by decreasing the ALT, AST, ALP and by increasing TP levels in serum.

Table 2 showed that Cadmium had significant deleterious effects on serum antioxidative status. Cadmium (Cd) at the doses of 5 mg/kg (Group B)had significantly (P<0.05) decreased the serum levels of superoxide dismutase (SOD), catalase (CAT), and glutathione (GSH) as compare to positive control (group A) whereas melondialdehyde (MDA) in serum had increased by the administration of cadmium alone indicating stress mediated lipid per-oxidation. The rats received Terminalia arjuna 200 mg/kg (Group C) had significantly reversed the situation as compared to group B, depicted that Terminalia arjuna alleviated the toxic effects of cadmium and the levels of glutathione,

Liver profile	ALT (nmol/ml)	AST (nmol/ml)	ALP (nmol/ml)	TP (mg/dl)
GROUPS	MEAN ± SD (LSD=19.23)	MEAN ± SD (LSD=5.55)	MEAN ± SD (LSD=8.23)	MEAN ± SD (LSD=1.05)
A	34.26 ± 2.05 b	31.71 ± 2.24b	82.65 ± 5.69c	6.22 ± 0.23a
B	106.53 ± 22.90 a	101.58 ± 3.05a	128.08 ± 6.38a	3.8 ± 0.50b
C	30.92 ± 1.16 b	28.26 ± 1b	104.54 ± 4.92b	6.24 ± 1.01a

Significance level =0.05

Table 1: Estimation of serum ALT, AST, ALP and total Protein

Stress profile	GSH (µg/ml)	SOD (µg/ml)	MDA (nmol/ml)	CAT (µmol/mol)
GROUPS				
	MEAN ± SD (LSD=1.15)	MEAN ± SD (LSD=2.89)	MEAN ± SD (LSD=8.72)	MEAN ± SD (LSD=4.96)
A	8.68 ± 0.54a	79.87 ± 1.62a	46.58 ± 1.52c	32.58 ± 3.19a
B	4.28 ± 0.41c	42.26 ± 2.64e	91.16 ± 9.14a	17.03 ± 3.36c
C	5.93 ± 0.58b	62.28 ± 1d	58.61 ± 3.79b	24.59 ± 3.51b

Significance level=0.05

Table 2: Estimation of serum GSH, SOD, MDA and Catalase

SOD and CAT were improved by decreasing the process of lipid peroxidation.

Discussion

It is well known that both aminotransferases (ALT and AST) are highly concentrated in the liver; ALT is localized solely in the cytoplasm, whereas AST is present both in the cytosol and mitochondria of hepatocytes [28]. Increased serum level of ALT, AST and ALP of rats of group B as compare to that of group A indicated that cadmium cause their release from the hepatocytes (Table1). Lowered total protein (TP) of group B as compare to that of group A was might be due to stoppage of protein synthesis and increased execration of proteins with cadmium (Table 1). Similar results were discussed by [29,30]. Our study showed that cadmium provoked apoptotic cell death in liver hepatocytes that was inverted by the phytochemicals in extract of Terminalia arjuna group C (Table1) in agreement with [31]. Administration of cadmium could cause cell lysis and release of cytoplasmic enzymes into the blood circulation, thereby leading to increased levels of these enzymes in the serum. This property is often used to assess the extent of cadmium-induced cellular damage. In the current study, elevated levels of AST and ALT were noted in response to cadmium induced toxicity. However, the level of enzymes significantly declined following concomitant administration of Terminalia arjuna extract. In the present study, we found that lipid per oxidation level was significantly elevated in plasma, of rats treated with cadmium as compared to control group thus significance increased oxidative stress. Similar results were supported by [32,33] who described that LPO is an early and sensitive effect of Cd exposure. Hassoun and Stohs [34] established that oxidative stress was induced following oral administration of cadmium chloride to rats. A parallel data had been described by Jurezuk et al. [35]. Additionally, Elizabeth et al, Jahangir et al and Eybl et al. [35-38] demonstrated that cadmium is considered to provoke lipid per oxidation and this has frequently been believed to be the main cause of its deleterious influence on membrane-dependent function.

An antioxidant should be fundamental component of an effective management of cadmium poisoning [39] as the results of present research showed that the mechanism of cadmium provoked damage, like other heavy metals, include the creation of reactive oxygen species and free radicals that alter the mitochondrial activity and genetic information [40,41]. Heavy metals cause their toxic effects directly or indirectly by producing cellular stress. Present research work and many previous studies have shown that cadmium metal has the capacity to produce free radicals and reactive oxygen species (ROS) consequential in depletion of enzyme activities, damage to lipid bilayer and DNA oxidation [42]. The reactive and free radical species include oxygen, carbon, sulfur and nitrogen radicals that are originating from super oxide radical, hydrogen peroxide and lipid peroxide [43].

Cd is unable to induce ROS directly because it cannot catalyze the fenton reaction but Cd induces oxidative stress indirectly. A number of studies have revealed the capability of Cd to replace Fe which is an active metal and run the fenton reaction thus increase in concentration of free Fe in cells enhance oxidative stress and lipid peroxidation by producing highly damaging hydroxyl radicals ($^{\circ}OH$) [14]. Many reports in animal models have illustrated that cadmium intoxication greatly increase the malondialdehyde (MDA) a product of lipid peroxidation [44]. MDA levels were found significantly high in plasma of rats treated with cadmium alone as compared to control group thus signifying increased oxidative stress. Manca et al, Abdul-Moniem and Ghafeer [31,33] who described that LPO is an early and sensitive effect of Cd exposure.

Acknowledgment

I acknowledge the efforts, support, love and guidelines of all my teachers, colleagues and friends throughout from my school times to University. Special thanks to talented, tremendously helpful, supportive and creative personality, my supervisorAssoc. Prof. Dr. Arif Malik and co-supervisor Prof. Dr. M.H. Qazi, who was a constant source of encouragement. Thanks for my wifewho was the first who motivated and support me. I am grateful to all those who supported me generously in completion of thesis especially brothers and friends Mr. Saeed Ismaeel and Mr. Abdul Manan.

References

1. Robbins J, Fleurentin C and Hefler A (2003) Hepatoprotective properties of crepisrueppelli and anisotesTrisules. Journal of ethanopharmacology76: 105-111.

2. Pradhan SC1, Girish C (2006) Hepatoprotective herbal drug, silymarin from experimental pharmacology to clinical medicine. Indian J Med Res 124: 491-504.

3. Agrwal SS (2001) Development of hepatoprotective formulation from plant sources. Pharmacology and therapeutics in the New Millennium. Narosa Publishing House, New Delhi, pp357-358.

4. Saleem MTS, Christina AJM, Chidambaranathan N, Ravi V, Gauthaman K (2008) Hepatoprotective activity of Anno-nasquamosa (Linn) on experimental animal model. Int J Applied Res Nat Pro 1: 1-7.

5. Nordberg G, Nogawa K, Nordberg M, Friberg L. Cadmium (2007) IHandbook on toxicology of metals. Academic Press, New York, USA, pp65-78.

6. Nair AR1, Degheselle O, Smeets K, Van Kerkhove E, Cuypers A (2013) Cadmium-Induced Pathologies: Where Is the Oxidative Balance Lost (or Not)? Int J MolSci 14: 6116-6143.

7. Satarug S1, Garrett SH, Sens MA, Sens DA (2010) Cadmium, environmental exposure, and health outcomes. Environ Health Perspect 118: 182-190.

8. Hogervorst J, Plusquin M, Vangronsveld J, Nawrot T, Cuypers A, et al. (2009) Current status of cadmium as an environmental health problem. ToxicolApplPharmacol 238: 201–208.

9. Goyer RA (1995) Nutrition and metal toxicity. Am J ClinNutr 61: 646S-650S.

10. Martelli A1, Rousselet E, Dycke C, Bouron A, Moulis JM (2006) Cadmium toxicity in animal cells by interference with essential metals. Biochimie 88: 1807-1814.

11. Cherian MG, Goyer RA (1978) Methallothioneins and their role in the metabolism and toxicity of metals. Life Sci 23: 1-9.

12. Thévenod F (2009) Cadmium and cellular signaling cascades: to be or not to be? ToxicolApplPharmacol 238: 221-239.

13. Bernard A (2008) Cadmium & its adverse effects on human health. Indian J Med Res 128: 557-564.

14. Cuypers A1, Plusquin M, Remans T, Jozefczak M, Keunen E, et al. (2010) Cadmium stress: an oxidative challenge. Biometals 23: 927-940.

15. Cannino G1, Ferruggia E, Luparello C, Rinaldi AM (2009) Cadmium and mitochondria. Mitochondrion 9: 377-384.

16. Lokendra S, Nameet K,Pankaj K (2009) Reactive oxygen species (ROS), oxidative damage and antioxidative defence systems with emphasis on herbal antioxidants and human and cattle health. Biochem Cell Arch 9:135-144.

17. Mathews CK, Van Holde KO and Ahern KG (2000) Biochemistry Pearson Education Inc. 551-557.

18. Nadkarni AK, Nadkarni KM (1954) Indian MateriaMedica. First ed. Popular Book Deport, Bomaby India, pp1198.

19. Bhattacharyya MH (2009) Cadmium osteotoxicity in experimental animals: mechanisms and relationship to human exposures. Toxicol Appl Pharmacol 238: 258-265.

20. Doorika P, Ananthi T (2012) Antioxidant and Hepatoprotective properties of Terminaliaarjuna Bark on Isoniazid Induced Toxicity in Albino rats. Asian J Pharm Tech 2: 15-18

21. Renugadevi J1, Prabu SM (2010) Cadmium-induced hepatotoxicity in rats and the protective effect of naringenin. Exp Toxicol Pathol 62: 171-181.

22. Anonymous (1996) Rendox manual procedure (4thEdn) Randox Laboratories Ltd, Diamond road Crumlin Co Antrim, United Kingdom.

23. Lowry OH, Rosebrough NJ, Farr AL, Randall RJ (1951) Protein measurement with the Folin phenol reagent. J BiolChem 193: 265-275.

24. Kakkar P, Das B, Viswanathan PN (1984) A modified spectrophotometric assay of superoxide dismutase. Indian J Biochem Biophys 21: 130-132.

25. Aebi H (1974) Catalase in Bergmeyer HU. Methods in Enzymatic Analysis. New York, Academic Press 3:276-286.

26. Ohkawa H, N Ohishi, K Yagi (1979) Assay for lipid peroxides in animal tissues by thiobarbituric acid reaction. J Anal Biochem. 95:351-358.

27. Moron MS, Depierre JW, Mannervik B (1979) Levels of glutathione, glutathione reductase and glutathione S-transferase activities in rat lung and liver. Biochim Biophys Acta 582: 67-78.

28. Rej R (1989) Aminotransferases in disease. Clin Lab Med 9: 667-687.

29. Shirish SP (2011) Protective effect of Terminalia arjuna against CCl4 induced liver damage in rats. Der Pharmacia Lettre 3: 84-90

30. Ilavarasan R, Mohideen S, Vijayalakshmi M and Manonmani G (2001) Hepatoprotective Effect of Cassia AngustifoliaVahl. Indian J pharm Science 63:504-507.

31. López E1, Arce C, Oset-Gasque MJ, Cañadas S, González MP (2006) Cadmium induces reactive oxygen species generation and lipid peroxidation in cortical neurons in culture. Free RadicBiol Med 40: 940-951.

32. Manca D1, Ricard AC, Trottier B, Chevalier G (1991) Studies on lipid peroxidation in rat tissues following administration of low and moderate doses of cadmium chloride. Toxicology 67: 303-323.

33. Abdel-Moneim WM,Ghafeer HH (2007) The Potential Protective Effect of Natural Honey Against Cadmium-Induced Hepatotoxicity And Nephrotoxicity. Mansoura J Forensic Med ClinToxicolXV: 2.

34. Elizabeth AM, Rosalyn DM, Jennifer AM, Rebecca RW, Beth AA (2003) Environmental cadmium levels increase phytochelatin and glutathione in lettuce grown in a chelator-buffered nutrient solution. Environ. Qual 32:1356-1364.

35. Hassoun EA1, Stohs SJ (1996) Cadmium-induced production of superoxide anion and nitric oxide, DNA single strand breaks and lactate dehydrogenase leakage in J774A.1 cell cultures. Toxicology 112: 219-226.

36. Jurczuk M1, BrzÃ³ska MM, Moniuszko-Jakoniuk J, GaÅ‚azyn-Sidorczuk M, Kulikowska-KarpiÅ„ska E (2004) Antioxidant enzymes activity and lipid peroxidation in liver and kidney of rats exposed to cadmium and ethanol. Food Chem Toxicol 42: 429-438.

Hepatoprotective and Antioxidative Effects of Terminalia Arjuna against Cadmium Provoked Toxicity...

47

37. Jahangir T1, Khan TH, Prasad L, Sultana S (2005) Alleviation of free radical mediated oxidative and genotoxic effects of cadmium by farnesol in Swiss albino mice. Redox Rep 10: 303-310.

38. Eybl V1, Kotyzová D, Leseticki L, Bludovská M, Koutenský J (2006) The influence of curcumin and manganese complex of curcumin on cadmium-induced oxidative damage and trace elements status in tissues of mice. J Appl Toxicol 26: 207-212.

39. El-Demerdash FM1, Yousef MI, Kedwany FS, Baghdadi HH (2004) Cadmium-induced changes in lipid peroxidation, blood hematology, biochemical parameters and semen quality of male rats: protective role of vitamin E and beta-carotene. Food Chem Toxicol 42: 1563-1571.

40. Patrick L (2003) Toxic metals and antioxidants: Part II. The role of antioxidants in arsenic and cadmium toxicity. Altern Med Rev 8: 106-128.

41. De-burbure, Buchet, Leroyer, Nisse, Haguenoer M, et al. (2006) Renal and neurologic Effects of cadmium, lead, mercury And arsenic in children: evidence of early Effects and multiple interactions at environmental Exposure levels. Environ. Health. Perspect114: 584-590.

42. Leonard SS1, Harris GK, Shi X (2004) Metal-induced oxidative stress and signal transduction. Free Radic Biol Med 37: 1921-1942.

43. Chen L1, Liu L, Huang S (2008) Cadmium activates the mitogen-activated protein kinase (MAPK) pathway via induction of reactive oxygen species and inhibition of protein phosphatases 2A and 5. Free Radic Biol Med 45: 1035-1044.

44. Yang JM1, Arnush M, Chen QY, Wu XD, Pang B, et al. (2003) Cadmium-induced damage to primary cultures of rat Leydig cells. Reprod Toxicol 17: 553-560.

9

Iguratimod Synergizes with Methotrexate to Exert Anti-Inflammatory and Bone-Protective Effect and Block the Progression of Collagen-Induced Arthritis in Mices

Qiong Luo[1], Yang Sun[1*], Biao Jin[1], Wei Zheng[1], Fenli Shao[1], Nan Hang[1], Yongqian Shu[2], Xiaomin Li[3], Yanhong Gu[2*] and Qiang Xu[1*]

[1]State Key Laboratory of Pharmaceutical Biotechnology, School of Life Sciences, Nanjing University, 22 Hankou Road, Nanjing 210093, China
[2]Department of Oncology, The First Affiliated Hospital with Nanjing Medical University, 300 Guangzhou Road, Nanjing 210029, China
[3]Department of Emergency, The First People's Hospital of Lianyungang, Lianyungang, Jiangsu 222002, China

Abstract

Rheumatoid Arthritis (RA) is an autoimmune disease characterized by chronic synovial inflammation and disability. The most widely used Disease-Modifying Antirheumatic Drug (DMARD) is methotrexate and it continues to be the gold standard. However, the use of high-dose methotrexate is associated with severe adverse effects. Iguratimod, which is currently used in clinics in China and Japan, is a novel oral DMARD for the treatment of RA. In this study, the effect of combination of methotrexate and iguratimod on murine Collagen-Induced Arthritis (CIA) and its mechanism was determined. Oral administration of iguratimod (3 mg/kg, 10 mg/kg) combined with methotrexate (1 mg/kg) potently blocked CIA development and delayed its progression, which was stronger than iguratimod or methotrexate used alone. Furthermore, infiltration of inflammatory cells into the synovium was remarkably inhibited by combination therapy and importantly, no bone erosion and joint destructions were observed in combination therapy group. In addition, combined administration of these two DMARDs suppressed production of cytokines (IL-17, IFN-γ, IL-6 and TNF-α) and antibodies (IgG and IgG2b) in serum, as well as humoral and cellular responses in CIA mice. Consistent with its effects in vivo, iguratimod combined with methotrexate significantly suppressed T and B cells responses in vitro. Taken together, our findings suggest that combination treatment with iguratimod and methotrexate should be an intriguing and preferable therapeutic strategy for treating RA.

Keywords: Iguratimod; Methotrexate; Rheumatoid arthritis; Collagen-induced arthritis; Combination therapy

Introduction

Rheumatoid Arthritis (RA) is a chronic systemic autoimmune disease with unclear etiology [1-4]. It is characterized by severe persistent synovitis that leads to the destruction of cartilage and bone, autoantibody production, and systemic inflammation [5,6]. Various cytokines, chemokines, effector cells, such as T- and B-lymphocytes, monocytes/macrophages, dendritic cells, Fibroblast-Like Synoviocytes (FLSs) and osteoclasts are involved in RA [7-11]. The therapeutic strategy of RA has undergone revolutionary changes [12,13]. Current drug therapies include two principal approaches: conventional Non-Steroidal Anti-Inflammatory Drugs (NSAIDs) and Disease-Modifying Antirheumatic Drugs (DMARDs) [14-16]. NSAIDs are only effective for controlling the symptoms of RA, such as pain, inflammatory, and stiffness, and the long-term disease progression can not be prevented by them [17]. However, unlike NSAIDs, DMARDs can not only improve symptoms but also interfere with the disease process [18,19]. DMARDs include methotrexate, sulfasalazine, hydroxychloroquine, and leflunomide. Recently, biological agents were introduced [17]. These biological-response modifiers include infliximab (inhibitor of TNF-α), anakinra (inhibitor of IL-1), abatacept (costimulation blocker), rituximab (anti-CD20 monoclonal antibody) and so on. However, its widespread use was limited by the high cost.

Methotrexate, a folic acid antagonist, has been the most widely used small molecular DMARD in the treatment of RA. It has been demonstrated effectiveness, high tolerability and low cost [17,20]. Methotrexate acts mainly on inhibiting the proliferation of rapidly dividing lymphocytes and other inflammatory cells [21]. Furthermore, methotrexate may diminish synovial collagenase gene expression [22], reduce toxic oxygen metabolites [23] and increase extracellular adenosine levels [24,25]. However, use of methotrexate has been limited by some toxicity problems, such as hepatitis, cirrhosis, cytopenias and interstitial pneumonitis [26]. Because the adverse effects are dose dependent, methotrex¬ate usually started in combination with other DMARDs in current management of RA. Iguratimod is an immunomodulatory compound and has been developed as a DMARD [27]. Our previous research had identified its unique antiarthritic mechanism which is different from the classical DMARDs. Iguratimod could block the IL-17 pathway in FLSs and then effectively treat CIA [28]. In the present study, we examined the effect of combination of iguratimod and methotrexate in a murine CIA model, and elucidated the possible mechanism.

Materials and Methods

Mice

Male DBA/1 mice were purchased from the Shanghai Experimental Animal Center, the Chinese Academy of Sciences. Mice used in

*Corresponding author: Yang Sun, School of Life Sciences, Nanjing University, 22 Hankou Road, Nanjing 210093 China, E-mail: yangsun@nju.edu.cn

Qiang Xu, School of Life Sciences, Nanjing University, 22 Hankou Road, Nanjing 210093 China, E-mail: molpharm@163.com

Yanhong Gu, Department of Oncology, The First Affiliated Hospital with Nanjing Medical University, 300 Guangzhou Road, Nanjing 210029 China, E-mail: njguyhphd@163.com

CIA model were 7-8 weeks of age. Animal welfare and experimental procedures were carried out strictly in accordance with the Guide for the Care and Use of Laboratory Animals (National Institutes of Health, the United States) and the related ethical regulations of our university. All efforts were made to minimize animals' suffering and to reduce the number of animals used.

Chemicals and reagents

Iguratimod was provided by Simcere Pharmaceutical (Nanjing, China) with purity more than 99%. Methotrexate, concanavalin A (Con A), lipopolysaccharide (LPS) and 3-(4, 5-dimethyl-2-thiazyl)-2, 5-diphenyl-2H-tetrazolium bromide (MTT) were purchased from Sigma-Aldrich (St. Louis, MO). Bovine type II collagen (CII) was purchased from Chondrex (Seattle, WA). ELISA kits for IL-17 and IFN-γ were purchased from Dakewe Biotech Co. Ltd (Shenzhen, China). Cytometric Bead Array (CBA) cytokine assay kit was purchased from BD Biosciences (San Jose, CA). All other chemicals were purchased from Sigma-Aldrich (St. Louis, MO).

Induction and assessment of CIA and drugs administration

Male DBA/1 mice (eight mice per group) were immunized on day 0 with an intradermal injection at the base of the tail of 100 μg bovine type II collagen (CII; Chondrex) emulsified in complete Freund's adjuvant (Chondrex). On day 21, mice were boosted by injection of 100 μg CII dissolved in incomplete Freund's adjuvant (Sigma). Mice were examined daily and scored for arthritis severity, with each paw assigned a clinical score as follows: 0, normal; 1, erythema and mild swelling confined to the ankle joint and toes; 2, erythema and mild swelling extending from the ankle to the midfoot; 3, erythema and severe swelling extending from the ankle to the metatarsal joints; 4, enclosing deformity with joint swelling. Hind paw thickness was measured with electronic plethysmometer (Paw Volume Meter).

For treatment, iguratimod and methotrexate were administered i.g. beginning on the day after the booster injection (day 22). The mice were randomly divided into 7 groups: Group 1, normal DBA/1J mice; Group 2, CIA mice with vehicle; Group 3, CIA mice with iguratimod, 3 mg/kg once a day; Group 4, CIA mice with iguratimod, 10 mg/kg once a day; Group 5, CIA mice with methotrexate, 1 mg/kg once every two days; Group 6, CIA mice with iguratimod plus methotrexate, iguratimod 3 mg/kg once a day, methotrexate 1 mg/kg once every two days; Group 7, CIA mice with iguratimod plus methotrexate, iguratimod 10 mg/kg once a day, methotrexate 1 mg/kg once every two days.

Radiographic assessment

At the end of the experiments, the mice were anesthetized and radiographs of the hind paws were obtained with a lumina XR system (Caliper IVIS Spectrum). Radiographic scoring criteria of each paw were assessed on the following scale: 0 = no bone damage, 1 = joint erosion and 2 = bone erosion and osteophyte formation.

Histopathology

Paws for histological analysis were removed from mice and immediately fixed in 4% paraformaldehyde. The paws were decalcified in EDTA, embedded in paraffin, sectioned, and stained with H&E. The sections were scored to assess joints inflammation on a scale of 0-4 under blinded conditions, according to the degree of hyperplasia in the synovial lining, mononuclear cell infiltration, and pannus formation. The maximum possible score per mouse was 8.

Quantitative real-time PCR

Total RNA was extracted from cells using Trizol Reagent (Invitrogen, Carlsbad, CA). One microgram of RNA was reversely transcribed to cDNA. The mRNA expression was determined by real-time PCR using iQ SYBR Green Supermix (Bio Rad). Mouse *Actb* gene was used as endogenous control for sample normalization. Results were presented as fold increases relative to the expression of mouse *Actb*. The primer sequences used in PCR were as follows: Actb, 5'- TGCT-GTCCCTGTATGCCTCT and 3'-TTTGATGTCACGCACGATTT; *Cxcl1*, 5'- CTTGCCTTGACCCTGAAGCTC and 3'- AGCAGTCT-GTCTTCTTTCTCCGT; *Cxcl2*, 5'- CCCCCTGGTTCAGAAAATCA and 3'- GCTCCTCCTTTCCAGGTCAGT; *Ccl2*, 5'- CCCAATGAG-TAGGCTGGAGA and 3'- AAGGCATCACAGTCCGAGTC; *Il6*, 5'- ACACATGTTCTCTGGGAAATCGT and 3'- AAGTGCATCATC-GTTGTTCATACA; *Rankl*, 5'- AGCACGAAAAACTGGTCGGG and 3'- AAGGGTTGGACACCTGAATGC; and *Mmp3*, 5'- ACTCTAC-CACTCAGCCAAGG and 3'- TCCAGAGAGTTAGACTTGGTGG.

Cytokine measurement

Serum were obtained from mice at the indicated time points and immediately centrifuged at 1500 g for 15 min. Samples were stored at -70°C until ready for used. Cytokine levels were measured using Cytometric Bead Array (CBA) cytokine assay kit (BD) and the amount of IFN-γ and IL-17 were determined using Quick EIA™ ELISA kits from Dakewe Biotechnology Company (Shenzhen, China).

Isolation of T cells and B cells

Mouse T lymphocytes were isolated from lymph nodes of C57/BL6 mice and B lymphocytes were isolated from spleens of C57BL/6 mice. All cells were purified using magnetic beads (Miltenyi Biotec, Auburn, CA) with more than 95% purity. For antigen-specific lymphocyte responses, T cells were isolated from lymph nodes and B cells were isolated from spleens of CIA mice. The cells were incubated in RPMI 1640 medium supplemented with 10% fetal bovine serum (FBS), 100 U/ml penicillin, and 100 μg/ml streptomycin under a humidified 5% (v/v) CO_2 atmosphere at 37°C.

Cell proliferation assay

Cells were cultured in 96-well plates at a density of 3×10^5 cells/well in RPMI 1640 medium (0.2 ml). Then the cells were treated with drugs and stimulated with 5 μg/ml of Con A for 24 h at 37oC in 5% CO_2/air. Then cell growth was evaluated with modified MTT assay. MTT (4 mg/ml in PBS, 20 μl per well) was added to each well. After 4 h of additional incubation, remove the culture media, 200 μl DMSO was added to dissolve the crystals. The absorption values at 570 nm were determined.

Measurement of cell apoptosis and CD23 expression with flow cytometry

Cell apoptosis was determined by Annexin V-FITC (fluorescein isothiocyanate) /PI (propidium iodide) staining. Samples were analyzed by FACS Calibur flow cytometer (Becton Dickinson, San Jose, CA). Annexin V^+/PI^- and Annexin V^+/PI^+ were considered as apoptotic cells in the early and late phase, respectively. Spleen cells (3×10^5) were stimulated with 1 μg/ml LPS with the addition of drugs simultaneously. The surface expression of CD23 was assessed after 24 h of culture. At the end of the culture period, the harvested cells were washed twice with buffer. Cells were stained with CD23 and B220 for 30 min at 4°C in the dark. Cells were then washed with buffer to remove the excess stains and analyzed in a FACS Calibur flow cytometer using Cell Quest software.

Statistics

Data are expressed as means ± SEM. Statistical analyses were performed using one-way analysis of variance (ANOVA) followed by Student's two-tailed t-test. P<0.05 was considered significant.

Results

Effects of the combination therapy with iguratimod and methotrexate on the development of CIA

According to our previous results, treatment with 30 mg/kg iguratimod resulted in a dramatic decrease in the arthritic scores and iguratimod at 10 mg/kg yielded a medium decrease in arthritic scores. In addition, treatment with 10 mg/kg methotrexate showed excellent antirheumatic properties, but with some adverse events. In this case, we chose 1 mg/kg methotrexate which could be well tolerated and 3 mg/kg plus 10 mg/kg iguratimod which showed mild antiarthritic properties for combined therapy. CIA was induced with type II collagen (CII) in CFA on day 0, then a booster injection with CII in IFA on day 21 in

male DBA/1J mice. As shown in Figure 1, CIA developed rapidly in vehicle-treated mice, and the incidence of arthritis achieved to 100% on day 25 post-immunization (Figures 1A and 1B). These CIA mice developed severe swelling, erythema and joint rigidity of the paws (Figures 1D and 1E). Treatment with iguratimod (3 mg/kg, 10 mg/kg) or methotrexate (1 mg/kg) only exhibited very weak inhibitory effects on the arthritic scores. In mice combined treated with iguratimod (3 mg/kg) and methotrexate (1 mg/kg), the onset of arthritis was delayed and the severity of CIA was attenuated compared with the vehicle mice. Furthermore, combination therapy with iguratimod (10 mg/kg) and methotrexate (1 mg/kg) showed excellent antirheumatic activities with reduction of scores in comparison with the vehicle group. Hind paw swelling was measured and the results correlated with that of the clinical scores (Figures 1D-1F). The body weights of each group were recorded every day (Figure 1C), and expressed as a change in weight from arthritis induction (day 21). In this study, we did not observe any adverse events, such as loss of appetite, lack of movement and weight loss, indicating that both iguratimod and methotrexate were well tolerated at our tested doses.

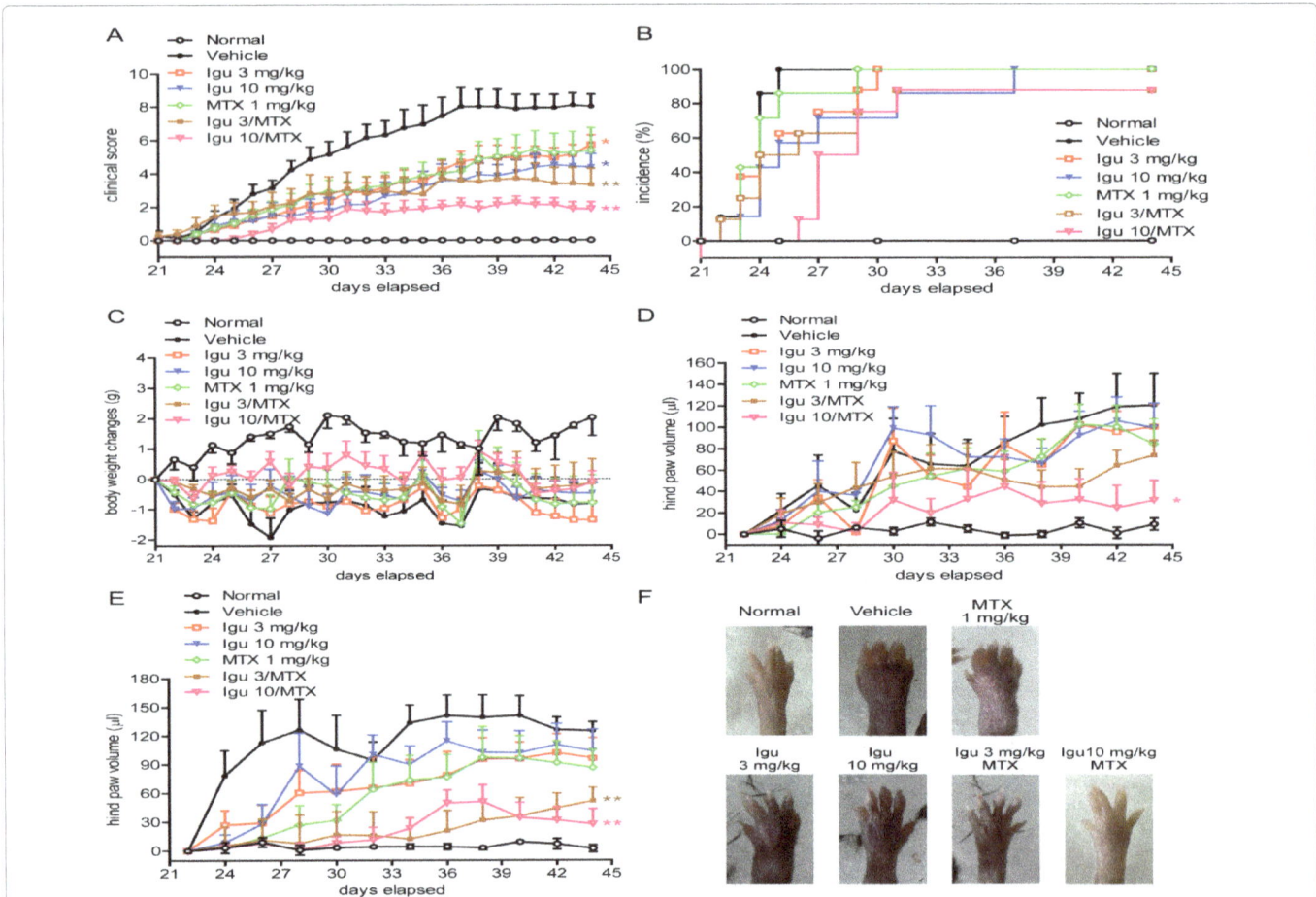

Figure 1: Effects of combination therapy with iguratimod and methotrexate on murine CIA. Male DBA/1J mice were immunized on day 0 with 100 μg of bovine type II collagen in complete Freund's adjuvant and were again a booster injection 21 days after. Iguratimod was given orally once daily from the day 22 and mice were treated with methotrexate orally once every two days. (A) The mean arthritis scores of CIA were shown. Values are given as the mean ± SEM of eight mice per group.*P< 0.05; **P< 0.01 versus vehicle. (B) The incidence of arthritis was shown. (C) Body weight changes in DBA/1J mice were measured and calculated. Values are given as the mean ± SEM of eight mice per group.*P< 0.05; **P< 0.01 versus vehicle. (D-E) Swelling of left (D) and right (E) hind paw in DBA/1J mice were measured and calculated as described in the materials and methods section. Values are given as the mean ± SEM of eight mice per group. *P< 0.05; **P< 0.01 versus vehicle. (F) Representative photos of hind paw in mice with CIA.

Iguratimod Synergizes with Methotrexate to Exert Anti-Inflammatory and Bone-Protective Effect and Block...

51

Effects of combination therapy on bone erosion in mice with CIA

In the radiographic evaluation of fore and hind paws, bone erosion, articular destruction and joint displacement were detected in vehicle-treated mice on day 44 (Figure 2A). However, oral administration of iguratimod and methotrexate displayed markedly protection against bone erosions and joint destructions as compared to vehicle group. Furthermore, no bone erosion was observed in mice treated with high dose of iguratimod (10 mg/kg) plus methotrexate. To confirm the protective effects, histological analysis was also carried out on the inflamed hind paws. The assessment revealed synovial hyperplasia, joint destruction and inflammatory cell infiltration of vehicle-treated mice (Figure 2B). In accordance with the effects on disease incidence and severity, combination therapy with iguratimod and methotrexate showed remarkable improvement in joint damage and inflammation as compared with those of the vehicle group. As shown in Figure 2B, cartilage and bone damage as well as inflammatory responses were significantly inhibited by the treatment of high dose iguratimod plus methotrexate.

Effects of combination therapy on local joint inflammation

The immunomodulatory effects of combination with methotrexate and iguratimod on proinflammatory cytokines, chemokines and tissue factors were further analyzed in inflamed paws. To evaluate whether the combination treatment suppressed the effector mechanisms of inflammation in CIA, the gene expression of various proinflammatory mediators was examined on day 44 by using quantitative real-time PCR. It was observed that combination therapy significantly decreased the mRNA levels of three major chemokines *Cxcl1, Cxcl2,* and *Ccl2*

compared to vehicle group in CIA. Also, growth factors associated with tissue destruction/remodeling were down-regulated by iguratimod or methotrexate treatment. The expressions of *Rankl* and *Mmp3* were significantly reduced in the joints from combination therapy group (Figure 3).

Effects of combination therapy on serum pro-inflammatory factors levels in CIA mice

To investigate the mechanism by which combination therapy controls CIA development and progression, we examined the levels of pro-inflammatory cytokines in CIA mice. As shown in Figure 4A, IL-17 production was significantly inhibited by the combination of iguratimod and methotrexate. Meanwhile, combination therapy showed mild inhibition against IFN-γ, TNF-α, and IL-6 levels. No difference was observed in the serum IL-10 between vehicle and combined treatment group. Not only decreased T cell response but also decreased B cell activity could play a role in the efficacy of DMARDs treatment. Therefore, antigen-specific B cell responses were examined. We measured the serum levels of total IgG or isotype-specific IgG2b anti-CII antibodies after treatment with different DMARDs. As shown in Figure 4B, treatment with methotrexate resulted in decreased levels of IgG and IgG2b antibodies. Furthermore, serum concentrations of IgG and IgG2b antibodies were significantly reduced by combination treatment of high dose iguratimod (10 mg/kg) plus methotrexate (Figure 4B).

Effects of combination therapy on antigen-specific responses in CIA mice

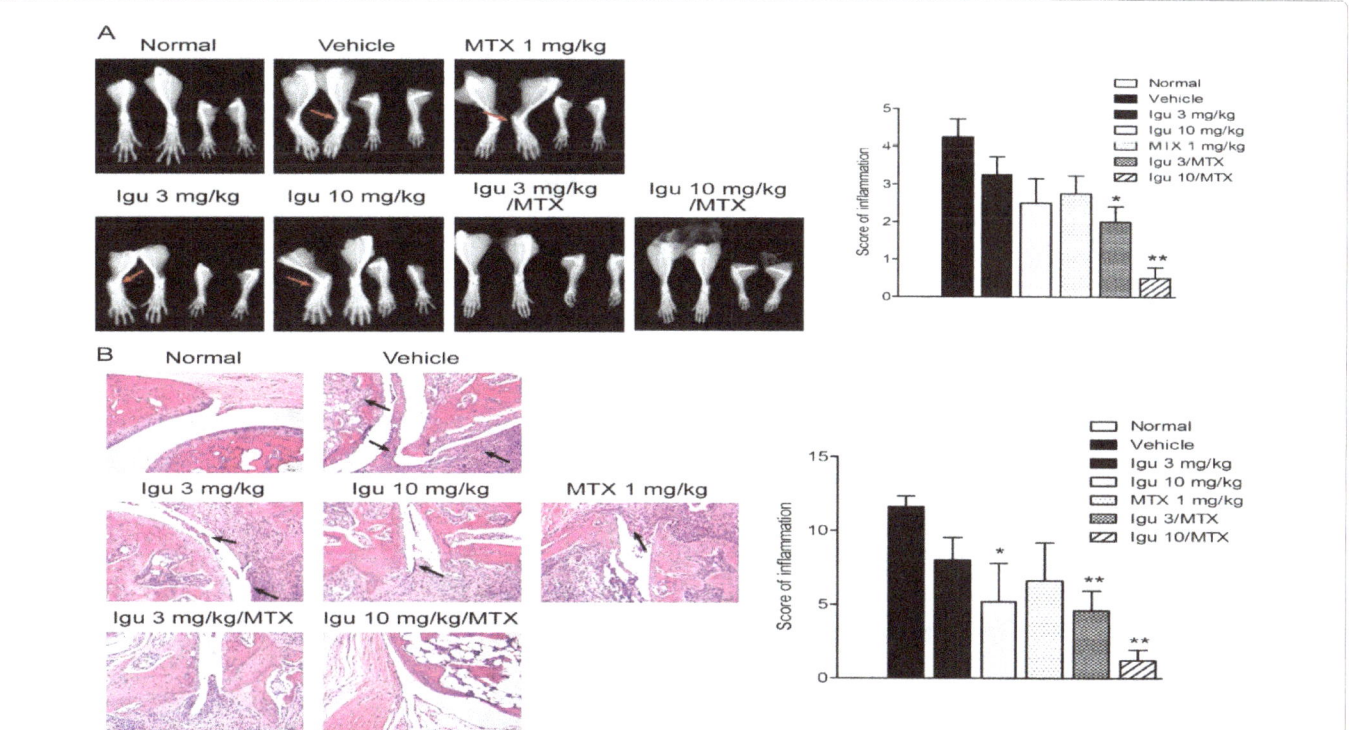

Figure 2: X-radiography and histopathology images of CIA mice. Arthritis joints from CIA mice were harvested at day 44. (A) Representative radiographs of the hind paws from CIA mice were shown. Arrows indicate areas of bone erosion. (B)Inflammatory infiltration scores were assessed by H&E staining. Arrows indicate areas of inflammation. Values are given as the mean ± SEM of eight mice per group. *P< 0.05; **P< 0.01 versus vehicle group.

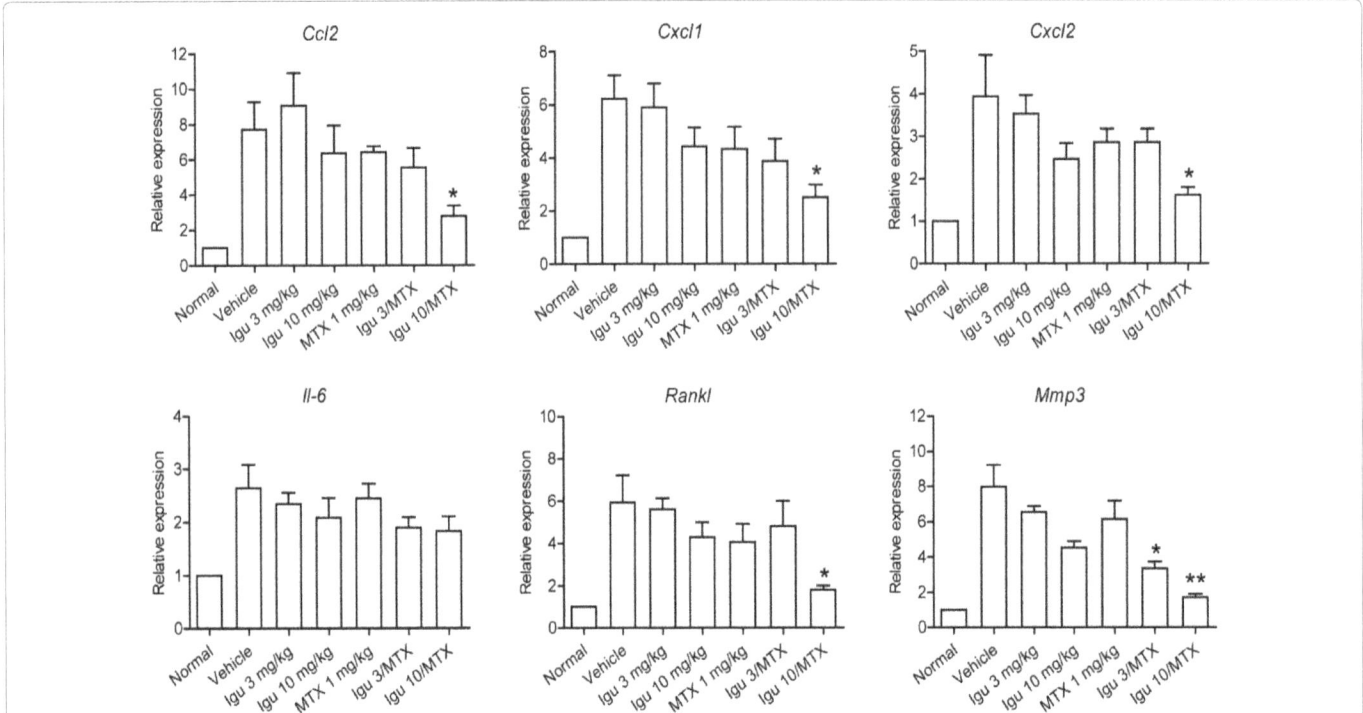

Figure 3: Effects of combination therapy with iguratimod and methotrexate on proinflammatory factors expression in CIA ankles. Total RNA was extracted from the ankle and metatarsal joints of mice in the naïve group, the control group and mice treated with drugs at day 44 post-immunization. The mRNA levels of *Ccl2, Cxcl1, Cxcl2, Il6, Rankl,* and *Mmp3* were measured by quantitative real-time RT-PCR. Values are given as the mean ± SEM of eight mice per group.*$P < 0.05$ versus vehicle group; **$P < 0.01$ versus vehicle group.

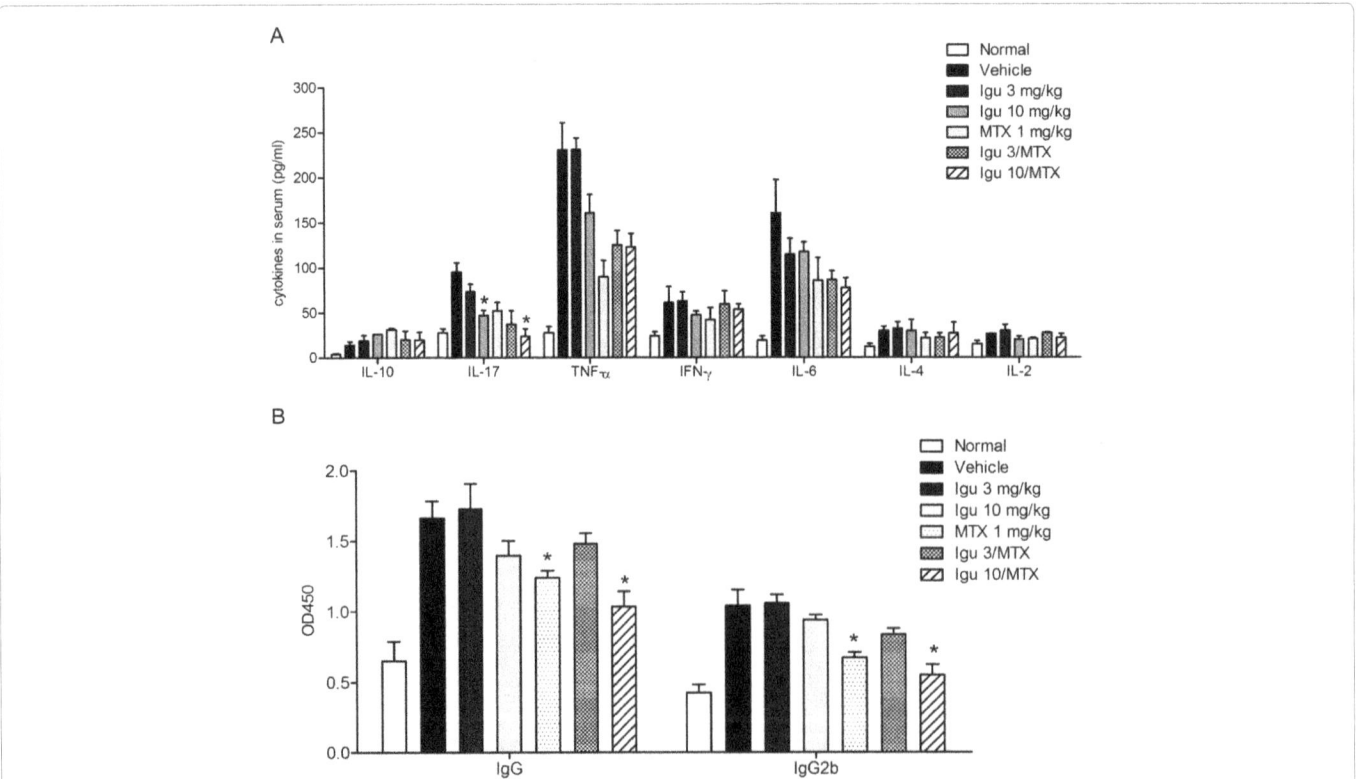

Figure 4: Effects of combination therapy with iguratimod and methotrexate on proinflammatory cytokines and antibodies production. Serum was obtained at peak clinical severity (day 44 post-immunization). (A) Cytokines in serum were measured by a Cytokine Bead Array(CBA). (B) Levels of total IgG and isotype-specific IgG2b anti-CII antibodies after treatment with iguratimod or methotrexate were determined by specific ELISA. Values are given as the mean ± SEM of eight mice per group.*$P < 0.05$ versus vehicle group.

Moreover, we evaluated antigen-specific responses of peripheral T cells isolated from CIA mice. As shown in Figure 5A and 5B, vehicle-, b iguratimod-, and methotrexate- treated mice exhibited comparable levels of serum cytokines, including IFN-γ and IL-17. However, combined treatment with iguratimod plus methotrexate resulted in significant reduction in the levels of IFN-γ and IL-17. Similar results were showed in antigen-specific T cell proliferation and B cell proliferation (Figure: 5 C and D). No significant difference was observed in CII-specific T cell proliferation or LPS-induced B cell proliferation between vehicle-, iguratimod-, and methotrexate-treated mice. However, combination with iguratimod and methotrexate markedly inhibited cell proliferation induced by denatured CII or LPS.

Effects of combination therapy on T cell responses

To examine the immunosuppressive potential in vitro, we evaluated the effects of combination therapy on the Con A-induced proliferation of T cells. MTT assay showed that iguratimod slightly inhibited T cell proliferation induced by Con A. The similar result was also seen in T cells treated with methotrexate. However, iguratimod in combination with methotrexate efficiently inhibited T cell proliferation induced by Con A. Subsequently, we determined whether the combination treatment could induce apoptosis of lymphocytes. We incubated T cells with iguratimod, methotrexate or iguratimod plus methotrexate in the presence of Con A for 24 h. Iguratimod did not influence the apoptotic cell counts relative to the untreated cells. However, cell apoptosis was detected when methotrexate was used. As shown in Figure 6B, combined incubation with iguratimod and methotrexate resulted in

significant apoptosis of 40% at 0.1 μM and 55% at 3 μM, respectively.

Effects of combination therapy on B cell responses

Given the reduction of antibodies on CIA mice, it seems likely that these drugs could regulate B cell activation or function. To explore this possibility, purified splenic B cells were stimulated with LPS in the presence of iguratimod, methotrexate or iguratimod plus methotrexate for 24 h, and then the proliferative response was assessed. As shown in Figure 7A, proliferation of LPS-stimulated B cells was inhibited by iguratimod in a dose-dependent manner. And the addition of methotrexate increased the inhibitory rate. Inhibition of B cell activation was also demonstrated by B cell activation marker CD23. Combination with iguratimod and methotrexate showed significant reduction of CD23 expression in the anti-B220-labeled B cells (Figures 7B and 7C). And culture supernatants from iguratimod plus methotrexate showed lower IgG and IgM levels compared with those from iguratimod (Figures 7D and 7E).

Discussion

Methotrexate, originally developed for leukemia therapy, has become to be the cornerstone of DMARD in the management of RA worldwide [29,30]. In RA, it is the first one to be chosen due to its excellent efficacy, tolerability, safety and cost [31]. However, for its dose-dependent adverse effects, methotrexate could be prescribed in combination with other synthetic or biological agents [32,33]. CIA has been widely used in preclinical studies as an animal model of RA, for evaluation of antiarthritic drugs [34]. In this study, the therapeutic

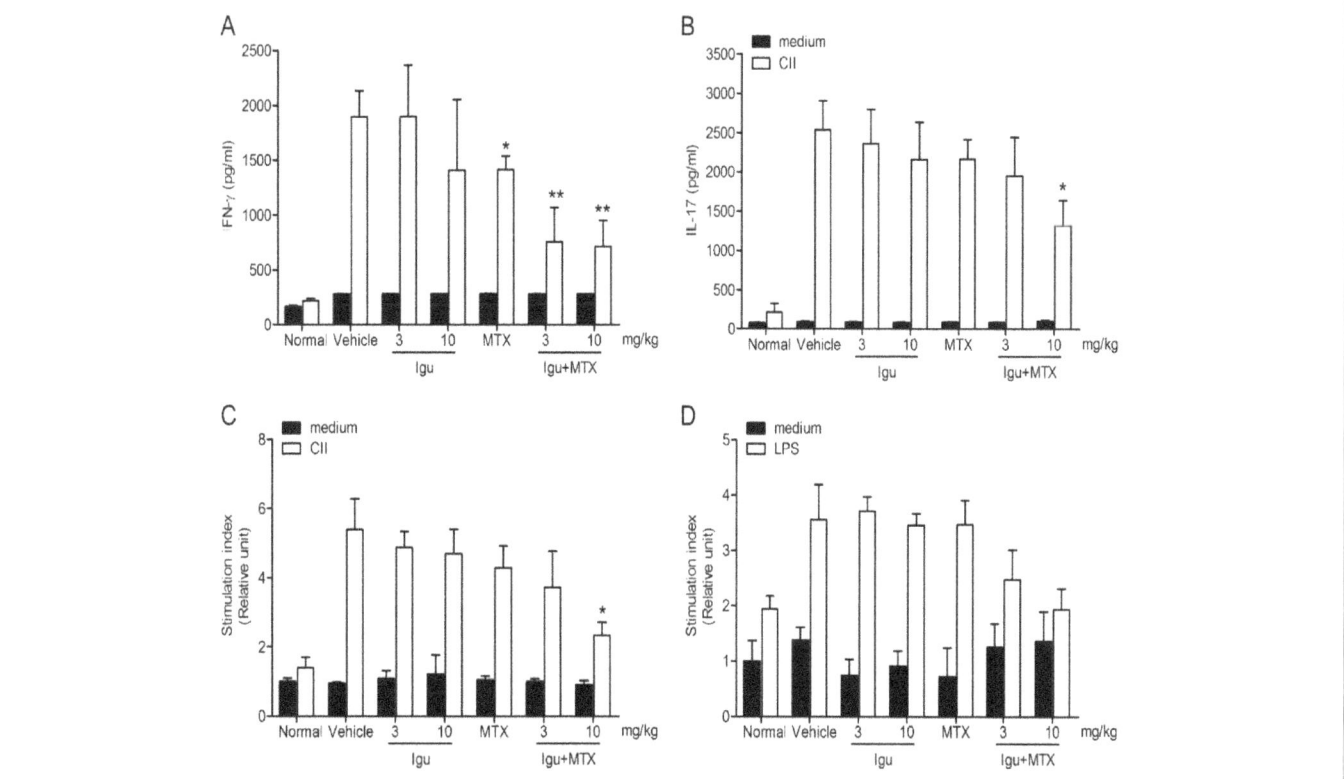

Figure 5: Effects of combination therapy with iguratimod and methotrexate on antigen-specific responses. (A-C) Regional lymph nodes were obtained from drug-treated or control CIA mice and single cell suspensions were restimulated with denatured CII (50 μg/ml) for 72 h. Supernatants (A-B) were determined by ELISA assays for indicated cytokines and proliferation (C) was examined by MTT. (D) Spleens were obtained from drug-treated or control CIA mice and single cell suspensions were restimulated with LPS (50 μg/ml) for 72 h. Proliferation was examined by MTT. Values are given as the mean ± SEM of eight mice per group.*P< 0.05; **P< 0.01 versus vehicle group.

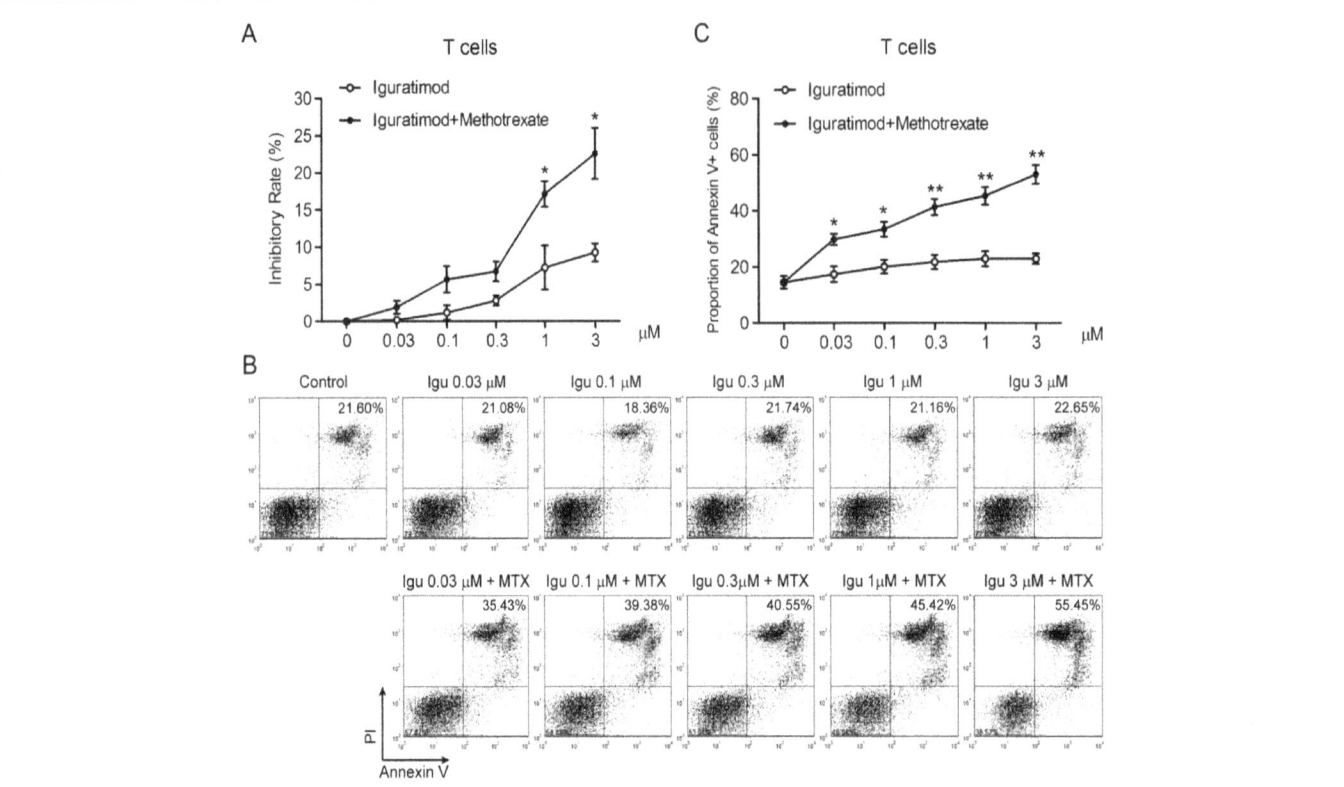

Figure 6: Effects of combination therapy with iguratimod and methotrexate on T cell responses. Lymph node cells (3×10^5) from naive mice were incubated for 24 h in the presence of 5 µg/ml Con A and 0.03-3 µM iguratimod alone or with 0.3 µM methotrexate. (A) Cell proliferation was measured at 540 nm by MTT uptake assay. (B-C) Cell apoptosis was measured by Annexin V/PI assay. Values are given as the mean ± SEM of three independent experiments.*$P < 0.05$; **$P < 0.01$ versus corresponding dose of iguratimodmonotherapy group.

effect of combination of iguratimod and methotrexate on CIA mice was investigated. It was indicated that the inflammation of joints, elevation of serum cytokines and antibodies levels, and bone destruction were all relieved through combination therapy. Evaluation of CIA in the present study has been performed on paw swelling, clinical scores, body weight, histopathology and X-radiography. Here we compared antiarthritic effects of iguratimod or methotrexate alone in CIA with combined iguratimod and methotrexate. Combination therapy was more efficacious to not only decrease clinical scores of disease but also reduce paw swelling than monotherapy. Histological and radiological analysis of joints further support that combination of iguratimod and methotrexate has strong anti-inflammatory effects as well as protective effects on joint tissue damage. The infiltration of inflammatory cells into the synovium plays a pivotal role in the progress of RA [1,35]. These cells release cytokines, chemokines, tissue factors, and metalloproteinases to lead to bone and cartilage destruction [36]. The gene expression of various proinflammatory mediators in inflamed paws was significantly reduced by combined iguratimod and methotrexate. Thus, in the present study of an animal model of RA, the combination therapy with iguratimod and methotrexate exerted stronger anti-arthritis effect than the monotherapy. There has been a randomized, double-blind, placebo-controlled trial reported, iguratimod was orally administered at doses of 50 mg/day and methotrexate was orally administered at doses of 8 mg/week for combination treatment [37]. Corresponding doses in mice were about 6.9 mg/kg/day and 1.2 mg/kg/week, respectively. In this case, the dosages of iguratimod and methotrexate we selected in our experiments were correlated to clinical studies. And the positive results and possible mechanism could be supportive for clinical trials. It is believed that the pathogenesis of

RA is closely related to dysregulation of T and B lymphocytes [36,38] and CIA is trigged by immune responses to type II collagen (CII). Therefore, pro-inflammatory cytokines and antibodies levels in serum of CIA mice were investigated. Efficacy in decreasing IL-17, IFN-γ, TNF-α, IL-6, IgG, and IgG2b productions was stronger in use of combined iguratimod and methotrexate than with use of iguratimod or methotrexate alone. Then CII and LPS were used to induce immune responses *ex vivo*. Iguratimod plus methotrexate treatment resulted in significant reduction in the levels of cell proliferation induced by denatured CII or LPS. Furthermore, CII induced elevations in IFN-γ and IL-17 levels were also suppressed in the combination treated CIA mice. Consequently, we employed in vitro models through T cell activation using Con A and B cell activation using LPS, respectively. It was found that monotherapy only slightly inhibited Con A induced proliferation but combination therapy showed stronger inhibitory effect than monotherapy group. Similar results were observed in Con A-induced apoptosis of T cells. Antibody response is of central importance because B cell-deficient mice do not develop the disease. In our study, proliferation and activation of LPS-stimulated B cells was significantly inhibited by iguratimod in a dose-dependent manner. And the addition of methotrexate remarkably enhanced the inhibitory effect on B cells. Taken together, the present study shows that combination treatment of iguratimod and methotrexate is superior to monotherapy in murine CIA, which can be expected to exert additive effects in alleviating the symptoms of RA. The mechanism of action was due to the inhibitory effects of iguratimod on fibroblast-like synoviocytes plus with the suppressive functions of methotrexate on T cells and B cells.

Conclusion

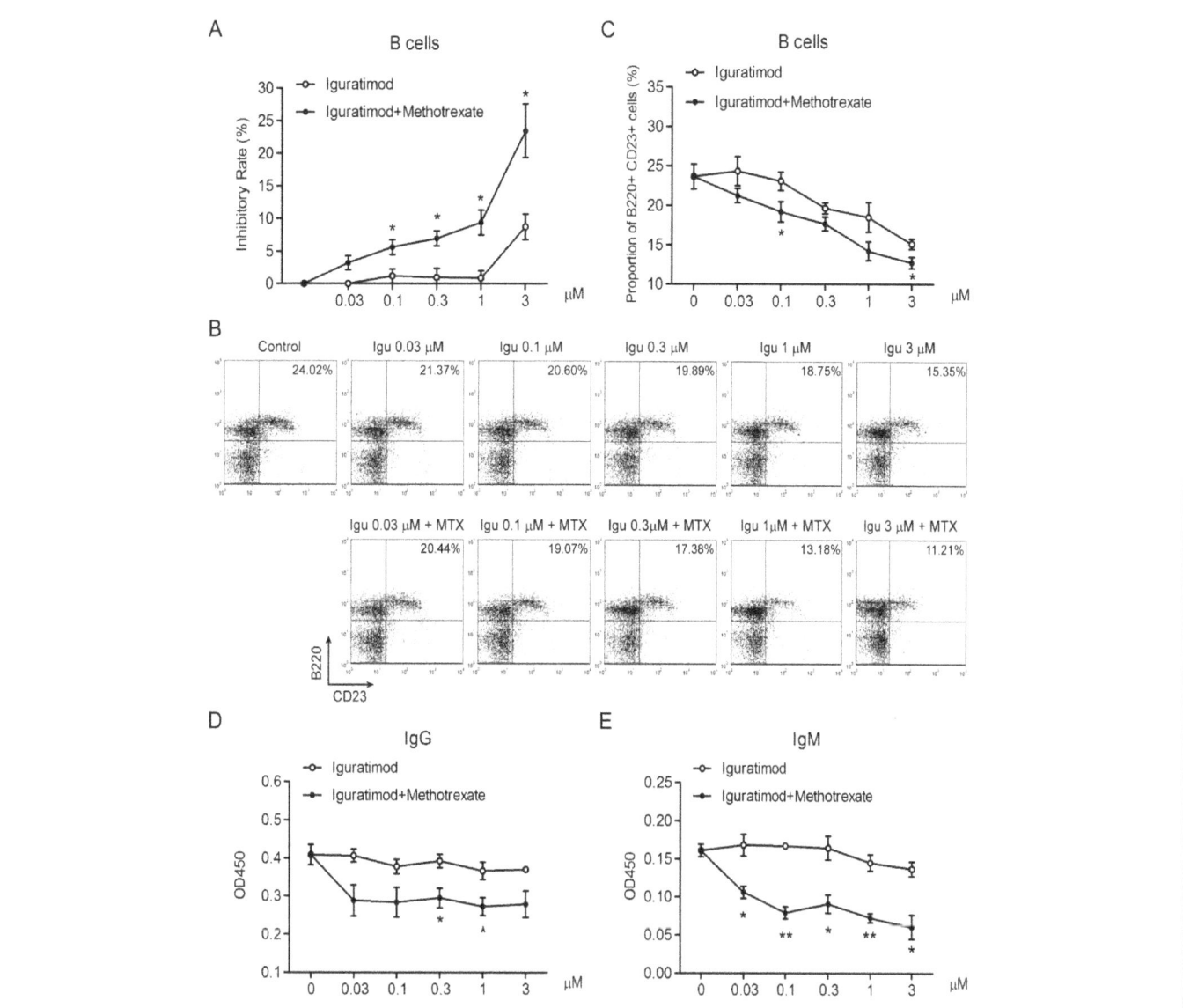

Figure 7: Effects of combination therapy with iguratimod and methotrexate on B cell responses. B cells from spleen (3×105) were stimulated with 1 µg/ml LPS for 24 h in the presence of and 0.03-3 µM iguratimod alone or with 0.3 µM methotrexate. (A) Cell proliferation was measured at 540 nm by MTT uptake assay. (B-C) Expression of CD23 was analyzed by flow cytometry. The production of IgG (D) andIgM (E) from supernatants was measured by ELISA assay. Values are given as the mean ± SEM of three independent experiments.*$P < 0.05$; **$P < 0.01$ versus corresponding dose of iguratimodmono therapy group.

These findings collectively suggest that combination therapy of iguratimod with methotrexate may be preferable of therapeutic value for the treatment of human RA.

Competing Interests

The authors declare that they have no competing interests.

Acknowledgment

We thank Simcere Pharmaceutical Company (Nanjing, China) for providing iguratimod. This work was supported by National Natural Science Foundation of China (Nos. 81273528, 81101563, and 91229109), Jiangsu Province Clinical Science and Technology Project (Clinical Research Center, BL2012008), and Ph.D. Programs Foundation of Ministry of Education of China (No. 20110091110016).

References

1. McInnes IB, Schett G (2007) Cytokines in the pathogenesis of rheumatoid arthritis. Nat Rev Immunol 7: 429-442.

2. Lanchbury JS (1993) Genetic aspects of rheumatoid arthritis. Clin Exp Rheumatol 11 Suppl 8: S9-11.

3. Winchester RJ (1981) Genetic aspects of rheumatoid arthritis. Springer Semin Immunopathol 4: 89-102.

4. Hyrich KL, Inman RD (2001) Infectious agents in chronic rheumatic diseases. Curr Opin Rheumatol 13: 300-304.

5. Smolen JS, Steiner G (2003) Therapeutic strategies for rheumatoid arthritis. Nat Rev Drug Discov 2: 473-488.

6. McInnes IB, Schett G (2011) The pathogenesis of rheumatoid arthritis. N Engl J Med 365: 2205-2219.

7. Zwerina J, Redlich K, Schett G, Smolen JS (2005) Pathogenesis of rheumatoid arthritis: targeting cytokines. Ann N Y Acad Sci 1051: 716-729.

8. Sweeney SE, Firestein GS (2004) Rheumatoid arthritis: regulation of synovial inflammation. Int J Biochem Cell Biol 36: 372-378.

9. Brennan FM, McInnes IB (2008) Evidence that cytokines play a role in rheumatoid arthritis. J Clin Invest 118: 3537-3545.

10. Gravallese EM (2002) Bone destruction in arthritis. Ann Rheum Dis 61 Suppl 2: ii84-86.

11. Mor A, Abramson SB, Pillinger MH (2005) The fibroblast-like synovial cell in rheumatoid arthritis: a key player in inflammation and joint destruction. Clin Immunol 115: 118-128.

12. Smolen JS, Aletaha D, Redlich K (2012) The pathogenesis of rheumatoid arthritis: new insights from old clinical data? Nat Rev Rheumatol 8: 235-243.

13. Jonsson B, Kobelt G, Smolen J (2008) The burden of rheumatoid arthritis and access to treatment: uptake of new therapies. Eur J Health Econ 8 Suppl 2: S61-86.

14. O'Dell JR (2004) Therapeutic strategies for rheumatoid arthritis. N Engl J Med 350: 2591-2602.

15. Abbott JD, Moreland LW (2004) Rheumatoid arthritis: developing pharmacological therapies. Expert Opin Investig Drugs 13: 1007-1018.

16. Nam JL, Winthrop KL, van Vollenhoven RF, Pavelka K, Valesini G, et al. (2010) Current evidence for the management of rheumatoid arthritis with biological disease-modifying antirheumatic drugs: a systematic literature review informing the EULAR recommendations for the management of RA. Ann Rheum Dis 69: 976-986.

17. Gaffo A, Saag KG, Curtis JR (2006) Treatment of rheumatoid arthritis. Am J Health Syst Pharm 63: 2451-2465.

18. Rachapalli SM, Williams R, Walsh DA, Young A, Kiely PD, et al. (2010) First-line DMARD choice in early rheumatoid arthritis--do prognostic factors play a role? Rheumatology (Oxford) 49: 1267-1271.

19. Smolen JS, Aletaha D, Koeller M, Weisman MH, Emery P (2007) New therapies for treatment of rheumatoid arthritis. Lancet 370: 1861-1874.

20. Kremer JM (1999) Methotrexate and leflunomide: biochemical basis for combination therapy in the treatment of rheumatoid arthritis. Semin Arthritis Rheum 29: 14-26.

21. Quéméneur L, Gerland LM, Flacher M, Ffrench M, Revillard JP, et al. (2003) Differential control of cell cycle, proliferation, and survival of primary T lymphocytes by purine and pyrimidine nucleotides. J Immunol 170: 4986-4995.

22. Genestier L, Paillot R, Quemeneur L, Izeradjene K, Revillard JP (2000) Mechanisms of action of methotrexate. Immunopharmacology 47: 247-257.

23. Phillips DC, Woollard KJ, Griffiths HR (2003) The anti-inflammatory actions of methotrexate are critically dependent upon the production of reactive oxygen species. Br J Pharmacol 138: 501-511.

24. Cronstein BN, Naime D, Ostad E (1993) The antiinflammatory mechanism of methotrexate. Increased adenosine release at inflamed sites diminishes leukocyte accumulation in an in vivo model of inflammation. J Clin Invest 92: 2675-2682.

25. Montesinos MC, Desai A, Delano D, Chen JF, Fink JS, et al. (2003) Adenosine A2A or A3 receptors are required for inhibition of inflammation by methotrexate and its analog MX-68. Arthritis Rheum 48: 240-247.

26. Alarcón GS, Tracy IC, Blackburn WD Jr (1989) Methotrexate in rheumatoid arthritis. Toxic effects as the major factor in limiting long-term treatment. Arthritis Rheum 32: 671-676.

27. Du F, Lü LJ, Fu Q, Dai M, Teng JL, et al. (2008) T-614, a novel immunomodulator, attenuates joint inflammation and articular damage in collagen-induced arthritis. Arthritis Res Ther 10: R136.

28. Luo Q, Sun Y, Liu W, Qian C, Jin B, et al. (2013) A novel disease-modifying antirheumatic drug, iguratimod, ameliorates murine arthritis by blocking IL-17 signaling, distinct from methotrexate and leflunomide. J Immunol 191: 4969-4978.

29. Malik F, Ranganathan P (2013) Methotrexate pharmacogenetics in rheumatoid arthritis: a status report. Pharmacogenomics 14: 305-314.

30. Romao VC, Canhao H, Fonseca JE (2013) Old drugs, old problems: where do we stand in prediction of rheumatoid arthritis responsiveness to methotrexate and other synthetic DMARDs? BMC Med 11: 17.

31. Aletaha D, Smolen JS (2002) The rheumatoid arthritis patient in the clinic: comparing more than 1,300 consecutive DMARD courses. Rheumatology (Oxford) 41: 1367-1374.

32. Mourao AF, Canhão H, Moura RA, Cascão R, Weinmann P, et al. (2011) Markers of progression to rheumatoid arthritis: discriminative value of the new ACR/EULAR rheumatoid arthritis criteria in a Portuguese population with early polyarthritis. Acta Reumatol Port 36: 370-376.

33. Mourao AF, Fonseca JE, Canhão H, Santos MJ, Bernardo A, et al. (2011) [Practical guide for the use of biological agents in rheumatoid arthritis - December 2011 update]. Acta Reumatol Port 36: 389-395.

34. Holmdahl R, Bockermann R, Bäcklund J, Yamada H (2002) The molecular pathogenesis of collagen-induced arthritis in mice--a model for rheumatoid arthritis. Ageing Res Rev 1: 135-147.

35. Vergunst CE, van de Sande MG, Lebre MC, Tak PP (2005) The role of chemokines in rheumatoid arthritis and osteoarthritis. Scand J Rheumatol 34: 415-425.

36. Firestein GS (2003) Evolving concepts of rheumatoid arthritis. Nature 423: 356-361.

37. Hara M, Ishiguro N, Katayama K, Kondo M, Sumida T, et al. (2013) Safety and efficacy of combination therapy of iguratimod with methotrexate for patients with active rheumatoid arthritis with an inadequate response to methotrexate: An open-label extension of a randomized, double-blind, placebo-controlled trial. Mod Rheumatol .

38. Chang BY, Huang MM, Francesco M, Chen J, Sokolove J, et al. (2011) The Bruton tyrosine kinase inhibitor PCI-32765 ameliorates autoimmune arthritis by inhibition of multiple effector cells. Arthritis Res Ther 13: R115.

10

Impact of Furfural and Kerosene Co-exposure through Inhalation in Lungs of Rats

Tabarak Malik[1*], Pandey DK[2] and Gupta GSD[3]

[1]Department of Biochemistry, Lovely Professional University-144402, India
[2]Department of Biotechnology, Lovely Professional University-144402, India
[3]Division of Petroleum Toxicology, Indian Institute of Toxicology Research- 226 001, India

Abstract

Furfural is being added to kerosene to check the adulteration of gasoline/high speed diesel oil. The possibility of a co-exposure of furfural and kerosene and the ability to exhibit the toxic effects of such a mixture were examined in view of the toxicity potential of the two alone and in combination with each other. A single inhalation exposure of rats to furfural was fully tolerated up to a concentration of 126 ppm. However, exposure to higher concentrations of furfural resulted in a dose dependent mortality. Exposure of rats to vapor of kerosene ranging from 426-1054 ppm did not show toxic signs and mortality up to a period of seven days. Simultaneous exposure of rats to furfural and kerosene vapors ranging in concentration from 35 ppm to 138 ppm showed a suppression of LC_{50} value of furfural. The LC_{50} was 105 ppm in rats exposed to furfural-kerosene vapors. Inhalation exposure of rats to ½ LC_{50} of furfural to 95 ppm, 1 hr daily, 5 days/week over a period of 28 days caused severe irritation of eyes and nose leading to lacrimation, perinasal and perioral wetness, labored breathing and mild nasal bleeding. Neither the body weight nor lung weight showed any change as compared to the control group. Activities of acid and alkaline phosphatase, glutamic pyruvic and glutamic oxaloacetic transaminases, succinic dehydrogenase, total sulfhydryl content and lactic acid content were evaluated.

Keywords: Furfural; Inhalation toxicology; Kerosene; Lactic acid; Succinic dehydrogenase

Introduction

The possibility of a co exposure of furfural and kerosene and the ability to exhibit the toxic effects were examined in view of the toxicity data profile available in the literature for the individual chemical entities. The toxicity data profile of kerosene has established its potential to produce skin, lung, liver and bone marrow changes in experimental animals. Likewise furfural is also known to be a moderately toxic chemical causing irritation of the eye and mucous membrane, disorders of the CNS and the biochemical injury of vital organs. It also resulted in pulmonary irritation, parenchymal injury irritation of eyes, nose, along with hyperplasia of the epithelium in the nasal cavities [1]. It was evident that a selective (cellular and/ or Cytochrome-P450 isozymes specific) enhancement of pulmonary mixed function oxidases by furfural stimulates its own pulmonary biotransformation and the oxidative metabolism which was facilitated by their enzymatic conjugation with glutathione. Metabolites and excretion of ^{14}C furfural in the rat and mouse indicated presence of furoylglycine and furan acrylic acid as the major urinary metabolites. There was only subtle difference in the metabolic profile as a function of dose size and species [2]. It is anticipated that public at large may get exposed to various types of kerosene mixtures with different chemical characteristics. The effects of two chemicals given simultaneously may produce a response that may be additive, synergistic, potentiating or antagonistic to their individual responses .Therefore, toxicological potential of furfural doped kerosene mixture was evaluated in lungs of rats on simultaneous co exposure of furfural and kerosene vapors through inhalation exposure. Such studies are expected to reveal the mechanism of toxic interaction of respective chemical entities in a chemical mixture.

Methods

Chemicals

All chemicals used in the study were of analytical grade, procured from Qualigens (India) Ltd, and Sigma chemicals (USA). Furfural (2-furfuraldehyde, CAS 98:01-1) max. Purity 99% was stored in an amber color sealed container under cold and dry conditions to avoid spontaneous and oxidative decomposition during storage. White kerosene was procured from the Lucknow Railway Workshop.

Animals

Adult male albino rats (avg. age 13weeks, and body weight 165.0 ± 5.0 gm.) were maintained at ITRC (Industrial Toxicology Research Centre) animal breeding facilities under 12hrs dark / light cycles at 25°C ± 2°C and 40-60% humidity. The study was approved from Institutional Animal Ethical Committee (IAEC). All rats were housed in stainless steel wired cages and provided with pelleted feed and fresh tap water *ad libitum* throughout the period of study.

Exposure of animals

The animals were divided into four groups: consisting of six rats each.

Group I; furfural alone (F)

Group II; Kerosene alone (K)

Group III; furfural and kerosene (K+F)

Group IV; Compressed air only (C)

Group I rats were exposed to 1/2 LC_{50} (single exposure) of furfural

*Corresponding author: Tabarak Malik, Department of Biochemistry, Lovely Professional University-144402, India, E-mail: malikitrc@gmail.com

essentially in the same manner as described earlier [1] using an all glass whole body exposure chamber (21 lit. capacity) under dynamic exposure condition (figure 1). The chamber concentration of furfural was 95ppm. Rats of group II were exposed to vapors of kerosene generated from 10.0 ml aliquot (426-1054ppm) using a similar set as for furfural, except that the temperature was raised to 220°C using a heating mantle in order to vaporize kerosene. The vapors were passed on to the main body of the chamber through a nebulizer. Group III rats were exposed to vapors of both, furfural and kerosene generated simultaneously. The mixed vapors were passed on through insulated glass tubes to prevent their condensation and delivered into a five-necked mixing chamber, maintained at 55°C to avoid condensation of the incoming vapors. The mixed vapors were then passed into main body of the chamber through a nebulizer along with a current of diluents air. Group IV rats were exposed to a current of compressed air only to serve as respective controls under identical specified experimental conditions. Monitoring of the chamber concentration was performed as described earlier [1] and final concentration was calculated according to NIOSH [3].

Gross observations and biochemical analysis

All rats were periodically examined for apparent signs of toxicity like irritation of eye and nose, lacrimation, external discharges / hemorrhages, general behavior, changes in fur coat and body weight and the rate of mortality. At the end of stipulated period of exposure, six rats from each group were killed by exsanguinations; lungs were surgically removed and cleaned free from arterial blood and other extraneous matter. Each lung was individually weighed and homogenized (20% w/v) in ice cold Tris buffer (0.1M, pH 7.2). The activity of Succinic Dehydrogenase (SDH) was estimated in 9000xg supernatant according to Slater and Bonner [4]. The total contents of lactic acid were estimated according to Huckabee [5] and, activities of acid and alkaline phosphatases and glutamic pyruvic and glutamic oxaloacetic transaminases by Wootton [6]. The total protein content of whole homogenate, and 9000xg fractions were estimated using Folin-Phenol reagent according to Lowry's method [7]. Glutathione content was estimated according to Jollow et al. [8].

Statistical Analysis

The group means and their standard errors for each observation in control and respective groups of exposed rats were calculated for statistical significance of results using student's t-test. P values less than 0.05 were considered significant.

Results

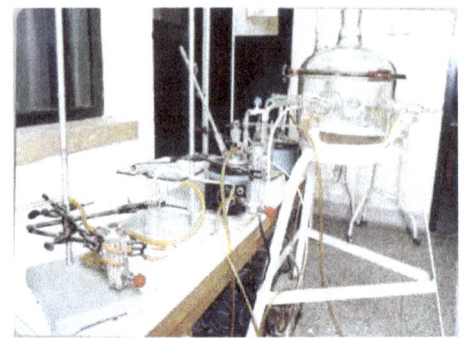

Figure 1: Inhalation assembly used for exposure of C-Compressed air only, F-furfural alone (95ppm), K-Kerosene alone (426-1054ppm), K+F-furfural and kerosene vapors (95ppm) and (426-1054ppm) respectively.

Gross observations and LC$_{50}$ Dose

Inhalation exposure of rats to furfural vapors caused severe irritation of eyes and nose leading to lacrimation, perinasal and perioral wetness and mild nasal bleeding. There was yellowish discoloration of furfural exposed rats felt respiratory difficulty but the body weights and lung weights were not significantly altered. A few rats also had mild nasal bleeding and corneal opalescence, which was recovered shortly after termination of the exposure. A single inhalation exposure of rats to furfural was fully tolerated up to a concentration of 126 ppm; however exposure to higher concentrations resulted in dose dependant mortality leading to 100% deaths at 221ppm. Accordingly, the LC$_{50}$ dose was found to be 189 ppm. Exposure of rats to vapors of kerosene ranging from 426-1054 ppm did not show toxic signs and mortality up to a period of 28 days. Simultaneous exposure of rats to furfural and kerosene vapors ranging in concentration from 35 ppm to 138ppm showed a suppression of LC$_{50}$ value of furfural by 56%. The LC$_{50}$ was 105ppm in rats exposed to furfural mixed kerosene vapors.

Autopsy

Animals that are exposed to furfural (Gr. I) and furfural kerosene mixture (Gr. III) exhibited congested lungs with one lobe heavily consolidated. Liver had no gross abnormality except a little darkening in color. Rats exposed to kerosene alone (Gr.II) did not show any abnormality.

Biochemical observation

Alkaline phosphatase activity was elevated in lungs of furfural exposed (F) and furfural and kerosene mixture exposed (K+F) rats (figure 2). The activities of acid phosphatase and Glutamic Pyruvic Transaminase (GPT) were unaltered (data not shown) in either group but that of Glutamic Oxaloacetic Transaminase (GOT) showed a significant inhibition in Furfural exposed group (F) (P<0.01). In Kerosene exposed group (K), however, they GOT activity was comparable to control (figure 3). Succinic Dehydrogenase (SDH) activity was inhibited in lung of furfural exposed group (F) of rats and was elevated in kerosene exposed group (K) of rats. The observed elevation was markedly suppressed in combined exposure group (K+F) of rats (P<0.01) though the values were still higher compared to control (figure 4). Lactic acid content in lungs of furfural exposed rats (F) showed significant increase (P<0.001) where as kerosene exposure resulted in depressed values. This depression was further aggravated in furfural mixed kerosene group (K+F) of rats (figure 5). Total sulfhydryls and glutathione contents did not alter significantly in either group (F), (K), or (K+F) (data not shown).

Discussion

The observed signs of furfural toxicity, viz; irritation of eyes and nose, lacrimation, external discharge, changes in fur coat etc. are in agreement with the reported findings [1]. Exposure to kerosene, on the other hand, did not reveal any gross changes of clinical significance at the reported concentrations. In close agreement to reported studies kerosene exposure alone did not result in any mortality, body weight changes and did not induce pathological changes in the lung of rats. A simultaneous exposure to vapors of furfural and kerosene in present studies resulted in a suppression of LC$_{50}$ value of furfural (189ppm) by 56% (105ppm) which could be an indication of either a synergistic and /or antagonistic effect of individual constituents. Support for such a phenomenon was further evident from the biochemical data in present studies. It was observed that activity of oxidative enzyme, Succinic Dehydrogenase (SDH) was suppressed with a concomitant

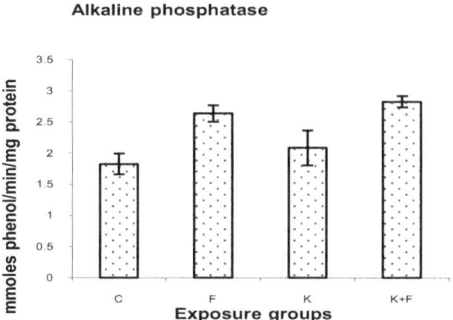

Figure 2: Alterations in alkaline phosphatase activity in lungs following inhalation exposure to furfural and kerosene vapours. The values are mean of 6 rats ± Standard Error as indicated by the bars. * *represents (p<0.001). C-Compressed air only, F-furfural alone (95ppm), K-Kerosene alone (426-1054ppm), K+F-furfural and kerosene vapors (95ppm) and (426-1054ppm) respectively.

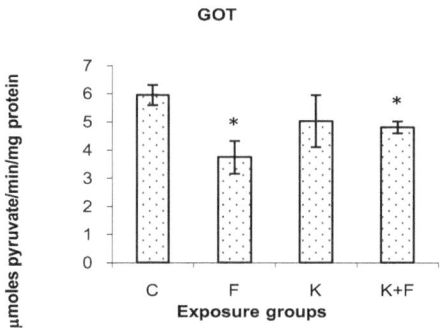

Figure 3: Alterations in glutamic oxaloacetic transaminase (GOT) activity in lungs following inhalation exposure to furfural and kerosene vapors. The values are mean of 6 rats ± Standard Error as indicated by the bars. * represents (p<0.01), C-Compressed air only, F-furfural alone (95ppm), K-Kerosene alone (426-1054ppm), K+F-furfural and kerosene vapors (95ppm) and (426-1054ppm) respectively.

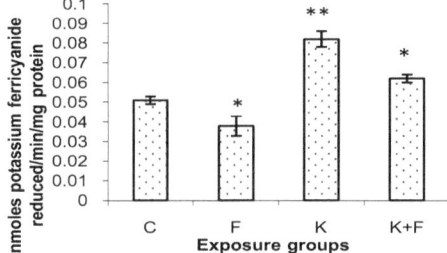

Figure 4: Alterations in succinic dehydrogenase activity in lung following inhalation exposure to furfural and kerosene vapors. The values are mean of 6 rats ± Standard Error as indicated by the bars. ** & * represents (p<0.001) & (p<0.01) respectively, C-Compressed air only, F-furfural alone (95ppm), K-Kerosene alone (426-1054ppm), K+F-furfural and kerosene vapors (95ppm) and (426-1054ppm) respectively.

increase in lactate concentration in the lung of rats exposed to vapors of furfural alone. Exposure to kerosene vapors, however, showed a reverse pattern suggesting that the two compounds may follow different pathways of metabolism and/or biotransformation [9,10]. However, on simultaneous exposure of rats to vapors of furfural and kerosene, the enhanced activity of SDH due to kerosene was suppressed with

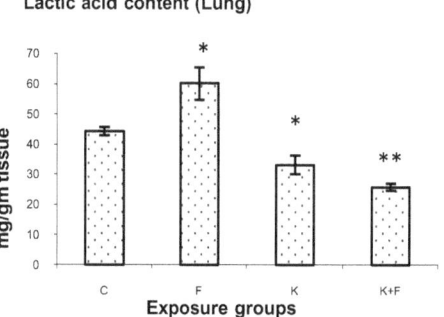

Figure 5: Alterations in lactic acid content in lungs following inhalation exposure to furfural and kerosene vapors. The values are mean of 6 rats ± Standard Error as indicated by the bars. * represents (p<.01) and ** (p<0.001), C-Compressed air only, F-furfural alone (95ppm), K-Kerosene alone (426-1054ppm), K+F-furfural and kerosene vapors (95ppm) and (426-1054ppm) respectively.

a concomitant decrease in lactate contents. A simultaneous decrease in lactate levels and an inhibition of GOT activity were also noticed. These findings are suggestive of an inhibition of cellular energy metabolism in lungs of furfural exposed rats with a simultaneous operation of non-oxidative pathways of metabolism. These findings are in agreement to those earlier reported by Danilov and Melnikova [11]. Changes in clinical enzymes viz; acid phosphatase and Glutamate Pyruvate Transaminase (GPT) in the lungs were not noticeable except mild elevations of alkaline phosphatase activity in lungs of furfural exposed rats. This is suggestive of a regenerative proliferation of type-II pneumocytes for which alkaline phosphatase is a marker enzyme [12]. Mild elevations in liver alkaline phosphatase activity may be suggestive of a possible damage to hepatocellular structure following furfural exposure. The activity was, however, unchanged in combined exposure group of rats. Ray et al. [13] had earlier shown changes in liver β-glucuronidase activity accompanied by alterations in secretory mechanism of liver as reflected by changes in serum protein pattern following s/c injection of 32 mg/kg body weight of furfural doped kerosene. The degree of lesion varies with the extent of exposure and results from toxic effects of kerosene hydrocarbons [14]. Present findings may possibly led us to explore the mode of action of individual chemical entities (furfural & kerosene) in a mixture on simultaneous exposure with particular reference to alterations in energy metabolism in the lungs using rat as an experimental model. The nature of such an interaction leading to suppression of oxidative metabolism could not be explained at the moment and needs further elucidation.

Acknowledgements

Thanks are due to Mr. Ram Surat & Mr. Abdul Aziz for rendering technical assistance and Mr. Lakshmi Kant for secretarial assitance.

References

1. Gupta GD, Misra A, Agarwal DK (1991) Inhalation toxicity of furfural vapours: an assessment of biochemical response in rat lungs. J Appl Toxicol 11: 343-347.

2. Parkash MK, Caldwell J (1994) Metabolism and excretion of [14C] furfural in the rat and mouse. Food Chem Toxicol 32: 887-895.

3. National Institute of Occupational Safety and Health (NIOSH) Manual of Analytical Methods (2nd Edn) Department of Health, Education & Welfare, USA, 1979.

4. Slater EC, Borner WD Jr (1952) The effect of fluoride on the succinic oxidase system. Biochem J 52: 185-196.

5. Huckabee WE (1966) Control of concentration gradients of pyruvate and lactate across cell membranes in blood. J Appl Physiol 9: 163-170.

6. Wootton IDP, King EJ, Freeman H (1982) Microanalysis in Medical Biochemistry. Churchill Livingstone London.

7. Lowry OH, Rosebrough NJ, Farr AL, Randall RJ (1951) Protein measurement with the folin phenol reagent. J Biol Chem 193: 265-275.

8. Jollow DJ, Mitchell JR, Zampaglione N, Gillette JR (1974) Bromobenzene-induced liver necrosis. Protective role of glutathione and evidence for 3,4-bromobenzene oxide as the hepatotoxic metabolite. Pharmacology 11: 151-169.

9. Rao GS, Kannan K, Goel SK, Pandya KP, Shanker R (1984) Subcutaneous kerosene toxicity in albino rats. Environ Res 35: 516-530.

10. Koschier FJ (1999) Toxicity of middle distillates from dermal exposure. Drug Chem Toxicol 22: 155-164.

11. Danilov VB, Melnikova EV (1976) New data on the mechanism of the biological effects of furfural. Probl Gig Organ Zdravookhr 5: 55-58.

12. Castranova V, Rabovsky J, Tucker JH, Miles PR (1988) The alveolar type II epithelial cell: a multifunctional pneumocyte. Toxicol Appl Pharmacol 93: 472-483.

13. Ray PK, Pandya KP, Dutta KK, Rao GS, Gupta GS (1987) Sub chronic Toxicity of Furfural Doped Kerosene. A Report from ITRC Lucknow.

14. Starek A, Kaminiski M (1982) Comparative studies on the toxicity of various dieelectrics, kerosene derivatives, used in the electroerosion technic. I. Morphological, cytoenzymatic and biochemical changes in the liver of rats chronically exposed to kerosene hydrocarbons. Med Pr 33: 239-253.

11

Induction of Activating Transcription Factor 6 via Activation of ERK and ROS-P38 MAPK is Related to Methylglyoxal-Induced Cytotoxicity in Human Retinal Pigment Epithelial Cells

Eun Jung Park[1], Young Sook Kim[1,2], Nu Ri Kang[1,2] and Jin Sook Kim[1,2]*

[1]*Korean Medicine Convergence Research Division, Korea Institute of Oriental Medicine (KIOM), 1672 Yuseongdae-ro, Yuseong-gu, Daejeon, South Korea*
[2]*Korean Medicine Life Science, University of Science Technology (UST), 217 Gajeong-ro, Yuseong-gu, Daejeon, South Korea*

Abstract

Methylglyoxal (MGO), a reactive α-oxoaldehyde produced by glucose metabolism, is elevated in several diabetic complications, including diabetic retinopathy. The breakdown of retinal pigment epithelial cells is implicated in the progression of diabetic retinopathy. Increased concentrations of MGO lead to retinal pigment epithelial cell death. In this study, we investigated the involvement of activating transcription factor 6 (ATF6) in MGO-mediated cytotoxicity in ARPE-19 cells. In response to high concentrations of MGO, unfolded protein response-related ATF6 was induced. Interestingly, the MGO also induced the generation of reactive oxygen species (ROS) and the phosphorylation of ERK and p38 MAPK. The induction of ATF6 was inhibited by ERK-specific and p38 MAPK-specific inhibitors (U0126 and SB202190) and by NAC, a well-known ROS scavenger. NAC also attenuated the phosphorylation of p38 MAPK. MGO induced cytotoxicity in the ARPE-19 cells, which was ameliorated by the inhibition of the ERK, p38 MAPK, and ROS pathways. Furthermore, the MGO-mediated cytotoxicity was inhibited by ATF6 siRNA. Taken together, these results clearly show that the induction of ATF6 via the ERK and ROS-p38 MAPK pathways is implicated in MGO-induced cytotoxicity in ARPE-19 cells.

Keywords: Diabetic retinopathy; Methylglyoxal; Activating transcription factor 6

Introduction

Diabetic retinopathy (DR), a major complication of diabetes, is a leading cause of vision loss among working-age adults in developed countries [1]. Recently, various structural and secretory dysfunctions of the retinal pigment epithelium (RPE) have been found in DR, and the breakdown of the RPE barrier plays a critical role in the induction of DR [2,3]. Therefore, the protection of the RPE is essential for retinal survival and, consequently, for visual function.

Methylglyoxal (MGO) is a highly reactive α-oxoaldehyde formed during glycolysis and generally metabolized by glyoxalase 1 (Glo-1) [4]. In diabetes, the chronic hyperglycemic condition induces the excessive formation of MGO [5]. MGO is major precursor of advanced glycation end products and has recently been shown to cause the induction of the receptor for advanced glycation end products [6,7]. Furthermore, the MGO-mediated accumulation of advanced glycation end products is closely correlated with DR [8].

The endoplasmic reticulum (ER) is a main organelle for protein synthesis and processing in eukaryotic cells [9]. ER stress, caused by the structural and functional disturbance of the ER, leads to the accumulation of misfolded or unfolded proteins and alterations in calcium homeostasis, triggering the unfolded protein response (UPR) [10]. Activating transcription factor 6 (ATF6) is one of the ER-resident UPR proteins. ATF6 is transported to the Golgi and processed by site-1 and site-2 proteases in response to stressful conditions [11]. Processed cytosolic ATF6 is translocated to the nucleus and controls the genes that encode ER-associated degradation components and XBP1 [12]. According to previous *in vivo* studies, ATF6 grains are observed in diabetic cataracts, and ATF6 is elevated in the retinal structures of db/db mice [13,14]. Also, ATF6 is induced by highly oxidized, glycated LDL in human retinal Müller cells, and ATF6 is translocated to the nucleus in retinal capillary pericytes [15,16]. However, there is no report on the role of ATF6 in eye disease, including DR. Therefore, we aimed to investigate the role of ATF6 in MGO-induced DR conditions in ARPE-19 cells.

Materials and Methods

Cell culture and reagents

ARPE-19 cells were obtained from the American Type Culture Collection (ATCC, Manassas, VA, USA). Cells were grown in Dulbecco's modified Eagle's medium/Ham's F-12 with 10% fetal bovine serum, 3 mM glutamine, and streptomycin/penicillin (100 mg/ml and 100 U/ml, respectively) in a 5% CO_2 incubator at 37°C. MGO and N-Acetyl-L-cysteine (NAC) were purchased form Sigma-Aldrich (St. Louis, MO, USA). SP600125, U0126, and SB202190 were obtained from Calbiochem (San Diego, CA, USA). Anti-ATF6 and actin antibodies were purchased from Santa Cruz Biotechnology (Santa Cruz, CA, USA). Anti-p-JNK, p-ERK, p-p38, JNK, ERK, and p38 antibodies were purchased from Cell Signaling Technology (Danvers, MA, USA).

Cell viability assay

The 3-(4,5-dimethylthiazol-2-yl)-2,5-diphenyltetrazolium bromide (MTT) assay was employed to measure cell viability. In brief, cells were

*Corresponding author: Jin Sook Kim, Korean Medicine Convergence Research Division, Korea Institute of Oriental Medicine (KIOM), 1672 Yuseongdae-ro, Yuseong-gu, Daejeon 305-811, South Korea, E-mail: jskim@kiom.re.kr

plated on 96-well plates and incubated with various concentrations of MGO with or without inhibitors. At the appropriate time, 20 μl MTT solutions (5 mg/ml) was added to each well and incubated for 4 h at 37°C. After incubation, the MTT solution was removed, and 100 μl DMSO was added to each well. Absorbance at 570 nm was measured in a microplate reader (BIO-TEK, Synergy HT, Winooski, VT, USA).

Western blotting

Cells were lysed with Laemmli sample buffer (Bio-Rad, Hercules, CA, USA), heated at 100°C for 5 min, and electrophoresed at 20 μg/lane on a denaturing SDS–polyacrylamide gel. Proteins were transferred to nitrocellulose membranes (GE Healthcare UK Ltd, Buckinghamshire, Germany) using a Bio-Rad tank blotting apparatus (Bio-Rad). Membranes were probed with specific targeting primary polyclonal antibodies, washed, and incubated with horseradish peroxidase-linked secondary antibodies. After the membranes were washed three times, signals were detected using EzWestLumiOne (Atto Corporation, Tokyo, Japan) and Fugifilm LAS-3000 (LAS-3000, Fuji Photo, Tokyo, Japan).

Measurement of reactive oxygen species (ROS) generation

The generation of ROS was measured by using 2',7'-dichlorofluorescein diacetate (DCF-DA) as a substrate (Invitrogen, Carlsbad, CA, USA). In brief, cells were incubated with 10 μM DCF-DA for 30 min before collection. For quantitative assessment of ROS generation, the cells were collected, suspended in PBS, and analyzed by the green fluorescence intensity from 10,000 cells with a FACSCalibur flow cytometer (Becton Dickinson, Franklin Lakes, NJ, USA). For image taking, DCF-DA-loaded cells were visualized using an Olympus IX81 microscope (Olympus, Tokyo, Japan).

siRNA transfections

The ATF6 siRNA duplexes used in this study were purchased from Dharmacon as siGENEOME SMART pool M-009917-01 (Thermo Fischer Scientific, Pittsburgh, PA, USA). Cells were transfected with siRNA oligonucleotides using Oligofectamine Reagent (Invitrogen, Carlsbad, CA, USA) according to the manufacturer's recommendations.

Densitometry

The band intensities were quantified using the open source software ImageJ 1.50b (Image Processing and Analysis in Java; http://imagej.nih.gov/ij/).

Statistical analysis

The data were statically analyzed with a Student's t-test. A p-value <0.05 was considered significant (SPSS for Window, version 22.0, IBM, Armonk, NY, USA).

Results

MGO decreases cell viability and induces ATF6 up-regulation in ARPE-19 cells

Previous reports have shown that the ER stress pathway activates many diabetic complications including DR [17-19]. Also, various ER stress-related factors such as CHOP and ATF4 are involved in the progression of DR [16,20]. In this study, we aimed to investigate how ATF6 participates in MGO-induced DR in ARPE-19 cells. First,

we treated ARPE-19 cells with MGO and observed the change in the expression level of ATF6 protein by using Western blotting. ATF6 protein expression levels were increased by 500 μM MGO (Figures 1A and 1B). MGO has cytotoxic activity as a well-known DR inducer [8]. To investigate the effect of MGO on cell viability in our system, ARPE-19 cells were treated with various concentrations (5-1000 μM) of MGO for 24 and 48 h. As shown in Figures 1C and 1D, cell viability was decreased by 500 and 1000 μM MGO, respectively. Furthermore, cell numbers were diminished, and morphological changes were also observed in the cells treated with 500 or 1000 μM MGO (Figure 1E).

Activation of ERK and p38 mediates MGO-induced ATF6 up-regulation and viability loss in ARPE-19 cells

According to several reports, the activation of MAPKs is involved in the induction of ATF6 [21-23]. We investigated the effect of MGO on MAPK phosphorylation in order to determine whether the activation of MAPKs is involved in MGO-induced ATF6 expression. The phosphorylation of JNK, ERK, and p38 peaked at 30 min after treatment with MGO (Figure 2A). Next, to test the role of individual MAPK pathways in MGO-induced ATF6 up-regulation and cytotoxicity, we examined the effects of SP600125 (an inhibitor of JNK), U0126 (an inhibitor of ERK), and SB202190 (an inhibitor of p38) on MGO-induced ATF6 expression and cell viability. As shown in Figure 2B, pre-treatment with U0126 and SB202190 slightly decreased the MGO-induced ATF6 up-regulation. However, SP600125, the JNK inhibitor, weakly increased ATF6 expression. Also, MGO-mediated cytotoxicity was partially restored by U0126 and SB202190 (Figure 2C). These results show that the induction of ATF6 and cytotoxicity might be partially mediated by the activation of the ERK and p38 signaling pathways in response to MGO in ARPE-19 cells.

ROS mediate MGO-induced ATF6 up-regulation and viability loss in ARPE-19 cells

MGO can generate ROS by reducing cellular glutathione levels [24]. To elucidate whether MGO generates ROS in ARPE-19 cells, the cells were incubated with DCF-DA, and relative green-fluorescence intensity was analyzed by flow cytometry and fluorescence microscopy. ROS were generated by 500 μM MGO in ARPE-19 cells (Figures 3A and 3B). To examine whether ROS generation might be involved in MGO-induced ATF6 expression in ARPE-19 cells, the cells were pre-treated with the ROS scavenger NAC and treated with MGO. ATF6 protein levels were then analyzed by Western blotting. As shown in Figure 3C, pre-treatment with NAC effectively suppressed MGO-induced ATF6. To further elucidate whether the ROS generation might participate in the activation of MAPK signaling pathways, cells were treated with NAC and MGO, and the phosphorylation states of ERK and p38 were subsequently checked. Interestingly, the MGO-induced phosphorylation of p38, but not that of JNK, was diminished by the NAC pre-treatment (Figure 3D). Furthermore, we tested the protective effect of NAC on the MGO-mediated reduction in cell viability. Pre-treatment with NAC completely ameliorated the MGO-mediated cytotoxicity (Figure 3D). Taken together, the results show that MGO-mediated ATF6 induction and viability reduction are induced by ROS and the activation of the p38 pathway in ARPE-19 cells.

ATF6 mediates MGO-induced cytotoxicity in ARPE-19 cells

To investigate how MGO-induced ATF6 regulates cell viability, ARPE-19 cells were transfected with control siRNA (siControl) and

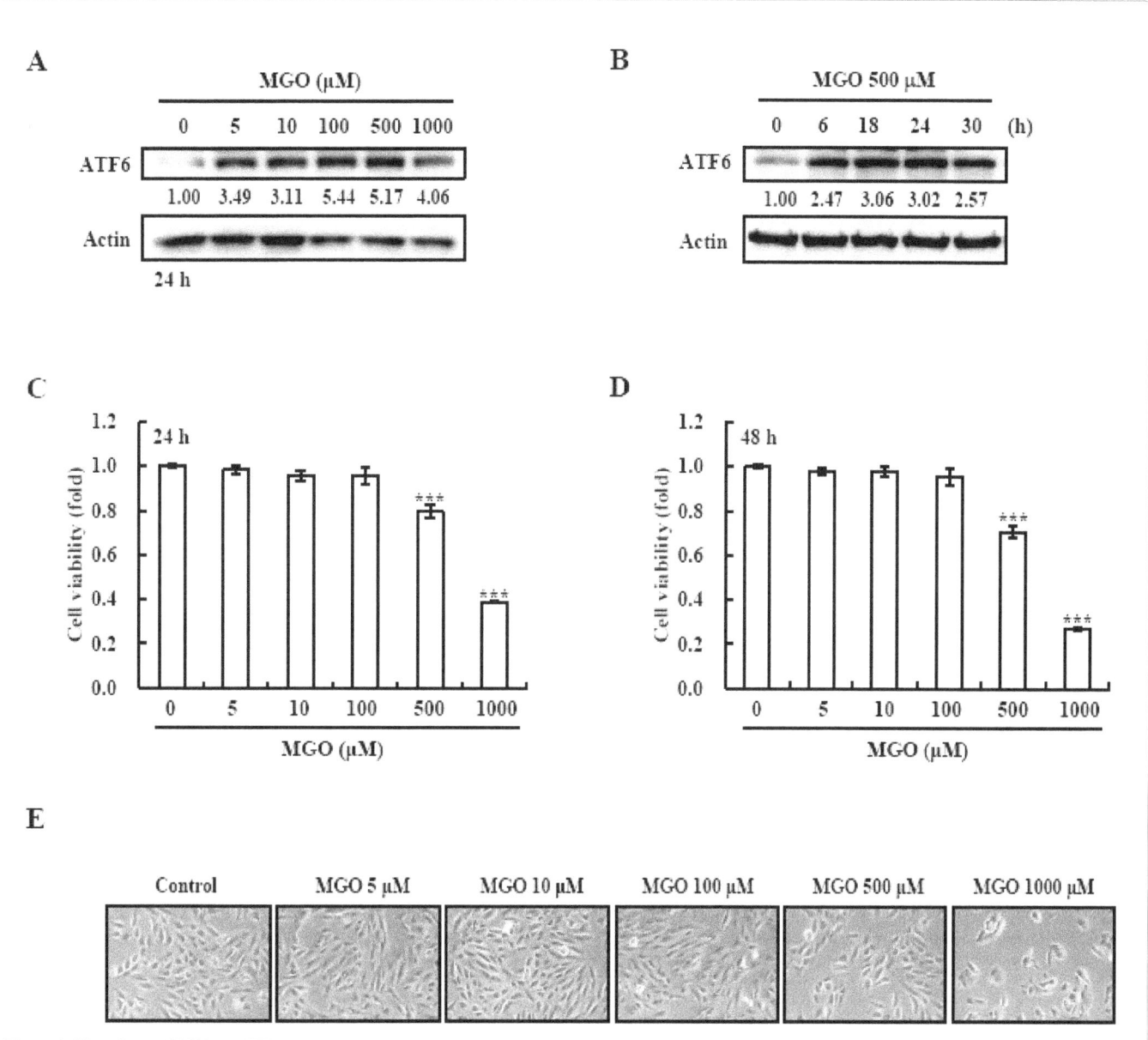

Figure 1: The effects of MGO on ATF6 protein expression levels, cell viability, and morphology in ARPE-19 cells. (A and B) ARPE-19 cells were seeded on 6-well culture plates and treated for 24 h with 5-1000 μM MGO or in a time-kinetic manner with 500 μM MGO, and the expression levels of ATF6 were observed by Western blotting. Actin served as a loading control. (C and D) ARPE-19 cells were seeded on 96-well culture plates and treated for 24 or 48 h with 5-1000 μM MGO, and cell viability was measured by MTT assay. (E) After treatment with 5-1000 μM MGO for 24 h, ARPE-19 cells were observed under an inverted microscope. Data are representative results from three independent experiments and expressed as mean ± SD. $^{***}P<0.001$ vs. control (n=8).

ATF6 siRNA (siATF6), and cell viability was measured in the presence or absence of MGO. A reduction in ATF6 protein level following transfection with siATF6 was identified by Western blotting (Figure 4A). MGO-mediated viability loss was partially ameliorated by the knockdown of ATF6 (Figure 4B). These result shows that the MGO-induced decrease in viability was mediated by ATF6 in ARPE-19 cells.

Discussion

In this study, we demonstrated for the first time that MGO induces cytotoxicity through the ERK-ATF6 and ROS-p38 MAPK-ATF6 pathways in ARPE-19 cells. The RPE is important for the maintenance of the visual system and is implicated in the pathogenesis of DR

[2,3]. As a diabetic condition, a high concentration of MGO induces apoptosis and cytotoxicity [25-27]. Similarly, our data show decreased cell viability with an increased concentration of MGO (Figure 1). Because the balance between cell survival and death in the RPE is highly associated with DR, these result show that the loss of ARPE-19 cells due to the excessive accumulation of MGO might be associated with the progression of DR.

According to previous reports, the ER stress marker CHOP plays an important role in MGO-mediated myocyte apoptosis, and MGO induces the UPR through the phosphorylation of UPR proteins (PERK and eIF2a) in human lens epithelial cells [28,29]. Also, the ER stress pathway activates many diabetic complications including DR, and

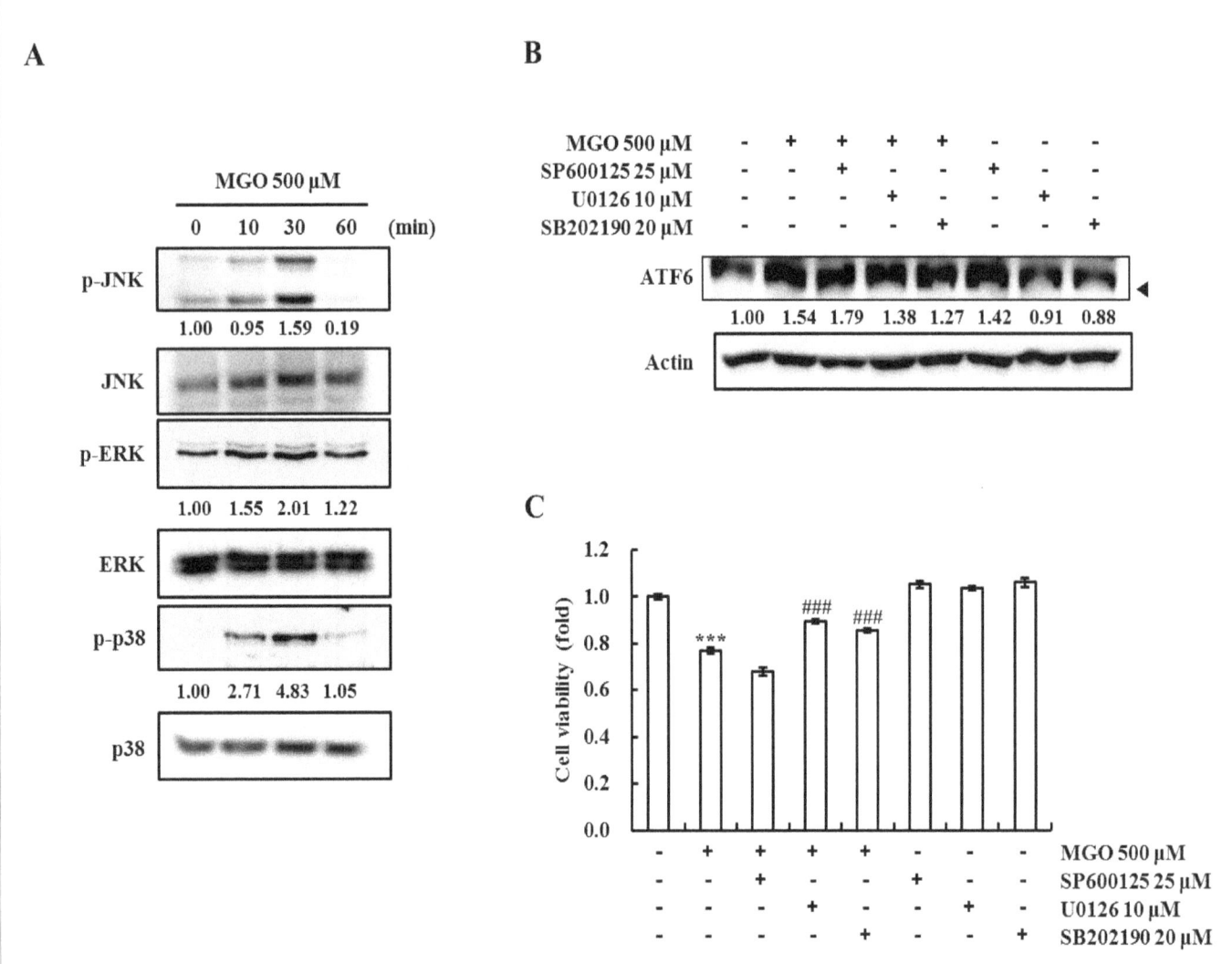

Figure 2: Involvement of MAPK pathways in MGO-mediated up-regulation of ATF6 and decreased viability in ARPE-19 cells. A) ARPE-19 cells were seeded on 6-well culture plates and treated for 10, 30, and 60 min with 500 µM MGO, and the phosphorylation levels of JNK, ERK, and p38 were determined by Western blotting using specific antibodies. The total form of JNK, ERK, and p38 served as a loading control. B) ARPE-19 cells were seeded on 6-well culture plates and treated for 24 h with 500 µM MGO in the presence or absence of JNK, ERK, and p38 inhibitors, and the expression levels of ATF6 were observed by Western blotting. C) ARPE-19 cells were seeded on 96-well culture plates and treated for 24 h with 500 µM MGO in the presence or absence of JNK, ERK, and p38 inhibitors, and cell viability was measured using the MTT assay. Data are representative results from three independent experiments and expressed as mean ± SD. ***$P<0.001$ vs. control; ###$P<0.001$ vs. MGO (n=8).

well-known ER stress-related factors (CHOP, ATF4, and GRP78/BiP) are involved in the progression of DR [16-20]. This is a novel finding that the induction of ATF6 occurs in MGO-treated RPE.

ER stress induces defense and restoration mechanisms using the UPR at early stages, but when the pro-survival UPR fails to overcome ER stress, it is sufficient to induce apoptosis and reduce cell viability [30]. Also, when ER stress is induced, ER-associated degradation is activated by ATF6, leading to cell survival, but ATF6 is also involved in the induction of cell death through the activation of pro-apoptotic CHOP [12,23,31-33]. Recent paper shows that MGO decreases RPE cell viability, resulting from the ER stress-dependent intracellular ROS formation, mitochondrial membrane potential loss, and intracellular calcium increase [34].

MAPK signaling is involved in the induction and activation of ATF6 [21-23]. In our data, the phosphorylation of JNK, ERK, and p38 MAPK was increased by MGO, but the induction of ATF6 was regulated by ERK and p38 MAPK (Figure 2). Furthermore, ROS generation is involved in cell death in several cell lines, and ROS generation is induced by MGO [5,7,24,27]. We also found that increased ROS were associated with the phosphorylation of p38, the induction of ATF6, and cytotoxicity in response to MGO in ARPE-19 cells (Figure 3). Therefore, the activation of ERK-ATF6 and ROS-p38-ATF6 by the excessive accumulation of MGO might be involved in the development of DR.

Acknowledgements

This research was supported by Grants (K16270) from the Korea Institute of Oriental Medicine (KIOM).

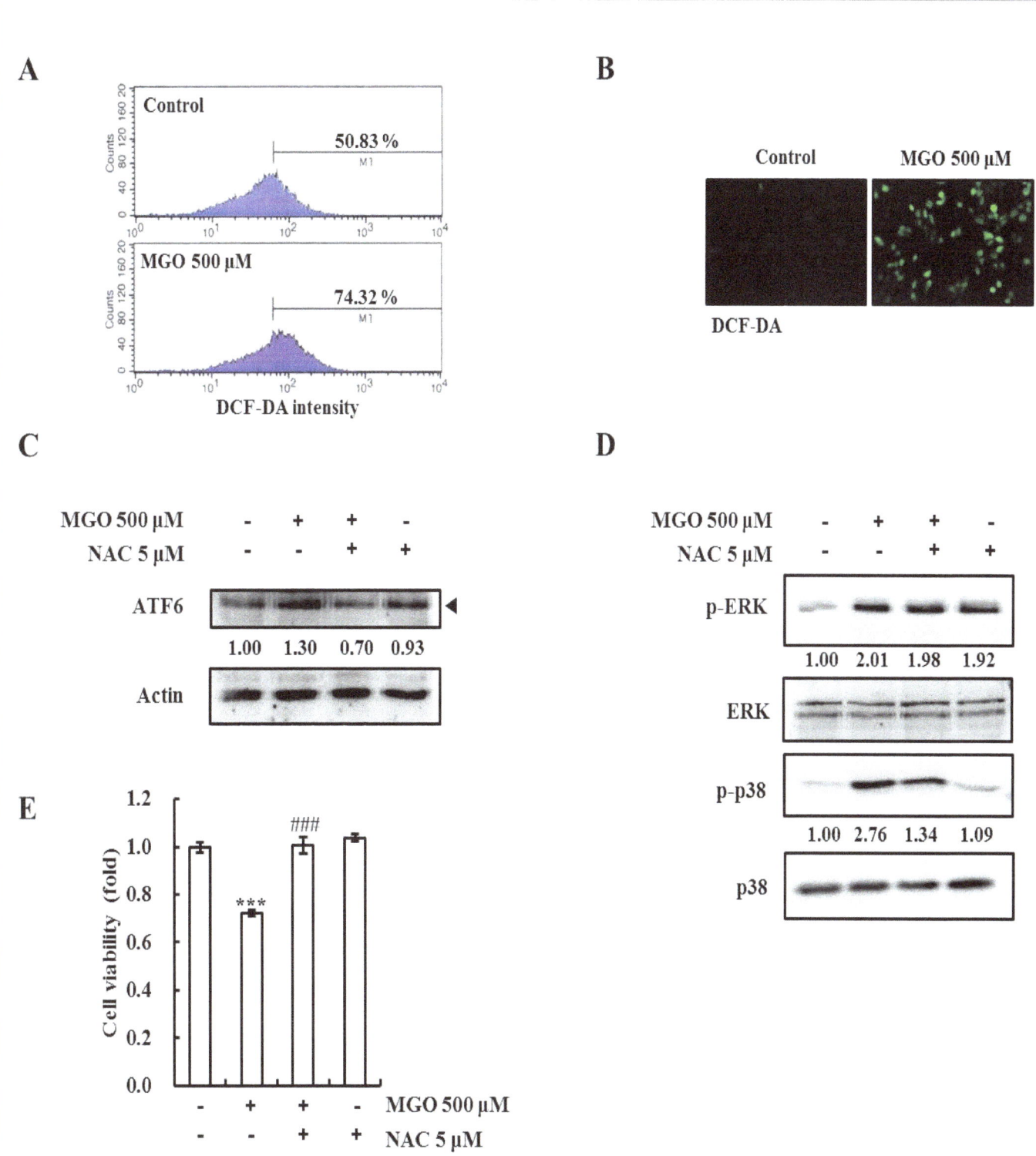

Figure 3: Involvement of ROS generation in MGO-mediated up-regulation of ATF6 and decreased viability in ARPE-19 cells. (A and B) ARPE-19 cells were seeded on 6-well culture plates and treated for 30 min with 500 μM MGO, and the DCF-DA-based ROS generation was determined using flow cytometry and fluorescence microscopy. C) ARPE-19 cells were seeded on 6-well culture plates and treated for 24 h with 500 μM MGO in the presence or absence of NAC, and the expression levels of ATF6 were observed by Western blotting. D) ARPE-19 cells were seeded on 6-well culture plates and treated for 30 min with 500 μM MGO, and the phosphorylation levels of ERK and p38 were determined by Western blotting. E) ARPE-19 cells were seeded on 96-well culture plates and treated for 24 h with 500 μM MGO in the presence or absence of NAC, and cell viability was measured by MTT assay. Data are representative results from three independent experiments and expressed as mean ± SD. ***P<0.001 vs. control; ###P<0.001 vs. MGO (n=8).

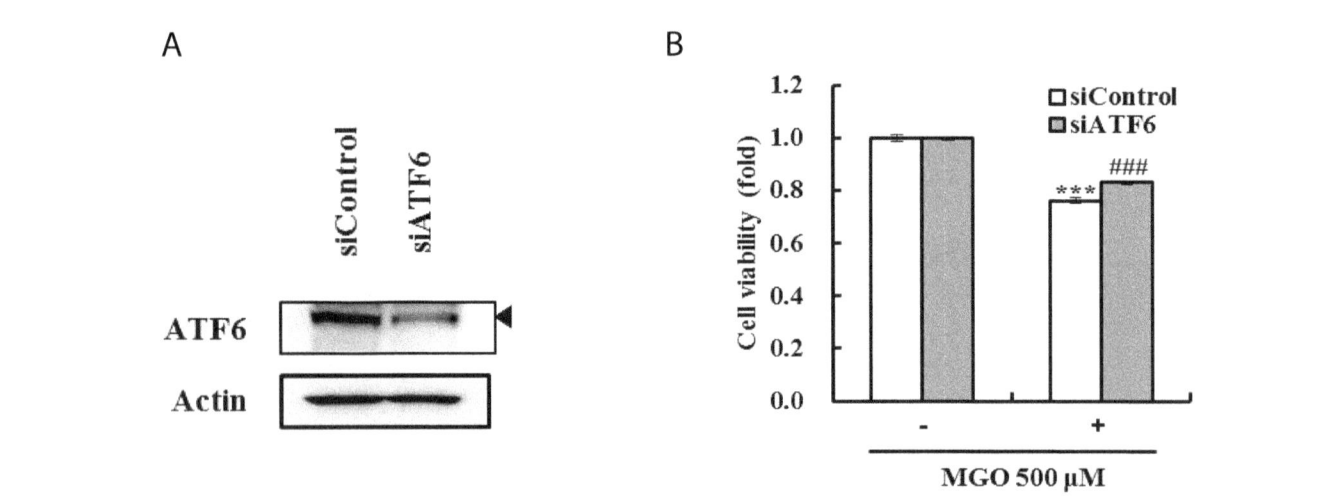

Figure 4: ATF6 is related to MGO-mediated decreased viability in ARPE-19 cells. (A and B) ARPE-19 cells were seeded on 6-well culture plates and transfected with control siRNA (siControl) or ATF6 siRNA (siATF6) with or without MGO after splitting. The cells were collected, the knockdown of ATF6 was observed by Western blotting, and cell viability was measured by MTT assay. Data are representative results from three independent experiments and expressed as mean ± SD. ***$P<0.001$ vs. control; ###$P<0.001$ vs. MGO (n=8).

References

1. Gargiulo P, Giusti C, Pietrobono D, La Torre D, Diacono D, et al. (2004) Diabetes mellitus and retinopathy. Dig Liver Dis 36: S101-S105.

2. Xu HZ, Song Z, Fu S, Zhu M, Le YZ (2011) RPE barrier breakdown in diabetic retinopathy: seeing is believing. J Ocul Biol Dis Infor 4: 83-92.

3. Simó R, Villarroel M, Corraliza L, Hernández C, Garcia-Ramírez M (2010) The retinal pigment epithelium: something more than a constituent of the blood-retinal barrier--implications for the pathogenesis of diabetic retinopathy. J Biomed Biotechnol 2010.

4. Piskorska D, Kopieczna-Grzebieniak E (1998) Participation of glyoxalases and methylglyoxal in diabetic complication development. Pol Merkur Lekarski 4: 342-344.

5. Thornalley PJ (1994) Methylglyoxal, glyoxalases and the development of diabetic complications. Amino Acids 6: 15-23.

6. Ramasamy R, Yan SF, Schmidt AM (2006) Methylglyoxal comes of AGE. Cell 124: 258-260.

7. Yao D, Brownlee M (2010) Hyperglycemia-induced reactive oxygen species increase expression of the receptor for advanced glycation end products (RAGE) and RAGE ligands. Diabetes 59: 249-255.

8. Stitt AW (2010) AGEs and diabetic retinopathy. Invest Ophthalmol Vis Sci 51: 4867-4874.

9. Hampton RY (2000) ER stress response: getting the UPR hand on misfolded proteins. Curr Biol 10: R518-R521.

10. Lindholm D, Wootz H, Korhonen L (2006) ER stress and neurodegenerative diseases. Cell Death Differ 13: 385-392.

11. Bernales S, Papa FR, Walter P (2006) Intracellular signaling by the unfolded protein response. Annu Rev Cell Dev Biol 22: 487-508.

12. Hetz C (2012) The unfolded protein response: controlling cell fate decisions under ER stress and beyond. Nat Rev Mol Cell Biol 13: 89-102.

13. Torres-Bernal BE, Torres-Bernal LF, Gutierrez-Campos RR, Kershenobich-Stalnikowitz DD, Barba-Gallardo LF, et al. (2014) Unfolded protein response activation in cataracts. J Cataract Refract Surg 40: 1697-1705.

14. Tang L, Zhang Y, Jiang Y, Willard L, Ortiz E, et al. (2011) Dietary wolfberry ameliorates retinal structure abnormalities in db/db mice at the early stage of diabetes. Exp Biol Med (Maywood) 236: 1051-1063.

15. Wu M, Yang S, Elliott MH, Fu D, Wilson K, et al. (2012) Oxidative and endoplasmic reticulum stresses mediate apoptosis induced by modified LDL in human retinal Muller cells. Invest Ophthalmol Vis Sci 53: 4595-4604.

16. Fu D, Wu M, Zhang J, Du M, Yang S, et al. (2012) Mechanisms of modified LDL-induced pericyte loss and retinal injury in diabetic retinopathy. Diabetologia 55: 3128-3140.

17. Oshitari T, Hata N, Yamamoto S (2008) Endoplasmic reticulum stress and diabetic retinopathy. Vasc Health Risk Manag 4: 115-122.

18. Ma JH, Wang JJ, Zhang SX (2014) The unfolded protein response and diabetic retinopathy. J Diabetes Res 2014: 160140.

19. Li B, Wang HS, Li GG, Zhao MJ, Zhao MH (2011) The role of endoplasmic reticulum stress in the early stage of diabetic retinopathy. Acta Diabetol 48: 103-111.

20. Chen Y, Wang JJ, Li J, Hosoya KI, Ratan R, et al. (2012) Activating transcription factor 4 mediates hyperglycaemia-induced endothelial inflammation and retinal vascular leakage through activation of STAT3 in a mouse model of type 1 diabetes. Diabetologia 55: 2533-2545.

21. Thuerauf DJ, Arnold ND, Zechner D, Hanford DS, DeMartin KM, et al. (1998) p38 Mitogen-activated protein kinase mediates the transcriptional induction of the atrial natriuretic factor gene through a serum response element. A potential role for the transcription factor ATF6. J Biol Chem 273: 20636-20643.

22. Luo S, Lee AS (2002) Requirement of the p38 mitogen-activated protein kinase signalling pathway for the induction of the 78 kDa glucose-regulated protein/immunoglobulin heavy-chain binding protein by azetidine stress: activating transcription factor 6 as a target for stress-induced phosphorylation. Biochem J 366: 787-795.

23. Tay KH, Luan Q, Croft A, Jiang CC, Jin L, et al. (2014) Sustained IRE1 and ATF6 signaling is important for survival of melanoma cells undergoing ER stress. Cell Signal 26: 287-294.

24. Beard KM, Shangari N, Wu B, O'Brien PJ (2003) Metabolism, not autoxidation, plays a role in alpha-oxoaldehyde- and reducing sugar-induced erythrocyte GSH depletion: relevance for diabetes mellitus. Mol Cell Biochem 252: 331-338.

25. Kim J, Son JW, Lee JA, Oh YS, Shinn SH (2004) Methylglyoxal induces apoptosis mediated by reactive oxygen species in bovine retinal pericytes. J Korean Med Sci 19: 95-100.

26. Fukunaga M, Miyata S, Liu BF, Miyazaki H, Hirota Y, et al. (2004) Methylglyoxal induces apoptosis through activation of p38 MAPK in rat Schwann cells. Biochem Biophys Res Commun 320: 689-695.

27. Heimfarth L, Loureiro SO, Pierozan P, de Lima BO, Reis KP, et al. (2013) Methylglyoxal-induced cytotoxicity in neonatal rat brain: a role for oxidative stress and MAP kinases. Metab Brain Dis 28: 429-438.

28. Palsamy P, Bidasee KR, Ayaki M, Augusteyn RC, Chan JY, et al. (2014) Methylglyoxal induces endoplasmic reticulum stress and DNA demethylation

in the Keap1 promoter of human lens epithelial cells and age-related cataracts. Free Radic Biol Med 72: 134-148.

29. Nam DH, Han JH, Lee TJ, Shishido T, Lim JH, et al. (2015) CHOP deficiency prevents methylglyoxal-induced myocyte apoptosis and cardiac dysfunction. J Mol Cell Cardiol 85: 168-177.

30. Wu J, Kaufman RJ (2006) From acute ER stress to physiological roles of the Unfolded Protein Response. Cell Death Differ 13: 374-384.

31. Karali E, Bellou S, Stellas D, Klinakis A, Murphy C, et al. (2014) VEGF Signals through ATF6 and PERK to promote endothelial cell survival and angiogenesis in the absence of ER stress. Mol Cell 54: 559-572.

32. Morishima N, Nakanishi K, Nakano A (2011) Activating transcription factor-6 (ATF6) mediates apoptosis with reduction of myeloid cell leukemia sequence 1 (Mcl-1) protein via induction of WW domain binding protein 1. J Biol Chem 286: 35227-35235.

33. Yoshida H, Okada T, Haze K, Yanagi H, Yura T, et al. (2000) ATF6 activated by proteolysis binds in the presence of NF-Y (CBF) directly to the cis-acting element responsible for the mammalian unfolded protein response. Mol Cell Biol 20: 6755-6767.

34. Chan CM, Huang DY, Huang YP, Hau SH, Kang LY, et al. (2016) Methylglyoxal induces cell death through endoplasmic reticulum stress-associated ROS production and mitochondrial dysfunction. J Cell Mol Med.

12

Inhibition of Tumors in Mice Models by a Synthetic Ceramide-analog AD2725

Qin JD[1,2]*, Weiss L[3], Zeira M[3], Yekhtin Z[3], Slavin S[3,4], Gatt S[2] and Dagan A[2,5]

[1]Department of Pediatrics, The University of Chicago, Chicago, USA
[2]Department of Biochemistry, Hebrew University School of Medicine, Jerusalem, Israel
[3]Department of Bone-Marrow Transplantation, Hadassah–Hebrew University of Medical Center, Jerusalem, Israel
[4]The International Center for Cell Therapy & Cancer Immunotherapy, Tel Aviv, Israel
[5]Department of Biochemistry and Molecular Biology, Institute for Medical Research Israel-Canada, Hebrew-University-Hadassah School of Medicine, Jerusalem, Israel

Abstract

A synthetic analog of ceramide (AD2725) elevated ceramide levels in MDA-MB-435 breast cancer cells inducing apoptosis and resulted in cell death. In animal studies, using a model of xenograft breast cancer cancer cells in nude mice, treatment with AD2725 resulted in a significant reduction of the tumor volume and weight, and a significantly prolonged survival of the treated mice. The analog also significantly elevated INF gamma and IL-12 cytokine levels and reduced the level of IL-10 in the plasma. These data indicate that use of suitable synthetic analogs that most probably elevate the ceramide levels may have beneficial anti-cancer therapeutic effects.

Keywords: Ceramide; Sphingolipids; Apoptosis; Cytokine; Breast cancer

Introduction

Apoptosis is recognized as an important mechanism by which cytotoxic agents induce tumor cell death [1,2]. One mechanism is using ceramide, as an intracellular, pro-apoptotic signaling molecule [3-5]. It is now clear that ceramide plays a central role in both apoptotic and mitogenic pathways [6,7]. Thus, generation of ceramide in cells initiates apoptosis and cell death while reduction of intracellular ceramide or increasing sphingosine-1-phosphate levels leads to drug resistance [8-12]. Ceramide is often generated in response to chemotherapeutic agents or radiation via hydrolysis of sphingomyelin [11,13]. Although the mechanism remains unclear, ceramide causes a disruption of mitochondria, leading to cell death by apoptosis [11,14-17]. Ceramide also reduces the vascular network that feeds the tumor [18]. In this study we used a synthetic ceramide-analog AD2725 to investigate the effects of chemotherapy while achieving an elevation of ceramide in the tumor cells. This study demonstrates that using a non-natural ceramide-like analog caused an elevation of intracellular ceramide level in MDA-MB-435 breast cancer cells, leading to their death by apoptosis and significantly prolonged the survival of tumor bearing mice.

Material and Methods

AD2646: $(2R,3R)$-2-(N-tetradecylamino)-3-(4-nitrophenyl)-1,3-propandiol; AD2673: $(2R,3R)$-2-amino-3-(4-tetradecanoylamino-phenyl)-1,3-propandiol, were synthesized by Dagan et al. [19] AD2725: $(2S,3R)$-2-(N-tetradecylamino)-3-phenyl-3-propanol, was synthesized as follows: One mille mole $(2S,3R)$-2-amino-3-phenyl-3-propanol was reacted with tetradecanal (1.2 mmol) in methanol/0.05 N acetic acid, 9:1 for 15 min and sodium cyanoborohydride ($NaCNBH_3$, 2 mmol) was added in portions during 1 h. The mixture was stirred overnight at room temperature, evaporated to dryness and the residue dissolved in dichloromethane/methanol, 2:1. Dilute HCl was added and following overtaxing, the upper phase was removed. The lower phase was washed two more times with dilute HCl and dried by adding $MgSO_4$. The solvent was collected, evaporated to dryness and the product was purified by column chromatography using increasing concentrations of methanol in dichloromethane. Product is 550 µmol (55% yields). AD2725 structure see Figure 1A.

Reagents

All chemical and solvents used were of analytical grade. Chemicals were purchased from Sigma Chemicals (St Louis, MO, USA). Thin layer chromatography plates were purchased from Whatman (Clifton, NJ, USA). Culture media and supplements were purchased from Beth Haemek, Israel.

Cell line

Breast cancer MDA-MB-435 cells were cultured at 37°C in an incubator with 5% CO_2 in air in RPMI-1640 medium, supplemented with 10% fetal calf serum, 1% penicillin-streptomycin, 1% glutamate and 4.5 g/L glucose. Once the cells grew to about 80% confluence, the medium was removed, fresh medium was added and incubation was continued.

Mice

Female CD1 nude mice (5-6 weeks old) weighing 20 g were purchased from the Harlan Laboratories, Israel. The animals were fed Purina chow and acidified water (pH 2.7) ad libitum, and maintained in an SPF animal facility at 21°C with a 12 h cycling of light. The animal studies were approved by The Ethics Committee of the Hebrew University-Hadassah School of Medicine.

Determining of cellular protein concentration and cell number

Cells were harvested, washed with PBS, trypsinized, suspended in PBS and sonicated for 10 seconds with a Microson XL probe sonicator (Misonix) at 40% output power. For quantifying the protein, a sample

*Corresponding author: Jingdong Qin, Ph.D., Department of Pediatrics, The University of Chicago, 5841 S Maryland Ave, Wyler MC4068, Chicago, IL, USA, E-mail: qjingdong@peds.bsd.uchicago.edu

(5 μl) was taken, interacted with Bradford reagent (250 μl) and the absorbance quantified at 595 nm. A culture sample was mixed with an equal volume of trypan blue, applied to a hemocytometer, and the numbers of live (unstained) and damaged or dead (blue) cells were determined.

Cell viability analysis

10^4 cells per 100 μl medium were seeded in each well in a 96-well plate, incubated overnight and varying concentrations of ceramide analogs in 100 μl medium containing 2 μl DMSO were added to the cultures. (The controls contained the same concentration of DMSO). An MTT solution was added and incubation was continued for 4 hours. The stop-solution [89% Isopropanol, 1% HCl (37%), 10% TtritonX-100] was then added and cell viability was determined at 570 nm.

Apoptosis determined by DNA fragmentation

1×10^6 MDA-MB-435 cells in 5 ml medium were seeded in a small flask and incubated for 24 h. The next day the medium was removed, new medium and 20 μM of AD2725 or AD2646 were added and incubation was continued for 24 h. On the third day, cells were harvested by trypsinization and the genomic DNA was extracted using the Sigma DNA extraction kit. Samples of DNA were then electrophoresed on a 1.5% agarose gel at 50 volts in TAE electrophoresis buffer for 2 hours. The DNA was detected by a UV-illuminator and pictures were taken.

Apoptosis determined by measuring activation of Caspase 3

Caspase-3 activity was assayed by Z-DEVD-R110 cleavage, using the EnzChek⁻ Caspase-3 Assay Kit #2 (Molecular Probes). Following incubation with the respective analogs, cells were collected, precipitated and washed with PBS. For each sample, 10^6 cells were lysed by incubating with 50 μl lysis buffer on ice for 30 min and cell debris was precipitated in a micro-centrifuge for 5 min at 5,000 rpm. The supernatants were incubated with 50 μM of the conjugated substrate Z-DEVD-R110 in a 100 μl reaction volume at room temperature for 30 min and the fluorescence of the released free R110 was measured at an excitation at 485 nm and emission at 535 nm using a FI.600 microplate fluorescence reader.

Quantification of cellular ceramide

MDA-MB-435 cells were incubated for 3 hours in the absence or presence of the ceramide analog AD2725 and AD2646 (20 μM) and 15 μM pyrene decanoic acid (P10), as a solution in 1 μl DMSO per ml reaction mixture. The cells were trypsinized, collected and washed twice with PBS. 2 ml PBS were added and the cell suspension was sonicated in a Microson XL probe sonicator (Misonix) for 10 seconds. A sample was taken for quantifying the cell protein using the Bradford procedure. To the rest were added 2 ml of dichloromethane-methanol, 1:1, stirred and centrifuged. The lower phase was collected and the upper one retreated with 1 ml of dichloromethane-methanol, 3:1. The two dichloromethane phases were combined and the solvent was evaporated to dryness under a stream of air. The residue was dissolved in dichloromethane-methanol, 1:1 and applied to the concentrating zone of a TLC silica gel plate having markers of P10 and P10-ceramide. The latter was developed in a mixture of dichloromethane-methanol-ammonia, 95:5:0.5. The P10-ceramide spots (viewed with an ultraviolet lamp) were scraped, dichloromethane-methanol, 1:1, was added, stirred sonicated in bath sonicator and centrifuged. The fluorescence of P10-ceremide was recorded in a spectrofluorometer (Perkin-Elmer LS5) using an excitation at 345 nm as an emission at 377 nm.

In vivo studies

CD1-Nude mice (5-6 week old) were irradiated with a total body irradiation (TBI) of 400 cGy and one day later injected with MDA-MB-435 cells.

Four types of experiments were performed:

1)   Breast cancer cells (4×10^6 cells in 0.1 ml medium) were injected intradermally into the left side of the flank and the next day the mice were injected i.p. with the analog AD2725.

2)   Breast cancer cells (4×10^6 cells in 0.1 ml medium) were injected intradermally into the left side of the flank and one week later the mice were injected i.p. with the analog AD2725.

3)   Breast cancer cells (5×10^6 cells in 0.2 ml medium) were injected intravenously into the lateral tail vein and two hours later the mice were injected i.p. with the analog AD2725.

4)   Breast cancer cells (5×10^6 cells in 0.2 ml medium) were injected intravenously into the lateral tail vein and the mice were given the analog AD2725 in the drinking water, starting day 0.

The tumor size was measured twice per week and the tumor volume was calculated from the formula: length × width^2 × π/6. Mice injected with saline or drunk regular water were used as controls. At the end of experiment, mice were sacrificed with CO_2; the tumors on the skin were removed and weighed. All organs of the mice were tested for presence of metastases.

Cytokine assay

The levels of cytokines in the plasma were assayed by ELISA assay. ELISA reagents were purchased as Opt. EIA Cytokine ELISA sets from BD Biosciences (San Diego, CA, USA) and the respective cytokines were analyzed according to the manufacturer's protocol as previously described [20].

Statistical analysis

Most results are based on experiments run in triplicates at least twice, except where indicated. Statistical analyses were performed by Student's t-test (except where indicated) and the results were considered statistically significant when $p<0.05$.

Results

Cytotoxic effects of the sphingolipid analogs

MDA-MB-435 cells (0.1×10^6 cells/ml, 100μl/well) were grown overnight in RPMI-1640 without FCS in 96-well plates, then incubated for 24 hours with increasing concentrations of three ceramide analogs AD2646, AD2673 and AD2725. The viability of cells were determined by the MTT assay, all the synthetic drugs exhibited cytotoxicity toward breast cancer cell line MDA-MB-435 based on a dose respond manner (Figure 1B), the estimated IC50 of AD2725 was 12.5 μM. Trypan blue staining results further showed that all the 3 synthetic analogs of ceramide severely damaged the breast cancer cells. AD2725 as a ceramide analog was used for a further study in vivo (average of 2 experiments, each one in triplicates).

Induction of apoptosis by the analogs

Caspase-3 analysis: MDA-MB-435 cells (1×10^6 cells/ml) were incubated for 3 hours with 20 μM AD2725, the cells were collected and induction of apoptosis was analyzed by the Caspase-3 activity procedure. As shown in Figure 1C, AD-2725 increased the Caspase-3 activity 4-5 fold relative to the control in which the cells were grown without the analogs (Figure 1C).

DNA laddering: In a small flask 2×10^5 of MDA-MB-435 cells/ml were seeded, 20 μM each of AD2725 and AD2646 were added and incubation for 24 hours. Cells were trypsinized and harvested; the genomic DNA was extracted, quantified and electrophoresed. Figure 1D shows the DNA electrophoresis on 1.5% agarose gel. DNA laddering was seen after 24 hours analogs treatment and without in control. In parallel experiments (not shown), the DNA laddering was not appeared after 6 hours when the concentration of the analogs was 20 μM, but when the concentration of AD2725 raised to 80 μM, considerable DNA fragments laddering was observed after 5 hours and was strengthened after 7 hours.

Quantification of cellular ceramide: As shown in HL-60 cell with ceramide analogs by Dagan et al. [19], incubation of MDA-MB-435 cells with AD2725 showed elevated cellular ceramide (Figure 2). This was measured by the conversion of pyrene-dodecanoic acid (P12) to pyrene dodecanoylsphingosine (P12-ceramide). In the current study, 6×10^6 MDA-MB-435 cells were incubated with 50 μM of P12 for 3 hours in the absence or presence of 20 μM of AD2646 or AD2725. The lipids were extracted, applied to a thin layer chromatography plate, and was developed in a mixture of chloroform–methanol–ammonia 95:5:0.5 (by volume). The P12-ceramide spots were visualized with a UV-lamp, and then were scraped, the lipid was extracted and the fluorescence was quantified in a spectrofluorometer., In Figure 2, the values of ceramides are presented as the fluorescent units divided by the cellular protein, indicating that AD2646 resulted in a 2.3 fold increase and AD2725 in a 2.6 fold P12-ceramide increased compared to the control.

Effect of AD2725 on the growth of MDA-MB-435 Xenografts: CD1-Nude mice were irradiated with 400 cGy TBI and following one day, each mouse was injected i.d. into one flank with 4×10^6 MDA-MB-435 cells in a volume of 0.1ml. After one day the mice were injected i.p. with 5 mg/kg of AD2725 in 10% CE saline daily. A control group (n=8) of mice was similarly treated with saline. As seen in (Figure 3A) after 25 days of daily injections, the tumors in AD2725 injected mice were significantly smaller than that of the controls. In another experiment the mice were injected i.d. with 4×10^6 MDA-MB-435 cells and when the tumors were palpated after a week, the ceramide analog AD2725 was injected i.p. for another 6 weeks. Also in these experiments there was a significant inhibition of the tumor growth, measured up to 25-50 days (Figure 3B).

Survival of nude mice injected i.v. with human breast cancer cells and treated with AD2725: CD1-Nude mice, 6 mice in each group, were irradiated with 400 cGy, and one day latter injected intravenously with 5×10^6 MDA-MB-435 cells and AD2725 (10 mg/kg) was administrated by intraperitoneal injections after two hours, and then continue 60 injections, starting day 0, 6 days per week. Figure 4A shows that all the treated mice by AD2725 survived till 80 days while the control mice started to die on 43 days and 2 mice of 6 died till 80 days. In another experiment, 8 mice in each group were injected with 5×10^6 breast cancer cells i.v. and the ceramide analog AD2725 was administered in the drinking water (10 mg/kg, starting day 0). The mice were followed up for 100 days. Figure 4B shows that mice treated with AD2725 in daily drink did not lose weight and survived more than 100 days. On the other hand 5 of the 8 mice in the control group died (Figure 4B).

Ceramide analog AD2725 effect on cytokine profile: Cytokine concentrations of IL-12, IFN-γ and IL10 were assessed by ELISA in sera from each group of mice. A significant reduction of IL10 was seen in AD2725 treated mice compared to the vehicle control (p<0.05). IFN- and IL-12 were significantly elevated in AD2725 treated mice compared to control (p<0.05) (Table 1).

Discussion

The accumulation of intracellular ceramide as a result of a) treatment by ceramide analogs *in vitro* [21], b) modification of endogenous ceramide metabolism [22], c) inhibition of the conversion of ceramide [23] and d) the induction of de novo ceramide synthesis [24] cause cancer cell death through apoptosis. Our results and those of others illuminate the potential therapeutic utility of ceramide to cancer. In this study, we show that the application of an analog of ceramide AD2725 has a cytotoxic effect on MDA-MB-435 breast cancer cells and 5 μM of AD2725 may reduce the number of cancer cells. These results are in agreement with other previous studies showing that ceramide can effectively induce apoptosis in tumor cells [25,26]. Moreover, in this study we show that AD2725 exhibited mitochondrial toxicity (IC50 12.5 μM) leading to cell death, we proposed that the mechanism of cell death is because of the accumulation of ceramide in mitochondria. The mechanism of ceramide induced apoptosis has been well established, the elevated ceramide in mitochondria is responsible for mitochondria dysfunction including loss of electron potential, cytochrome C release and prerequisites for caspase activation [27,28].

In agreement with these data, our results show a significant inhibition of growth of the human breast cancer cells MDA-MB-435 *in vivo* as xenograft in nude mice. The mice that were injected i.v. with tumor cells and drank water with AD2725 did not lose weight and survived more than 100 days, whereas 60% of the control died within this period. Same as our previously study in TSU-Pr1 prostate cancer model [29], we found mice injected i.v. with MDA-MB-435 cells and treated i.p. with AD2725 showed a remarkable reduction of metastases in internal organs of the survivors, whereas all control mice died with developed metastases tumors (data not show). Measuring the cytokine

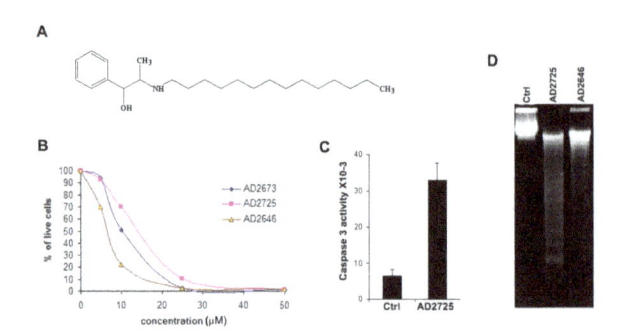

Figure 1: Structures of AD2725, effects of the analogs AD2725, AD2646 and AD2673 on viability of MDA-MB-435 cells and induction of cell apoptosis. A: The chemical structures of the non-natural ceramide analogs AD2725. B: Effects of AD2725 on viability of tumor cell MDA-MB-435. MDA-MB-435 Cells (10^ 5/well) were plated overnight in serum free medium, and then were incubated with increasing concentrations of AD AD2725, AD2646 and AD2673 for 24 hours. The cells were collected and the number of viable cells determined, cell damage/death was determined by trypan blue staining as described in Materials and Methods. C and D: Inductions of apoptosis were measured by Caspase-3 activity and DNA laddering. MDA-MB-435 cells were incubated for 3 hours with 20 μM of AD2725. The cells were collected and apoptosis was analyzed by quantification of Caspase-3 activity (C): MDA-MB-435cells were incubated with AD2646 or AD2725 for 24 hours with 20 μM of the analogs; DNA was extracted and treated as described in Materials and Methods (D): Lane1: Control without analog; Lane2: with AD2725 and Lane3: AD2646 treatment.

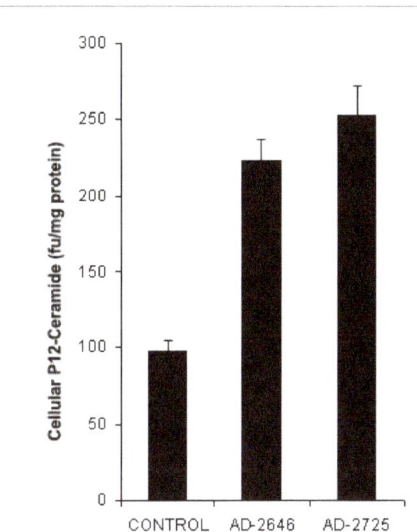

Figure 2: Elevation of cellular ceramide following incubation with the analogs. MDA-MB-435cells were incubated for 3 hours with 20 µM of AD2646 or AD2725 in the presence of 50 µM pyrene dodecanoic acid (P12). The cells were collected, the lipids extracted, applied to thin layer chromatography plates and the P-12-ceramide was quantified as described in materials and methods.

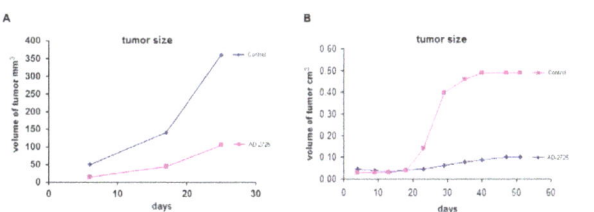

Figure 3: Inhibition of subcutaneous growth of MDA-MB-435 tumor in CD1 NUDE mice. A: CD1 NUDE mice were injected intradermally into one flank with 5 × 10⁶ MDA-MB-435cells, and next day the mice were injected i.p. with the analog AD2725 near the tumor site with 10 mg/kg of AD2725 in 10% Cremophor, control group mice were injected by Cremophor-ethanol (vehicle). B: MDA-MB-435cells (5 × 10⁶ cells in 0.2 ml medium) was injected i.d. into one flank of mice, when the tumors were palpable after one week; the mice were injected daily i.d. near the tumor site with 10 mg/kg of AD2725 in 10% Cremophor and 10% ethanol. The tumor size was measured twice per week and the tumor volume was calculated form the formula: length × width² × π/6. Tumor sizes were determined as described in materials and methods.

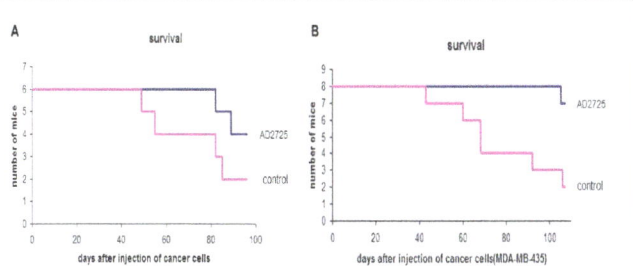

Figure 4: Survival of CD1 Nude female mice injected intravenously with MDA-MB-435 cells followed by intraperitoneal injections and daily water drinking with AD2725. A: MDA-MB-435cells (5 × 10⁶) were injected i.v. and 2 hours later the mice were treated with the analog AD2725. Daily i.p. injections of AD2725 were continued for 23 days, followed by 7 bi-daily injections. Survival of the mice was followed for 7 more weeks without injections. B: MDA-MB-435 cells (5 × 10⁶ cells in 0.2ml medium) were injected i.v. into the lateral tail vein and the mice were given AD2725 in the drinking water, starting day 0.

In vivo treatment of Mice	Number of Mice		Cytokine evaluated	pg/ml Median	pg/ml Range
AD2725	4	Plasma	IL-10	10	10-660
Vehicle	4	Plasma	IL-10	372	19-820
AD2725	4	Plasma	IL-12	217	122-3800
Vehicle	4	Plasma	IL-12	15	10-1080
AD2725	6	Plasma	IF N gamma	115	10-240
Vehicle	7	Plasma	IF N gamma	10	10-185

Table 1: Cytokine levels in the plasma from untreated and AD2725 treated mice.

levels in the plasma revealed a significant reduction in IL-10 level in the AD2725 treated mice and a huge elevation in IL-12 and IFN-γ. IFN-γ plays a crucial role in enhancing tumor cell cytotoxicity and this has been showed in T cells mediated breast cancer (MCF-7) cells killing [30]. Preclinical studies demonstrat that IL-12 promotes specific anti-tumor immunity in several types of tumors [30]. Those results that IL-12 induced production of IFN-γ and suppression of IL-10 are in agreement with ours. Ceramide down-regulates LPS-stimulated production of IL-5, IL-10, and IL-13 [31]; the pro-inflammatory cytokine (eg. TNF--∝) mediated synthesis of ceramide can be inhibited by IL-10 and IL-13 through the activation of PI3-kinase [29]. Elevating Th1 related cytokines and reducing Th2 related IL-10 is responsible for eradication of tumor cells, vaccination with breast cancer cells that were transfected by pcDNA-IL-12 induced a Th1 dominant immune response and resulted in IL-12 secretion and tumor regression in mice [30]. Eguchi et al. [32] suggested that IL-12 stimulates non-specific killing, they showed that transduction of the IL-12 gene to MC38 significantly reduced tumorigenicity in immunocompetent mice. Lee et al. [33] showed that herbal prescription also significantly inhibited liver tumor metastasis and caused a marked increase of Th1 cytokine (IFN-γ) and a decrease of Th2 cytokine (IL-4) stimulated by Concanavalin A. Tsung et al. [34] demonstrated that IL-12 played an essential role in the induction of Th1 response against tumors and showed that IL-12 caused complete regression of 10-days s.c. tumors (4-8 mm) with activation of NO synthase and induction of macrophages. In addition, Park et al. and Cohen et al. [35,36] summarized that healthy women with a family history of breast cancer have shown decreased immune responses, such as low NK cell activity and low Th1-cytokine production.

In light of these results, we suggest that administration of ceramide analog AD2725 elevates ceramide in MDA-MB-435 breast cancer cells leading to apoptosis and growth inhibition of tumor. In addition, we propose that ceramide analogs AD-2725 can react as immune-modulators and create a shift of Th2 to Th1. Th1 cells and Th1 associated cytokines can create anti-tumor response which leads to a suppression of tumor growth and induces cell death.

References

1. Kaufmann SH, Earnshaw WC (2000) Induction of apoptosis by cancer chemotherapy. Exp Cell Res 256: 42-49.

2. Hannun YA (1997) Apoptosis and the dilemma of cancer chemotherapy. Blood 89: 1845-1853.

3. Mullen TD, Obeid LM (2012) Ceramide and Apoptosis: Exploring the Enigmatic Connections between Sphingolipid Metabolism and Programmed Cell Death. Anticancer Agents Med Chem 12: 340-363.

4. Hannun YA, Luberto C, Mao C, Obeid LM (2015) Bioactive Sphingolipids in Cancer Biology and Therapy.

5. Mathias S, Peña LA, Kolesnick RN (1998) Signal transduction of stress via ceramide. Biochem J 335: 465-480.

6. Kolesnick RN, Krönke M (1998) Regulation of ceramide production and apoptosis. Annu Rev Physiol 60: 643-665.

7. Morad SA, Cabot MC (2013) Ceramide-orchestrated signalling in cancer cells. Nat Rev Cancer 13: 51-65.

8. Hannun YA, Luberto C (2000) Ceramide in the eukaryotic stress response. Trends Cell Biol 10: 73-80.

9. Jaffrézou JP, Laurent G, Levade T (2002) Ceramide in regulation of apoptosis. Implication in multitoxicant resistance. Subcell Biochem 36: 269-284.

10. Hannun YA, Obeid LM (2002) The Ceramide-centric universe of lipid-mediated cell regulation: stress encounters of the lipid kind. J Biol Chem 277: 25847-25850.

11. Hannun YA, Obeid LM (2008) Principles of bioactive lipid signalling: lessons from sphingolipids. Nat Rev Mol Cell Biol 9: 139-150.

12. Kunkel GT, Maceyka M, Milstien S, Spiegel S (2013) Targeting the sphingosine-1-phosphate axis in cancer, inflammation and beyond. Nat Rev Drug Discov 12: 688-702.

13. Kolesnick R, Fuks Z (2003) Radiation and ceramide-induced apoptosis. Oncogene 22: 5897-5906.

14. Hannun YA (1996) Functions of ceramide in coordinating cellular responses to stress. Science 274: 1855-1859.

15. Yu J, Novgorodov SA, Chudakova D, Zhu H, Bielawska A, et al. (2007) JNK3 signaling pathway activates ceramide synthase leading to mitochondrial dysfunction. J Biol Chem 282: 25940-25949.

16. Gudz TI, Tserng KY, Hoppel CL (1997) Direct inhibition of mitochondrial respiratory chain complex III by cell-permeable ceramide. J Biol Chem 272: 24154-24158.

17. Ganesan V, Perera MN, Colombini D, Datskovskiy D, Chadha K, et al. (2010) Ceramide and activated Bax act synergistically to permeabilize the mitochondrial outer membrane. Apoptosis 15: 553-562.

18. Stover TC, Sharma A, Robertson GP, Kester M (2005) Systemic delivery of liposomal short-chain ceramide limits solid tumor growth in murine models of breast adenocarcinoma. Clin Cancer Res 11: 3465-3474.

19. Dagan A, Wang C, Fibach E, Gatt S (2003) Synthetic non-natural sphingolipid analogs inhibit the biosynthesis of cellular sphingolipids, elevate ceramideand induce apoptotic cell death. Biochim Biophys Acta 1633: 161-169.

20. Ji YH, Weiss L, Zeira M, Abdul-Hai A, Reich S, et al. (2003) Allogeneic cell-mediated immunotherapy of leukemia with immune donor lymphocytes to upregulate antitumor effects and downregulate antihost responses. Bone Marrow Transplant 32: 495-504.

21. Shabbits JA, Mayer LD (2003) Intracellular delivery of ceramide lipids via liposomes enhances apoptosis in vitro. Biochim Biophys Acta 1612: 98-106.

22. Lucci A, Han TY, Liu YY, Giuliano AE, Cabot MC (1999) Modification of ceramide metabolism increases cancer cell sensitivity to cytotoxics. Int J Oncol 15: 541-546.

23. Lafont E, Milhas D, Carpentier S, Garcia V, Jin ZX, et al. (2010) Caspase mediated inhibition of sphingomyelin synthesis is involved in FasL-triggered cell death. Cell Death Differ 17: 642-654.

24. Rath G, Schneider C, Langlois B, Sartelet H, Morjani H, et al. (2009) De novo ceramide synthesis is responsible for the anti-tumor properties of camptothecin and doxorubicin infollicular thyroid carcinoma. Int J Biochem Cell Biol 41: 1165-1172.

25. Mimeault M (2002) New advances on structural and biological functions of ceramide in apoptotic/necrotic cell death and cancer. FEBS Lett 530: 9-16.

26. Kester M, Kolesnick R (2003) Sphingolipids as therapeutics. Pharmacol Res 47: 365-371.

27. Birbes H, El Bawab S, Obeid LM, Hannun YA (2002) Mitochondria and ceramide: intertwined roles in regulation of apoptosis. Adv Enzyme Regul 42: 113-129.

28. Bose A, Baral R (2007) IFNalpha2b stimulated release of IFNgamma differentially regulates T cell and NK cell mediated tumor cell cytotoxicity. Immunol Lett 108: 68-77.

29. Qin JD, Weiss L, Slavin S, Gatt S, Dagan A (2010) Synthetic, non-natural analogs of ceramide elevate cellular ceramide, inducing apoptotic death to prostate cancer cells and eradicating tumors in mice. Cancer Invest 28: 535-543.

30. Shi M, Su L, Hao S, Guo X, Xiang J (2005) Fusion hybrid of dendritic cells and engineered tumor cells expressing interleukin-12 induces type 1 immune responses against tumor. Tumori 91: 531-538.

31. Chiba N, Masuda A, Yoshikai Y, Matsuguchi T (2007) Ceramide inhibits LPS-induced production of IL-5, IL-10, and IL-13 from mast cells. J Cell Physiol 213: 126-136.

32. Eguchi J, Hiroishi K, Ishii S, Mitamura K (2003) Interferon-alpha and interleukin-12 gene therapy of cancer: interferon-alpha induces tumor-specific immune responses while interleukin-12 stimulates non-specific killing. Cancer Immunol Immunother 52: 378-386.

33. Lee SJ, Saiki I, Hayakawa Y, Nunome S, Yamada H, et al. (2003) Antimetastatic and immunomodulating properties of a new herbal prescription, Bojung-bangam-tang. Int Immunopharmacol 3: 147-157.

34. Tsung K, Meko JB, Peplinski GR, Tsung YL, Norton JA (1997) IL-12 induces T helper 1-directed antitumor response. J Immunol 158: 3359-3365.

35. Park NJ, Kang DH (2006) Breast cancer risk and immune responses in healthy women. Oncol Nurs Forum 33: 1151-1159.

36. Cohen M, Klein E, Kuten A, Fried G, Zinder O, et al. (2002) Increased emotional distress in daughters of breast cancer patients is associated with decreased natural cytotoxic activity, elevated levels of stress hormones and decreased secretion of Th1 cytokines. Int J Cancer 100: 347-354.

13

Integrin-Linked Kinase Inactives the Wnt Pathway through Connexin

Youping Yang[1], Hongxia Lin[2], Yangli Zhu[2], Hongwei Wu[2], Ruoyan Wang[2], Jianmin Zhang[2], Linghui Zeng[3], Ximei Wu[3#] and Rongbiao Ying[2*]

[1]The first People's Hospital of Wenling, Wenling, Zhejiang, 317500, China
[2]Taizhou Cancer Hospital, Wenling, Zhejiang, 317500, China
[3]Zhejiang University, Hangzhou, Zhejiang, 310058, China
[#]These authors have equally contributed.

Abstract

One of the hallmarks of cancers is the silencing of tumor suppressor genes and certain signaling pathways. The Wnt pathway is activated in many types of cancers, leading to tumor progression and metastasis. Here we demonstrated that integrin-linked kinase (ILK) plays a critical role in the suppression of the Wnt pathway via decreasing Wnt3a-induced stabilization of β-catenin, which leaded to the block of the functional gap-junctional intercellular communications (GJIC). Inhibition of ILK in prostate cells resulted in the inactivation of the Wnt pathway components GSK3β and inactivation of Lef1 transcription with concomitant inducing of connexins, which forming channels between adjacent cells. In line with the above changes, over-expression of connexin 43 (Cx43) also inhibited the activity of Lef1 transcription factor induced by Wnt3a media and the transcription of target genes of Wnt signaling. Together, our data demonstrates a role for ILK as a regulator of Wnt pathway through Cx43 which is a negative feedback regulation of Wnt signaling and ILK may be a potential cancer therapeutic target.

Keywords: ILK; Wnt signaling; Connexin 43; Prostate tumor cells

Abbreviations: ILK: Integrin-Linked Kinase; Cx43: Connexin 43; Gjs: Gap Junctions; GJIC: Intercellular Communication via Gap Junctions; Lef-1: Lymphoid Enhancer-Binding Factor-1; TCF: T Cell Factors

Introduction

Tumor progression, metastatic potential and response to therapy depend on complex genetic, epigenetic and tumor micro environmental interplay. Secreted signaling molecules of the Wnt family have been widely investigated and found to have a prominent role to induce human malignant diseases, such as breast and prostate cancer [1-3]. In the presence of Wnt stimulation, β- catenin at Thr41, Ser37 and Ser31 sites are dephosphorylated [4], resulting in accumulation of unphosphorylated β-catenin in the cytoplasm. The stabilized β-catenin enters the nucleus, which consequently activates transcription of downstream target genes via lymphoid enhancer-binding factor-1 (Lef-1) and T cell factors (TCF) [5,6]. Integrin-linked kinase (ILK) is an integrin associated actin and tublin cytoskeletal interacting effector, which is involved in the regulation of cell survival, proliferation, and migration [7,8]. ILK coordinates several signaling pathways, and it has been shown to activate Pi3Kinase/Akt, Wnt, TGF-β and epithelial-mesenchymal transition signaling in various types of cancer cells [9-11]. Moreover, siRNA-mediated silencing of ILK in MDA-MB-231, PC3, and other cell lines examined result in inhibition of Ser473-Akt phosphorylation and induction of apoptosis [12,13], and the small-molecule inhibitors of ILK, QLT0267 and T315 [14,15] , exhibit antitumor efficacy in vitro and/or in vivo in various types of cancer cells, in part, by targeting Akt activation. To form an organized multi-cellular structure, the cells within tissues and organs are connected via specialized junctions [16]. The four types of junctions between cells are the adherent junctions, tight junctions, desmosomes and gap junctions (GJs) [17]. Gap junctions are membrane-spanning channels that allow for the movement of small molecules across cell membranes [18,19]. Intercellular communication via gap junctions (GJIC) plays important roles in regulating cell growth and differentiation and in maintaining tissue homeostasis [20,21]. This type of cell communication is often impaired during cancer development, and several members of the connexin protein family have been shown to act as tumor suppressors [16,22,23]. A gap junction may consist of up to several thousand intercellular channels. One channel is formed by two hemi channels called connexins, with each composed of six connexin protein subunits.

The connexin protein family comprises 21 members in humans, of which the best studied isoform is connexin 43 (Cx43) [17,21]. One potential regulator of gap junction expression and function that might have important implications for developmental processes as well as for normal function in adult stages is the Wnt family genes. However, the effect of ILK on GJIC remains elusive. Hence in the present study, we tried to determine whether ILK regulate Cx43 expression and function in prostate tumor cells and the mechanism.

Materials and Method

Cell culture, transfection and infection

All the cell lines used in the present study were obtained from ATCC (Manassas, VA). Wnt3a-expressing and control L cells were used for the production of biologically active Wnt3a conditional media (Wnt3a) and control L media (L), respectively. PC3 cells were maintained in DMEM/F12 1:1 with 10% bovine serum (Life Technologies) according to instructions, DU145 cells were maintained in the DMEM. Wnt3a- and L- conditioned media were used at 1:1 dilution in normal growth media. Cells were harvested by trypsinization, re-suspended in culture media, and transfected with various siRNA or plasmids using Lipofectamine Plus (Invitrogen) according to the manufacturer's instructions. Lentivirus expressing shRNA-ILK or Cx43 was produced as below, and diluted 1:1 with growth media before use. For viral infections, cells were incubated with the virus for 12 hours before switched to growth media.

Lentivirus packaging

To generate shRNA lentivirus, shRNA vectors were co-transfected

*Corresponding author: Rongbiao Ying, Taizhou Cancer Hospital, Wenling, Zhejiang, 317500, China,
E-mail: yingrongbiao@163.com

into HEK293T cells with the packaging plasmids pMDL, pREV and pVSVG using Lipofectamine. Supernatants were collected 48 hrs after transfection, and passed through 0.45 μm nitrocellulose filters. PC3 cells were infected with viral supernatants diluted 1:1 with growth media and supplemented with 5 mg/ml polybrene. Lentivirus of over-expression pLVX vectors were co-transfected into HEK293T cells with the packaging plasmids pMD2G and pSPAX and collected the supernatants using the same method.

Luciferase assay

For Lef1 transcriptional activity assays, the indicated cells were plated on 24-well dishes in triplicates and co-transfected with 500 ng of a 10:1 mixture of Lef1 reporter and Renilla. After 24 hrs, the cells were cultured in the media in presence of either L or Wnt3a media for 48 hrs. In some cases, the cells were co-transfected with siRNA oligonucleotides. The luciferase activity was assayed using the dual luciferase reporter assay system (Promega).

Quantitative RT-PCR

PC3 cells were seeded in 6-well plates. At confluence, cells were infected with lentivirus and stimulated with L or Wnt3a media for 48 hrs. Total RNA was extracted using TRIzol reagent (Takara Biotechnology). Messenger RNA levels of ILK, Cx43, Cx32, c-MYC and CyclinD1 were determined by quantitative RT-PCR according to the manufacturer's instructions.

Western blot analysis

Cellular lysates were prepared and proteins were resolved by sodium dodecylsulfate- polyacrylamide gel electrophoresis. Proteins were transferred to PVDF membranes. The blots were blocked with 3% bovine serum albumin for 1 h at room temperature and probed with rabbit anti-human antibodies against p-glycogen synthase kinase (GSK) 3β, GSK3β, ILK, GAPDH.

Immunoprecipitation

PC3 cells were plated 1×10^4 cells/cm^2 overnight, after a variety of treatments. Cytosolic and nuclear fractions of cells were prepared by using NE-PER Nuclear and Cytoplasmic Extraction Reagents (Thermo Scientific, Waltham, MA, USA) as per the manufacturer's instructions. β-Actin and Lamin-B were used as the internal standards for the cytosolic and nuclear fractions, respectively.

Statistical analysis

With the exception of western blot analysis, graphical data are presented as mean values ± standard error (SD). P-values were calculated using unpaired Student's t-tests comparing control with treated cells. Statistically significant differences are indicated within the text and by asterisks. Data are representative of at least three independent experiments.

Results

Inhibition of ILK activity decreased Wnt3a-induced activation of Lef1 transcriptional activity

The Wnt signaling pathway is required during embryonic development and for the maintenance of homeostasis in adult tissues. However, aberrant activation of the pathway is implicated in a number of human disorders, including cancer of the gastrointestinal tract, breast, liver, melanoma, and hematologic malignancies. To determine a potential role of ILK in canonical Wnt pathway, we initially examined

activity of the Lef1 transcription factor in different human cancer cell lines. As shown in (Figure1A and 1B) Lef1-luciferase activity induced by Wnt3a media was suppressed significantly upon siRNA-mediated knockdown of ILK expression in PC3 and DU145 prostate tumor cells, indicating that inhibition of ILK leads to Lef1 inactivation in these cell lines. In contrast, over-expression of ILK significantly induced the Lef1-luciferase activity by 2 fold (Figure 1C and 1D). These data suggest that inhibition of ILK negates canonical Wnt signaling, in line with this observation, over-expression of ILK induced canonical Wnt signaling in either the presence or absence of Wnt3a.

Inhibition of ILK activity decreased Wnt3a-induced stabilization of β- catenin

Given that β-catenin is the central signal transducer of the Wnt signaling pathway, we next examined the effect of the inhibition of ILK activity on β-catenin protein content, and Wnt3a-induced stabilization of β-catenin in prostate tumor cells. Wnt3a induced the β-catenin protein levels in cytosolic and nuclear fractions by 1.5 and 3.0 fold in PC3 cells, respectively. Whereas knockdown of ILK decreased nuclear fraction of β-catenin by 67% in the presence of Wnt3a and had no obvious effect on the basal levels of cytoplasmic β-catenin (Figure 2A). Silencing of ILK also reduced nuclear β-catenin protein levels in response to recombinant Wnt3a protein in DU145 cells (Figure 2B). β-catenin stabilization is considered as the key factor in the activation of the downstream components of Wnt signaling pathway. Phosphorylation of β-catenin at Ser45 by casein kinase-1 (CK1) and at Thr41, Ser37, and Ser33 by GSK3β regulates its stabilization in the cytosol, and the phosphorylated β-catenin is recognized by E3 ubiquitin ligase and undergoes proteolytic degradation. To determine the role of ILK in the stabilization of β-catenin, we assessed changes in β-catenin

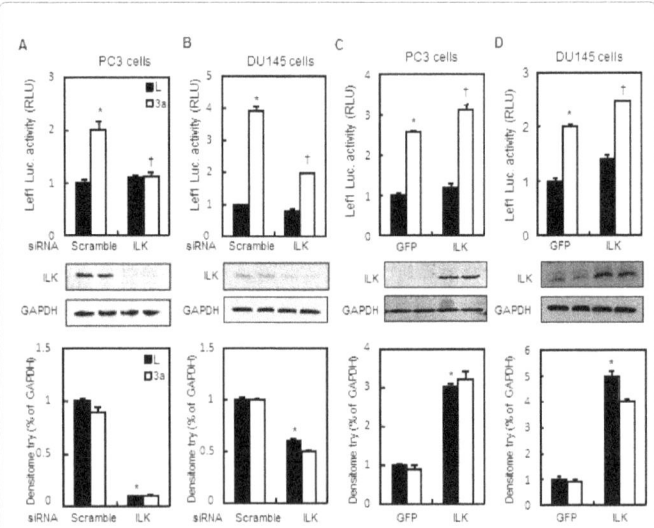

Figure 1: Silencing ILK leaded to functional inactivation of Lef1 in prostate cells. (A, B) Silencing ILK affected the Lef1 luciferase activity. Co-transfected indicated cells with the Lef1 luciferase, Renilla luciferase plasmids and respective siRNAs, non-silencing control (scramble) or siRNAs against ILK (siILK). After 24 hrs, PC3 and DU145 cells were further cultured for 24 hrs in the presence of L or Wnt3a conditional media. Upper panel, representative western blots of ILK, lower panel, histogram representing ILK. (C, D) Over-expression of ILK affected the Lef1 luciferase expression in the presence of L (-) or Wnt3a (+) conditional media. After co-transfection with the reporter constructs, cells were infected with lentivirus respective expression of GFP or ILK, then cultured for 24 hrs in conditional media.*p<0.05 vs. L media and control siRNA (or GFP), †p<0.05 vs. Wnt3a media and control siRNA(or GFP).

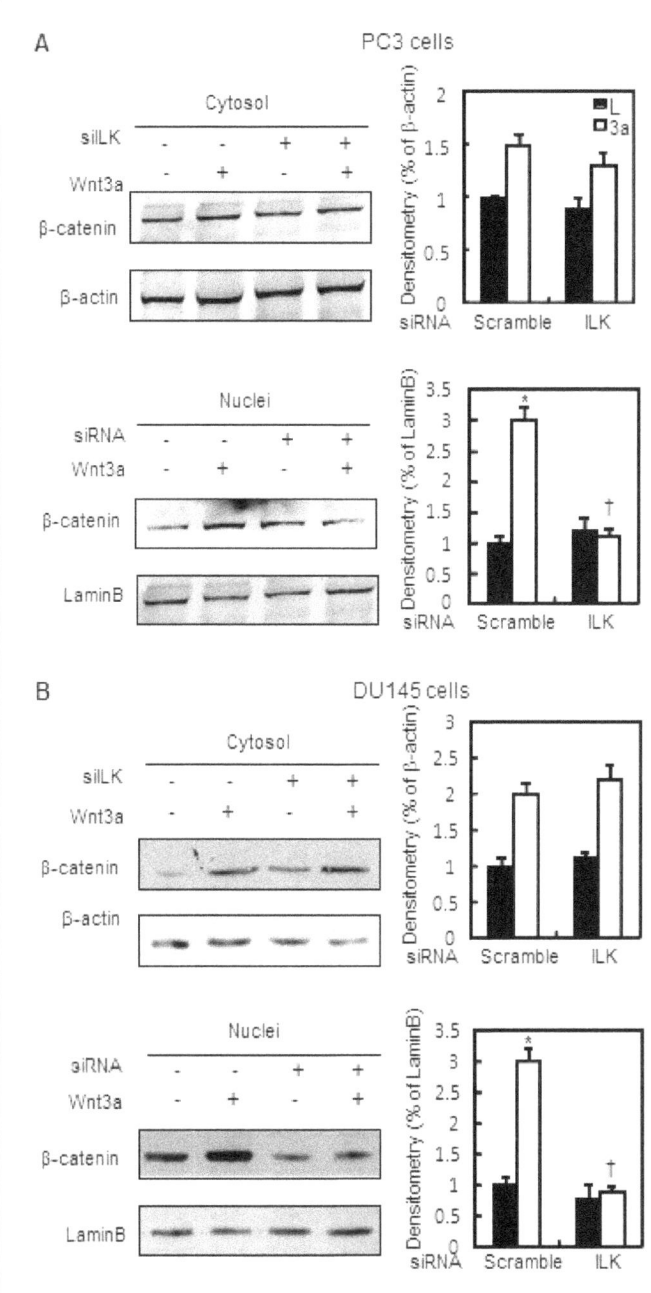

Figure 2: β-Catenin levels in prostate cells effected by ILK in the presence or absence of Wnt3a. (A) Silencing ILK reduced β-catenin protein levels in nuclear fractions of PC3 cells. Western blot analyses of β-catenin levels in cytosolic and nuclear fractions of PC3 cells transfected with siRNA in the presence of L(−) or Wnt3a (+) conditional medium for 24 h. Left panel, representative western blots of β-catenin, right panel, histogram representing. (B) Silencing ILK reduced β-catenin protein levels in nuclear fractions of DU145cells. The signal from the first band was defined as 1.

Then, we performed reporter assays and co-immunoprecipitation to confirm GSK3β signaling as a downstream event of ILK signals in the regulation of β-catenin stabilization. GSK3β inhibitor, SB216763, increased Lef1-luciferase activity but showed no significant effect in PC3 cells expressing ILK siRNA (Figure 3B). Furthermore, protein complexes precipitated with a ILK antibody contained an abundance of GSK-3β as well as ILK as expected, suggesting that physical interactions exist between endogenous ILK and GSK-3β (Figure 3C).

Taken together, these observations suggest that inhibition of ILK may suppress canonical Wnt signaling through inducing GSK3β-mediated phosphorylation of β-catenin at Thr41, Ser37, and Ser33 sites.

Effects of ILK inhibition on growth and migration of prostate cancer cells

Our above results have indicated that ILK is involved in Wnt/β-catenin signaling, to examine the role of ILK in growth of prostate cancer cells, we tested the expression of canonical Wnt signaling target genes in the presence or absence of Wnt3a in PC3 cells. Wnt3a not only increased mRNA levels of CyclinD1 and c-Myc (Figure 4B and 4C), but also increased the expression of connexin 43 (Cx43) and Cx32, encoded gap junctions (Figure 4D and 4E). These observations suggest that ILK

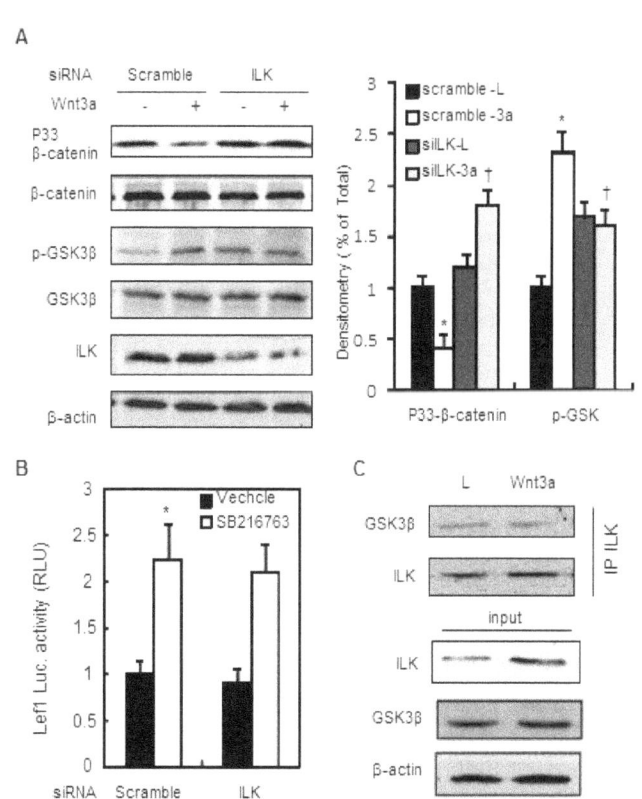

Figure 3: Stabilization of β-catenin affected by ILK in PC3 cells. (A) Silencing ILK affected the activation of GSK3β and stabilization of β-catenin in PC3 cells. After transfected with respective siRNAs and further cultured for 48 hrs, cells were stimulated with L or Wnt3a media for 1 hrs. Left panel, representative western blots of β-catenin and GSK3β, right panel, histogram representing. (B) Effects of GSK3β inhibitor on Lef1 luciferase activities in PC3 cells transfected with siRNAs in the presence of L orWnt3a conditional medium. (C) Co-immunoprecipitation of endogenous GSK3β and ILK. After Wnt3a treatments, PC3 cells were subjected to immunoprecipitation and western blot analyses by using the indicated antibodies. The signal from the first band was defined as 1. *p<0.05 vs. L media and vehicle treatment.

phosphorylation in PC3 cells. The levels of β-catenin phosphorylation at Ser33 sites in PC3 cells transfected with ILK or control (Scramble) siRNA were examined in either the presence or absence of Wnt3a media. Phosphorylation of β-catenin at Ser33 was reduced in response to Wnt3a (50%) but induced by siILK (Figure 3A). Parallel to the changes of phosphorylation levels of β- catenin, Wnt3a increased the GSK3β phosphorylation at Ser9 while siILK attenuated it.

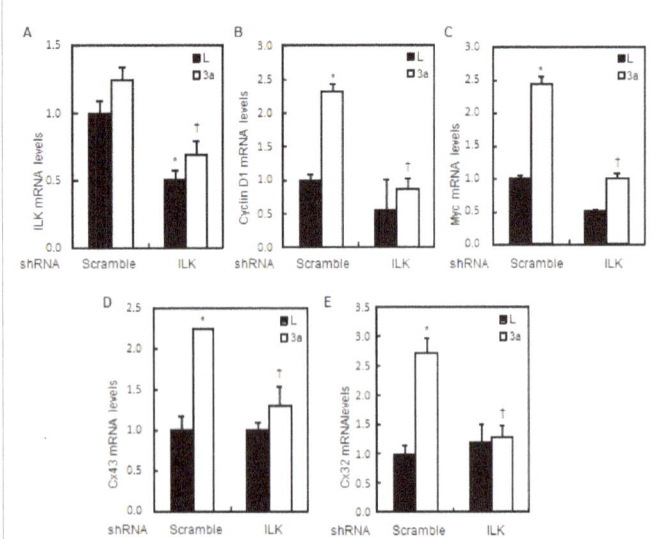

Figure 4: The expression levels of canonical Wnt signaling target genes. (A) The efficiency of knockdown of ILK. Infected PC3 cells by respective lentivirus, and then cultured for 48hrs. (B and C) The mRNA levels of target genes of Wnt pathway affected by ILK. (D and E) The mRNA levels of Connexin tested by RT-PCR. *p<0.05 vs. L media and control lentivirus, †p<0.05 vs. Wnt3a media and contro lentivirus.

may be associated with intercellular communication via gap junctions. Proliferation rate was examined to detect the effect of inactivation of Wnt pathway in prostate cells. As shown in Figure 5A, the growth curves were shown that the proliferation of the cells treated with Wnt3a media was increased compared to the cells treated with L media after 24 hrs of culture, whereas the proliferation of PC3 cells infected by ILK-shRNA-expressing (shILK) lentiviruses slowdown. To assess the role of ILK in cell migration, we performed the wound-healing assay. Scrape wounds were introduced into confluent monolayers of PC3 cells and wound closure rates monitored at 24 hourly intervals in the PC3 cells infected with shILK lentiviruses, whereas significant increase in closure rates occurred in PC3 cells infected with scramble-shRNA-expressing (scramble) lentiviruses (Figure 5B). Thus, inhibition of ILK reduced cell proliferation and migration in prostate cells, these may be associated with the change of intercellular communication via gap junctions.

Cx43 constrain growth of prostate cancer cells by interfering with the Wnt/β-catenin pathway

Impairment of gap junctional intercellular communication, caused by mutations or loss of function of connexins, especially Cx43 which is expressed in several tissues and organs, like heart, gonads, lens and skin, is involved in a number of diseases. Our above results have indicated that ILK is involved in Wnt/β-catenin signaling and affects the mRNA levels of Cx43 in prostate cells. In order to examine the role of connexin in tumor progression, we tested the effect of Cx43 on proliferation. Wnt3a promoted PC3 cells proliferation slightly, whereas cells ectopically expression of Cx43 slowed down the proliferation compared with control (Figure 6A). The mRNA levels of CyclinD1, the target genes of Wnt/β-catenin signaling were induced by Wnt3a media but attenuated by over-expression of Cx43 (Figure 6B). Then we examined the apoptosis affected by Cx43 in PC3 cells. Western blotting results showed that over-expression of Cx43 induced the levels of caspase3 and caspase9 (Figure 6C). These observations raise the possibility that ILK affected the PC3 cells proliferation and vitality due to the abnormal expression of Cx43.

Discussion

ILK has received much attention in light of the mechanistic link between aberrant ILK up-regulation and tumor progression in many types of human malignancies including breast, colon, liver, ovary, pancreas, prostate, stomach, and thyroid [24-26]. ILK is well known as a critical regulator in the surviving of cancer cell through the Akt pathway [27]. In addition, the Wnt pathway plays an important role in the maintenance of the balance of the cell number and in the promotion of tumor genesis [28-30]. Recently accumulative data suggest two different roles of ILK in the regulation of the Wnt signaling pathway in mammalian cells [10,28]. Firstly, as an intermediate regulator in

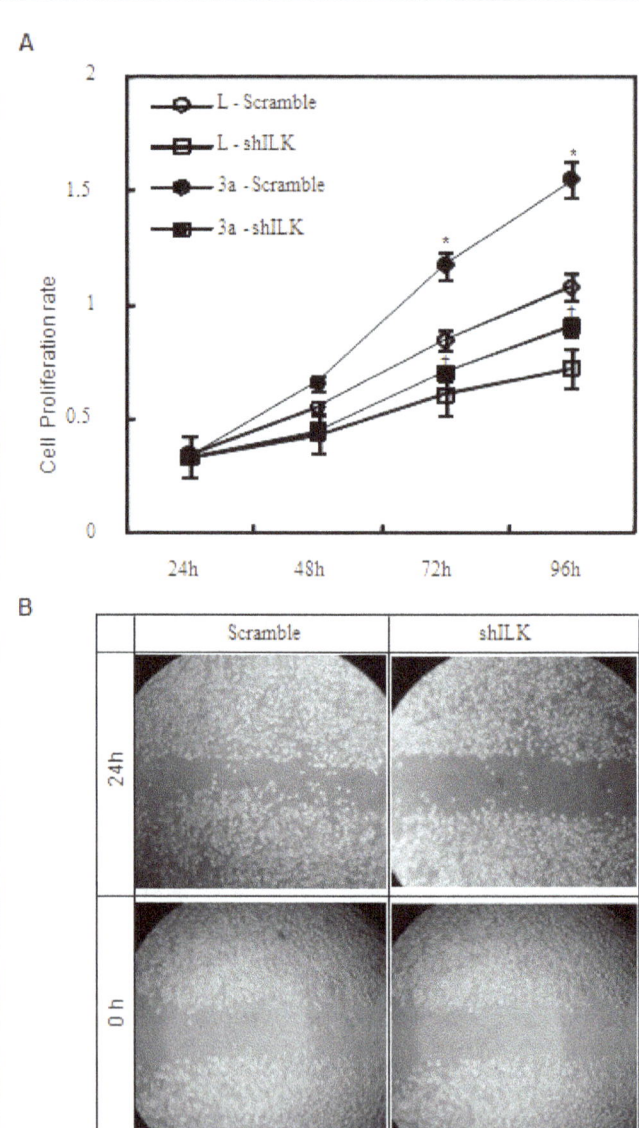

Figure 5: Effects of ILK inhibition on growth and migration of prostate cancer cells. (A) Cell proliferation interfered by siILK. All cells were infected by respective lentivirus, control (scramble) or silencing ILK (shILK), and seeded in 96-well plates, each well containing approximately 2 × 103 cells. After 24, 48, 72 or 96 hrs stimulated with condition media, cells were incubated with CCK8 for 1 hrs and tested the OD. (B) Silencing ILK affected the migration of PC3 cells. PC3 cells infected by respective lentivirus were plated in 6-well plates, and made a straight scratch using a pipette tip, after all the cultures are confluent. *p<0.05 vs. L media and control lentivirus, †p<0.05 vs. Wnt3a media and control lentivirus.

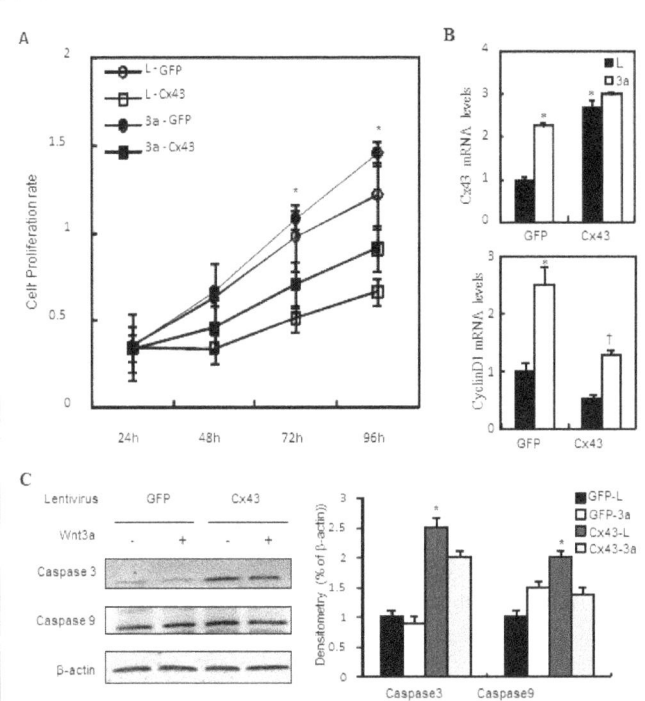

Figure 6: Cx43 constrained growth of PC3 cells. (A) Cell proliferation interfered by Cx43. Infected cells were seeded in 96-well plates, and stimulated with condition media for 24, 48, 72 or 96 hrs. (B) mRNA levels of CyclinD1 and Cx43 affected by Cx43 lentivirus. Infected PC3 cells with lentivirus, control (GFP) or over-expression of Cx43 (Cx43), and then stimulated with conditional media for 48hrs. (C) Ectopic expression of Cx43 enhanced levels of apoptosis. PC3 cells were infected with respective lentivirus and stimulated by conditional media for 48hrs. Left panel, representative western blots of Caspase3 and Caspase9, right panel, histogram representing. *p<0.05 vs. L media and control lentivirus, †p<0.05 vs. Wnt3a media and control lentivirus.

the acute stabilization of β-catenin by Wnt3a, ILK may play role in the multi-protein β-catenin destruction complex [31,32]. Secondly, there is a more pronounced effect of ILK inhibition on the nuclear accumulation of β-catenin [33]. Thus, ILK could also play a role in nuclear localization of β-catenin. Our research indicated ILK was able to induce inhibitory phosphorylation of GSK-3β, which modulates activities of transcription factors Lef1/Tcf, including activator protein β-catenin and supported this notion in prostate cells such as PC3 and DU145.

The communication between cells and their microenvironment induces activation or inactivation of intracellular signaling pathways and the survival of tumor cells depend on their ability to adapt to their environment [34]. Impaired gap junction intercellular communication was observed in cancer cells nearly 50 years ago [35]. In the normal colonic epithelial tissue, three connexin isoforms, connexin 26 (Cx26), Cx32 and Cx43, have been shown to be expressed at the protein level [36]. Colorectal cancer development is associated with loss of connexins expression or re-localization of connexins from the plasma membrane to intracellular compartments. It has been reported that ILK activates the expression of YB-1, which facilitates EMT through the translational activation of Snail and other EMT- inducing transcription factors [37,38]. This premise is supported by the finding that genetic knockdown or pharmacological inhibition of ILK could inhibit EMT, in part, through the suppression of Snail expression in PC3 and MDA-MB-468 cells [38,39]. However, to date the role of ILK as an intermediate regulator of GJIC is not clear. Our data suggest

ILK inhibits the level of connexins in PC3 cancer cells. These results raise the possibility that ILK promotes tumor progression through blocking the GJIC. We have observed that there is a more pronounced effect of ILK promoting tumor progression. Some data pointed that Wnt3a induced the expression of Cx43 [40,41]. In this paper we found ectopically expression of Cx43, the target gene of Wnt pathway in PC3 cells inhibit the proliferation which is consistent with the results down regulation of ILK. Our hypothesis is that inhibition or genetic depletion of ILK down-regulate the expression of Cx43, and reducing the gap junction communication, resulting the change of tumor progression. Our data suggest a novel mechanism of regulation of the Wnt pathway by ILK in tumor cells. With this work, we have provided new insights of Wnt pathway and provided data suggesting that ILK is a potential therapeutic target of inhibiting tumor cell growth through Cx43.

Acknowledgement

This work was supported by the National Natural Science Foundation of Zhejiang Province (LY12H16005 to YPY).

References

1. Park JH, Kwon HY, Sohn EJ, Kim KA, Kim B, et al. (2013) Inhibition of Wnt/Î²-catenin signaling mediates ursolic acid-induced apoptosis in PC-3 prostate cancer cells. Pharmacol Rep 65: 1366-1374.

2. Prasad CP, Gupta SD, Rath G, Ralhan R (2007) Wnt signaling pathway in invasive ductal carcinoma of the breast: relationship between beta-catenin, dishevelled and cyclin D1 expression. Oncology 73: 112-117.

3. Verras M, Sun Z (2006) Roles and regulation of Wnt signaling and beta-catenin in prostate cancer. Cancer Lett 237: 22-32.

4. Willert K, Shibamoto S, Nusse R (1999) Wnt-induced dephosphorylation of axin releases beta-catenin from the axin complex. Genes Dev 13: 1768-1773.

5. Ishitani T, Ninomiya-Tsuji J, Matsumoto K (2003) Regulation of lymphoid enhancer factor 1/T-cell factor by mitogen-activated protein kinase-related Nemo-like kinase-dependent phosphorylation in Wnt/beta-catenin signaling. Mol Cell Biol 23: 1379-1389.

6. Wodarz A, Nusse R (1998) Mechanisms of Wnt signaling in development. Annu Rev Cell Dev Biol 14: 59-88.

7. Boulter E, Van Obberghen-Schilling E (2006) Integrin-linked kinase and its partners: A modular platform regulating cell-matrix adhesion dynamics and cytoskeletal organization. Eur J Cell Biol 85: 255-263.

8. O'Meara RW, Michalski JP, Anderson C, Bhanot K, Rippstein P, et al. (2013) Integrin-linked kinase regulates process extension in oligodendrocytes via control of actin cytoskeletal dynamics. J Neurosci 33: 9781-9793.

9. Janji B, Melchior C, Vallar L, Kieffer N (2000) Cloning of an isoform of integrin-linked kinase (ILK) that is upregulated in HT-144 melanoma cells following TGF-beta1 stimulation. Oncogene 19: 3069-3077.

10. Oloumi A, Syam S, Dedhar S (2006) Modulation of Wnt3a-mediated nuclear beta-catenin accumulation and activation by integrin-linked kinase in mammalian cells. Oncogene 25: 7747-7757.

11. Persad S, Attwell S, Gray V, Delcommenne M, Troussard A, et al. (2000) Inhibition of integrin-linked kinase (ILK) suppresses activation of protein kinase B/Akt and induces cell cycle arrest and apoptosis of PTEN-mutant prostate cancer cells. Proc Natl Acad Sci U S A 97: 3207-3212.

12. Chen Z, Xing YQ, Xu C (2012) siRNA-mediated downregulation of the integrin-linked kinase alters the proliferation and apoptosis in retinoblastoma cells. Zhonghua yan ke za zhi (Chinese journal of ophthalmology) 48: 159-163.

13. Gao J, Zhu J, Li HY, Pan XY, Jiang R, et al. (2011) Small interfering RNA targeting integrin-linked kinase inhibited the growth and induced apoptosis in human bladder cancer cells. Int J Biochem Cell Biol 43: 1294-1304.

14. Kalra J, Warburton C, Fang K, Edwards L, Daynard T, et al. (2009) QLT0267, a small molecule inhibitor targeting integrin-linked kinase (ILK), and docetaxel can combine to produce synergistic interactions linked to enhanced cytotoxicity, reductions in P-AKT levels, altered F-actin architecture and improved treatment outcomes in an orthotopic breast cancer model. Breast Cancer Res 11: R25.

15. Santos ND, Habibi G, Wang M, Law JH, Andrews HN, et al. (2007) Urokinase-type Plasminogen Activator (uPA) is Inhibited with QLT0267 a Small Molecule Targeting Integrin-linked Kinase (ILK). Transl Oncogenomics 2: 85-97.

16. Martin PE, George CH, Castro C, Kendall JM, Capel J, et al. (1998) Assembly of chimeric connexin-aequorin proteins into functional gap junction channels. Reporting intracellular and plasma membrane calcium environments. J Biol Chem 273: 1719-1726.

17. Saez JC, Berthoud VM, Branes MC, Martinez AD, Beyer EC (2003) Plasma membrane channels formed by connexins: their regulation and functions. Physiol Rev 83: 1359-1400.

18. Gruijters WT (2003) Are gap junction membrane plaques implicated in intercellular vesicle transfer? Cell Biol Int 27: 711-717.

19. Murray SA, Nickel BM, Gay VL (2009) Gap junctions as modulators of adrenal cortical cell proliferation and steroidogenesis. Mol Cell Endocrinol 300: 51-56.

20. Kjenseth A, Fykerud T, Rivedal E, Leithe E (2010) Regulation of gap junction intercellular communication by the ubiquitin system. Cell Signal 22: 1267-1273.

21. Sirnes S, Lind GE, Bruun J, Fykerud TA, Mesnil M, et al. (2015) Connexins in colorectal cancer pathogenesis. Int J Cancer 137: 1-11.

22. McLachlan E, Shao Q, Wang HL, Langlois S, Laird DW (2006) Connexins act as tumor suppressors in three-dimensional mammary cell organoids by regulating differentiation and angiogenesis. Cancer Res 66: 9886-9894.

23. Solan JL, Lampe PD (2009) Connexin43 phosphorylation: structural changes and biological effects. Biochem J 419: 261-272.

24. Persad S, Dedhar S (2003) The role of integrin-linked kinase (ILK) in cancer progression. Cancer Metastasis Rev 22: 375-384.

25. Tan C, Cruet-Hennequart S, Troussard A, Fazli L, Costello P, et al. (2004) Regulation of tumor angiogenesis by integrin-linked kinase (ILK). Cancer Cell 5: 79-90.

26. Teo ZL, McQueen-Miscamble L, Turner K, Martinez G, Madakashira B, et al. (2014) Integrin linked kinase (ILK) is required for lens epithelial cell survival, proliferation and differentiation. Exp Eye Res 121: 130-142.

27. Edwards LA, Thiessen B, Dragowska WH, Daynard T, Bally MB, et al. (2005) Inhibition of ILK in PTEN-mutant human glioblastomas inhibits PKB/Akt activation, induces apoptosis, and delays tumor growth. Oncogene 24: 3596-3605.

28. Naves MA, Requião-Moura LR, Soares MF, Silva-Júnior JA, Mastroianni-Kirsztajn G, et al. (2012) Podocyte Wnt/ss-catenin pathway is activated by integrin-linked kinase in clinical and experimental focal segmental glomerulosclerosis. J Nephrol 25: 401-409.

29. Nusse R (1992) The Wnt gene family in tumorigenesis and in normal development. J Steroid Biochem Mol Biol 43: 9-12.

30. Smalley MJ, Dale TC (2001) Wnt signaling and mammary tumorigenesis. J Mammary Gland Biol Neoplasia 6: 37-52.

31. Oloumi A, McPhee T, Dedhar S (2004) Regulation of E-cadherin expression and beta-catenin/Tcf transcriptional activity by the integrin-linked kinase. Biochim Biophys Acta 1691: 1-15.

32. Xie D, Yin D, Tong X, O'Kelly J, Mori A, et al. (2004) Cyr61 is overexpressed in gliomas and involved in integrin-linked kinase-mediated Akt and beta-catenin-TCF/Lef signaling pathways. Cancer Res 64: 1987-1996.

33. Tan C, Costello P, Sanghera J, Dominguez D, Baulida J, et al. (2001) Inhibition of integrin linked kinase (ILK) suppresses beta-catenin-Lef/Tcf-dependent transcription and expression of the E-cadherin repressor, snail, in APC-/- human colon carcinoma cells. Oncogene 20: 133-140.

34. Serrano I, McDonald PC, Lock F, Muller WJ, Dedhar S (2013) Inactivation of the Hippo tumour suppressor pathway by integrin-linked kinase. Nat Commun 4: 2976.

35. Goodenough DA (1978) Gap junction dynamics and intercellular communication. Pharmacol Rev 30: 383-392.

36. Martin PE, Blundell G, Ahmad S, Errington RJ, Evans WH (2001) Multiple pathways in the trafficking and assembly of connexin 26, 32 and 43 into gap junction intercellular communication channels. J Cell Sci 114: 3845-3855.

37. Gil D, Ciołczyk-Wierzbicka D, Dulińska-Litewka J, Zwawa K, McCubrey JA, et al. (2011) The mechanism of contribution of integrin linked kinase (ILK) to epithelial-mesenchymal transition (EMT). Adv Enzyme Regul 51: 195-207.

38. Serrano I, McDonald PC, Lock FE, Dedhar S (2013) Role of the integrin-linked kinase (ILK)/Rictor complex in TGFβ-1-induced epithelial-mesenchymal transition (EMT). Oncogene 32: 50-60.

39. Kiefel H, Bondong S, Pfeifer M, Schirmer U, Erbe-Hoffmann N, et al. (2012) EMT-associated up-regulation of L1CAM provides insights into L1CAM-mediated integrin signalling and NF-ĸB activation. Carcinogenesis 33: 1919-1929.

40. Du WJ, Li JK, Wang QY, Hou JB, Yu B (2008) Lithium chloride regulates connexin43 in skeletal myoblasts in vitro: possible involvement in Wnt/beta-catenin signaling. Cell Commun Adhes 15: 261-271.

41. Liu X, Liu W, Yang L, Xia B, Li J, et al. (2007) Increased connexin 43 expression improves the migratory and proliferative ability of H9c2 cells by Wnt-3a overexpression. Acta Biochim Biophys Sin (Shanghai) 39: 391-398.

14

Low Serum Zinc and Increased Acid Phosphatase Activity in Type 2 Diabetes Mellitus with Periodontitis Subjects

Pushparani DS*

Department of Biochemistry, SRM Dental College, SRM University, Ramapuram, Chennai-600089, Tamil Nadu, India

Abstract

Micronutrient zinc plays a major role in influencing the periodontal conditions in Type 2 diabetes mellitus (T2DM) subjects. In the developed countries nearly 40% of the people are zinc deficient among the T2DM. Now it is estimated that nearly 2 billion subjects in the developing world may be zinc deficient. The periodontal diseases are highly prevalent and can affect up to 90% of the world wide population. Many chronic diseases have been associated with periodontal disease which results in adverse pregnancy outcomes, cardiovascular disease, stroke, pulmonary disease, and diabetes, but the causal relations have not been established. Zinc in human play an important role in cell mediated immunity and was also an antioxidant and anti-inflammatory agent. Zinc helps in the stabilization of lysosomal membranes. The increased acid phosphatase activity might be a result of destructive processes in alveolar bone in advanced stages of periodontal disease. In light of the available data, the study aimed to show how low serum zinc and increased level of lysosomal enzyme, acid phosphatase affect the subjects of Type 2 diabetes mellitus with periodontitis.

Keywords: Acid phosphatase; Inflammation; Periodontitis; Type 2 diabetes mellitus; Zinc

Introduction

Type 2 diabetes mellitus (T2DM) is one of the most challenging health concerns of the 21st century. It is a chronic disease reaching epidemic levels in both developed and developing countries. According to International Diabetes Federation (IDF), Diabetes Atlas, sixth edition, the prevalence of T2DM is increasing at an alarming rate, affecting 382 million people worldwide in 2013 and this would rise to 592 million in 2035 [1]. The West Pacific Region is home to one quarter of the world's population, and China now has the largest patient population with diabetes as well as Pacific Islands countries with the highest prevalence rates. The incidence of periodontitis is rapidly increasing worldwide and is still a significant problem for many patients with T2DM [2]. The expression of a range of immune mediators, such as C-reactive protein (CRP) and the inflammatory cytokines interleukin (IL)-1, IL-6 and tumour necrosis factor (TNF)-α, are often reported in T2DM [3]. The possible for the dietary components to modulate inflammatory processes are found to be a new approach in the management of T2DM [4].

Periodontitis is considered as one of the main, oral health problems encountered in patients with diabetes mellitus. Periodontitis affects approximately 50% of adults and over 60% of over 65 year olds, with severe periodontitis impacting 10–15% of populations [5,6]. Periodontal disease is a microbially initiated chronic inflammatory disease, in which dysregulated immune-inflammatory processes are responsible for the majority of host tissue destruction, and ultimately tooth loss [7]. Periodontal disease is associated with increased incident diabetes risk, poor glycemic control, and diabetic complications, probably due to the higher levels of systemic proinflammatory mediators that exacerbate insulin resistance [8,9].

Polymorphonuclear leukocytes (PMNLs) are the primary defence cells of the periodontium. In uncontrolled diabetes, reduced PMNL function and defective chemotaxis can give rise to impaired host defences and development of disease [10]. Plenty of microbial antigens stimulate both humoral antibody-mediated and cell mediated immune responses are usually safety, but a continual microbial task in the use of the fore mentioned risks results in the malfunction of both soft and hard tissues, mediated by cytokine and prostanoid flows. Both the host and bacteria in the periodontal biofilm liberate proteolytic enzymes that damage tissue [11]. They release chemotactic factors that hire polymorphonuclear leucocytes into the tissues; if continual, these cells discharge various enzymes that break down tissues. Once a periodontal pocket forms and becomes packed with bacteria, the situation becomes mostly permanent and produce pro-inflammatory cytokines and mediators [12,13]. Peripheral blood monocytes from diabetic subjects produce elevated levels of tumor necrosis factor-alpha (TNF-α) in response to antigens from Porphyromonas gingivalis compared to monocytes from non-diabetic controlsubjects [14]. During phagocytosis, the granular (lysosomal) enzymes are released from polymorphonuclear cells into the extracellular medium.

Gingival epithelial cells function as an innate host defense system to prevent intrusion by periodontal bacteria. However, persistent contact of sub-gingival bacterial biofilm with gingival crevices induces bacterial penetration into periodontal tissues. Immunofluorescence and immunehistochemical techniques have revealed the existence of *Porphyromonas gingivalis, Aggregatibacter actinomycetemcomitans, Prevotella intermedia,* and *Actinomycesnaes lundii* in gingival tissues [15]. In addition, intra cellular localization of several periodontal bacteria, including *P. gingivalis, A. actinomycetemcomitans, Tannerella forsythia,* and *Treponemadenticola* has been identified.

Acid phosphatases (EC 3.1.3.2) are generally classified as non-specific enzymes and often occur in multiple molecular forms [16]. It is one among the hydrolytic enzymes associated with lysosomes of cells from a variety of tissues. They differ in molecular size and cellular localisation, as well as in substrate specificity and susceptibility to

***Corresponding author:** Pushparani DS, Department of Biochemistry, SRM Dental College, SRM University, Ramapuram, Chennai-600089, Tamil Nadu, India, E-mail: ds_pushpa@yahoo.com*

inhibitors. There is also a particular class of ACPs that require metal ions for activity [17]. The Zn^{2+} dependent ACP has been detected in several animal tissues and species [18]; two main molecular forms, differing in tissue distribution, have been found. Brain, heart, skeletal muscle, erythrocytes, lung, spleen, and stomach contain a 62 kDa molecular form of the Zn^{2+} dependent ACP, whereas liver contains a higher molecular weight form of the enzyme. The small intestine and kidney contain both high and low molecular weight forms [19].

Zinc is required by all cell types, playing crucial catalytic, structural and regulatory roles, by binding to a zinc proteome estimated in humans to contain approximately 3000 members [20]. Crystallographic studies have demonstrated the presence of zinc in the crystal of insulin. There are several reasons to suspect, that abnormal zinc metabolism could play a role in the pathogenesis of diabetes mellitus and some of its complications. Several human studies confirmed that diabetes had an effect on disrupting Zn homeostasis. A defect in Zn homeostasis may affect the signal transduction response to insulin and by reducing the production of cytokines, which lead to beta-cell death during the inflammatory process in the pancreas [21]. Under normal conditions Zn is found throughout the pancreas, where it forms an integral component of the insulin crystalline structure [22], serving to stabilize the insulin granule by rendering it less soluble [23].

Zinc interacts with general metabolism of protein, carbohydrate and lipid, as well as on taste, smell, appetite regulation and food consumption. This micronutrient participates both in the synthesis and actions of these hormones, which are intimately linked to bone metabolism. In vitro studies have shown that Zn stimulates osteoblastic bone formation [24]. The basic mechanisms of action of this trace element are intimately linked to the structure and action of countless enzymes involved in many different metabolic processes. In this respect, when Zn specifically acts on cartilage growth it is involved in multiple enzymatic reactions which make this a multi factorial event. Zn could decrease the extent of oxidative damage by decreasing free radical production at the ligand-binding site; and through its role in the Cu–Zn superoxide dismutase enzyme [25,26]. In animals, Zn supplementation lowers elevated blood glucose in genetically obese mice [27] and reduces the extent of lipid peroxidation and atherosclerotic plaques in rabbits on a high-cholesterol diet even though these animals are not Zn deficient [28]. The interaction between glycemic markers and serum zinc levels in humans is unclear. Therefore, with the available data, the present study aimed to study the relationship between serum zinc and acid phosphatase level in type 2 diabetes mellitus with periodontitis.

Material and Methods

Study participants

The study consisted of a total of 600 subjects in the age group of 25 to 56 years. The subjects were divided into four groups, consisting of 150 participants in each group as:

Group I: Control healthy subjects

Group II: T2DM without periodontitis

Group III: T2DM with periodontitis

Group IV: Non-DM with periodontitis

Group I subjects were selected from a generalised population. Group II subjects for the studies were enrolled from the SRM Speciality Hospital, India and group III and group IV subjects were selected from the outpatients attending the Department of Periodontology and Oral Implantology, SRM Dental College, India. The study plan was approved by the Institutional Ethical Committee of Medical and Health Sciences, SRM University, India and an informed written consent was obtained from all the participants.

Clinical assessments

Relevant clinical history and physical examination were recorded for all the subjects. Six milliliters of fasting blood sample was withdrawn from ante-cubital vein under aseptic precautions and collected into the vials for assessment of various parameters. All subjects were submitted blood collection, number of teeth present and missing, pathological migration, and probing depth (PPD) and clinical attachment level (CAL) evaluation.

Patients with diabetes mellitus were under diabetic diet and did not take nutritional supplements and any drugs that are known to interfere with the serum levels of studied metals during the period of study. The healthy controls were not on any kind of prescribed medication or dietary restrictions.

Inclusion and exclusion criteria

All periodontitis individuals included under the category of periodontitis should have more than 30% of the sites with Clinical attachment level (CAL) ≥ 3mm and pocket depth (PD) ≥ 5 mm, at least 2 teeth in each quadrant with the condition of 20 teeth in all the subjects. Diabetic subjects should have T2DM, diagnosed by a physician by means of the oral glucose tolerance test, for at least the past 5 years.

Type 2 diabetic patients having vascular complications as diabetic nephropathy, neuropathy and retinopathy were excluded from the study. Smokers, alcoholics, drug abused, patients who had periodontal therapy six months prior to the study, patients under antibiotics and having systemic disease other than diabetics, taking hormone drugs, lipid lowering drugs, hypotensive diuretics, oral contraceptives, and pregnant women, were excluded from the study.

Basic measurements and assays

BMI was calculated based on measures of body weight and height as weight in kilograms divided by height in meters squared. The systolic and diastolic blood pressure was determined as the mean of two measurements. Blood samples were collected after an overnight fast for each subject. Serum was obtained by centrifuging the blood at 1500 rpm for 10 minutes. HbA1c was analyzed by the high-performance liquid chromatography method (Biosystems S.A, Costa Brava, Spain) and results are expressed in percentage, with a reference value of 5 to 7%. Serum glucose was measured by the glucose oxidase-peroxidase (GOD-POD) method, using the reagent kit purchased from Merck Specialities Private Limited, India.

Serum zinc was estimated, using the Nitro-PAPS (pyridylazo-N-propyl-N-sulfopropylamino-Phenol) method, and the values expressed in µg/dl. Acid phosphatase (ACP) was analysed by the technique described by Gutman and Gutman [29], using di sodium phenyl phosphate as the substrate. The incubations were performed at 37°C for 1 hour, and the reaction was stopped by adding 10% trichloroacetic acid. After removal of the precipitate, the concentration of ACP was determined by the differences in extinction at 620 nm against the reagent blank in a spectrophotometer. This difference in extinction was used as a measure of enzyme activity. The enzyme activity was expressed as micromoles of substrate hydrolysed/ min/ L.

Statistical analysis

Data were presented as mean ± SD (standard deviation). An

unpaired Student's t test and Newman-Keuls multiple comparison test were used to evaluate the differences between groups. Correlations between various variables are done using Pearson's correlation equations. The statistical significance was taken as $p<0.05$. All statistical analysis was performed, using the statistical software package, Winks SDA 7.0.5 (Windows Kwik Stat).

Results

The demographic characteristics within group I (healthy controls), group II (T2DM without periodontitis), group III (T2DM with periodontitis) and group IV (Non-DM with periodontitis) are shown in Table 1.There were no statistical differences in the mean of the systolic blood pressure, and diastolic blood pressure among the four groups. The mean (± SD) percentages of HbA1c levels was found to be 7.74 ± 1.31 in group II and 8.38 ± 1.17 in group III and are statistically significant when compared to control. However, T2DM patients with periodontitis had significantly higher HbA1c than T2DM patients without periodontitis and there was no significant difference between the Group IV and Group I (control) subjects.

The clinical parameters descriptive statistics are shown in Table 2. The mean FBG level was significantly elevated in the group II and group III subjects, when compared to group I and group IV. As expected the mean levels of periodontal probing depth (PPD) and clinical attachment level (CAL), were significantly greater than 4 mm in T2DM with periodontitis and in Non-DM with periodontitis, when compared to healthy subjects.

The serum concentration of zinc in groups I, II, III and IV is shown in Figure 1. According to the Newman-Keuls Multiple Comparison test, the means levels of the serum zinc of group III was lesser than the means of all other groups. At $p<0.05$, the means of group III was significantly different when compared to other groups. Our data show that T2DM with periodontitis (106.8 ± 31.83) individuals have lower zinc than those without this disease. The serum zinc level in T2DM without periodontitis (157.2 ± 45.8, group II) and Non-DM with periodontitis (135.7 ± 51.39, group IV) which are found to be significantly higher when compared to control (113.4 ± 12.65, group I).

The expression of Acid phosphatase was found to be ten times

Parameters	Control Group I	T2DM without periodontitisGroup II	T2DM with periodontitisGroup III	Non-DM withperiodontitisGroup IV
No of subjects	150	150	150	150
Gender (M/F)	80/70	78/72	77/73	75/75
Age, years	35.46 ± 10.74	46.26 ± 10.02***	44.42 ± 10.37***	41.66 ± 10.45***
Duration of diabetes, years	-	8.39 ± 5.35	8.70 ± 4.82	-
HbA1c %	5.20 ± 0.51	7.74 ± 1.31***	8.38 ± 1.17***	5.14 ± 0.56 NS
BMI, kg/m²	22.72 ± 1.5	23.32 ± 1.49**	24.07 ± 1.51**	23.93 ± 1.12**
Systolic blood pressure(mm Hg)	119.5 ± 4.65	126.4 ± 5.70NS	128.8 ± 5.09NS	126.7 ± 8.39NS
Diastolic blood pressure(mm Hg)	72.93 ± 2.10	75.14 ± 1.78NS	79.05 ± 3.03NS	76.47 ± 4.52NS

Values are expressed as Mean ± SD; except for gender (Male, M / Female, F). Glycosylated hemoglobin, HbA1c; Body mass index, BMI. Differences were considered significant at ***$p<0.0001$; **$p<0.001$for parameters of group II, III, IV vs group I and NS, non-significant

Table 1: Demographic characteristics of the study population within the four groups.

Parameters	Control Group I	T2DM without periodontitis Group II	T2DM with periodontitis Group III	Non-DM withperiodontitisGroup IV
No of subjects	150	150	150	150
Gender (M/F)	80/70	78/72	77/73	75/75
FBG, mg/dl	95.28 ± 12.51	183.7 ± 57.16***	176.7 ± 59.12***	96.88 ± 12.67NS
PPD, mm	1.45 ± 0.13	1.42 ± 0.17NS	4.61± 0.51***	4.67 ± 0.46***
CAL, mm	0.708 ± 0.27	0.64 ± 0.49NS	4.91± 0.37***	4.62 ± 0.58***

Values are expressed as Mean ± SD; except for gender (Male, M / Female, F). Fasting blood glucose, FBG; Periodontal probing depth, PPD; Clinical attachment level, CAL. Differences were considered significant at ***$p<0.0001$; **$p<0.001$; *$p<0.05$ for parameters of group II, III, IV vs group I and NS, non-significant.

Table 2: Clinical characteristics of the study population.

Parameters	Control Group I		T2DM without periodontitis Group II		T2DM with periodontitis Group III		Non-DM withperiodontitis Group IV	
	r	p	r	p	r	p	r	P
Zinc								
HbA1c	0.024	0.809	0.000	0.100	0.024	0.813	0.0816	0.420
FBG	−0.107	0.390	0.006	0.446	0.216	0.002*	0.133	0.333
PPD	0.266	0.437	0. 030	0.766	-0.123	0.445	-0.112	0.266
CAL	−0.033	0.331	0.039	0.693	0.065	0.257	0.125	0.214
Acid phosphatase								
HbA1c	-0.139	0.167	-0.045	0.655	0.009	0.924	-0.129	0.199
FBG	-0.141	0.160	0.170	0.049*	-0.023	0.813	0.039	0.696
PPD	-0.008	0.936	-0.003	0.976	0.193	0.054	-0.028	0.777
CAL	-0.038	0.702	0.032	0.746	-0.327	0.000*	-0.062	0.537

Pearson coefficient ratio, r; Glycosylated hemoglobin, HbA1c; Fasting blood glucose, FBG; Periodontal probing depth, PPD; Clinical attachment level, CAL, *significant p value.

Table 3: Pearson correlation between Zinc and Acid phosphatase with other independent variables in the 4 groups.

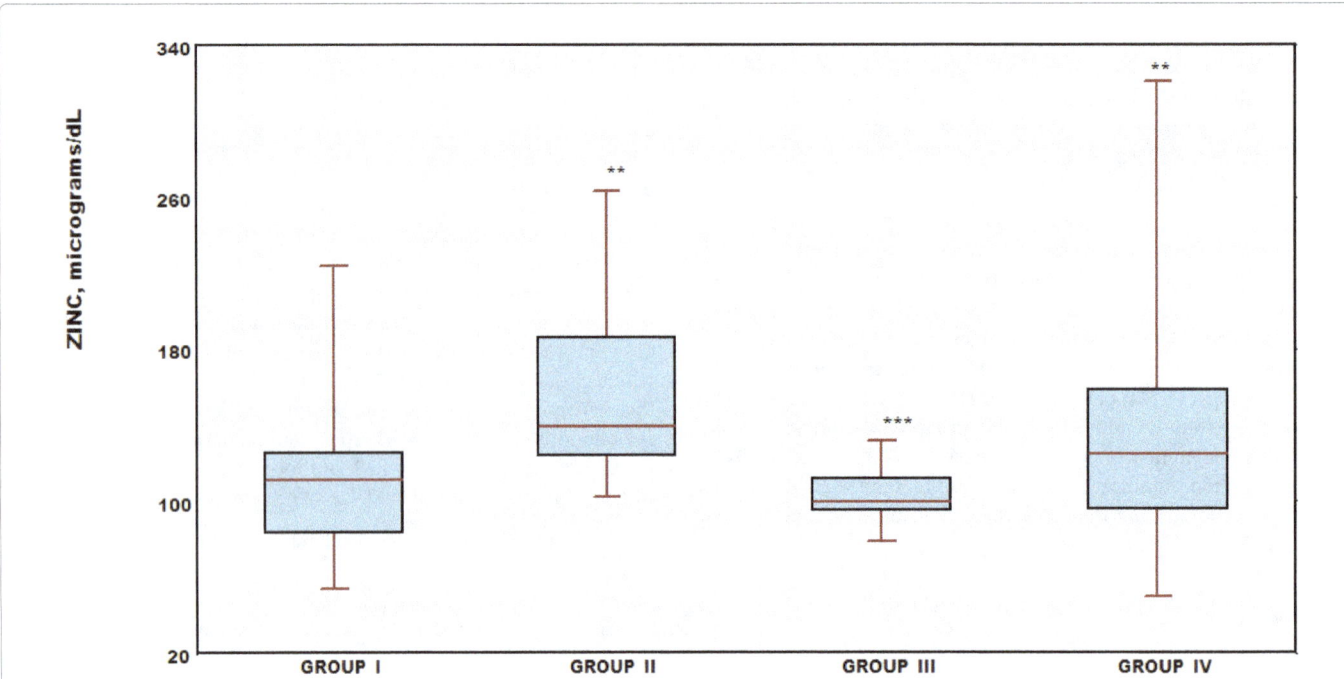

Figure 1: Serum zinc level in the healthy control (group I), T2DM without periodontitis (group II), T2DM with periodontitis (group III) andNon-DM with periodontitis (group IV). The box represents the mean, mean ± SD and the range. Differences were considered significant at *** $p < 0.0001$; ** $p < 0.001$ when compared to control.

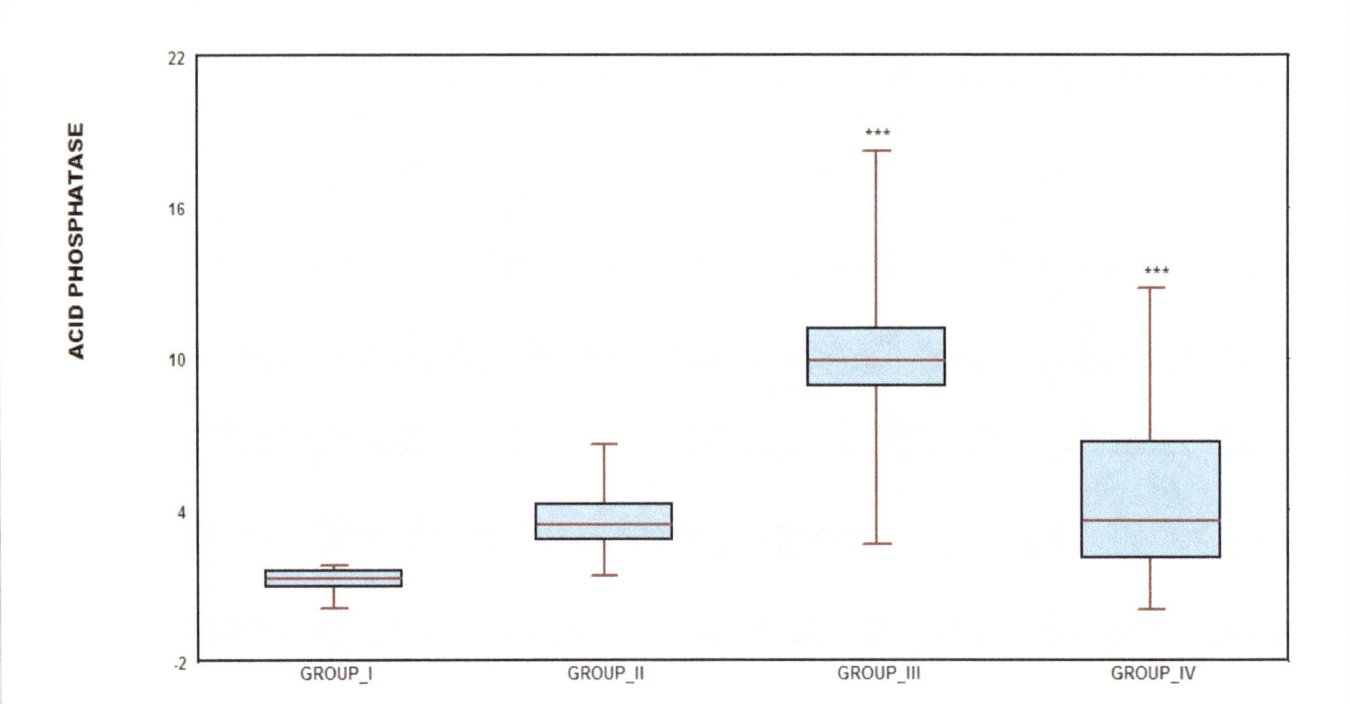

Figure 2: Serum Acid phosphatase (micromoles/min/L) in the healthy control (group I), T2DM without periodontitis (group II), T2DM with periodontitis (group III) and Non-DM with periodontitis (group IV). Differences were considered significant at *** $p < 0.0001$ when compared to control.

increased in group III whereas the levels were found to be elevated three times in group II, and four times in the group IV subjects (Figure 2). We found a significant positive correlation between serum zinc and acid phosphatase among the group II (T2DM without periodontitis),

and group IV (Non-diabetes with periodontitis) but no correlation with group I and group III (T2DM with periodontitis) (Figure 3a-3d). In T2DM without periodontitis (group II), ACP showed positive correlation with FBG. Among the T2DM with periodontitis (group

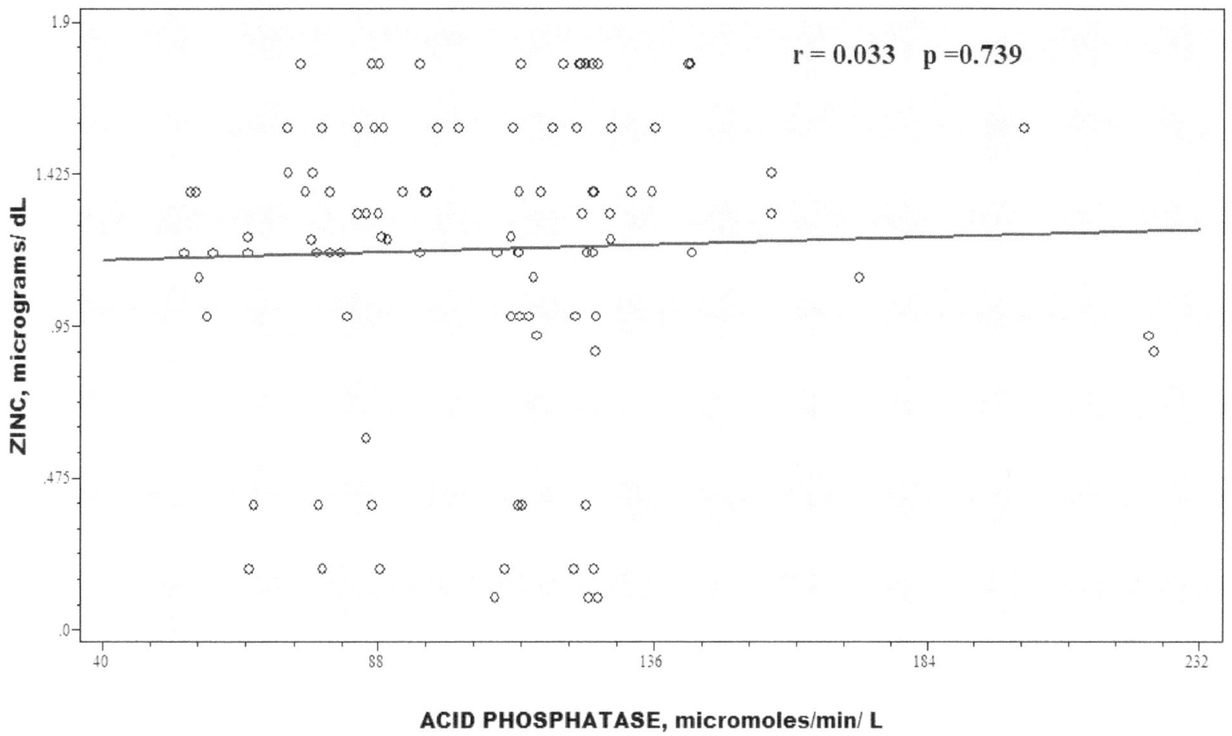

Figure 3a: Pearson's correlation plots showing the relationship between serum Zinc and Acid phosphatase in Control healthy individuals.

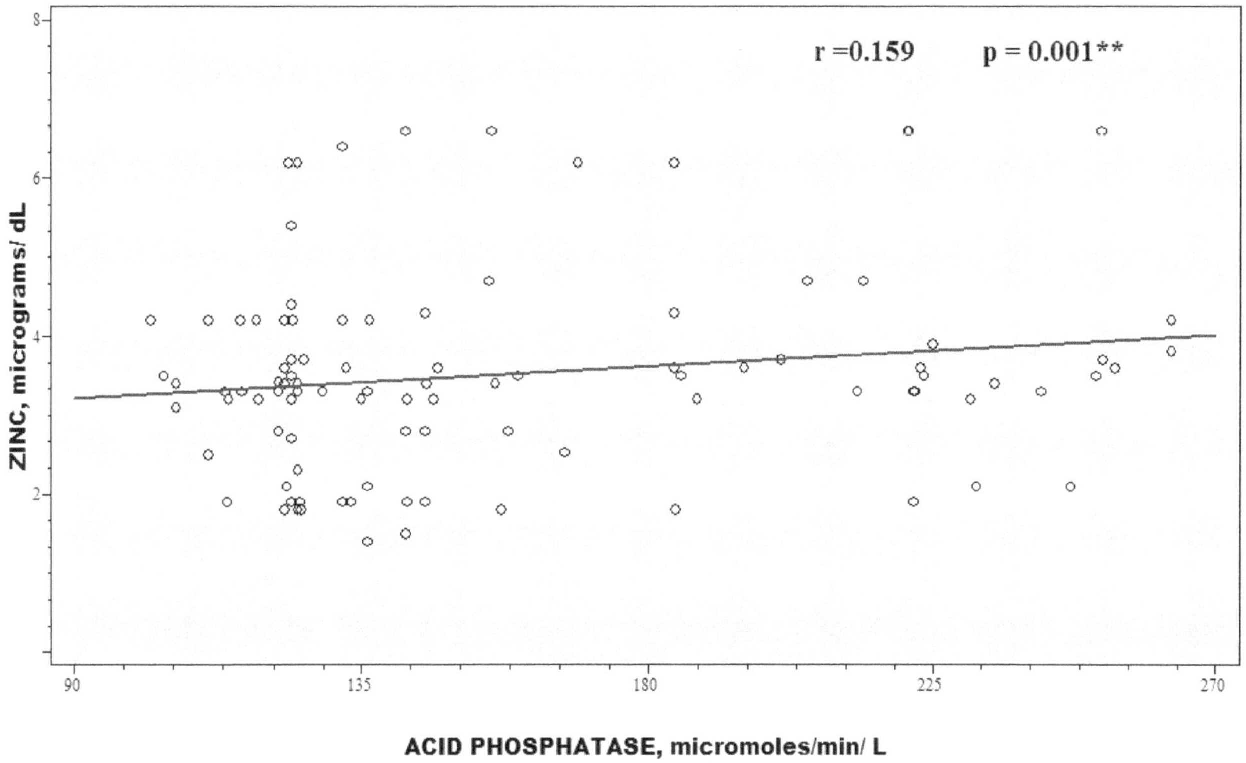

Figure 3b: Pearson's correlation plots showing the relationship between serum Zinc and Acid phosphatase in T2DM without periodontitis.

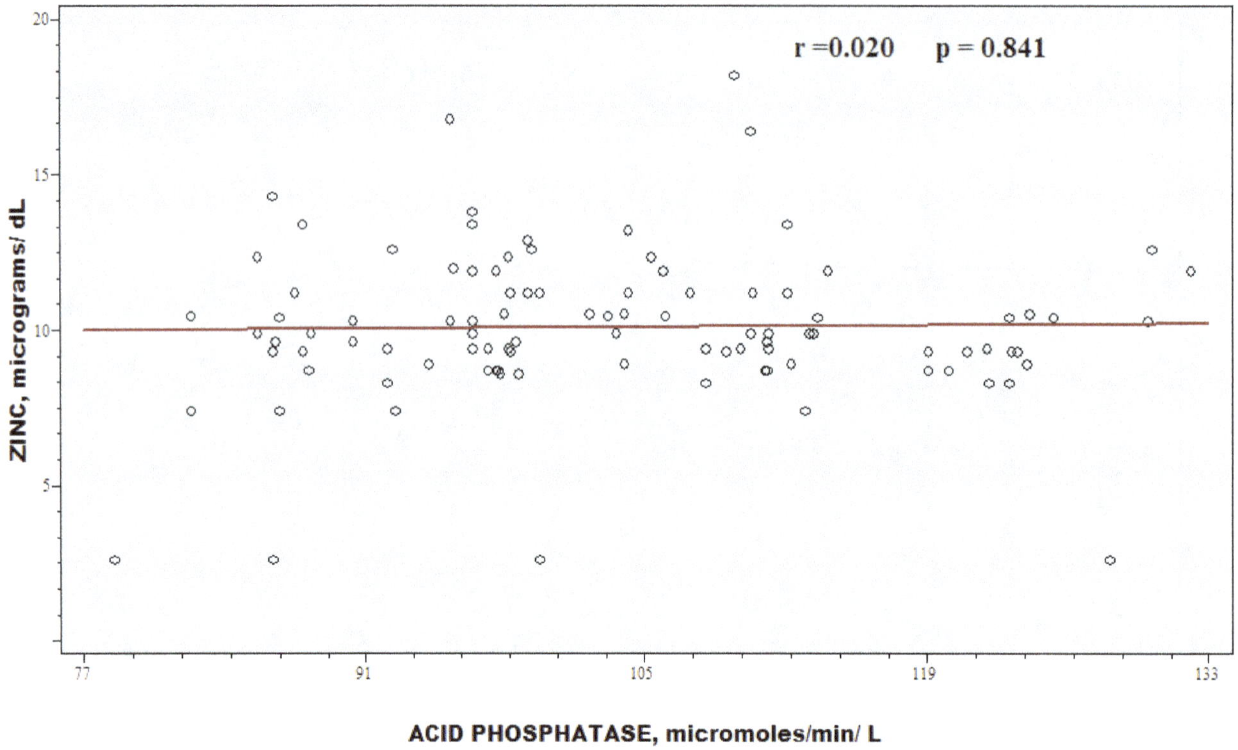

Figure 3c: Pearson's correlation plots showing the relationship between serum Zinc and Acid phosphatase in T2DM with periodontitis.

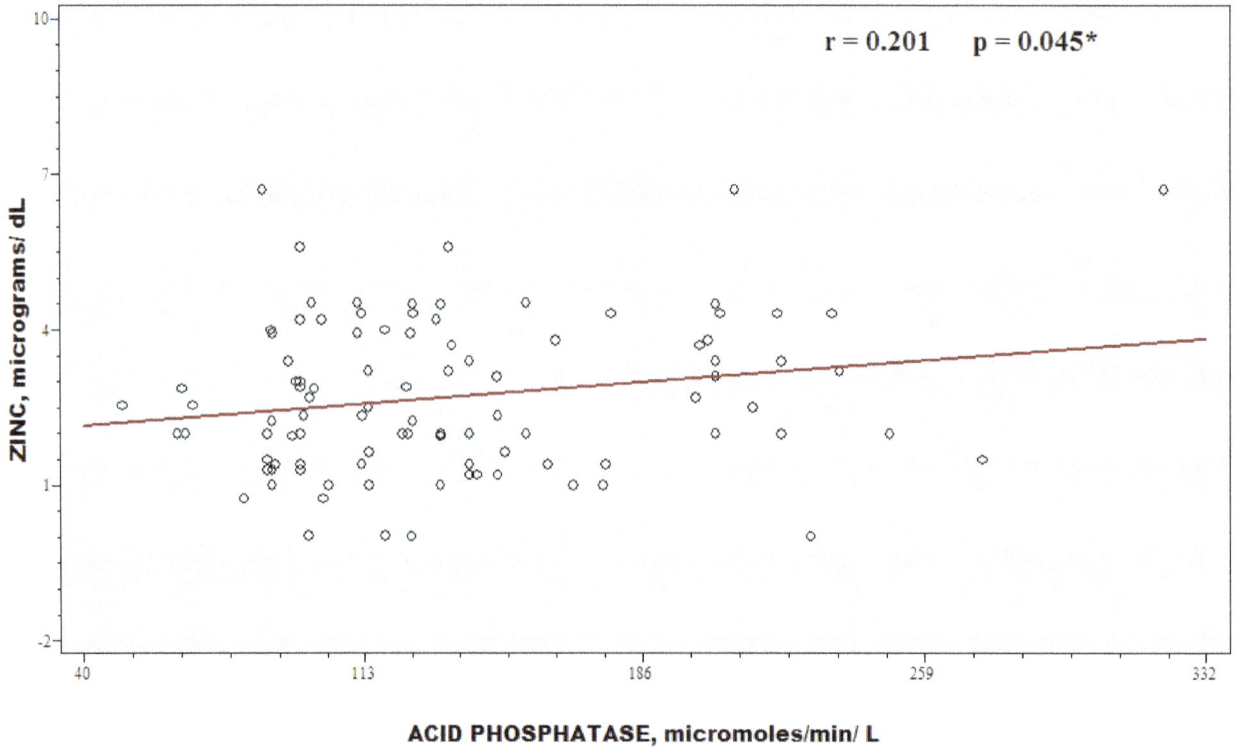

Figure 3d: Pearson's correlation plots showing the relationship between serum Zinc and Acid phosphatase in Non-DM with periodontitis.

III), ACP showed positive correlation with PPD and it showed negative correlation with CAL, and zinc correlated positively with fasting blood glucose (Table 3).

Discussion

Antioxidants play a role as defenders against occurred damages by metal-mediated free radicals. Zinc acts as an antioxidant for the decrease of oxidative stress [30]. Usually the serum Zn concentration is used to determine the Zn status, but the serum Zn concentration is not only decreased in real Zn deficiency, but also in stress [31]. During stress, serum Zn is redistributed from the serum into the liver. The protective effects of zinc against increased rates of lipid peroxidation could be due to its capability to combine and strengthen cellular membranes against lipid peroxidation and disintegration. Another probable protective mechanism of metallothionein is its ability to release Zn for binding at sites on membrane surfaces, displacing adventitious iron thereby inhibiting lipid peroxidation. A substitute protective mechanism of Zn may be its capacity to induce metallothionein synthesis. The high sulfhydryl content enables metallothionein to efficiently scavenge oxy-radicals [32]. Furthermore, the suggested outcome of Zn in causing the SH-rich metallothionein synthesis may preserve the SH-residue in many functional proteins. Therefore, Zn may protect the structural and functional integrity of the SH dependent enzymes including those regulating glucose metabolism.

Acid phosphatase (ACP) activity is widespread throughout nature. It has been widely investigated amongst the lysosomal enzymes, and has often been used as a lysosomal marker. Enzyme reactions are inhibited by metals which may form a complex with the substrate, combine with the protein-active groups of the enzymes, or react with the enzyme-substrate complex. This ACP is transported to lysosomes as an integral protein with the lysosomal targeting signal contained in the cytoplasmic tail [33]. Metals play a central role in life processes of living organisms. Essential metals are catalysts in biochemical reactions function as stabilizers of protein structures and serve in maintaining an osmotic balance. High concentrations of most metals essential and non-essential are toxic for living cells. Zinc can act as co-factors for several enzymes. At pH 5.5, the Zn ion is an essential activator, since the enzyme shows no activity in the absence of this ion. Metal treatment may affect cell and/or mitochondrial membrane permeability, lysosome membrane stability, protein unfolding and/or precipitation, enzyme inhibition, irreversible conformational changes and mutations in nucleic acids [34].

In our study, the ACP level was found to be increased significantly to about ten times (10.09 ± 2.46) among the T2DM with periodontitis (group III) when compared to control (1.18 ± 0.47). We also observed that the ACP level was increased in to about three times in group II (3.50 ± 1.27) and four times (4.38 ± 3.15) in group IV subjects. This finding is in agreement to the findings of Agoda and Glew [35] who found elevated activity of ACP in diabetes mellitus. When comparison was done between diabetes with and without periodontitis, a statistically significant increase was found in diabetes with periodontitis group. But the level of enzyme concentration is increased three times in group II and four times in group IV. This gives for the evidence that, the increased activity of this enzyme in diabetes with periodontitis may be as a result of decreased serum Zn in group III.

ACP was found to be elevated in diabetes mellitus. We found higher activity of acid phosphatase in T2DM with periodontitis [36] which would indicate that in these patients the activation process is not restricted to the enzymes capable of degrading mucopolysaccharides

and gycloproteins and the levels of ACP correlate with measurements of disease severity or activity. Hydrolysis of a variety of orthophosphate esters as well as transphosphorylation reactions is catalyzed by enzymes from many sources. One of the possible explanations for this relation could be that the insufficient influx of glucose into cells owing to the lack of insulin led to the decreased synthesis of adenosine triphosphate (ATP).

The presence of acid phosphatase in serum arises from various sources, including erythrocytes, leukocytes, platelets, kidneys, spleen and liver, each of which contribute molecular variants (isoenzymes) of ACP that are specific to the organ or cells of origin. It was observed that zinc correlated positively with ACP among the group II and group IV subjects. The correlation between ACP activity and zinc concentration may reflect a common origin of these two substances, or binding of Zn by acid phosphatise [37]. Various studies have shown that ACP, which is an important marker of phagocytic activity in phagocytes (activated macrophages and neutrophils).

Results obtained in the present study indicate a close and complex relationship between lysosomal and antioxidant responses to metals. These elements in fact could exert their toxicity both through a direct and indirect pathway, the effects of which are not easy to distinguish. The direct effect of zinc could be related to the binding of these elements to the lysosomal membrane, to the increased loading of metal-binding proteins within the lysosomal compartment, as well as to the removal of antioxidant compounds (through oxidation or mixed complexes formation) and inhibition of antioxidant enzymes. Further, metals could have an indirect effect mediated by the formation of oxy radicals. These reactive species could enhance lysosomal damage by promoting the peroxidation of membranes and in the meantime would further reduce the antioxidant cellular defenses. In this respect, it could be speculated that lysosomal damage is at least in part dependent on the efficiency of antioxidant mechanisms. In fact, as more of these defenses are depleted, the more severe will be the indirect effects of zinc metal on lysosomal membranes.

ACP is among the enzymes associated with bone metabolism. It is present in neutrophils and considered a lysosomal marker. Desquamated epithelial cells, macrophages and several bacteria, including Actinobacillus, Capnocytophaga and Veillonella, also produce this enzyme. The increased activity might be a consequence of destructive processes in alveolar bone in advanced stages of development of periodontal disease [38]. The demise associated with tissue can cause a discharge of lysosomal enzymes, with a destruction of the nearby tissue. The extracellular ACP found in gingival fluid could represent an accumulation of lysosomal enzyme from the rapidly desquamating epithelial cells of the crevicular epithelium or from connective tissue cells. It may have a bacterial origin and for that reason they play a role in the formation of pathological pocket [39]. Among its isozymes circulating L-tartrate-resistant acid phosphatase has been shown to be a sensitive marker for evaluation of osteoclastic function. Bone histology and biochemical markers of bone formation and resorption in the diabetic animal models indicated a decreased osteoblast activity combined with normal or decreased osteoclast activity [40].

Human ACP is normally found at low concentrations. However, pronounced changes in their synthesis occur in particular diseases, where unusually high or low enzyme expression is seen as part of the patho-physiological process [41]. In our study, the result of ACP is highly increased in T2DM with periodontitis when compared to other groups. Different forms of ACP are found in different organs, and their serum levels are used as a diagnostic tool for many diseases. Therefore, decreased zinc and elevated level of ACP may be a contributing factor for the progression of T2DM with periodontitis. Pro- and anti-inflammatory processes are crucial in the different phases of wound healing and their disturbances interfere with tissue homeostasis and wound healing.

Acknowledgement

The author would like to thank the Management, Dean and Vice-Principal of SRM Dental College, SRM University, Ramapuram, Chennai, for supporting and providing all the laboratory facilities to carry out the experimental work.

References

1. Patterson C, Guariguata L, Dahlquist G, Soltész G, Ogle G, et al. (2014) Diabetes in the young - a global view and worldwide estimates of numbers of children with type 1 diabetes. Diabetes Res Clin Pract 103: 161-175.

2. Costanian C, Bennett K, Hwalla N, Assaad S, Sibai AM (2014) Prevalence, correlates and management of type 2 diabetes mellitus in Lebanon: findings from a national population-based study. Diabetes Res Clin Pract 105: 408-415.

3. Fernández-Real JM, Vendrell J, García I, Ricart W, Vallès M (2012) Structural damage in diabetic nephropathy is associated with TNF-Î ± system activity. Acta Diabetol 49: 301-305.

4. Gupta S, Gambhir JK, Kalra O, Gautam A, Shukla K, et al. (2013) Association of biomarkers of inflammation and oxidative stress with the risk of chronic kidney disease in Type 2 diabetes mellitus in North Indian population. J Diabetes Complications 27: 548-552.

5. Fox CH (1992) New considerations in the prevalence of periodontal disease. Curr Opin Dent 2: 5-11.

6. White D, Pitts N, Steele J, Sadler K, Chadwick B (2011) Diseases and related disorders - a report from the Adult Dental Health Survey 2009. London: NHS Information Centre for Health and Social Care.

7. Eke PI, Dye BA, Wei L, Thornton-Evans GO, Genco RJ, et al. (2012) CDC Periodontal Disease Surveillance workgroup: James Beck (University of North Carolina, Prevalence of periodontitis in adults in the United States: 2009 and 2010. J Dent Res 91: 914-920.

8. Lalla E, Papapanou PN (2011) Diabetes mellitus and periodontitis: a tale of two common interrelated diseases. Nat Rev Endocrinol 7: 738-748.

9. Chang PC, Lim LP (2012) Interrelationships of periodontitis and diabetes: A review of the current literature. Journal of Dental Sciences 7: 272-282.

10. Duarte PM, Napimoga MH, Fagnani EC, Santos VR, Bastos MF, et al. (2012) The expression of antioxidant enzymes in the gingivae of type 2 diabetics with chronic periodontitis. Arch Oral Biol 57: 161-168.

11. Kinane DF, Preshaw PM, Loos BG; Working Group 2 of Seventh European Workshop on Periodontology (2011) Host-response: understanding the cellular and molecular mechanisms of host-microbial interactions--consensus of the Seventh European Workshop on Periodontology. J Clin Periodontol 38 Suppl 11: 44-48.

12. Kim EK, Lee SG, Choi YH, Won KC, Moon JS, et al. (2013) Association between diabetes-related factors and clinical periodontal parameters in type-2 diabetes mellitus. BMC Oral Health 13: 64.

13. Salvi GE, Collins JG, Yalda B, Arnold RR, Lang NP, et al. (1997) Monocytic TNF alpha secretion patterns in IDDM patients with periodontal diseases. J Clin Periodontol 24: 8-16.

14. Guzman S, Karima M, Wang HY, Van Dyke TE (2003) Association between interleukin-1 genotype and periodontal disease in a diabetic population. J Periodontol 74: 1183-1190.

15. Sardi JC, Duque C, Camargo GA, Hofling JF, Gonçalves RB (2011) Periodontal conditions and prevalence of putative periodontopathogens and Candida spp. in insulin-dependent type 2 diabetic and non-diabetic patients with chronic periodontitis—A pilot study. Archives of oral biology 56: 1098-1105.

16. Hayman AR, Cox TM (2003) Tartrate-resistant acid phosphatase knockout mice. J Bone Miner Res 18: 1905-1907.

17. Panara F, Angiolillo A, Fagotti A, Di Rosa I, Francesca S, et al. (1992) Acid phosphatases in mammalian tissues. Evidence for the existence of a 57 kDa Zn(2+)-dependent acid phosphatase form. Int J Biochem 24: 1619-1623.

18. Minkin C (1982) Bone acid phosphatase: tartrate-resistant acid phosphatase as a marker of osteoclast function. Calcif Tissue Int 34: 285-290.

19. Togawa T, Takada M, Aizawa Y, Tsukimura T, Chiba Y, et al. (2014) Comparative study on mannose 6-phosphate residue contents of recombinant lysosomal enzymes. Molecular Genetics and Metabolism 111: 369–373.

20. Plum LM, Rink L, Haase H (2010) The essential toxin: impact of zinc on human health. Int J Environ Res Public Health 7: 1342-1365.

21. Mocchegiani E, Giacconi R, Malavolta M (2008) Zinc signalling and subcellular distribution: emerging targets in type 2 diabetes. Trends Mol Med 14: 419-428.

22. Pushparani DS, Anandan SN, Theagarayan P (2014) Serum zinc and magnesium concentrations in type 2 diabetes mellitus with periodontitis. J Indian Soc Periodontol 18: 187-193.

23. Roussel AM, Kerkeni A, Zouari N, Mahjoub S, Matheau JM, et al. (2003) Antioxidant effects of zinc supplementation in Tunisians with type 2 diabetes mellitus. J Am Coll Nutr 22: 316-321.

24. Yamaguchi M, Weitzmann MN (2011) Zinc stimulates osteoblastogenesis and suppresses osteoclastogenesis by antagonizing NF-Î°B activation. Mol Cell Biochem 355: 179-186.

25. Maret W, Sandstead HH (2006) Zinc requirements and the risks and benefits of zinc supplementation. J Trace Elem Med Biol 20: 3-18.

26. Rungby J (2010) Zinc, zinc transporters and diabetes. Diabetologia 53: 1549-1551.

27. Capdor J, Foster M, Petocz P, Samman S (2013) Zinc and glycemic control: a meta-analysis of randomised placebo controlled supplementation trials in humans. J Trace Elem Med Biol 27: 137-142.

28. Foster M, Petocz P, Samman S (2013) Inflammation markers predict zinc transporter gene expression in women with type 2 diabetes mellitus. J Nutr Biochem 24: 1655-1661.

29. Gutman AB, Gutman EB (1938) An "Acid " Phosphatase Occurring In The Serum Of Patients With Metastasizing Carcinoma Of The Prostate Gland. J Clin Invest 17: 473-478.

30. Myers SA, Nield A, Myers M (2012) Zinc transporters, mechanisms of action and therapeutic utility: implications for type 2 diabetes mellitus. J Nutr Metab 2012: 173712.

31. Jagdish K, Mehul S, Nehal S (2010) Effect of Hesperidin on serum glucose, HbA1c and oxidative Stress in myocardial tissue in experimentally induced myocardial infarction in diabetic rats. Pharmacognosy Journal 2: 185-189.

32. Lal M, Sudha K, Beena VS,Gayathri MR (2013) Influence of modified levels of plasma modified levels of plasma magnesium, Cu, Zn and Iron levels on thiols and protein status in diabetes mellitus and diabetic retinopathy. International Journal of Analytical Pharmaceutical and Biomedical Sciences 2: 67-72.

33. Moustafa SA (2004) Zinc might protect oxidative changes in the retina and pancreas at the early stage of diabetic rats. Toxicol Appl Pharmacol 201: 149-155.

34. Bull H, Murray PG, Thomas D, Fraser AM, Nelson PN (2002) Acid phosphatases. Mol Pathol 55: 65-72.

35. Fujimoto S, Okano I, Tanaka Y, Sumida Y, Tsuda J, et al. (1996) Zinc-ion-dependent acid phosphatase exhibits magnesium-ion-dependent myo-inositol-1-phosphatase activity. Biol Pharm Bull 19: 882-885.

36. Kwapiszewski R, Kwapiszewska K, Kutter JP, Brzozka Z (2015) Three-layer poly(methyl methacrylate) microsystem for analysis of lysosomal enzymes for diagnostic purposes. Anal Chim Acta 853: 702-709.

37. Pushparani DS, Nirmala S (2013) Comparison of Acid phosphatase and β D-Glucuronidase Enzyme Levels in Type 2 Diabetes Mellitus with and without Periodontitis. IJSER 4: 1164-1168.

38. Yoshie H, Tai H, Kobayashi T, Oda-Gou E, Nomura Y, et al. (2007) Salivary enzyme levels after scaling and interleukin-1 genotypes in Japanese patients with chronic periodontitis. J Periodontol 78: 498-503.

39. Heitz-Mayfield LJ (2005) Disease progression: identification of high-risk groups and individuals for periodontitis. J Clin Periodontol 32 Suppl 6: 196-209.

40. Tomita S, Komiya-Ito A, Imamura K, Kita D, Ota K, et al. (2013) Prevalence of Aggregatibacter actinomycetemcomitans, Porphyromonas gingivalis and Tannerella forsythia in Japanese patients with generalized chronic and aggressive periodontitis. Microbial Pathogenesis 61-62: 11-15.

41. Funhoff EG, Bollen M, Averill BA (2005) The Fe(III)Zn(II) form of recombinant human purple acid phosphatase is not activated by proteolysis. J Inorg Biochem 99: 521-529.

15

Metformin Improves Carbohydrate Metabolism and Minimizes Walker Tumor Growth in Young Rats

Oliveira AG and Gomes-Marcondes MCC*

Department of Structural and Functional Biology, Institute of Biology, State University of Campinas – UNICAMP Campinas, Brazil

Abstract

Cancer cachexia occurs in more than 50% of cancer patients and is characterized by body weight loss, particularly lean body mass. Metformin is a drug that is widely prescribed to type 2 diabetes patients, in whom studies have shown a lowered cancer risk. This study was conducted to analyze the effects of Walker 256 tumor cells on muscle glucose uptake and glycogen storage, as well as to examine the modulatory effect of metformin treatment on tumor growth and energy store in tumor-bearing rats. Wistar rats were distributed into 4 groups: control (C), metformin (M), tumor-bearing (W) and tumor-bearing treated with metformin (WM). Metformin was orally administered (33 mg/kg/day by gavage), and all animals were sacrificed when the relative tumor mass reached 10%. Metformin reduced muscle spoliation in the WM group, while the W group exhibited a 10% reduction in lean mass. The tumor mass ratio was markedly decreased in the WM group compared to the W group (23%, p < 0.05). Muscle and liver glycogen storage were significantly reduced in the W group, whereas metformin treatment led to an increase in glycogen storage in the M and WM groups. Liver alkaline phosphatase activity increased in both the tumor-bearing groups, but the WM group had 11% lower activity than the W group. Muscle GLUT4 expression increased in both the metformin-treated groups, and metformin treatment did not affect citrate synthase activity, which was decreased in both the tumor-bearing groups. These results suggest that metformin can attenuate the tumor effects on glucose metabolism and improve the host welfare, which is jeopardized during cancer cachexia.

Key words: Cancer; Walker 256 tumor; Metformin; Glycogen storage; Glucose metabolism.

Introduction

Cachexia has been described as a complex metabolic syndrome that may be associated with other illnesses and is characterized by the loss of muscle, which may or may not be associated with a loss of fat mass [1].

The cachexia process depends on the tumor type, especially in lung and gastrointestinal cancer, and is responsible for up to 20% of all cancer deaths [2]. Therefore, the waste of lean body mass is the most important factor for worse prognosis [3] and is highly correlated with morbidity and mortality in cancer patients [1]. Cancer patients also exhibit metabolic changes in glucose metabolism [4], such as decreased glucose uptake by peripheral tissues, even though glucose utilization by the tumor cells is greatly increased [5].

Metformin (dimethylbiguanide) (M) is currently the most commonly used drug to treat patients with type 2 diabetes mellitus (T2DM), and it has been prescribed to more than 120 million people [6]. T2DM patients treated with metformin take 500-2550 mg daily, and some observational studies have shown that metformin-treated T2DM patients have reduced cancer mortality and morbidity [7]. Although the molecular mechanism by which metformin acts is not exactly known, metformin stimulates cell signaling through insulin receptor (IR), resulting in reduced insulin resistance and decreased serum insulin levels [8].

The Walker 256 (W) tumor has been extensively used as a model to study cachexia [9]. In young rats, Walker neoplastic cells grow extremely fast, causing cachexia in less than 15 days and altering the host glucose metabolism [10]. Although the most important factor in clinical treatment is the maintenance of lean mass, the lipid and carbohydrate stores are also essential.

Thus, the aim of this study was to analyze the modulatory effects of metformin on Walker 256 tumor evolution and to evaluate the muscle and liver tissue responses, focusing on glucose metabolism and its role in the cachexia state, in tumor-bearing rats treated with the same metformin dose typically used in T2DM treatment.

Materials and Methods

Chemicals

All chemical were purchased from Sigma-Aldrich (St. Louis, MO, USA), unless otherwise noted.

Animals and tumor implants.

Forty eight male Wistar rats (4 weeks old (100–120 g)) were obtained from the animal facility at CEMIB/State University of Campinas and were housed in collective cages under controlled temperature (22 ± 2°C) and light cycle conditions (12 h light/dark). The animals were allowed a semi-purified control diet (AIN-93G) [11] and water *ad libitum*. Walker 256 cells were originally obtained from Christ Hospital (USA) and were maintained in our laboratory through consecutive subcutaneous or intra peritoneal passages. The Walker cell suspension (1x10^6 cells) was implanted in the subcutaneous right flank. Control rats were injected with 0.9% sodium chloride. The experimental protocol (#895-1) was approved by the Ethical Committee of the State University of Campinas.

*Corresponding author: Gomes-Marcondes MCC, Department of Structural and Functional Biology, Institute of Biology, State University of Campinas – UNICAMP Campinas, Brazil, E-mail: cintgoma@unicamp.br

Metformin treatment and experimental procedures

Metformin was dissolved in the drinking water (100 mg/L) and 33 mg/kg body weight was given daily by gavage administration; treatment began at the time of tumor implantation. The metformin concentration was estimated using allometric scaling [12] from human data and using the initial recommended dose for T2DM patients (500 mg/day). Forty eight animals were distributed into 4 groups: control (C), Walker 256 tumor-bearing (W), metformin-treated (M) and tumor-bearing treated with metformin (WM) (n = 12 rats per group). Tumor weight was measured using the formula $TW = - 0.079768 + 0.000456 \times L \times W \times T$, where L is the length, W is the width and T is the thickness of the tumor; all parameters were measured using a caliper rule. When the tumor mass reached 10% of the body mass, the animals were subjected to overnight fasting (12 h) and were then sacrificed by cervical dislocation. Blood samples were collected by cardiac puncture to determine serum glucose, lactate and insulin levels. Gastrocnemius muscle and liver samples were collected for glycogen content assay and histochemistry.

In vitro assay for cell viability

W 256 cells isolated from animals bearing Walker tumors were cultured in 199 medium supplemented with 10% fetal bovine serum, 10,000 units/mL penicillin and 10,000 μg/mL streptomycin (LGC Biotecnologia, SP, Brazil) at 37°C in a humid incubator with 5% CO_2. The cells were seeded at a density of 1×10^4 cells per well in 96-well plates and treated with 0 (control), 10, 10^2, 10^3, 10^4 or 10^5 μM metformin for 24, 48 or 72 h. Cell viability was determined using an MTT assay [13] and quantified using a spectrophotometer with a 570 nm filter after solubilization of the formazan with DMSO.

Glucose tolerance test (GTT)

Before sacrifice (2 h), the overnight fasted animals were subjected to an intragastric gavage with 2 g/kg glucose solution, and blood samples were collected by caudal vena bleeding. A serum glucose assay was performed with samples taken at 0 min, 30 min, 60 min, 90 min, and 120 min after glucose intake. The glucose concentration was quantified by enzymatic reaction based on glucose-oxidase [14].

Periodic acid-Schiff (PAS) stain

Muscle and liver samples were fixed in 4% paraformaldehyde in 0.1 M phosphate buffer (10.9 g/L, Na_2HPO_4; 3.2 g/L, $NaHPO_4$, pH 7.4) for 24 h and embedded in paraffin wax. The paraffin wax-embedded samples were cut into 5 μm sections for histochemistry analysis using PAS stain. The integrated optical density (IOD) of the PAS positive images was determined by analyzing 20 fields (300 μm^2 each) from one slide; at least 3 animals were quantified per group using the Image J software (National Institutes of Health, USA).

Citrate synthase activity

Samples of gastrocnemius muscle were collected and immediately frozen in liquid nitrogen. The samples were kept at -80°C until homogenization in homogenizing buffer (2 mM EDTA in 175 mM KCl, pH 7.4). The samples were centrifuged at 16,000 g for 20 min and the citrate synthase activity was accessed using a colorimetric method [15]. All samples were tested for linearity up to 4 min of reaction and the values were normalized to total muscle protein concentration [16].

Lactate concentration

Blood samples were clarified by centrifugation at 1,000 g for 10 min

and analyzed for lactate concentration using an enzymatic ultra-violet based assay [17] (Bioclin, MG, Brazil).

Alkaline phosphatase activity

Liver samples were collected, immediately frozen in liquid nitrogen and kept at -80°C until homogenization in cold phosphate-buffered saline (pH 7.4) supplemented with 0.1% Triton X-100. The homogenates were centrifuged at 16,000 g for 20 min and the alkaline phosphatase activity was measured using a colorimetric assay [18] the values were normalized to total liver protein content.

Immunoblotting

Gastrocnemius samples were homogenized in 100 mM Tris, 10 mM $Na_4P_2O_7$, 10 mM FNa, 1 mM Na_3VO_4, 10 mM EDTA, 2 mM PMSF, 0.1 mg/mL aprotinin, 0.1% Triton-X100, pH 7.4, and were centrifuged at 16,000 g for 20 min. Protein concentration was measured using a colorimetric method [16] and the sample was added to 2X loading buffer. The protein sample (40 μg) was resolved by SDS-PAGE in a 10% resolving gel and electroblotted onto a PVDF membrane (EMD Millipore, Billerica, MA, USA). The proteins were revealed using primary antibodies against GAPDH (1:1000) and GLUT4 (1:500) and secondary anti-rabbit (1:10000) and anti-goat (1:10000) antibodies (Santa Cruz biotechnology, CA, USA) after reaction with a chemiluminescent reagent (Thermo Fisher Scientific, Rockford, IL USA). The band intensity was quantified using the Image J software (National Institutes of Health, USA).

Insulin concentration

The serum insulin concentrations of the blood samples were evaluated using an ELISA kit (# EZRMI-13K) according to the manufacturer's instructions (EMD Millipore, Billerica, MA, USA).

Statistical analysis

The results were expressed as the mean + SEM. Comparisons within control and tumour-bearing groups were performed using one-way ANOVA [15] followed by Bonferroni's multiple comparison post-hoc test (Graph Pad Prism software, v3.00 for Windows 98, USA). A nonparametric t test was used when two groups were compared (W group versus WM group). Data were considered statistically significant when the P value was less than 5%.

Results

Effects of tumor growth

Table 1 shows that the tumor-bearing animals developed the cachectic state. Body weight was decreased by 10% in the W animals compared to the C group, whereas the WM group exhibited a non-significant reduction in body weight. Body mass gain was decreased in both the tumor-bearing groups W (34%) and the WM (30%) group, as was the carcass mass (18% in W and 17% in WM). In the in vitro experiments with W 256 cells, metformin treatment resulted in a reduction in cell viability when added at higher concentrations (from 10^3 to 10^5 μM); after 72 h exposure, treatment with 10^3 μM metformin led to a 40% decrease in cell viability (Figure 1A). The relative tumor mass (tumor mass to body weight ratio) was decreased by 23% in animals treated with metformin, compared to the W group (Figure 1B). The relative liver mass was increased in both tumor-bearing groups (W and WM = 17%) compared to the C group. The relative adrenal mass was increased in both tumor-bearing groups (W and WM = 22%) compared to the C group. Gastrocnemius mass decreased by 21% in the W group compared to C, whereas WM exhibited a 10% reduction in muscle Compared to the M group; however, the muscle protein content did not vary among the groups. Serum glucose was highly decreased in both tumor-bearing groups (W = 48%; WM = 41%) (Table 1). The serum insulin level was reduced by 18% in the tumor-bearing group compared to the C group; however, the metformin treatment also decreased the insulin content by 32% and 48% in the M and WM groups, respectively. The serum lactate concentration increased 31% in the W group, but increased only 14% in the WM animals compared to the control group (Table 1).

Tumor growth decreased blood glucose levels

GTT analysis showed that the area under curve decreased in both tumor-bearing groups (W = 36%; WM = 28%) (Table 1). Serum glucose levels decreased in both the tumor-bearing groups (W = 48%; WM = 47% C); conversely, the GTT results showed that metformin was not able to minimize the difference in glycemia between the WM and C groups (Table 1). Serum glucose was decreased by 10% in the M group compared to the C group, demonstrating that metformin was able to stimulate glucose uptake in peripheral tissues (Table 1); however, the area under the curve from the GTT analysis showed similar values for both the M and C groups.

Tumor growth negatively affects liver glycogen storage while metformin treatment modulates this phenotype

Glycogen storage, as assessed by PAS staining, decreased by 28% in the W group compared to C, whereas it was similar in WM and increased by 26% in M (Figure 2A and 2B). Glycogen storage increased by 44% in WM (Figure 2A and 2B) as compared to the W group. The alkaline phosphatase activity in the liver increased in both tumor-bearing groups as compared to the C group; however, this enzyme activity was further reduced in the WM group than in the W group (W = 40%; WM = 25%) (Figure 2C). When comparisons were made between the two tumor-bearing groups, the alkaline phosphatase activity in the WM group was 11% lower than in the W group and was statistical similar to C (Figure 2C).

Tumor growth affects the gastrocnemius muscle and metformin treatment improves its energy storage

The muscle glycogen storage was decreased by 40% in the W animals compared to the C animals, and this reduction was not statistically

significant. On the other hand, in both metformin-treated groups, glycogen storage was greatly increased (2.3-fold in M; 1.1-fold in WM) when compared with C (Figure 3A and 3B). Comparison between the tumor-bearing groups showed that glycogen storage was increased 2.5 times in the WM group compared to the W group. GLUT4 expression was similar in the W and C groups, whereas it increased in the metformin-treated groups, by 13% in M and 17% in WM (Figure 3C). Comparison between the tumor-bearing groups showed that GLUT4 expression in the WM group was 14% higher than in the W group (Figure 3C). Citrate synthase activity in both tumor-bearing groups decreased approximately 23% when compared with C (Figure 3D).

Discussion

We showed that metformin treatment could improve the host cachectic state, enhance the liver and muscle responses, and minimize Walker tumor evolution. We also showed that Walker tumor growth led to a loss of body mass associated with other metabolic changes in the tumor-bearing rats, demonstrating that this type of tumor can lead to damaging effects on the host. The most important point of this paper is that we treated the tumor-bearing animals with metformin at the same dose used to treat T2DM patients, showing that at even a common dose, this treatment could improve the host responses (carbohydrate metabolism) and also reduce the relative tumor mass.

Most of the tumor cells use glucose anaerobically, even under normal oxygen conditions. This feature was previously described by Otto Warburg, who demonstrated that neoplastic cells had greater glycolytic activity than normal cells, even in normoxia [19]. The increasing anaerobic use of glucose is not due to just one reason but can be associated with mutations in mitochondrial genes, increased expression of low Km hexokinase isoforms, oncogenic signals such as *ras* and *src* and expression of hypoxia-inducible factor (HIF) [20]. The increased glucose consumption provides the neoplastic cells with precursors for DNA, protein and lipid synthesis, as well as increases the serum lactate concentration. Solid and fast growing tumors, such as Walker 256 carcinoma, need to overcome the absence of vascularization to keep growing, and, for this reason, the use of glucose anaerobically can provide the ATP necessary to maintain metabolic reaction, as well as to convert pyruvate into lactate to regenerate NAD+.

Lactate produced by neoplastic cells is responsible for the decrease in the pH of the tumor microenvironment, which plays a crucial role in the activation of HIF. This activation is responsible for the stimulation

	C (n = 12)	W (n = 12)	M (n = 12)	WM (n = 12)
Initial body mass (g)	108.3 ± 4.4	105.8 ± 4.0	112.0 ± 4.1	108.4 ± 3.9
Final body mass (g)	199.6 ± 5.2	179.2 ± 5.6*	204.8 ± 4.3	184.7 ± 3.7
Mass gain (%)	85.7± 3.1	56.8± 3.7*	84.2± 3.4	58.7± 4.2*
Carcass mass (g)	165.5 ± 5.5	135.0 ± 4.1*	164.5 ± 5.2	136.1 ± 3.2*
Relative liver mass (%)	5.2± 0.2	6.1 ± 0.1*	5.2± 0.2	6.1± 0.2*
Relative muscle mass (%)	0.66± 0.04	0.52 ± 0.01*	0.60± 0.02	0.54± 0.01*
Muscle protein (µg/µL)	6.7 ± 0.37	5.8 ± 0.32	6.9 ± 0.46	6.7± 0.60
Relative adrenal mass (%)	0.027± 0.002	0.033± 0.002*	0.027± 0.001	0.034± 0.003*
Liver protein (µg/µL)	5.25± 0.16	5.09± 0.03	5.01± 0.02	5.01± 0.03
Serum glucose (mg/dL)	89.8± 4.8	46.6± 4.8*	81.1± 5.1	47.5± 3.9*
GTT -area under curve (mg/dL x 90 min)	7336± 336	4417± 393*	7397± 468	5341± 483*
Serum insulin (ng/mL)	0.563± 0.036	0.463± 0.069	0.384± 0.082	0.287± 0.057*
Serum lactate (mg/dL)	19.69± 0.96	25.83± 0.57*	19.84± 0.42	22.42± 0.51**

Legend: C: control; W: Walker 256 tumor-bearing; M: metformin-treated; WM: Walker 256 tumor-bearing and treated with metformin. The results are expressed as the mean ± SEM. *P < 0.05 versus the C group; ** P<0.05 versus the W group.

Table 1: Tumor growth effects on body and organ growth

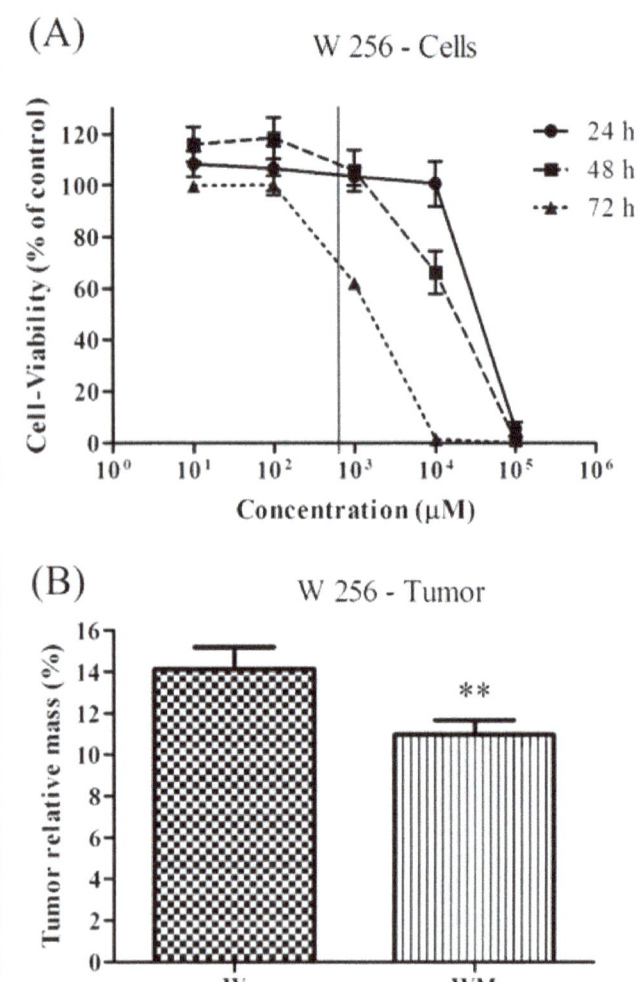

Figure 1: Effects of metformin on cell viability and tumor growth. (A) Dose-response curve for metformin treatment of W256 cells cultured in vitro for 24, 48 and 72 h. The vertical line shows the same metformin concentration used in the in vivo experiments (600 µM). The results represent the mean ± SEM of three independent experiments. (B) Relative tumor mass in the W and WM groups. Legend: W - tumor-bearing group; WM - tumor-bearing rats treated with metformin. The minimum number of animals used per group was 8. The columns represent the mean ± SEM. ** P<0.05 versus the W group.

of angiogenesis, glucose uptake, glycolysis, growth factor signaling, apoptosis, invasion and metastasis [21]. As a matter of fact, our data could suggest that metformin treatment was able to attenuate HIF activation, leading to a reduced tumor mass in relation to the carcass weight. In parallel, tumor evolution results in increased adrenal gland activity, as adrenocorticotrophic hormone (ACTH) is enhanced in these tumor-bearing groups; the increase in ACTH leads to increases in both corticosterone and catecholamine hormones, which results in disposable serum glucose (energy mobilization). Although, metformin treatment improved glycogen storage, in this case, the metformin treatment was not able to reverse the increase in ACTH (1.9-fold increase in W group and 1.7-fold increase in WM). Tumor growth with increased Cori cycle activity can result in energy expenditure [22] and contributes, at least in part, to cachexia. The Cori cycle is a pathway in the liver that converts lactate into glucose, resulting in a net loss of 4 ATP molecules for each glucose molecule. Metformin was able to reduce the relative tumor mass, as it was significantly lower in the metformin administered

tumor-bearing rats than the non-administered tumor-bearing ones. Meanwhile, we also found that metformin inhibited tumor proliferation and cell viability based on the cell culture data, confirming the lower tumor mass to body weight ratio. The reduced tumor mass most likely led to a decrease in the serum lactate concentration in the WM group, which should result in less substrate for the Cori cycle, thus attenuating the tumor growth effects in host tissues, such as liver and muscle. Many studies have confirmed that neoplastic cells produce high lactate levels and consume large amounts of glucose, as confirmed by measuring the lactate dehydrogenase activity and glucose uptake [23]. In this work, we did not measure the activity of this enzyme; however, in our previous work, we showed that this enzyme had increased activity in the tumor-bearing rats. These findings suggest that metformin likely altered the lactate dehydrogenase activity of the tumor cells, and, once the Walker tumor induces host cachexia, reducing the tumor activity most likely benefited the host carcass. It is known that Walker 256 induces cachexia likely through cachexia mediators, which are released by the tumor itself or the host, such as IL-6, TNF-α and proteolysis-inducing factor (PIF) (2); in our previous work, we have observed higher levels of these factors in Walker tumor-bearing animals [24,25]. It is possible that the decreased tumor growth caused by metformin treatment was associated with a decreased release of these cachexia mediators, thus attenuating the tumor effects on the host carcass. A recent study shows that high doses of metformin (500 mg/kg/day) can lead to an efficient decrease in tumor growth in vivo and *in vitro* [26]. In our previous experiment, we also found reduced Walker tumor growth following treatment with 500 mg/kg/day metformin (data not shown). In this study, we demonstrated that even low doses (similar dose given in T2DM patient, corresponding to 600 µM) can be effective at attenuating the tumor growth rate and its effects in the host body *in vitro* and in vivo.

Additionally, glycogen storage increased in the muscle and liver tissue in the tumor-bearing metformin-treated animals. We suggest that the increased GLUT4 expression stimulated by metformin could be responsible for its increased translocation to the cellular membrane,

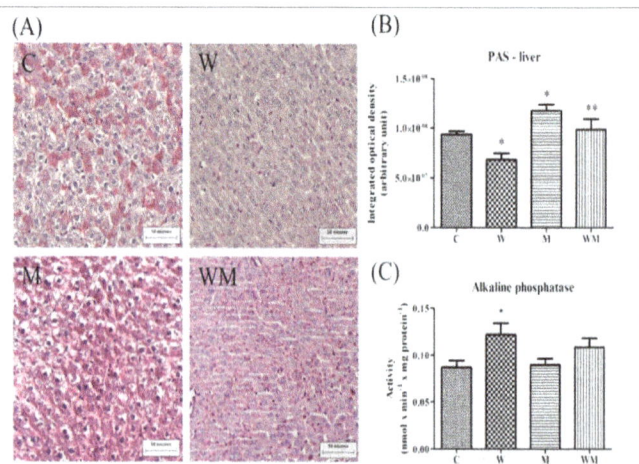

Figure 2: Effects of tumor growth and metformin in the liver of young Walker tumor-bearing rats, showing the glycogen content in the liver by staining the histological sections with PAS (5 µm, purple dye) (A), quantification of glycogen content in the PAS stained images (B), and liver alkaline phosphatase activity (C). Legend: C - control group; W - tumor-bearing group; M - metformin-treated group; WM - tumor-bearing rats treated with metformin. The minimum number of animal used per group was 8. The histology magnification was 200x. The columns represent the mean ± SEM. * P < 0.05 versus the C group. ** P<0.05 versus the W group

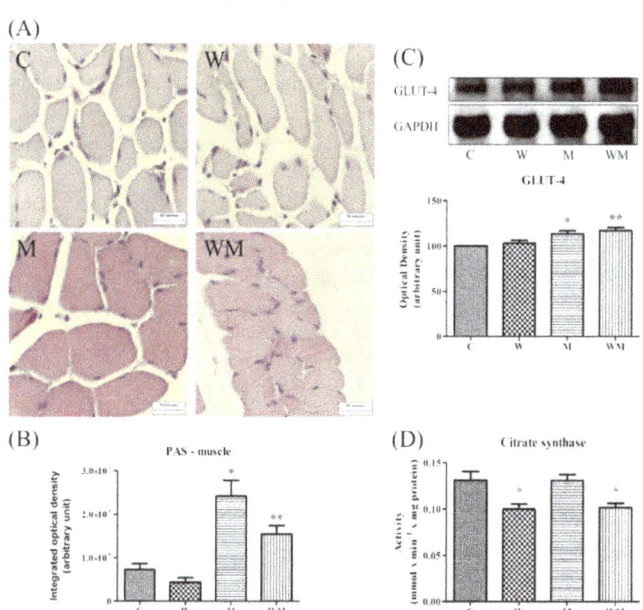

Figure 3: Effects of tumor growth and metformin in the gastrocnemius muscle of young tumor-bearing rats, showing the muscle glycogen storage in the histological sections (5 µm, purple dye) (A), quantification of the glycogen content measured in in the PAS stained images (B), representative image of GLUT4 immunoblot analysis and quantification of GLUT4 expression in the gastrocnemius muscle (C), and citrate synthase activity in the gastrocnemius muscle (D). Legend: C - control group; W - tumor-bearing group; M - metformin-treated group; WM - tumor-bearing rats treated with metformin. The minimum number of animal used per group was 8. The histology magnification was 200x. The columns represent the mean ± SEM. * P < 0.05 versus the C group. ** P<0.05 versus the W group.

leading to increased glucose uptake by the muscle, even under conditions of low insulin. Studies have shown that metformin is able to stimulate the AMP-activated protein kinase (AMPK) [27]. Although the mechanisms remain unclear, one of the roles of AMPK is to stimulate glucose transport through the cellular membrane by stimulating GLUT4 translocation in muscle and lipid cells [28]. Our study is in accordance with the literature, as both metformin-treated groups demonstrated an increase in GLUT4 expression, possibly leading to higher glucose transport in the muscle, which most likely enhanced the muscle glycogen storage. Conversely, other studies reported no changes in glycogen content and synthesis in the muscle because AMPK is activated by metformin. The increased glycogen content in the muscle of both metformin-treated animals may be beneficial to save energy, especially under the catabolic conditions established in the tumor-bearing rats. We verified that there was low citrate synthase activity in both tumor bearing groups, and we suggested the catabolic state found in the host could be associated with a low oxidative capacity of skeletal muscle to minimize energy wasting.

Metformin also increased glucose storage as glycogen in the liver, although the levels did not reach the levels observed in the gastrocnemius muscle. Metformin was able to decrease hepatic gluconeogenesis [27], allowing the glucose that was taken up by hepatocytes to be stored as glycogen. Glycogen storage increased significantly in both metformin-treated groups when compared to their respective controls, suggesting that metformin treatment could preserve the energy store that is important in this catabolic state. Alkaline phosphatase activity can be used to test liver function [29], which could be impaired during this catabolic state due to tumor development, as we observed an increase

in liver weight in both tumor-bearing rats. During cancer evolution, the increased liver weight is the first phenotype that was observed, and this may be a consequence of higher activity cell and synthesis, particularly of C-reactive protein [20], as our previous work showed that tumor-bearing animals had high levels of C-reactive protein. The decreased tumor growth caused by metformin treatment can be responsible for the decreased alkaline phosphatase activity in hepatic cells, indicating the tumor effects on the host were as pronounced as in tumor-bearing group without metformin. This fact suggests that even a common metformin dosage (the same dose used to treat T2DM patients) could result in benefits, as metformin improved energy storage, as well as the tissue response of both the liver and muscle, and also enhanced the muscle glucose transporter, which was associated with decreased tumor growth. Further studies are underway in our laboratory to determine how metformin could counteract the tumor effects on carbohydrate metabolism in parallel with body mass wasting during cancer-induced cachexia. In conclusion, this study shows that low-dose metformin treatment minimized tumor development, as a possible antitumoral agent, and was beneficial to the cachectic state in tumor-bearing rats by improving carbohydrate metabolism.

Acknowledgments

This work was supported by a grant from Fundação de Amparo a Pesquisa do Estado de São Paulo – FAPESP, #2010/11328-9 and Conselho Nacional de Desenvolvimento Científico e Tecnológico – CNPq, # 304604/2010-0. A.G.O. is a research fellow supported by Fundação de Amparo a Pesquisa do Estado de São Paulo, Grant #2008/07737-0, São Paulo, Brazil. The manuscript was edited for proper English language, by native English speaking editors at American Journal Experts (Certificate Verification Key: 22F1-3B08-B193-9A76-11B9.

Disclosure statement

The authors declare that they have no competing interests.

References

1. Evans WJ, Morley JE, Argilés J, Bales C, Baracos V, et al. (2008) Cachexia: A new definition. Clinical Nutrition 27: 793-799.

2. Tisdale MJ (2010) Cancer cachexia. Current opinion in gastroenterology 26 :146-151.

3. Tisdale MJ (2002) Cachexia in cancer patients. Nat Rev Cancer 2:862-871.

4. Albrecht JT, Canada TW (1996) Cachexia and anorexia in malignancy. HematolOncolClin North Am 10:791-800.

5. Adekola K, Rosen ST, Shanmugam M (2012) Glucose transporters in cancer metabolism. CurrOpinOncol 24:650-654.

6. Viollet B, Guigas B, Sanz Garcia N, Leclerc J, Foretz M, et al.(2012) Cellular and molecular mechanisms of metformin: an overview. ClinSci (Lond) 122:253-270.

7. Libby G, Donnelly LA, Donnan PT,Alessi DR, Morris AD, et al. (2009)New Users of Metformin Are at Low Risk of Incident Cancer: A cohort study among people with type 2 diabetes. Diabetes Care 32:1620-1625.

8. Cantrell LA, Zhou C, Mendivil A, Malloy KM, Gehrig PA, et al. (2010) Metformin is a potent inhibitor of endometrial cancer cell proliferation--implications for a novel treatment strategy. GynecolOncol 116:92-98.

9. Freitas JJS, Pompeia C, Miyasaka CK, Curi R. (2001) Walker-256 tumor growth causes oxidative stress in rat brain. J Neurochem 77:655-663.

10. Vicentino C, Constantin J, AparecidoStecanella L, Bracht A, Yamamoto NS (2002) Glucose and glycogen catabolism in perfused livers of Walker-256 tumor-bearing rats and the response to hormones. Pathophysiology 8: 175-182.

11. Reeves PG, Nielsen FH, Fahey GC (1993) Ain-93 Purified Diets for Laboratory

Rodents - Final Report of the American Institute of Nutrition Ad Hoc Writing Committee on the Reformulation of the Ain-76a Rodent Diet. J Nutr 123:1939-1951.

12. Mahmood I (2007) Application of allometric principles for the prediction of pharmacokinetics in human and veterinary drug development. Adv Drug Deliver Rev 59:1177-1192.

13. Mosmann T (1983) Rapid colorimetric assay for cellular growth and survival: application to proliferation and cytotoxicity assays. J Immunol Methods 65:55-63.

14. Trinder P (1969) Determination of Blood Glucose Using 4-Amino Phenazone as Oxygen Acceptor. J ClinPathol 22: 246.

15. Srere PA. [1] Citrate synthase: [EC 4.1.3.7. Citrate oxaloacetate-lyase (CoA-acetylating)]. In: John ML, editor. Method Enzymol. Volume 13: Academic Press; 1969. p. 3-11.

16. Bradford MM (1976) A rapid and sensitive method for the quantitation of microgram quantities of protein utilizing the principle of protein-dye binding. Anal Biochem72:248-254.

17. Westgard JO, Lahmeyer BL, Birnbaum ML (1972) Use of the Du Pont "automatic clinical analyzer" in direct determination of lactic acid in plasma stabilized with sodium fluoride.ClinChem 18:1334-1338.

18. Martins MJ, Negrao MR, Hipolito-Reis C (2001) Alkaline phosphatase from rat liver and kidney is differentially modulated. ClinBiochem 34:463-468.

19. Pelicano H, Martin DS, Xu RH, Huang P (2006) Glycolysis inhibition for anticancer treatment. Oncogene 25:4633-4646.

20. Tisdale MJ (2009) Mechanisms of cancer cachexia.Physiol Rev 89:381-410.

21. Brahimi-Horn MC, Pouyssegur J (2005) The hypoxia-inducible factor and tumor progression along the angiogenic pathway. Int Rev Cytol242:157-213.

22. Roh MS, Ekman LG, Jeevanandam M, Brennan MF (1985) Elevated energy expenditure in hepatocytes from tumor-bearing rats. J Surg Res 38:407-415.

23. Holroyde CP, Gabuzda TG, Putnam RC, Paul P, Reichard GA (1975) Altered glucose metabolism in metastatic carcinoma. Cancer research 35:3710-3714.

24. Salomao EM, Toneto AT, Silva GO, Gomes-Marcondes MC (2010) Physical exercise and a leucine-rich diet modulate the muscle protein metabolism in Walker tumor-bearing rats.Nutr Cancer 62:1095-1104.

25. Goncalves EM, Salomao EM, Gomes-Marcondes MC (2013) Leucine modulates the effect of Walker factor, a proteolysis-inducing factor-like protein from Walker tumours, on gene expression and cellular activity in C2C12 myotubes. Cytokine 64:343-350.

26. Rocha GZ, Dias MM, Ropelle ER, Osorio-Costa F, Rossato FA, et al. (2011) Metformin amplifies chemotherapy-induced AMPK activation and antitumoral growth. Clin Cancer Res 17:3993-4005.

27. Shaw RJ, Lamia KA, Vasquez D, Koo SH, Bardeesy N, et al. (2005) The kinase LKB1 mediates glucose homeostasis in liver and therapeutic effects of metformin. Science 310:1642-1646.

28. Lee JO, Lee SK, Jung JH, Kim JH, You GY, et al. (2011) Metformin induces Rab4 through AMPK and modulates GLUT4 translocation in skeletal muscle cells. J Cell Physiol 226:974-981.

29. Nair KG, Deepadevi KV, Arun P, Kumar VM, Santhosh A, et al. (1998) Toxic effect of systemic administration of low doses of the plasticizer di-(2-ethyl hexyl) phthalate [DEHP] in rats. Indian J ExpBiol 36:264-272.

16

Methanol Extracts of Medicinal Plants Used for Oral Healthcare in Cameroon

Ashu Michael Agbor*

Universite des Montagnes, Dental surgery, Bangangte, Cameroon

Abstract

Background: Traditional healers in Cameroon are actively involved in oral healthcare and traditional herbs are used for management of oral diseases. However the analysis of phytoconstituents of medicinal plants used for oral healthcare in Cameroon has not been done. The objective of the study was to determine the phytoconstituents of medicinal plants used for oral healthcare in Cameroon.

Methods: Samples of fresh plants used for dental treatment collected from South west and litorral regions of Cameroon that were free from diseases were obtained from the traditional healers.The plants were dried and the dried powder was macerated with intermediate stirring for 48 hours in methanol before filtering with Whattman filter paper. The filtrate was evaporated to dryness of solvent using the rotative evaporator in order to obtain the concentrated extracts of each plant sample. The plant extracts were then qualitatively tested for the presence of phytochemicals such as alkaloids, flavonoids, saponins, terpenoids, steroids and tannins using the standard procedures.

Results: All the six (6) plants were found to be rich in at least one of the secondary metabolites. Steroids, terpenoids and flavonoids were found in all the plants samples. Alkaloids were present in *Ageratum conyzoides* and *Carica papaya*. Tannins were present in *Ageratum conyzoides, Emilia coccinea, Gossypium sp* and *Carica papaya*. Saponins were present in *Ageratum conyzoides, Carica papaya* and *Momordica charantia*. Phlobatannins was present in *Emilia coccinea, Gossypium sp, Carica papaya* and *Spilanthes africana*. Cardiac glycosides were present in *Emilia coccinea, Carica papaya,* and *Momordica charantia. Carica papaya* contained all these phytochemicals.

Conclusion: This study revealed the presence of active secondary metabolites in herbs used for different dental treatment. The clinical trial of phytochemicals on the oral conditions is necessary to determine their pharmacological activity.

Keywords: Cameroon; Ethnomedicinal plants; Oral health; Phytochemicals; Traditional healer

Introduction

Plant chemicals used for medicinal purposes which can be derived from any part of the plant like bark, leaves, fruits, flowers, roots, seeds are largely the secondary metabolites [1]. These secondary metabolites are derived biosynthetically from plant primary metabolites and are not directly involved in the growth, development, or reproduction of plants. They are usually produced in specific groups of plant families or specific tissues, cells or developmental stages throughout plant development [2,3]. The seconday metabolites play a key role in maintaining plant fitness as they function in the protection of plants against microbial (bacteria, fungi and viral) infections, herbivory (slugs and snails, arthropods, and vertebrates), UV radiation, attraction of pollinators and frugivores, allelopathy, and signaling [2,4]. They also serve as drugs, drug precursors, drug prototypes, templates for synthetic modification, and pharmacological probes [4].

Knowledge of the chemical constituents of plants is desirable because such information will be of value for the synthesis of complex chemical substances [5]. Such phytochemical screening of various plants is reported by many workers [6-8] in other aspects of medicine but not in dentistry.

Green plants synthesize and preserve a variety of biochemical products, many of which are extractable and used as chemical feed stocks or as raw material for various scientific investigations [9].

Medicinal herbs have been used in one form or another under indigenous systems of medicine [10]. It has been mentioned that the complete phytochemical investigations of medicinal plants should be carried out [8], because these secondary metabolites are commercially important and are responsible for medicinal activity of the plant [8,9].

Plants contain secondary metabolites such as alkaloids, flavonoids, steroids, phenolics, terpenes, volatile oils etc. as well as other substance that are important for radical scavenging effects as well as their potential antibacterial, estrogenic and anti-cancer activities [1].

Few reports have been made on the use of medicinal plants in the treatment of dental diseases. These reports have been reported mostly from India and Africa [11-15]. The use of *Argemone maxicana, Azadirachta indica* and *Ocimum basilicum* in dental health care has been reported by Singh and Dhakre [11]. Sadangi et al. [15] have reported 10 species of medicinal plants used in the treatment of ear and mouth diseases by the tribal people of Kalahandi district.

Medicinal plants extracts have been shown to exibit antibacterial activity against various oral microflora [16-18]. The anti-inflammatory, antioxidants, antibacterial, astringent and other useful properties of several plants and plant parts have reported [19]. These properties are considered valuable in the treatment of diverse dental and oral diseases.

Medicinal plants consitutue a significant proportion of traditional medical practices for oral diseases in Cameroon [20]. However the analysis of phytoconstituents of medicinal plants used for oral

***Corresponding author:** Ashu Michael Agbor, Universite des Montagnes, Dental surgery, Bangangte, Cameroon, E-mail: agborasm@yahoo.com healthcare in Cameroon has not been done. The objective of the study was to determine the phytoconstituents of common medicinal plants used for oral healthcare in Cameroon.

Materials and Methods

There are many plant materials that have been identified to treat dental problems but specific plants with significant clinical qualities needed phytochemical analysis.

Selection and identification of plants

Plants analysed during this study were selected specifically based on the frequency of usage by traditional healers and also by specific significant clinical role. Prior to the analysis of these plants, they were identified at the Department of Botany of University of Dchang and Confirmed at the National Herbarium at Yaounde. The following groups of plants were selected to be analyzed;

One plant used for atraumatic tooth extractions, three plants used for dental pain relief, one plant used for tooth bleaching, one plant used for mouth washing/ halitosis. The plants were identified and coded for analytical purposes

Sample collection: Samples of fresh plants used for dental treatment in Cameroon that were free from any plant disease were obtained from the traditional healers at the beginning of the rainy season. The plants were dried and one (1) kg of each dried plant was checked for any mould or dust after which was sent to the laboratory for analysis.

Phytochemical screening: They were also sterilized on a hot air oven and each material was wrapped with aluminium foil before sterilization.

Extraction of plant materials: Different amount of dried powder obtained from each plant material was macerated with intermediate stirring for 48 hours in methanol before filtering. After filtration with Whattman filter paper, the residue was thrown away and the filtrate was evaporated to dryness of solvent using the rotative evaporator in order to obtain the concentrated extracts of each plant sample which was weighed and stored in clean flask in a refrigerator until usage.

Screening of different plant extracts: The different plant extracts were qualitatively tested for the presence of phytochemicals such as alkaloids, flavonoids, saponins, terpenoids, steroids and tannins using the standard procedures as previously described [21-24].

Test for alkaloids

Drangendoff's reagent was used; as such 10 mg of each plant extract in 5 mL of 1% ethanolic HCl and 5 drops of Drangendoff's reagent were added. The formation of orange precipitate incates the presence of alkaloids.

Test for flavonoids

The method adopted for this study is the one in which 5 mL of diluted ammonia solution was added to a portion of extract dissolved in ethanol, followed by addition of concentrated sulphuric acid. A yellow colouration was observed in each extract, indicating the presence of flavonoids.

Test for steroids

Two mL of acetic anhydride was added 10 mg ethanolic extract of each sample with 2 mL of concentrated sulphuric acid. The colour changing from violet to blue indicated the presence of steroids.

Test for terpenoids/terpenes

The Salkowski test was used. Ten milli gram of each extract was dissolved in chloroform, and 4 mL concentrated sulphuric acid was carrefully added to form a layer. A redish brown colouration of the inter-face was formed to show positive result for the presence of terpenoids or terpenes.

Test for saponins

The persistent frothing test for saponin was used. To 50 mg of each extract was added 5 mL of distilled water. The mixture was vigorously shaken and heated to boil for a stable persistent froth. The frothing was mixed with 4 drops of olive oil and shaken vigorously for the formation of emulsion thus indicating the presence of saponins.

Test for tannins

About 15 mg of each extract contained in test tube was dissolved in ethanol and 3 drops of Ferric Chloride solution was added. A deep browrish green or a blue-black colouration indicates a positive test for tannins.

Test for phlobatannins

Deposition of red precipitate when an aqueous extract of each plant sample was boiled with 2% hydrochloric acid was taken as evidence for the presence of phlobatannins.

Test for cardiac glycosides

The Keller-Killani test was used. About 10 mg of each plant extract dissolved in ethanol was treated with 2 mL of glacial acetic acid containing 2 drops of ferric chloride solution. This was underlayed with 1.5 mL of concentrated sulphuric acid. A brown ring of the interface indicates a deoxysugar characteristic of cardenolides (cardic glycosides). A violet ring appears below the brown ring, while in the acetic acid layer a greenish ring was observed.

Results

This study revealed the presence of phytochemicals considered as active medicinal chemical constituents in the studied plants. Table 1 shows the total weight percentage yield of the crude extracts of the six plants. Important medicinal phytochemicals such as alkaloids, tannins, saponins, steroids, phlobatannins, terpenoids, flavonoids, and cardiac glycosides were present in the samples. The phytochemical analysis showed that all the six (6) plants are rich in at least one of the secondary metabolites such as alkaloids, tannins, saponins, steroids, phlobatannins, terpenoids, flavonoids, and cardic glycosides. Steroids,

Plant code	Plant part used	Amount of dry powder used (g)	Amount of extract obtained (g)	Yield (%)
Ag	Aerial part	34	1.5	4.41
Emi	Aerial part	46.5	5.5	11.83
Cot	Leaves	43	3.9	9.06
Cari	Leaves	87	3.4	3.90
Spi	Aerial part	28	2.9	10.35
Mor	Aerial part	6.5	0.4	6.15

Ag: *Ageratum conyzoides* (Asteraceae)
Emi: *Emilia coccinea* (Asteraceae)
Spi: *Spilanthes africana* (Asteraceae)
Cot: *Gossypium sp*, Coton (Malvaceae)
Car: *Carica papaya* (Caricaceae)
Mor: *Momordica charantia* (cucubitaceae)

Table 1: Percentage yeild of extracts.

Plants	Alkaloids	Tannins	Saponins	Steroids	Phlobatannins	Terpenoids	Flavonoids	Cardiac glycosides
Ag	+	+	+	+	-	+	+	-
Emi	-	+	-	+	+	+	+	+
Cot	-	+	-	+	+	+	+	-
Car	+	+	+	+	+	+	+	+
Spi	-	-	-	+	+	+	+	-
Mor	-	-	+	+	-	+	+	+

+: indicates presence of phytochemicals, -: indicates absence of phytochemicals.
Ag: *Ageratum conyzoides* (Asteraceae)
Emi: *Emilia coccinea* (Asteraceae)
Spi: *Spilanthes africana* (Asteraceae)
Cot: *Gossypium sp*, Coton (Malvaceae)
Car: *Carica papaya* (Caricaceae)
Mor: *Momordica charantia* (Cucubitaceae)

Table 2: Qualitative analysis for phytoconstituents of crude extracts of the six plants.

terpenoids and flavonoids were found in all the plants samples in this study. Alkaloids were present in *Ageratum conyzoides* and *Carica papaya*. Tannins were present in *Ageratum conyzoides*, *Emilia coccinea*, *Gossypium sp* and *Carica papaya*. Saponins were present in *Ageratum conyzoides*, *Carica papaya* and *Momordica charantia*. Phlobatannins were present in *Emilia coccinea*, *Gossypium sp*, *Carica papaya* and *Spilanthes africana*. Cardic glycosides were present in *Emilia coccinea*, *Carica papaya*, and *Momordica charantia*. *Carica papaya* contained all these phytochemicals (Table 2).

Discussion

Even though a more recent figure is not available, the WHO has estimated that up to 80% of the population in Africa and the majority of the populations in Asia and Latin America use herbs for their primary healthcare need [25]. In industrialized countries, plant-based traditional medicines or phyto-therapeuticals are often termed complementary or alternative medicine (CAM), and their use has increased steadily over the last 10 years [26]. The tradition of herbs use in the treatment of diseases are usually handed from generation to generation in many communities and the repository of the knowledge is predominantly with the traditional healers which is not documented or transfered.The knowledge of the chemical constituents of plants is desirable because such information will be of value for the synthesis of complex chemical substances [5]. It has been mentioned that the complete phytochemical investigations of medicinal plants should be carried out because these secondary metabolites are commercially important and are responsible for medicinal activity of the plant [27].

Argiratum conizoides (king plant) is one of the common plants called African panacea or the king of plants in Cameroon because it treats several diseases. This study showed that the plant has many secondary metabolites like alkaloids, tannin, saponins, terpenoids and flavonoids. The result is similar to that carried out by Onuoha and colleagues [27] where all secondary metabolites were present except flavonoids.It is used in Cameroon for calming down pain and for tooth extractions by traditional healers. Its analgesic property is attributed to the ability of alkaloids to inhibit pain in dental caries. The fibrinolytic and heamostatic properties of this plant explain why it is used for tooth extraction.These properties need to be investigated in future. The plant has been found to be effective against septic wounds micro-organisms *(S. aureus and E. coli)* [7] and other oral micro-organisms actinomycetes and *P. gingivalis*. It has also been found to have strong cytotoxic effects similar to that of vincristine [28,29]. Huge amount of phenolics and flavonoids present in the plant might be responsible for its promising cytotoxic activity [30,31] and the possible mechanism of cytotoxicity is due to its poisonous effect

on cell mitosis [29].This cytotoxic property calls for precautions when the plant is being used.

Emilia coccinea is used to calm down toothache in Cameroon. The leaves are also eaten raw and can be mixed with guinea corn and lime juice to serve as a remedy for sore throat [32,33]. The leaves are also used for cleaning wounds and the roots for diarrhoea. In Nigeria, the leaves are eaten cooked as salad or spinach and the fresh juice of the leaves is a remedy for sore eyes. According to earlier reports, [34] *Emilia coccinea* is used medicinally for the treatment of syphilis, hernia, gonorrhoea, ulcer, craw-craw, abscesses of the breast, ringworm, lice, measles, cough etc. The bioactivities of *Emilia coccinea* have been confirmed in various laboratories, these include antidiarrhoeral, antimicrobial and fungicidal activity [35] due to its rich constituents of secondary metabolites. In this study the plant extracts contained Tannins, steriods, Phlobatannins, tepenes, Flavonoids and Cardic glycosides. Alkaloids and saponins were absent.This is consistent with a phytochemical analysis done in Nigeria by Edeoga and colleagues [32] which demostrated that all phytochemicals were present except Phlobatannins. According to previous studies, the phytochemical screening of *E. coccinea* has revealed the presence of some secondary metabolites including alkaloid, cardiac glycoside [36].

Cotton *(Gosipium barbadense)* leaves are boiled into a hot tea, used for gaggling to calm down toothache. It is also used as an adjuvant with *Ageratum conyzoides* for tooth extractions.It contained tannins, steriods, phlobatannins, terpenes and flavonoids. Alkaloids, cardiac glycosides and saponins were absent. Apena and coleagues in Nigeria showed that leaf extracts of *G. barbadense* contained tannins, phlobatinins, cardiac glycosides and flavonoids, but saponins and anthraquinones were absent [37,38]. They also found out that leaf extracts also contained alkaloids such as quinoline, indole and morphine [39,40]. Some species of *Gosipium* have been shown to possess antibacteria, antiinflamatory, wound healing and anti-cancer properties [39,40]. An infusion of the leaf is taken as an antedote for colds and bronchitis and the young shoots pulped for palpitations and as dressings for wounds and in the treatment of systematic diarrhoeas [39]. A number of bioactive triterpenoid and sesquiterpenoid aldehydes compound have been isolated and characterized from this and related species [38].

Whitish latex of *Carica papaya* is applied directly to the affected areas of the toothache to cure toothache while the decoction of its fresh unripe fruits and infusions of its leaves is used for treating mouth sore and oral thrush. *Carica papaya* analysis in this study contained all secondary metabolites tested.This result is similar to other studies [41]. In addition, it contains phytochemicals such as vitamins, enzymes, protiens, alkaloids, lectins, saponins, flavonoids, sterols, minerals and glycosides [41,42]. In addition, it contains phytochemicals such as vitamins, enzymes, proteins, alkaloids, lectins, saponins, flavonoids, sterols, minerals and glycosides [41,43]. Alkaloids present in *C. papaya* could be responsible for its antibacterial activity and are also used as analgesics and narcotics for pain relief [41].

Chitinase is the anti-fungal enzyme extracted from the plant; the recombinant papya chitinase has anti-bacterial properties [41]. Capaine, an extract from the seeds and leaves has anti-helmethic properties, boost immunity and also act as cardiac depressant [41]. Flavonoids, glycosides and cardiac glycosides found in the extracts are suggestive of their antioxidant property. Flavonoid glycosides are reported to be antioxidants and used as anti-inflammatories in the treatment of capillary fragility [43] which is applicable to diseases like gingivitis.

The seed and the pulp of *Carica papaya* have been shown to treat more than 20 diseases and studies revealed it's bacteriostatic against common oral microorganisms like *Staphylococcus* spp [41]. The latex of *Carica papaya* has been shown to reduce the growth of *Candida albican* by 60%; the fruits when used as topical ulcers dressing have been found to promote desloughing, granulation and healing [41]. These properties make it suitable for the treatment of mouth sores such as apthus ulcers.

Spilanthes africana is another plant that is widely used by traditional healers in Cameroon. It is also used as a mouth wash for instant treatment of halitosis due to its peppermint taste and for the treatment of minor bone fractures of the teeth and the alveolar bone; when applied directly to the cavity, it alleviates toothache. *Spilanthes acmella* Murr (Compositae) is the well known "toothache plant", also commonly used as a spice. It has a long history of use as a folklore remedy, e.g. for toothache, rheumatism and fever [44]. In this study *Spilanthes africana* was found to contain steroids, phlobatannins, terpenoids, and flavonoids. Sterols are responsible for the antiinflamatory and analgesic properties of this plant. The use of *Spilanthes spp* in the treatment of toothache by direct application by traditional healers had been documented in India [45]. Analgesic and anti-Inflammatory activities of different *Spilanthes* species has made it useful for the treatment of toothache, mucositis and sore throat and to relieve pain from boils, cut wounds, and other types of wounds in traditional medicine [45]. Besides, it has been found to be specific against several microorganisms responsible for oro-facial pathologies. *Spilanthes* had been found also to have anti -pyretic, anti-cancer, anti-fungal and anti-oxidant activities [45].

Momordica charantia (Cucurbitaceae), the aerial part of the plant is used in Cameroon as an adjuvant in tooth extraction, post extraction management of extraction socket and also for tooth bleaching. The leave extracts is widely used for toothache and post extraction dressing by traditional healers. In the current study, *M.charantia* was found to contain, saponins, steroids, terpenoids, flavonoids and cardiac glycosides. It has been shown to be widely used to treat several diseases because of its anthelminitic, anti-viral, anti-ulcer and antimicrobial activities [46]. Its antibacterial activity has been demonstrated against *Bacillus subtilis*, *Escherichia coli*, *Pseudomonas aeruginosa* and *Staphyalococcus aureus* [47] which form part of the natural and pathogenic oral flora. It has also been found to exibit some antifertility, antihyperglycemic [47] and hypoglycemic activities [48]. Its steroids contents have been attributed to its antiglycermic and analgesic activities [47] while terpenes for its antimicrobial and anti-oxidant activities. Extensive studies on the antidiabetic properties of this plant have been done, but more studies are required in the area of oral health care.

Conclusion

This study revealed that all the medicinal plants studied had huge quantities of secondary metabolites that may be responsible for their medicinal use. More detailed research is needed for these plants because of their multiple uses.

Acknowledgement

We wish to acknowledge Dr. Razak abdul a.k.a Petit Alhaji for his openness and for providing most of the plants used for this study.

References

1. Sukirtha K, Growther L (2012) Antibacterial, antifungal and phytochemical analysis of selected medicinal plants. J Nat Prod Plant Resour 2: 644-648.

2. Pichersky E, Gang DR (2000) Genetics and biochemistry of secondary metabolites in plants: an evolutionary perspective. Trends Plant Sci 5: 439-445.

3. Dixon RA (1999) Plant natural products: the molecular genetic basis of biosynthetic diversity. Curr Opin Biotechnol 10: 192-197.

4. Li J, Ou-Lee TM, Raba R, Amundson RG, Last RL (1993) Arabidopsis Flavonoid Mutants Are Hypersensitive to UV-B Irradiation. Plant Cell 5: 171-179.

5. Savithramma N, Linga Rao M, Suhrulatha D (2011) Screening of medicinal plants for secondary metabolites. Middle-East J Sci Res 8: 579-584.

6. Siddiqui S, Verma A, Rather AA, Jabeen F, Meghvansi MK (2009) Preliminary phytochemicals analysis of some important medicinal and aromatic plants. Advances in Biological Research 3: 188-195.

7. Ashok PK, Kanimozhi M (2010) Phytochemical screening and antimicrobial activity from five Indian medicinal plants against humanpathogens. Middle-East Journal of scientific research 5: 157-162.

8. Chitravadivu C, Manian S, Kalaichelvi K (2009) Qualitative analysis of selected medicinal plants, Tamilnadu, India. Middle-East J Sci Res 4: 144-146.

9. Joy PP, Thomas J, Mathew S, Skaria BP (2001) Medicinal Plants. In: Bose TK, Kabir J, Das P, Joy PP (eds.) Tropical Horticulture. Naya Prokash, Calcutta, India 2: 449-632.

10. Knoll-Kohler E, Stiebel J (2002) Amine fluoride gel affects the viability and the generation of superoxide anions in human polymorphonuclear leukocytes: an in vitro study. European Journal of Oral Sciences 110: 296-301.

11. Singh D, Dhakre JS (1989) Some medicinal plants of Mathura district (U. P.) Mendel 6: 60-66.

12. Jadhav D (2006) Plant sources used for the treatment of different types of fevers by Bhil Tribe of Ratlam district, Madhya Pradesh, India. J Econ Taxon Bot 30: 909-911.

13. Elujoba AA, Odeleye OM, Ogunyemi CM (2005) Traditional Medical Development for medical and dental primary Health care Delivery System in Africa. Afr J Trad CAM 2: 46-61.

14. Aharoni A, Galili G (2011) Metabolic engineering of the plant primary-secondary metabolism interface. Curr Opin Biotechnol 22: 239-244.

15. Sadangi N, Padhy RN, Sahu RK (2005) A contribution to medico- ethnobotany of kalahandi district, orissa on ear and mouth disease. Anc Sci Life 24: 160-163.

16. Dinesh MD, Uma MS, Anjali VM, Meenatchisundaram NS, Shanmugam V (2013) Inhibitory properties of aqueous extracts of selected indigenous medicinal plants against dental caries causing Streptococcus mutans and Streptococcus mitis. Afr J Basic Appl Sci 5: 8-11.

17. Pathak A, Sardar A, Kadam V, Rekadwak B, Karuppayil MS (2012) Efficiency of some medicinal plants against human dental pathogens. Indian J Natural Products and Resources 3: 123-127.

18. Jenkinson HF, Lamont RJ (2005) Oral microbial communities in sickness and in health. Trends Microbiol 13: 589-595.

19. Bhardwaj A, Bhardwaj SV (2012) Ethno-dentistry: popular medicinal plants used for dental diseases in India. J Intercult Ethnopharmacol 1: 62-65.

20. Agbor AM, Naidoo S (2011) Knowledge and practice of traditional healers in oral health in the Bui Division, Cameroon. J Ethnobiol Ethnomed 7: 6.

21. Sofowora EA (1993) Medicinal plants and traditional medicine in Africa. Spectrum Books, Ibadan, Nigeria 289.

22. Harborne JB (1998) phytochemical methods. A guide to modern techniques of plant analysis. 3rd ed Chapman and Hall Int Ed NY 40 - 137.

23. Trease GE, Evans WC (2002) Phytochemicals. In: Pharmacognosy (15thedn.) Saunders Publishers, London, pp. 42-44, 221- 229, 246- 249, 304-306, 331-332, 391-393.

24. Tang CS (2005) Phytochemistry of Medicinal Plants. Phytochem of Medicinal and Pharmacology 99: 787-794.

25. Salim AA, Chin YW, Kinghorn AD (2008) Bioactive molecules and medicinal plants. In: Ramawat KG, Merillon JM (eds) Drug discovery from plants, Springer, New York, USA 1-24.

26. Sneader W (1996) Drug Prototypes and their Exploitation, John Wiley & Son, Chichester, UK.

27. Onuoha OG, Ayo JA, Osuagwu V, Iruolaje F (2013) Investigation of the antibacterial activity of Ageratum Conyzoides extract on microorganisms isolated from septic wound. Topcls Journal of Herbal Medicines 2: 182-188.

28. Nasrin F (2013) Antioxidant and cytotoxic activities of Ageratum conyzoides stems. Int Current Pharmaceutical J 2: 33-37.

29. Okwori AEJ, Dina CO, Junaid S, Okeke IO, Adetunji JA, et al. (2007) Antibacterial activities of Ageratum conyzoides extracts on selected bacterial pathogens. Int J Microbiol 4: 1937- 1949.

30. Moreira MD, Picanço MC, Barbosa LC, Guedes RN, Barros EC, et al. (2007) Compounds from Ageratum conyzoides: isolation, structural elucidation and insecticidal activity. Pest Manag Sci 63: 615-621.

31. Edeoga HO, Okwu DE, Mbaebie BO (2005) Phytochemical constituents of some Nigerian medicinal plants. Afr J Biotechnol 4: 685-688.

32. Ogbebor N, Adekunle AT (2005) Inhibition of conidial germination and mycelia growth of Corynespoa casiicola (Berk and Curt) of rubber (Hevea brasilieusis Muella Arg) using extract of some plants. Afr J Bitechnol 4: 996-1000.

33. Ndip RN, Malange Tarkang AE, Mbullah SM, Luma HN, Malongue A, et al. (2007) In vitro anti-Helicobacter pylori activity of extracts of selected medicinal plants from North West Cameroon. J Ethnopharmacol 114: 452-457.

34. Ayitey-Smith E (1989) Prospects and Scope, Plant Medicine in Health Care. Ghana University Press 29.

35. Mensah JK, Ihenyen J, Iyamu M (2013) Phytochemical and antimicrobial properties of Emilia coccinea (Cass.) Asian J Contemp Sci 2: 26-31.

36. Odugbemi T (2008) Outlines and pictures of Medicinal plants from Nigeria. University of Lagos press, Nigeria 283-285.

37. Essien EE, Aboaba SO, Ogunwande IA (2011) Constituents and antimicrobial properties of the leaf essential oil of Gossypium barbadense (Linn.). J Med Plants Res 5: 702-705.

38. Sultana A (2012) Gossypium herbaceum Linn: An Ethnopharmacological Review. JPSI 1: 1-5.

39. Velmurugan C, Venkatesh S, Sandhya K, Lakshmi BS, Vardhan RR, et al. (2012) Wound healing activity of methanolic extract of leaves of Gossypium herbaceum. Cent Eur J Exp Biol 1: 7-10.

40. Apena A, Atole C, Chinweike-Umeh SN, Usigbe UE, Ojekunle MO, et al. (2004) The nutritive potentials of cotton (Gossypium barbadense) Leaves. Nig Food J 22: 160-163.

41. Krishna KL, Paridhavi M, Patel JA (2008) Review on nutritional, medicinal and pharmacological prpoperties of Carica papaya. Natural Products Radiance 7: 364-373.

42. Imaga NA, Gbenle GO, Okochi VI, Adenekan S, Duro-Emmanuel T, et al. (2010) Phytochemical and antioxidant nutrient constituents of Carica papaya and Parquetina nigrescens extracts. Sci Res Essays 5: 2201-2205.

43. Iwu MM (1993) Handbook of African Medicinal Plants. CRC Press, USA 141-142.

44. Paulraj J, Govindarajan R, Palpu P (2013) The Genus Spilanthes Ethnopharmacology, Phytochemistry, and Pharmacological Properties: A Review. Advances in Pharmacological Sciences. 2013: 1-22.

45. Prachayasittikul S, Suphapong S, Worachartcheewan A, Lawung R, Ruchirawat S, et al. (2009) Bioactive metabolites from Spilanthes acmella Murr. Molecules 14: 850-867.

46. Farnsworth NR, Bunyapraphatsara N (1992) Thai medicinal plants recommended for primary health care system; Prachachon, Bangkok.

47. Sharma S, Tandon S, Semwal B, Singh K (2011) Momordica charantia Linn: A Comprehensive Review on Bitter Remedy. Journal of Pharmaceutical Research And Opinion 1: 42-47.

48. Raman A, Lau C (1996) Anti-diabetic properties and phytochemistry of Momordica charantia L. (Cucurbitaceae). Phytomedicine 2: 349-362.

17

Mono-Methyl Selenium and Cancer Therapy: Current Status and Future Translational Research Needs

Barrow K, Jiang C and Lü J*

Department of Biomedical Sciences, School of Pharmacy, Texas Tech University Health Sciences Center, 1300 South Coulter Street, Amarillo, TX79106, USA

Abstract

The human clinical trials with seleno-methionine (SeMet) for prostate cancer prevention and selenized-yeast (contains mostly SeMet) for the prevention of non-small cell lung cancer and prostate cancer in North America conclusively rejected the use of these selenium (Se) forms for cancer prevention in human populations with adequate Se intake. Nevertheless, solid mechanism-based preclinical studies with other Se forms have suggested the potential for their use at pharmacological doses as adjuvant treatment alone and especially as chemo-enhancers for combination cancer therapy. Of the distinct pools of Se metabolites, the mono-methylated Se (MM-Se) has many desirable attributes for cancer therapy, affecting a multitude of crucial molecules and signaling pathways in cancer epithelial cells, vascular endothelial cells and microenvironment. Inorganic selenite/selenide in excess of selenoprotein synthesis can lead to DNA single strand breaks, which implicate possible genotoxicity to normal cells and are therefore unattractive for long-term use. In this paper, we review animal studies with MM-Se such as methylseleninic acid and Se-methylselenocysteine as well as inorganic Se for inhibition of xenograft tumors of several organ sites as single therapy and those using MM-Se to enhance the therapeutic efficacy of cancer chemotherapeutic drugs and to reduce the dose-limiting toxicities of such modalities. We present and critique potential mechanisms of action for such applications and future improvement. Since Se-methylselenocysteine was the only MM-Se with a published human pharmacokinetic study, we discuss future research directions to enable clinical translation studies.

Abbreviations: AR: Androgen Receptor; ER: Estrogen Receptor; Se: Selenium; MM-Se: Mono-Methyl(Ated)-Selenium; DMDSe: Di-Methylselenide; GPx3: Glutathione Peroxidase 3; Ph-SeGPx: Phospholipid Glutathione Peroxidase; MSeA: Methylseleninic Acid; MSeC: Se-Methylselenocysteine; MSeCN: Methylselenocyanate; SeCys: Selenocysteine; Se-GPx: Glutathione Peroxidase; Sel-P or SEPP1: Selenoprotein P; Sel-W: Selenoprotein W; SeMe: Selenomethionine; TDI: Thyroixine Deiodinase; Trx: Thioredoxin; TrxR: Thioredoxin Reductase; GR: Glutathionine Reductase

Introduction and Scope of Review

By now, several well-designed human clinical trials in North America have conclusively dismissed using seleno-methionine (SeMet) or SeMet-rich selenized-yeast for cancer prevention in human populations with adequate Se intake [1-4]. These failures to show preventive efficacy of SeMet and Se-yeast have cast shadow on the potential utility of other and newer forms of Se (e.g., mono-methylated Se, MM-Se) for cancer chemoprevention. Many reviews have been published discussing the reasons for the failure [5-8]. Based on the well-documented metabolic and biochemical differences between SeMet and the MM-Se [9,10], as well as the preclinical efficacy outcomes [11], we have argued that the failure of SeMet cannot be equated to all Se forms are ineffective for cancer chemoprevention [12]. We have recently articulated two major lessons from these trials [13]: 1) Antioxidant hypothesis was tested in wrong subjects/patient populations; 2) Se agent selection was not supported by cell culture and animal efficacy data.

Whereas the major focal point of Se research for the last two decades has been on the cancer preventive efficacy of SeMet and Se-Yeast in human trials, several groups, including those of Y. Rustum and C. Ip at Roswell Park Cancer Institute and ours, have studied the possible cancer therapeutic application, especially of the MM-Se forms distinct from SeMet. In this paper, we review animal studies with MM-Se such as methylseleninic acid (MSeA) and Se-methylselenocysteine (MSeC) as a single agent in "adjuvant therapy" context and those using MM-Se to enhance therapeutic efficacy of chemotherapy drugs in a number

of cancers and to reduce dose-limiting toxicities of such drugs. We examine and contrast pertinent studies with inorganic Se forms such as selenite and selenite in the context of cancer therapy. In addition, we present and critique potential mechanisms of action for therapeutic applications and for their further refinements. Furthermore, we discuss the current status of human studies with MM-Se and suggest future research directions to enable clinical translation studies. Because we focus on endogenous Se metabolism and MM-Se metabolites, we will not discuss Se-substituted derivatives of S-containing drugs or aromatic synthetic Se compounds. Readers interested in these topics are referred to following expert reviews [8,14].

Active Anti-Cancer Metabolite Theory

Se deficiency is not a health concern in the USA. As a result, most animal models and cell culture studies since the mid-1980s have dealt with chemotherapeutic or chemopreventive levels of Se and have focused on the cancerous cells as the targets of its anti-cancer effects. Most animal models have shown cancer chemopreventive activity of Se intake that is 20-50 times greater than the nutritional requirement [10]. It had been proposed decades ago that cancer chemoprevention by Se in nutritionally adequate subjects was independent of the antioxidant activity of plasma or tissue glutathione peroxidase (SeGPx) [10,15]. This paradigm was based on the observation that the dietary level of

***Corresponding author:** Junxuan Lü, Department of Biomedical Sciences, Texas Tech University Health Sciences Center School of Pharmacy, 1300 South Coulter Street, Amarillo, TX79106, USA,
E-mail: junxuan.lu@ttuhsc.edu

Se (2 ppm or greater as selenite or other Se forms) needed to achieve a significant cancer preventive activity in rodent animal models far exceeded that required (i.e., 0.1 ppm or mg/kg) to support maximal SeGPx in the blood (glutathione peroxidase 3, GPx3) or the target tissues from which the experimental cancers arose. This view has been extended to the other selenoproteins identified subsequently in the past 2 decades, including phospholipid glutathione peroxidase (Ph-SeGPx or GPx4), selenoprotein P (Sel-P or SEPP1), selenoprotein W (Sel-W), thyroixine de-iodinases (TDI) and thioredoxin reductases (TrxRs) [9,16,17]. The studies with transgenic suppression of selenoproteins (increased prostate and colon cancer risk with decreased SeGPxs in the presence of adequate dietary selenium) and the TrxR1 knockdown transfectant cells (decreased lung cancer growth with knocked down TrxR1) indicate likely contradicting roles of these proteins as regulators of cancer risk in the nutritional range of Se intake [18].

Metabolically, excess Se beyond the need for selenoprotein synthesis (hydrogen selenide is co-translationally incorporated into the selenocysteine (SeCys)-containing selenoproteins) is methylated into methylselenol, which is further methylated and excreted as dimethylselenide (volatile through breath) and trimethylselenonium (urine) or converted into selenosugars (Figure 1). Although SeMet is the most abundant natural MM-Se, it is predominantly incorporated into general proteins in place of methionine (non-specific substitution) or metabolized to SeCys through a trans-selenation pathway similar to the transulfuration pathway from methionine to cysteine. The efficiency of the latter pathway will be dependent on the metabolic capacity of the cell types and organs. Liver and hepatocytes are expected to be well equipped with the metabolic enzymes, whereas in general non-hepatic tumor cells in culture would be expected to be limited in this ability.

Ip and Ganther [10,19] proposed that the active anti-cancer Se metabolites were likely MM-Se species (presumably methylselenol) and the cancer chemopreventive efficacy of a given Se compound might depend on the rate of its metabolic conversion to the active MM-Se form(s). Circumstantial evidence was obtained by comparing the efficacy of forms of Se that fed into different Se metabolite pools, with precursors of methylselenol displaying greater preventive efficacy than those for hydrogen selenide or dimethylselenide in the chemically induced rodent mammary carcinogenesis model [20,21]. Extending on the methylselenol structure-activity theme, subsequent work had shown that the alkyl-selenol and allyl-selenol precursor compounds were more active against mammary carcinogenesis than methylselenol precursors on an equal molar basis of dietary Se intake [22,23]. However, these structure-activity studies have not been extended beyond the mammary carcinogenesis model for assessing the general applicability of the methylselenol hypothesis in other organ sites.

In cell culture models, studies by us and others focusing on the levels of Se exposure in therapeutic range have shown that MM-Se compounds that are putative precursors to the methylselenol pool induce numerous cellular, biochemical and gene expression responses that are distinct from those induced by the forms of Se that enter the hydrogen selenide pool [9,16]. These major cellular and biochemical effects have been summarized and detailed in earlier reviews [9,16]. We updated newer findings from the last decade and schematically present them in Figure 1.

Hydrogen selenide pool

Sodium selenite and sodium selenide, which feed into the hydrogen selenide (H_2Se) pool, rapidly (within minutes to a few hours of Se exposure) induce DNA single strand breaks (SSBs), S phase or G_2/M cell cycle arrest and lead to subsequent cell death by apoptosis, autophagy and necrosis [9]. Sodium selenide and SeCys could recapitulate the DNA SSB induction and the apoptosis effects of selenite in the model system [24]. A superoxide dismutase mimetic compound, copper dipropylsalicylate, blocked DNA SSBs and apoptosis, indicating that selenite per se did not trigger these events [25]. Studies have provided further support for ROS (superoxide generation) as intermediates for activating p53 Ser-15 phosphorylation in apoptosis induced by selenite in LNCaP prostate cancer cell model [26,27]. Published data from our group indicated that selenite given by daily oral dosage of 3 mg/kg body weight to tumor bearing nude mice increased DNA SSBs in peripheral blood nucleated cells whereas, the same dosage of MSeA or MSeC lacked this effect [11]. Further studies in animal models and in humans are necessary to confirm the in vivo genotoxicity of selenite.

The methylselenol pool

Our group has shown that MM-Se methylselenol precursors such as methylselenocyanate (MSeCN) and MSeC induced apoptosis of mammary tumor epithelial cells and leukemia cells without the induction of DNA single strand breaks (SSBs) [24,28,29]. Furthermore, MSeA-induced cancer cell apoptosis was caspase-dependent, whereas selenite-induced cell death was independent of these death proteases in DU145 prostate cancer cells with mutant P53. MM-Se led to G_1 arrest [28-33], inhibitory effects on cyclin-dependent kinases [33,34] and protein kinase C [35]. In terms of genotoxicity implications, a daily oral dosage of 3 mg per kg body weight, MSeA and MSeC significantly suppressed human DU145 xenograft growth without increasing DNA SSBs in the peripheral blood nucleated cells of the host mice whereas the same dosage of selenite caused increased DNA SSBs and was ineffective for suppressing xenograft growth [11].

Direct demonstration of methylselenol intra-cellular cytotoxicity through adenoviral delivery of bacterial Pseudomonas putida methioninase (Ad-METase) gene into cancer cells was carried out by R. Hoffman's group in vitro and in vivo, when SeMet was provided as substrate to enzymatically produce methylselenol [36]. In METase-transduced tumor cells, the cytotoxicity of SeMet is increased by 3 orders of magnitude compared with non-infected cells. A strong bystander effect occurred because of methylselenol release from METase-producing cells and uptake by surrounding tumor cells. They showed that methylselenol damaged the mitochondria via oxidative stress and caused cytochrome c release into the cytosol, thereby activating the caspase cascade and apoptosis. In animal xenograft model, they showed that Ad-METase/SeMet treatment profoundly inhibited tumor growth in mice and significantly prolonged their survival. The same group [37] also investigated the combination of SeMet/Ad-METase gene therapy with doxorubicin in a nude mice model with H460 lung cancer cell xenograft. Doxorubicin was administered by intraperitoneal injection (i.p.) twice per week at a dose of 2 mg/kg body weight and SeMet of 1 μmole (i.e., 79 μg) per mouse by intratumoral injection daily, starting the day after the adenovirus infection. After two weeks of treatment, the control- and the doxorubicin-treated tumors had increased by ten times. The tumors in mice treated by SeMet/Ad-METase grew 5.8 times, and those in mice receiving a combination of doxorubicin and SeMet/Ad-METase grew only 2.5 times. It was also determined that the tumor doubling time of the respective individual treatment was around 2-3 days but was increased to 10 days by the combination treatment.

Our group demonstrated that methylselenol generated from SeMet via METase added directly to cell culture medium efficiently induced cell apoptosis [32] in human umbilical vein endothelial cells (HUVECs) and the DU145 human prostate cancer cells. Exposure of

DU145 cells to methylselenol generated in the sub-micromolar range of substrate SeMet led to caspase-mediated cleavage of poly(ADP-ribose) polymerase (cPARP), nucleosomal DNA fragmentation, and morphologic apoptosis, recapitulating MSeA effects cited above. Biochemically, METase/SeMet-generated methylselenol also inhibited phosphorylation of protein kinase AKT and extracellularly regulated kinases 1/2 (ERK 1/2) as did MSeA. In the HUVECs, methylselenol exposure resulted in G_1 arrest action similar to MSeA in mitogen-stimulated G_1 progression during mid-G_1 to late G_1. This stage-specificity was also mimicked by inhibitors of phosphatidylinositol 3-kinase. In the last 5 years, Zeng and coworkers in a number of publications [38-40] followed up this means of generating methylselenol in other cancer cell culture models and examined cell cycle and molecular changes. Overall, these findings indicate that methylselenol is one of the proximal active metabolites.

Beside apoptosis, we and others have shown that MM-Se compounds exert a rapid inhibitory effect on the expression of key molecules of cancer and angiogenesis. For example, sub-apoptotic concentrations of MSeA inhibited the expression and secretion of the angiogenic factor VEGF in several cancer cell lines [41]. MSeA also inhibited the expression of matrix metalloproteinase (MMP)-2 in the vascular endothelial cells [41,42]. These effects plus a potent inhibitory effect on the cell cycle progression of vascular endothelial cells [31,32] indicate that methylselenol can be a key inhibitor of angiogenic switch regulation in early lesions and in tumors [9]. MSeA and methylselenol released by METase from SeMet inhibited androgen receptor (AR) expression and its signaling to prostate specific antigen (PSA) [43-45] as well as PSA stability [43]. MSeA has also been shown to inhibit estrogen receptor (ER) signaling in breast and endometrial cancer cells [46-49] and as a novel suppressor of aromatase expression [50]. Specifically, the expression of the aromatase gene, CYP19, is controlled in a tissue-specific manner by the alternate use of different promoters. In obese postmenopausal women, increased peripheral aromatase is primarily attributed to the activity of the glucocorticoid-stimulated promoter, PI.4, and the cAMP-stimulated promoter, PII. MSeA effectively suppressed aromatase activation by dexamethasone (a synthetic glucocorticoid), and forskolin (a specific activator of adenylate cyclase). Unlike the action of aromatase inhibitors, MSeA suppression of aromatase activation is not mediated via direct inhibition of aromatase enzymatic activity. Rather, it is attributable to a marked down-regulation of PI.4- and PII-specific aromatase mRNA expression, and thereby a reduction of aromatase protein.

In primary human fibroblast cell culture MSeA was shown to induce cellular senescence, an irreversible arrest of cell proliferation, more potently than other Se forms by W. Cheng's group [51,52]. They found that MSeA, MSeC and selenite at concentrations less than or equal to their respective LD_{50} induced senescence only in the noncancerous cells MRC-5 (lung fibroblasts) and CRL1790 (colon fibroblasts), not in cancer cell lines. They showed that this senescence induction by MSeA was dependent on ATM kinase activity and wild type p53 in the MRC-5 cells, as inhibition or genetic silencing of ATM or p53 decreased induction of senescence.

In addition to apoptosis and senescence induction, MSeA was shown by our group to induce autophagy in some but not all pancreatic cancer cell lines [53]. Effort to attenuate autophagy signaling led to increased apoptosis in MSeA-treated cells, consistent with a generalized notion that drug-induced autophagy confers survival advantage to the cancer cells. Our finding stresses the multiple-targeting nature of MSeA exposure and the cellular fate will be determined by the balance of these, oftentimes opposing, signaling pathways.

Extending on the MM-Se specificity theme, MSeA, MSeC and dimethylselenide (DMDSe) were observed to stimulate the cell surface expression of ligands for the lymphocyte receptor NKG2D in Jurkat T cells [54], specifically inducing the expression of MICA/B major histocompatibility complex class I related chain genes, which are up-regulated in stressed cells for immune system recognition. MSeA and DMDSe up-regulated the maximum MICA/B response at 5 µM, On the other hand, selenite, selenate, SeMet, selenocysteine and hydrogen selenide had no effect on the cell surface expression of MICA/B. At the transcription level, MSeA and MSeC induced the mRNA levels of MICA/B and ULBP2, whereas selenite did not. The work suggests MM-Se could improve NKG2D-based cancer immune therapy.

Methylselenol ←→ MSeA redox cycle through thioreduxin reductase (TrxR)

Gromer and Gross [55] examined Ganther's speculation [19] that methylselenol and MSeA might exert their effects by inhibition of the selenoenzyme TrxR via the irreversible formation of a diselenide bridge. Failing to find such Se entity, they showed that MSeA did not act as an inhibitor of mammalian TrxR but was an excellent substrate, which was reduced by TrxR according to the equation 2 NADPH + 2 H$^+$ + CH$_3$SeO$_2$H → 2 NADP$^+$ + 2 H$_2$O + CH$_3$SeH. They identified the Se-containing product of this reaction by mass spectrometry using silver to trap the reactive methylselenol. Nascent methylselenol was found to efficiently reduce both H$_2$O$_2$ and glutathione disulfide GSSG. They found that MSeA was a poor substrate for human glutathione reductase (GR, not a selenoprotein) and the catalytic selenocysteine residue of mammalian TrxR was essential for MSeA reduction to methylselenol.

R. Gopalakrishna's group showed [56] that MSeA, but not methylselenol, inactivated protein kinase C (PKC) isoforms which depending on the type, site and extent of modification could be involved in either tumor progression or promotion. MSeA was shown to inactivate pure PKC enzyme activity, which could be reversed by the TrxR system or thiol agents, but methylselenol did not. In two prostate cancer cell lines (DU145 and LNCaP) under serum-starved conditions, MSeA (5 µM) caused the reduction in PKC activity as early as 5 to 15 minutes. PKC activity recovered slightly by 2 hours but not to the level of the control activity. The extent of inactivation in these cell lines were observed to be less than in that of the pure PKC enzyme possibly due to TrxR-mediated MSeA←→MSeH redox cycling to remove MSeA from the site of action. The increase in PKC inactivation, in particular the promitogenic and prosurvival PKCepsilon isoenzyme was observed to be associated with increased apoptosis and cell growth inhibition. For other protein kinase enzymes, for example, protein kinase A, 10 times higher MSeA was required to inactivate. The inactivation of PKC was further enhanced when MSeA was made from methylselenol by the PKC-bound phospholipid peroxides within close proximity to PKC thioclusters. As low as nanomolar Se resulted in the oxidation of the catalytic unit of PKC by the MSeA-methylselenol redox cycle, highlighting the specificity of MSeA in inactivating PKC.

In a subsequent paper by the same group [57], MSeA was shown in submicromolar concentrations to prevent the transformation of prostate epithelial cells. However, micromolar levels of MSeA were required to prevent cell growth, invasion and cause apoptosis in prostate cancer cells. MSeA sensitivity was inversely correlated to PKCepsilon levels, with PKCepsilon ectopic over-expression resulting in minimum MSeA induction of epithelial cell transformation and prostate cancer cell apoptosis. In addition, resistance to MSeA treatment was linked to increased TrxR expression and inhibition of TrxR increased the cancer cells' sensitivity to MSeA. These studies suggest that both PKCepsilon and TrxR can negate the efficacy of MSeA.

Therefore, it could be that methylselenol, MSeA and their redox cycling intermediates, especially in localized protein microenvironment of thioclusters, may provide specific targeting niches to negatively regulate enzymatic activities involved in cancer promotion or growth. Retrospectively, many of the reported activities that we and others attributed to the "methylselenol" pool should be recast in the framework of dynamic MSeA:MSeH redox cycling balances (Figure 1).

In vivo "molecular targets" of MM- Se in cancer models

Our group examined the impact of acute Se treatments (i.e., daily single oral gavage of 2 mg Se /kg of body weight for 3 days) of female Sprague-Dawley rats bearing 1-methyl-1-nitrosourea-induced mammary carcinomas to increase the probability of detecting *in vivo* apoptosis and the associated gene/protein changes in the malignant epithelial cells [58]. Whereas control carcinomas doubled in volume in 3 days, MSeC and selenite treatments caused regression in approximately half of the carcinomas, accompanied by a 3- to 4-fold increase of apoptosis and approximately 40% inhibition cancerous epithelial cell proliferation. The mRNA levels of growth arrest-DNA damage inducible 34 (*gadd34*), *gadd45*, and *gadd153* genes were, contrary to expectation [29], not higher in the Se-treated carcinomas than in the gavage- or diet restriction-control groups. The Gadd34 and Gadd153 proteins were localized in the non-epithelial cells and not induced in the cancer epithelial cells of the Se-treated carcinomas. On the other hand, both Se forms decreased the expression of cyclin D1 and increased levels of p27Kip1 and c-Jun NH2-terminal kinase activation in a majority of the mammary carcinomas. In addition, the lack of induction of *gadd* genes *in vivo* by MSeA was confirmed in a human prostate xenograft model in athymic nude mice. In summary, these experiments showed the induction of cancer epithelial cell apoptosis and inhibition of cell proliferation by Se *in vivo* through the potential involvement of cyclin D1, p27Kip1, and c-Jun NH2-terminal kinase pathways. They cast doubt on the three *gadd* genes as mediators of Se action *in vivo*.

Using the transgenic adenocarcinoma mouse prostate (TRAMP) model, our group established the efficacy of MSeA and MSeC against prostate carcinogenesis and characterized potential mechanisms [12]. Eight-week-old male TRAMP mice (C57B/6 background) were given a daily oral dose of water, MSeA, or MSeC at 3 mg Se/kg body weight and were euthanized at either 18 or 26 weeks of age. By 18 weeks of age, the genitourinary tract and dorsolateral prostate weights for the MSeA- and MSeC-treated groups were lower than for the control (P < 0.01). At 26 weeks, 4 of 10 control mice had genitourinary weight > 2 g, and only 1 of 10 in each of the Se groups did. In addition, Se treatment resulted in delayed lesion progression, increased apoptosis, and decreased proliferation without appreciable changes of T-antigen expression in the dorsolateral prostate of Se-treated mice. Decreased serum insulin-like growth factor I when compared with control mice was observed in the Se-treatment groups as well. In another experiment, giving MSeA to TRAMP mice from 10 or 16 weeks of age increased their survival to 50 weeks of age, and delayed the death due to synaptophysin-positive neuroendocrine carcinomas and synaptophysin-negative prostate lesions and seminal vesicle hypertrophy. Wild-type mice receiving MSeA from 10 weeks did not exhibit decreased body weight or genitourinary weight or increased serum alanine aminotransferase compared with the control mice. Therefore, these Se compounds were effective in the inhibition of this model of prostate carcinogenesis.

Our proteomic analyses suggest unique potential molecular targets for each of these chemoprevention-active MM-Se forms with little "protein targets" overlap between MSeA and MSeC [59] and they are not interchangeable. Additionally, we detected a possible adverse prostate cancer risk profile for MSeC through onco-proteins such as fatty acid synthase. These data, when considered in the framework of dynamic MSeA:MSeH redox cycling, would be reasonable pending on the entry point of MM-Se to fuel the redox cycle. Whether such findings are present in mammary and other organ sites should be examined to assess the generalizability. Further investigations of the tissues/organs exposed to these two MM-Se forms in higher mammal species such as dogs and primates may help to predict and inform the potential adverse impacts of each form for human translation.

MM-Se forms are superior to SeMet or selenite in a therapy context

Whereas both MSeC and MSeA have been shown to inhibit mammary carcinogenesis in the 1990's (21, 60), their anti-cancer efficacy in prostate or other non-mammary organs has only recently been tested. In several *in vivo* models, the MM-Se compounds in comparison with SeMet or selenite were more efficacious in reducing tumor sizes and reducing molecular markers. Our group has shown that the orally administered MSeA and MSeC dose-dependently (1 and 3 mg Se/kg) inhibit the *in vivo* growth of DU145 human prostate cancer xenograft in athymic nude mice whereas selenite and SeMet are not active [11]. Each Se was given by a daily single oral dose regimen starting the day after the subcutaneous inoculation of cancer cells (resembling residual and disseminated cancer cells in an adjuvant chemotherapy context). In the same study, MSeA was observed to be more active than MSeC against PC-3 xenograft growth. In terms of tolerability, all four Se compounds at the tested doses of 3 mg per kg or lower did not adversely affect the body weight of the mice. Selenite treatment did however increase DNA single-strand breaks in peripheral lymphocytes, whereas the other Se forms did not. The measurement of Se content in the tissue showed that SeMet treatment led to 9.1-fold more liver Se retention and approximately 3.6 times higher than mice treated with an equal dose of methyl-Se, even though this form of Se was least effective in reducing the DU145 or PC-3 xenograft growth. The observed massive tissue Se accumulation (non-specific incorporation in place of Met into proteins) and the lack of anti-cancer potency agreed well with earlier work with SeMet in conventional rodent models [21,61]. In summary, MSeA exhibited superior *in vivo* "adjuvant" therapy efficacy against two human prostate cancer xenograft models over SeMet and selenite, without the genotoxic property of selenite.

Yan and Demars have shown that MSeA at 2.5 mg Se/kg provided in AIN93G diet significantly reduced pulmonary metastatic yield when compared with the controls (p<0.05), SeMet did not have such an effect [62] using Lewis lung carcinoma (LLC) in male C57BL/6 mice. Mice were fed AIN93G control diet or that diet supplemented with MSeA or SeMet at 2.5 mg Se/kg for 4 weeks at which time they were injected intramuscularly or subcutaneously with 2.5 × 10^5 LLC cells. Experiments were terminated 2 weeks later for mice injected intramuscularly or 2 weeks after surgical removal of primary tumors from mice subcutaneously injected with cancer cells. Dietary supplementation with MSeA significantly reduced pulmonary metastatic yield when compared with the controls (p < 0.05) in both models; however, SeMet did not. MSeA significantly decreased plasma concentrations of urokinase-type plasminogen activator (p<0.05) and plasminogen activator inhibitor-1 (p<0.05) and vascular endothelial growth factor (p<0.05), fibroblast growth factor (p<0.05) and platelet-

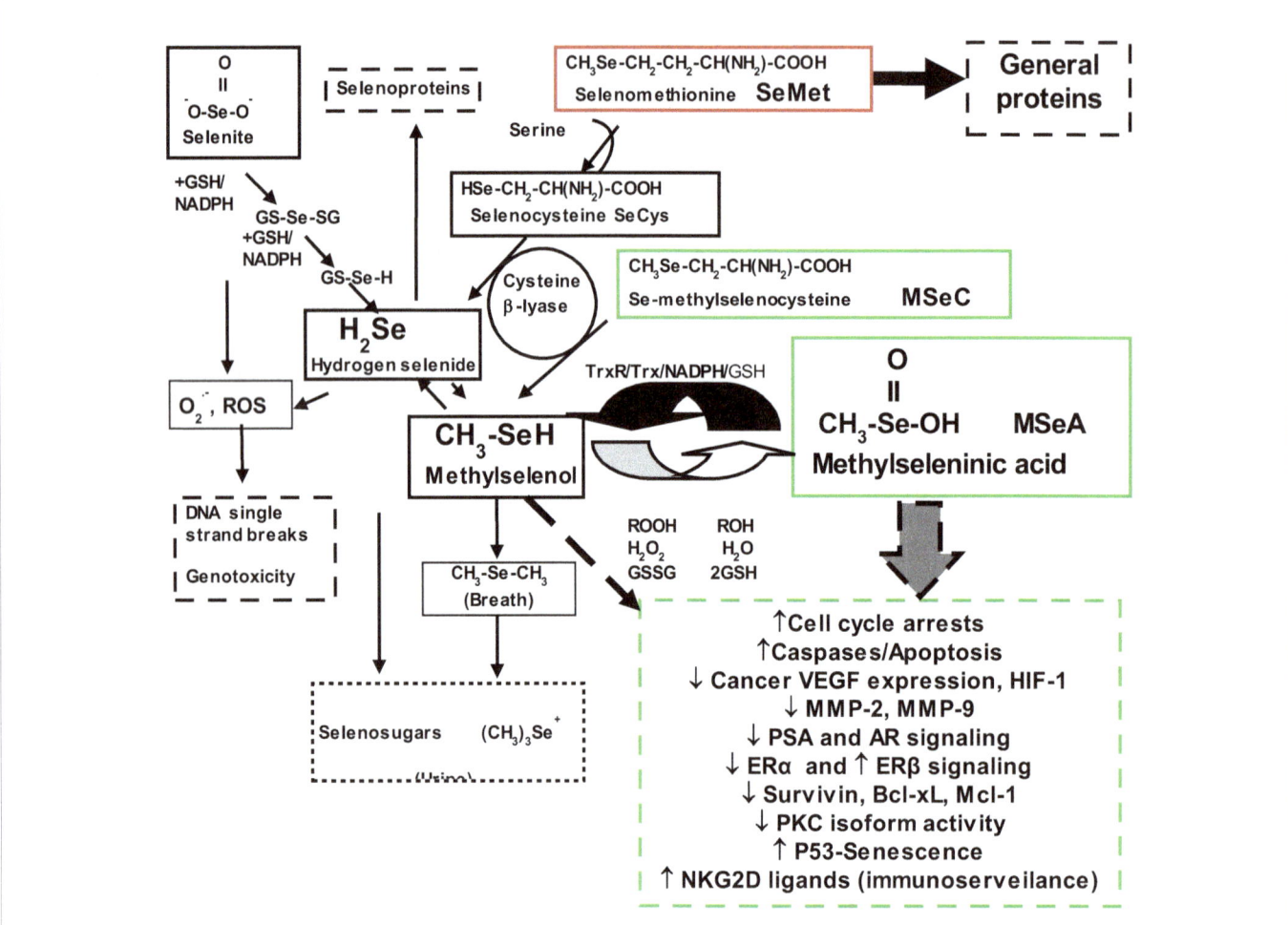

Figure 1: Possible metabolism of MM-Se and inorganic selenite and bio-activities of MM-Se in cancer therapy For selenoamino acids, tissue cysteine β-lyases release hydrogen selenide and methylselenol from selenocysteine (SeCys) and methylselenocysteine (MSeC), respectively. Methylselenol (CH3SeH, or CH3Se- at physiological pH) pool may be selectively enriched by precursor compounds including MSeC, methylseleninic acid (MSeA), methylselenocyanate (MSeCN) or functional foods such as Se-garlic, bypassing the hydrogen selenide (H2Se) pool. Selenomethionine (SeMet) leads to massive tissue accumulation of Se due to its non-specific incorporation into general proteins in place of Met. Selenite undergoes reductive metabolism involving GSH/NADPH, can cause DNA damage, likely through reactive oxygen species (ROS). Selenate is almost inert in cell culture studies. Cell culture studies have supported a redox cycle between methylselenol and MSeA, involving thioredoxin (Trx) and Trx reductases (TrxR), NADPH as well as ROS/hydrogen and phospholipid peroxides. Given MSeC by itself was little active against cultured cancer cells (most of them lacking cysteine β-lyase), anti-cancer bioactivities attributed to a given MM-Se were more likely consequences of composite actions of methylselenol:MSeA redox duet and their intermediates.

derived growth factor-BB (p < 0.05), SeMet did not affect any of the aforementioned measurements. These results demonstrate that MSeA reduces spontaneous metastasis of LLC in mice, perhaps through inhibition of the urokinase plasminogen activator system and reducing angiogenesis.

Combination therapy applications of MM-Se vs. SeMet in animal models

A few studies in the last decade have resulted in a renewed interest in the therapeutic potential of Se as an enhancer of existing treatment modalities. Y. Rustum's group [63] used athymic nude mice bearing human non-small cell carcinoma HNSCC (FaDu and A253) and colon carcinoma (HCT-8 and HT-29) xenografts to evaluate the potential role of Se compounds as selective modulators of the toxicity and anti-tumor activity of selected anticancer drugs: fluorouracil, oxaliplatin, cisplatin, taxol and doxorubicin with particular emphasis on irinotecan, a topoisomerase I poison. They showed that a sub-lethal dose of Se either as MSeC or SeMet was highly protective against toxicity induced

by these chemotherapeutic agents. Furthermore, MSeC significantly increased the cure rate (no detectable tumor at the transplant site for up to 3 months after treatment was terminated) of xenografts bearing human tumors that are sensitive (HCT-8 and FaDu) and resistant (HT-29 and A253) to irinotecan. An increased cure rate (100%) was achieved in nude mice bearing HCT-8 (20% with irinotecan alone) and FaDu xenografts (30% with irinotecan alone) treated with the MTD of irinotecan (100 mg/kg/week for 4 weeks) when combined with MSeC. Administration of higher doses of irinotecan (200 and 300 mg/kg/week for 4 weeks) was required to achieve high cure rate for HT-29 and A253 xenografts. Administration of these higher drug doses was possible due to selective protection of normal tissues by Se. The observed *in vivo* protective action against drug toxicity was highly dependent on the schedule of Se, which required a minimum of 3 days ahead of the first drug treatment.

In their next study [64], the effect of MSeC on the pharmacokinetic and pharmacogenetic profiles of genes relevant to irinotecan metabolic pathway to identify possible mechanisms associated with the observed combinational synergy was evaluated. Nude mice bearing tumors (FaDu and A253) were treated with MSeC, irinotecan, and their combination. Samples were collected and analyzed for plasma and intra-tumor concentration of irinotecan and its active form 7-ethyl-10-hydroxyl-camptothecin (SN-38) by high-performance liquid chromatography. After MSeC treatment, the intra-tumor concentration of SN-38 increased to a significantly higher level in A253 than in FaDu tumors and was associated with increased expression of carboxyesterase CES1 (involved in the de-esterification of irinotecan) in both tumor models. MSeC/irinotecan treatment, compared with irinotecan alone, resulted in a significant decrease in levels of ABCC1 and DRG1 (multi-drug resistant associated proteins, drug efflux pumps) in FaDu tumors and an increase in levels of CYP3A5 and TNFSF6 (involved in increased drug metabolism and inducing apoptosis respectively) in A253 tumors. No statistically significant changes induced by MSeC/irinotecan were observed in the levels of other investigated variables (transporters, degradation enzymes, DNA repair, and cell survival/death genes).

In a subsequent paper [65], the Rustum group further examined the basis for MSeC in increasing the therapeutic index of irinotecan against human tumor xenografts using the FaDu and A253 models. A MSeC minimum effective dose of 0.01 mg/day for 28 days to the maximum tolerated dose (MTD) of 0.2 mg/day for 28 days was established for enhancing efficacy, with treatment beginning 7 days prior to irinotecan treatment. From the lower MseC doses to the MTD, the mice's cure rate in the combination with irinotecan was increased. On its own, MSeC did not have any effect on the cure rate but reduced tumor growth by as much as 30%. The highest plasma Se concentration was achieved 1 hour after a single dose and 28 days after daily treatment of MSeC. The ability of FaDu tumors to retain Se was significantly better than A253 tumors, and the highest Se concentration in normal murine tissue was achieved in the liver. Peak plasma and tissue Se concentrations were functions of the dose and duration of MSeC treatment. The MSeC-dependent increase in Se level in normal murine tissues may contribute to the protective effect against irinotecan toxicity observed in those tissues. Intra-tumoral total Se concentration was not found to be predictive of the combination therapy response rates. These authors pointed out a critical need to develop a method to measure the active metabolites of MSeC, rather than total Se.

The same group [66] demonstrated that one mechanism of selectivity was the differential impact of MSeC on the content of irinotecan and its active metabolite SN-38 between tumors of HNSCC and the normal tissue. In this situation, the *in vivo* synergy between MSeC and irinotecan is influenced by treatment schedule. For the FaDu tumors, the concurrent combination (MSeC and irinotecan administered for 2 hours) resulted in no increase in the enhancement of irinotecan's response rate. However, the sequential combination of MSeC administered for 7 days before irinotecan resulted in 65% increase in irinotecan's response rate. These findings were also seen in the A253 xenografts. The combination of MSeC/irinotecan enhanced tumor vessel maturation, intra-tumor concentration of SN-38 and apoptotic death of tumor cells. Normal tissue drug concentrations were not impacted by MSeC treatment. Their finding is of clinical relevance for using MSeC to decrease tumor drug resistance and achieve higher active metabolite of irinotecan to ultimately enhance cure rates.

Our group established the enhancement of paclitaxel efficacy by MSeA in androgen receptor-negative PCa [67]. In nude mice, the paclitaxel and MSeA combination inhibited growth of the DU145 subcutaneous xenograft with the equivalent efficacy of a four-time higher dose of paclitaxel alone. MSeA decreased the basal and paclitaxel-induced expression of Bcl-XL and survivin *in vitro* and *in vivo*. Ectopic expression of Bcl-XL or surviving attenuated MSeA/paclitaxel-induced apoptosis. The sensitization effect of MSeA on paclitaxel has been confirmed in a triple-negative breast cancer xenograft model [68]. The synergism was attributable to more pronounced induction of caspase-mediated apoptosis, arrest of cell cycle progression at the G_2/M checkpoint, and inhibition of cell proliferation. Treatment of SCID mice bearing MDA-MB-231 triple-negative breast cancer xenografts for four weeks with MSeA (4.5 mg/kg/day, orally) and paclitaxel (10 mg/kg/week, through (i.p.) resulted in a more pronounced inhibition of tumor growth compared with either agent alone. The combination of MSeC with estrogen receptor positive breast cancer chemotherapy drug tamoxifen also resulted in synergistic tumor growth inhibition in the MCF-7 breast xenograft tumors in ovariectomized female athymic nude mice [69]. Sustained-release estradiol was implanted into the ovariectomized mice, which allowed the MCF-7 tumors to grow. Tamoxifen pellets were also implanted subcutaneously while MSeC was administered by i.p. after the tumors reached 100 mm³. For the tumors in mice given estradiol implant, tamoxifen and MSeC had the greatest suppression, while each agent on its own had some suppression. At termination of the study, cell proliferation and angiogenesis were reduced as early as seven days by MSeC.

Y. Dong's group aimed to exhibit the efficacy of MSeA and a recently approved androgen receptor antagonist drug MDV3100 (Enzalutamide) both *in vitro* and *in vivo* as well as the MSeC and MDV3100 combination *in vivo* [70]. Using prostate cancer 22Rv1 cells in androgen-deprived conditions, dihydrotestosterone (DHT)-stimulated trans-activating activity of the androgen receptor was suppressed by the combination of MSeA and MDV3100 in the most statistically significant manner as compared to each individual agent. In addition, the mRNA levels of the androgen receptor downstream targets PSA and KLK2 had the most pronounced inhibition both with and without DHT with the MDV3100 and MSeA combination. The effect of these two compounds in inhibiting cell growth was found to be synergistic with the combination treatments producing combination indexes of less than 1. In the 22Rv1 tumor xenograft model, however, the results were quite different. The MDV3100 dose used was 10 mg/kg and 3 mg Se/kg/day for both MSeC and MSeA. The tumor growth of the animals being treated with both MSeA and MDV3100 showed no difference from the group treated only with MDV3100. On the other hand, the group treated with the combination of MSeC and MDV3100 had the smallest tumors, with them being significantly smaller than any of the single agent treatments. The authors offered the explanation that the lack of MSeA and MDV3100 efficacy in vivo might be due to MSeA and MDV3100 conjugation when prepared in the same dosing solution.

Cisplatin (CDDP) use in oncology is largely limited by its severe side effects including gastrointestinal toxicity and nephrotoxicity. For testing the utility of sodium selenosulfate to attenuate CDDP side effect, Li and co-workers treated mice by i.p. with 9 μmol sodium selenosulfate/kg for 11 days [71]. On days 5 and 7, they gave the mice an injection of CDDP of 8 mg/kg 1 hour after sodium selenosulfate treatment. Sodium selenosulfate decreased the incidence of diarrhea as a measure of gastrointestinal toxicity from 88% to 6%. Such a prominent protective effect promoted them to evaluate the safety potential of long-term sodium selenosulfate application in comparison with sodium selenite. Mice were administered with each Se for 55 days at the doses of 12.7 and 19 μmole/kg (1.0 mg and 1.5 mg Se/kg by i.p. injection). The low-dose sodium selenite caused growth suppression and hepatotoxicity which were aggravated by the high-dose, leading to 40% mortality rate, but no toxic symptoms were observed in the two sodium selenosulfate groups. Their results suggest sodium selenosulfate at an innocuous dose can markedly prevent CDDP-induced gastrointestinal toxicity while improving cancer "cure" rate.

Potential mechanisms of efficacy enhancement

Using androgen-independent and p53 non-functional prostate cancer cell culture models, our group investigated the Se specificity and signaling pathways underlying the enhancement action on apoptosis-induced by different classes of chemotherapeutic drugs [72]. DU145 and PC3 human AR-negative PCa cells were exposed to minimal apoptotic doses of Se and/or the topoisomerase I inhibitor SN38 (irinotecan active metabolite), the topoisomerase II inhibitor, etoposide or the microtubule inhibitor paclitaxel/taxol. The results showed that sublethal MSeA increased the apoptosis potency of SN38, etoposide, or paclitaxel by several folds higher than the expected sum of the apoptosis induced by MSeA and each drug alone. The combination treatment did not further enhance JNK1/2 phosphorylation that was induced by each drug in DU145 cells. The JNK inhibitor SP600125 substantially decreased the activation of caspases and apoptosis induced by MSeA combination with SN38 or etoposide and completely blocked these events induced by MSeA/paclitaxel. A caspase-8 inhibitor completely abolished apoptosis and caspase-9 and caspase-3 cleavage, whereas a caspase-9 inhibitor significantly decreased caspase-3 cleavage and apoptosis but had no effect on caspase-8 cleavage. None of these caspase inhibitors abolished JNK1/2 phosphorylation. In contrast to MSeA, selenite did not show any enhancing effect on the apoptosis induced by these drugs. The results support the enhancing effect was primarily through interactions between MSeA and JNK-dependent targets to amplify the caspase-8-initiated activation cascades in a p53-defective background.

In a follow up study, our group established the enhancement of paclitaxel efficacy by MSeA *in vivo*, and investigated Bcl-XL and survivin as molecular targets of MSeA to augment apoptosis in PCa [67]. MSeA decreased the basal and paclitaxel-induced expression of Bcl-XL and survivin *in vitro* and *in vivo*. Ectopic expression of Bcl-XL or survivin attenuated MSeA/paclitaxel-induced apoptosis. Along the line of suppression of survival molecules, MSeA was shown to enhance ABT-737 apoptosis in several cancer cell lines: breast, prostate and colon cancer cell lines [73]. Potential mechanisms were attributed to the decreased Mcl-1 (prosurvival molecule) expression by MSeA both at the basal level and due to ABT-737 induction, in addition to the re-activation of Bad, a pro-apoptotic protein after its inactivation by ABT-737 by MSeA. The synergistic effect was dependent on Bax expression in the model system, suggesting a central role of mitochondria apoptosis.

Rustum's group examined synergistic activity in the clonal TRAMP cell line C2G by MSeC and docetaxel [74]. Cells were treated with combinations of MSeC and/or docetaxel concurrently or sequentially with 24 hours MSeC pretreatment. It was observed that the concurrent administration of MSeC and docetaxel in this cell line did not enhance docetaxel's efficacy. On the other hand, the 24 hour pretreatment of MSeC enhanced docetaxel's cell growth inhibition synergistically. Using this treatment scheme, caspase-3 activity was significantly increased as early as 30 minutes. The caspase inhibitor z-VAD-fmk significantly attenuated the increased apoptosis induced by the combination treatment, indicating that the synergistic apoptosis is caspase-dependent. Survivin was decreased significantly by the combination treatment as compared to each drug individually.

In several breast cancer cell lines, MSeA with tamoxifen synergistically increased the caspase-mediated apoptosis as observed by the increased cleavage of caspases -7, -8 and -9 and PARP [75]. Cytochrome c and Bim were also increased due to MSeA treatment. The inhibition of the caspases by the general caspase inhibitor completely blocked MSeA induced apoptosis on its own and with tamoxifen. Specific caspase -8 and -9 inhibition suggested that the cleavage of caspase 9 was needed for the cleavage of caspase-8 by MSeA.

In cell culture models, the MSeA-specific enhancement action on drug-induced apoptosis was also found with tumor necrosis factor-related apoptosis-inducing ligand (TRAIL). Yamaguchi et al. [76] demonstrated that the concomitant treatment with TRAIL and MSeA produced synergistic effects on the induction of apoptosis in androgen-dependent LNCaP and androgen-independent DU145 prostate cancer cells. MSeA rapidly down-regulated the expression of the cellular FLICE inhibitory protein, a negative regulator of death receptor signaling. In addition, they demonstrated that the synergistic effects of MSeA and TRAIL resulted from the activation of the mitochondrial pathway-mediated amplification loop. MSeA also effectively blocked TRAIL-mediated BAD phosphorylation at Ser^{112} and Ser^{136} in DU145 cells and was accompanied by induction of the mitochondrial permeability transition and the release of cytochrome c and Smac/DIABLO proteins from the mitochondria and into the cytosol. These results suggest that MSeA may help to enhance efficacy of and overcome resistance to drug-induced or TRAIL-mediated apoptosis in prostate cancer cells.

Whereas p53 was not required for the enhancement effect of MSeA on apoptosis induced by drugs or TRAIL as discussed above [72,76], our group has shown a critical role of p53 and Bax/mitochondria pathway of caspases to mediate selenite's ability to enhance apoptosis induced by TRAIL in the LNCaP cells [27]. Selenite induced a rapid generation of superoxide and p53 Ser-15 phosphorylation, an indicator of DNA damage. It also increased Bax abundance and translocation into the mitochondria. Selenite and TRAIL combined treatment led to synergistic increases of Bax abundance and translocation into mitochondria, loss of mitochondrial membrane potential, cytochrome c release and the cleavage activation of caspases-9 and -3. Inactivating p53 with a dominant negative mutant abolished apoptosis without affecting superoxide generation, whereas a superoxide dismutase mimetic agent blocked p53 activation, Bax translocation to mitochondria, cytochrome c release and apoptosis induced by selenite/TRAIL. In support of Bax as a crucial target for crosstalk between selenite and TRAIL pathways, introduction of Bax into p53-mutant DU145 cells enabled selenite to sensitize these cells for TRAIL-induced apoptosis. The results indicate that selenite induces a rapid superoxide burst and p53 activation, leading to Bax up-regulation and translocation into mitochondria, which restores the crosstalk with stalled TRAIL signaling for a synergistic caspase-9/3 cascade-mediated apoptosis execution.

It is therefore possible that the p53 functional status of the cancer may influence the choice of Se forms to provide the most enhancement of efficacy to be balanced with an optimal reduction of side effects. Since the risk for selenite-induced DNA damage and genotoxicity in the treatment of a cancer patient is less of a concern than for primary prevention use, the combined use of selenite and methyl Se with chemotherapeutic drugs may target a broader spectrum of cancers.

Rustum's group investigated the role of MSeC on increased drug delivery via tumor vascular maturation in mice with FaDu head and neck squamous cell carcinoma (HNSCC) xenografts after 2 weeks of oral MSeC treatment [77]. Changes in microvessel density (CD31), vascular maturation (CD31/alpha-smooth muscle actin), perfusion (Hoechst 33342/DiOC7), and permeability (dynamic contrast-enhanced magnetic resonance imaging) were determined at the end of the 14-day treatment period. Double immunostaining of tumor sections revealed a marked reduction (approximately 40%) in microvessel density accompanying tumor growth inhibition following MSC treatment along with a concomitant increase in the vascular maturation index (approximately 30% > control) indicative of increased pericyte coverage of microvessels. Hoechst 33342/DiOC7 staining showed improved vessel functionality, and dynamic contrast-enhanced magnetic resonance imaging using the intravascular contrast agent, albumin-GdDTPA, revealed a significant reduction in vascular permeability following MSC treatment. They found a 4-fold increase in intratumoral doxorubicin levels with MSC pretreatment compared with administration of doxorubicin alone. Similar conclusion was reached with a different drug irinotecan [66] in that its efficacy was influenced by treatment schedule with MSeC and associated with enhancement of tumor vessel maturation, intra-tumor concentration of active metabolite SN-38 and apoptotic death of tumor cells. Normal tissue drug concentrations were not impacted by MSeC.

This group further examined the mechanism of enhanced irinotecan efficacy by MSeC in HNSCC with respect to the angiogenic master regulator hypoxia inducible factor 1 (HIF-1) [78]. MSeA-induced down regulation of or shRNA knockdown of HIF-1α, which is the upstream-regulator of VEGF and carbonic anhydrase IX (CAIX), resulted in the increased cell death under hypoxic but not normoxic conditions. In the animal model, the combination treatment of irinotecan and MSeC in treating the parental xenografts in comparison with the HIF-1α knockdown tumors treated with only irinotecan resulted in similar therapeutic efficacy, supporting a role of HIF-1a as a target of MSeA to enhance therapeutic effect.

In a separate study from the Rustum group [79], the phase II drug conjugating enzyme Ugt1a, which metabolizes lipophilic molecules into water soluble metabolites, was observed to be necessary for MSeC's protective efficacy against toxicity caused by irinotecan in rats. In the Ugt1a mutant rats, the maximum tolerated doses of irinotecan were lower than wild-type rats. This was specific for irinotecan as no differences were observed for docetaxel and cisplatin which are not substrates for Ugt1a.

In summary, MM-Se compounds (likely through methylselenol: MSeA redox cycle) enhance therapeutic efficacy through several potential mechanisms of action, ranging from increased tumor vascular maturity and drug delivery and retention, reduction in the expression of prosurvival molecules, increased caspase-mediated apoptosis, to improved tolerance to toxicity of the chemotherapeutic drugs, which usually have dose-limiting toxicity (Figure 2). These results indicate that there is a possible role for MM-Se compounds in enhancing the therapeutic efficacy of the current approved drugs and their efficacy, scheduling optimization and mechanisms of action should be further investigated.

Translational studies involving Se for cancer therapy

The observed improvement of MTD for a number of chemotherapeutic drugs in rodent models by MSeC and SeMet led Rustum and co-workers [80] to conduct a phase I study to determine the impact of a fixed, non-toxic high dose of SeMet on the MTD of irinotecan in cancer patients. SeMet was given orally as a single daily dose containing 2.2 mg of Se starting 1 week before the first dose of irinotecan. The Se dosage was 11 times higher than that used in the Clark study [81] or SELECT. Irinotecan was given by i.v. once weekly every 6 weeks (one cycle) for 4 cycles. The starting dose of irinotecan was 125 mg/m²/week. Escalation (by 30% each time) occurred in

cohorts of three patients until the MTD was defined. Pharmacokinetic studies were done for Se, irinotecan and irinotecan's metabolites. The results showed that three of four evaluable patients at dose level 2 of irinotecan (160 mg/m²/week) had dose-limiting diarrhea. None of the six evaluable patients at dose level 1 (125 mg/m²/week irinotecan) had dose-limiting toxicity. One patient with a history of irinotecan-refractory colon cancer achieved a partial response. SeMet displayed a long half-life of prolonged accumulation towards steady-state concentrations. SeMet did not significantly change the pharmacokinetics of irinotecan or any of its metabolites. However, the co-administration of SeMet significantly reduced the irinotecan biliary index, which has been associated with gastrointestinal toxicity. It was also shown that the plasma concentrations of Se were sub-optimal. The authors concluded that SeMet at the dose and schedule used did not allow for the safe escalation of irinotecan beyond the previously defined MTD of 125 mg/m². Disease stabilizations were noted in this highly refractory population. Given the outcomes of SELECT and HGPIN (Progression From High-Grade Prostatic Intraepithelial Neoplasia to Cancer) studies (3, 4), the lack of effects is not surprising in hindsight. Considering the better action profiles of MM-Se than SeMet discussed above, it will be very interesting to consider MSeC and MSeA for future trials.

This group also performed a study to determine the recommended dose of SeMet amongst seven tested doses in combination with irinotecan to achieve selenium concentrations of over 15 µM after 1 week of SeMet loading [80]. A total of 31 patients were enrolled and evaluated for treatment-related toxicity. They all had a confirmed solid tumor for which therapy was not available for treatment. SeMet was administered twice a day orally during the loading phase in the form of 400 or 800 µg capsules with dosages from 3200 to 7200 µg. Irinotecan was adminsterd after a week of SeMet treatment at a fixed dose of 125 mg/m² once weekly. In spite of the Se concentrations surpassed 15 µM, SeMet did not offer any protection against irinotcan toxicity.

An Australian group assessed the safety, tolerability and pharmacokinetics of sodium selenate in men with castration-resistant prostate cancer [82]. Patients were defined to have castration-resistant prostate cancer and eligible for the study, after anti-androgen therapy had been stopped for at least 4 weeks before the trial and serum PSA levels were at least 5 µg/L having increased 3 successive times, 2 weeks apart in the presence of castrate levels of serum testosterone. Sodium selenate was administered daily for 3 weeks. Initially, the sodium selenate was given at a fixed dose (one patient each at 5, 10, 15 and 30 mg), however, after observing the short half-life in serum, the same total daily dose was administered in three separate doses throughout the day in order to generate steady state plasma levels of sodium selenate. During the two years of enrollment, 19 patients were enrolled with a mean age of 72. 12 of these patients completed the treatment for 12 weeks. Of the other 7, 4 withdrew from the study due to disease progression, 1 with grade 3 fatigue, another with concomitant grade 3 diarrhea, muscle cramps and acute renal impairment. These three patients were all in the 90 mg dose group, receiving 30 mg sodium selenate trice daily. The only serious adverse event that could have been due to sodium selenate was in the patient that experienced acute renal impairment (increased creatinine level from 90 mmol/L to 260 mmol/L). From the patient's medical records, it was noted that they had a prior history of underlying kidney disease, even though the immediate cause could not be determined. Therefore, sodium selenate's role in this occurrence could not be ruled out.

Due to the short half-life in the single dose treatments, the recommended phase II dose of 20 mg trice daily, showed a half-life

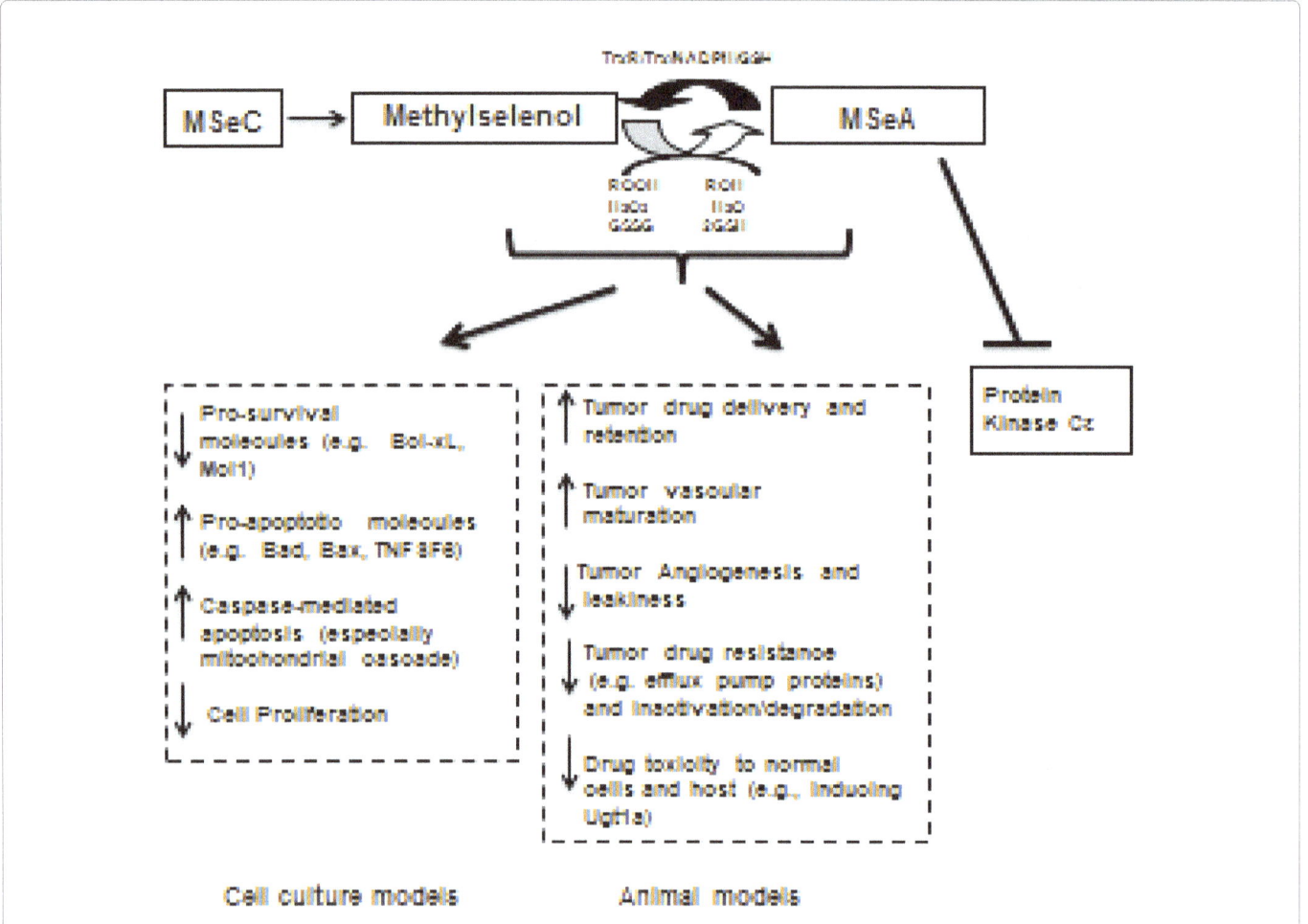

Figure 2: Possible mechanisms of how MM-Se enhances cancer chemotherapy The two precursors of methylselenol, MSeC and MSeA, enter methylselenol: MSeA redox cycle at opposite ends. Cell culture studies employed MSeA almost exclusively. Mechanisms studies in animal studies were based on MSeC, and occasionally MSeA. Although MSeA not methylselenol had been demonstrated to specifically inactivate PKCepsilon, the observed bioactivities potentially contributing to enhanced chemotherapy efficacy of a given MM-Se were more likely consequences of composite actions of methylselenol: MSeA redox duet and their intermediates.

of 2.9 hours and tmax of 2.5 hours. Selenite was the major metabolite in the plasma and reached steady-state levels by three weeks. On the other hand, while selenite was hardly detected in the urine after 24 hours, selenate, SeMet and other methyl selenium species were the major selenium compounds identified. As a surrogate marker of tumor progression, PSA was monitored throughout the study. One patient had a 57% reduction in PSA and two patients' tumor stabilized for 28 and 41 weeks. For all other patients who completed the 12-week scheduled treatment, the mean doubling time of PSA increased from 2.2 to 4.0 months. As this study was not designed in order to assess the efficacy of sodium selenate, its probable role in the treatment of CRPC and other cancers should be further examined. It is not surprising that humans tolerated super-high doses of selenate (compared to 200 ug SeMet used in SELECT and other trials) when considering that selenate was almost biologically inert in cell culture models.

The FDA approval of Investigational New Drug IND status for MM-Se is required for human studies in the US. Preclinical short and long term toxicology studies of MSeC have been conducted by the National Cancer Institute through the Division of Cancer Prevention (DCP) Rapid Access to Preventive Intervention Development (RAPID) Program [83]. Male and female CD rats received daily gavage doses of 0, 0.5, 1.0, or 2.0 mg Se/kg/day (0, 3, 6, or 12 mg/m²/day). Also, both male and female beagle dogs received daily gavage doses of 0, 0.15, 0.3, or 0.6 mg Se/kg/day (0, 3, 6, or 12 mg/m²/day) for 28 days. In the rats, MSeC induced dose-related hepatomegaly in both sexes; mild anemia, thrombocytopenia, and elevated liver enzymes were observed in high dose females only. In the middle and high dose females, there was a statistically significant observed decrease in hematocrit, hemoglobin, mean RBC volume and platelet count. Microscopic pathology included hepatocellular degeneration (high dose males, all doses in females), arrested spermatogenesis (high dose males), and atrophy of corpora lutea (middle and high dose females). In dogs, MSeC induced mild anemia in middle and high dose males, and in high dose females. Reduced hematocrit and RBC count were observed in the middle and high dose dogs and reduced hemoglobin in only the high dose males. Toxicologically significant microscopic lesions in dogs were seen only in the liver (peliosis and vacuolar degeneration in high dose males, midzonal necrosis in males in all dose groups). Based on liver pathology seen in female rats in all dose groups, the no observed adverse effect level (NOAEL) for MSeC in rats is <0.5 mg Se/kg/day. Based on alterations in hematology parameters and liver morphology in male dogs in all dose groups, the NOAEL for MSeC in dogs is < 0.15 mg Se/kg/day. Taking the NOAEL of dogs as reference (~ 0.1 mg/kg), an equivalent value extrapolated to humans for a 70 kg person is 7,000 µg Se/day.

Roswell Park investigators led by J. Marshall conducted and published the first-in-human single-dose pharmacokinetics of MSeC in men [84]. In this randomized and double-blinded study, subjects received either a single dose of MSeC at 1 of 3 different concentrations or the placebo. In the first wave, 5 subjects received 400 µg of Se and 1 received placebo; in the second wave, 5 subjects received 800 µg of Se and 1 received placebo; in the third wave, 5 subjects received 1,200 µg of Se and 1 received placebo. The results show that the most distinct concentration curve is for the 1,200 µg dose, although the curve of the 800 µg dose slightly exceeds that of the 400 µg dose and that of the 400 µg dose exceeds that of placebo. For those receiving Se, t_{max} are similar, ranging between 3 and 5 hours for the 400 through 1,200 µg cohorts. The mean Se C_{max} increases in a dose–response fashion from 10 for placebo to 22.8, 30.75, and 63.2 ng/mL (~0.8 µM) for 400, 800, and 1,200 µg dose subjects, respectively. There were 25 grade 1 adverse events reported, with no association between the administration or dose of MSeC to the adverse event experienced. As a result, no evidence of toxicity could be established. Similar studies should be planned and conducted for MSeA given the significant differences in rodent proteomic profiles of these two MM-Se highlighted earlier [59,85].

Conclusions and future directions

Mechanistic studies have indicated that the forms of Se are critical for therapy, depending on their entry into two distinct Se metabolite pools that exert diverse and differential effects on signaling pathways, leading to proliferative arrest and cell death/apoptosis. In cell culture models, MM-Se (the methylselenol-MSeA redox duet) have many desirable attributes of cancer chemoprevention and therapy, including targeting key signaling pathways, angiogenic switch regulators, invasion and metastasis molecules and in general cancers as well as sex hormone signaling in gender-specific cancers. The hydrogen selenide pool in excess of selenoprotein synthesis can lead to DNA single strand breaks and genotoxicity to normal cells. In several animal models, the MM-Se compounds used alone exhibited greater (adjuvant) therapeutic efficacy in treating several cancer types, for example breast and prostate cancer models than SeMet. Their utility as chemoenhancer by improving the efficacy of approved drug modalities is promising and more preclinical animal efficacy studies are warranted. Several potential mechanisms include suppression of prosurvival molecules and increased caspase activation, enhanced drug uptake and retention, and decreased toxicity of chemodrugs to host (Figure 2). Accumulating data support MSeC and MSeA as more meritorious candidates than SeMet or selenite for future clinical investigations of cancer therapeutic efficacy, especially in the combination with chemotherapies, and perhaps biotherapies and radiotherapy. Our proteomic analyses of prostate and their lesions from MSeA vs. MSeC-treated mice indicated these forms are non-exchangeable. Therefore, their safety and efficacy should be each rigorously studied and compared in animal models, preferably higher mammals than rodents, to provide solid scientific choice of a preferable form for human translation.

Acknowledgements

We regret the inability to cite many worthy papers due to space limitations. We thank Jinhui Zhang, PhD and Michael Melkus, PhD for help and valuable contributions. This work was supported by US National Cancer Institute R01 grant CA172169.

References

1. Karp DD, Lee SJ, Keller SM, Wright GS, Aisner S, et al. (2013) Randomized, double-blind, placebo-controlled, phase III chemoprevention trial of selenium supplementation in patients with resected stage I non-small-cell lung cancer: ECOG 5597. J Clin Oncol 31: 4179-4187.

2. Algotar AM, Stratton MS, Ahmann FR, Ranger-Moore J, Nagle RB, et al. (2013) Phase 3 clinical trial investigating the effect of selenium supplementation in men at high-risk for prostate cancer. Prostate 73: 328-335.

3. Marshall JR, Tangen CM, Sakr WA, Wood DP Jr, Berry DL, et al. (2011) Phase III trial of selenium to prevent prostate cancer in men with high-grade prostatic intraepithelial neoplasia: SWOG S9917. Cancer Prev Res (Phila) 4: 1761-1769.

4. Lippman SM, Klein EA, Goodman PJ, Lucia MS, Thompson IM, et al. (2009) Effect of selenium and vitamin E on risk of prostate cancer and other cancers: the Selenium and Vitamin E Cancer Prevention Trial (SELECT). JAMA: the journal of the American Medical Association 301: 39-51.

5. El-Bayoumy K (2009) The negative results of the SELECT study do not necessarily discredit the selenium-cancer prevention hypothesis. Nutr Cancer 61: 285-286.

6. Hatfield DL, Gladyshev VN (2009) The Outcome of Selenium and Vitamin E Cancer Prevention Trial (SELECT) reveals the need for better understanding of selenium biology. Mol Interv 9: 18-21.

7. Christensen MJ (2014) Selenium and prostate cancer prevention: what next--if anything? Cancer Prev Res (Phila) 7: 781-785.

8. Sharma AK, Amin S (2013) Post SELECT: selenium on trial. Future Med Chem 5: 163-174.

9. Lu J, Jiang C (2005) Selenium and cancer chemoprevention: hypotheses integrating the actions of selenoproteins and selenium metabolites in epithelial and non-epithelial target cells. Antioxid Redox Signal 7:1715-1727.

10. Ip C (1998) Lessons from basic research in selenium and cancer prevention. J Nutr 128: 1845-1854.

11. Li GX, Lee HJ, Wang Z, Hu H, Liao JD, et al. (2008) Superior in vivo inhibitory efficacy of methylseleninic acid against human prostate cancer over selenomethionine or selenite. Carcinogenesis 29: 1005-1012.

12. Wang L, Bonorden MJ, Li GX, Lee HJ, Hu H, et al. (2009) Methyl-selenium compounds inhibit prostate carcinogenesis in the transgenic adenocarcinoma of mouse prostate model with survival benefit. Cancer Prev Res (Phila) 2: 484-495.

13. Lu J, Jiang C, Zhang J (2014) Cancer Prevention with Selenium: costly lessons and difficult but bright future prospects. In: Kong A-NT, editor. Inflammation, Oxidative Stress and Cancer: CRC Press Taylor Francis pp 477-494.

14. el-Bayoumy K, Upadhyaya P, Chae YH, Sohn OS, Rao CV, et al. (1995) Chemoprevention of cancer by organoselenium compounds. J Cell Biochem Suppl 22: 92-100.

15. Combs GF Jr, Gray WP (1998) Chemopreventive agents: selenium. Pharmacol Ther 79: 179-192.

16. Lu J, Hu H, Jiang C (2009) Regulation of signaling pathways by selenium in cancer. In: Surh YJD, Z.; Cadenas, E.; Packer, L., editor. Dietary Modulation of Cell Signaling pathways (Book): CRC Press pp 42.

17. Ip C, Dong Y, Ganther HE (2002) New concepts in selenium chemoprevention. Cancer Metastasis Rev 21: 281-289.

18. Hatfield DL, Tsuji PA, Carlson BA, Gladyshev VN (2014) Selenium and selenocysteine: roles in cancer, health, and development. Trends Biochem Sci 39: 112-120.

19. Ganther HE (1999) Selenium metabolism, selenoproteins and mechanisms of cancer prevention: complexities with thioredoxin reductase. Carcinogenesis 20: 1657-1666.

20. Ip C, Ganther HE (1990) Activity of methylated forms of selenium in cancer prevention. Cancer Res 50: 1206-1211.

21. Ip C, Hayes C, Budnick RM, Ganther HE (1991) Chemical form of selenium, critical metabolites, and cancer prevention. Cancer Res 51: 595-600.

22. Ip C, Vadhanavikit S, Ganther H (1995) Cancer chemoprevention by aliphatic selenocyanates: effect of chain length on inhibition of mammary tumors and DMBA adducts. Carcinogenesis 16: 35-38.

23. Ip C, Zhu Z, Thompson HJ, Lisk D, Ganther HE (1999) Chemoprevention of mammary cancer with Se-allylselenocysteine and other selenoamino acids in the rat. Anticancer Res 19: 2875-2880.

24. Lu J, Jiang C, Kaeck M, Ganther H, Vadhanavikit S, et al. (1995) Dissociation of the genotoxic and growth inhibitory effects of selenium. Biochem Pharmacol 50: 213-219.

25. Lu J (2001) Apoptosis and angiogenesis in cancer prevention by selenium. Adv Exp Med Biol 492: 131-145.

26. Zhao R, Xiang N, Domann FE, Zhong W (2006) Expression of p53 enhances selenite-induced superoxide production and apoptosis in human prostate cancer cells. Cancer Res 66: 2296-2304.

27. Hu H, Jiang C, Schuster T, Li GX, Daniel PT, et al. (2006) Inorganic selenium sensitizes prostate cancer cells to TRAIL-induced apoptosis through superoxide/p53/Bax-mediated activation of mitochondrial pathway. Mol Cancer Ther 5: 1873-1882.

28. Lu J, Pei H, Ip C, Lisk DJ, Ganther H, et al. (1996) Effect on an aqueous extract of selenium-enriched garlic on in vitro markers and in vivo efficacy in cancer prevention. Carcinogenesis 17: 1903-1907.

29. Kaeck M, Lu J, Strange R, Ip C, Ganther HE, et al. (1997) Differential induction of growth arrest inducible genes by selenium compounds. Biochem Pharmacol 53: 921-926.

30. Jiang C, Wang Z, Ganther H, Lü J (2002) Distinct effects of methylseleninic acid versus selenite on apoptosis, cell cycle, and protein kinase pathways in DU145 human prostate cancer cells. Mol Cancer Ther 1: 1059-1066.

31. Wang Z, Jiang C, Ganther H, Lü J (2001) Antimitogenic and proapoptotic activities of methylseleninic acid in vascular endothelial cells and associated effects on PI3K-AKT, ERK, JNK and p38 MAPK signaling. Cancer Res 61: 7171-7178.

32. Wang Z, Jiang C, Lü J (2002) Induction of caspase-mediated apoptosis and cell-cycle G1 arrest by selenium metabolite methylselenol. Mol Carcinog 34: 113-120.

33. Zhu Z, Jiang W, Ganther HE, Thompson HJ (2002) Mechanisms of cell cycle arrest by methylseleninic acid. Cancer Res 62: 156-164.

34. Sinha R, Medina D (1997) Inhibition of cdk2 kinase activity by methylselenocysteine in synchronized mouse mammary epithelial tumor cells. Carcinogenesis 18: 1541-1547.

35. Sinha R, Kiley SC, Lu JX, Thompson HJ, Moraes R, et al. (1999) Effects of methylselenocysteine on PKC activity, cdk2 phosphorylation and gadd gene expression in synchronized mouse mammary epithelial tumor cells. Cancer Lett 146: 135-145.

36. Miki K, Xu M, Gupta A, Ba Y, Tan Y, et al. (2001) Methioninase cancer gene therapy with selenomethionine as suicide prodrug substrate. Cancer Res 61: 6805-6810.

37. Gupta A, Miki K, Xu M, Yamamoto N, Moossa AR, et al. (2003) Combination efficacy of doxorubicin and adenoviral methioninase gene therapy with prodrug selenomethionine. Anticancer Res 23: 1181-1188.

38. Zeng H, Briske-Anderson M, Idso JP, Hunt CD (2006) The selenium metabolite methylselenol inhibits the migration and invasion potential of HT1080 tumor cells. J Nutr 136: 1528-1532.

39. Zeng H, Wu M, Botnen JH (2009) Methylselenol, a selenium metabolite, induces cell cycle arrest in G1 phase and apoptosis via the extracellular-regulated kinase 1/2 pathway and other cancer signaling genes. J Nutr 139: 1613-1618.

40. Zeng H, Cheng WH, Johnson LK (2013) Methylselenol, a selenium metabolite, modulates p53 pathway and inhibits the growth of colon cancer xenografts in Balb/c mice. J Nutr Biochem 24: 776-780.

41. Jiang C, Ganther H, Lu J (2000) Monomethyl selenium--specific inhibition of MMP-2 and VEGF expression: implications for angiogenic switch regulation. Mol Carcinog 29: 236-250.

42. Jiang C, Jiang W, Ip C, Ganther H, Lu J (1999) Selenium-induced inhibition of angiogenesis in mammary cancer at chemopreventive levels of intake. Mol Carcinog 26: 213-225.

43. Cho SD, Jiang C, Malewicz B, Dong Y, Young CY, et al. (2004) Methyl selenium metabolites decrease prostate-specific antigen expression by inducing protein degradation and suppressing androgen-stimulated transcription. Mol Cancer Ther 3: 605-611.

44. Dong Y, Lee SO, Zhang H, Marshall J, Gao AC, et al. (2004) Prostate specific antigen expression is down-regulated by selenium through disruption of androgen receptor signaling. Cancer Res 64: 19-22.

45. Zhao H, Whitfield ML, Xu T, Botstein D, Brooks JD (2004) Diverse effects of methylseleninic acid on the transcriptional program of human prostate cancer cells. Mol Biol Cell 15: 506-519.

46. Lee SO, Nadiminty N, Wu XX, Lou W, Dong Y, et al. (2005) Selenium disrupts estrogen signaling by altering estrogen receptor expression and ligand binding in human breast cancer cells. Cancer Res 65: 3487-3492.

47. Shah YM, Kaul A, Dong Y, Ip C, Rowan BG (2005) Attenuation of estrogen receptor alpha (ERalpha) signaling by selenium in breast cancer cells via downregulation of ERalpha gene expression. Breast Cancer Res Treat 92: 239-250.

48. Shah YM, Al-Dhaheri M, Dong Y, Ip C, Jones FE, et al. (2005) Selenium disrupts estrogen receptor (alpha) signaling and potentiates tamoxifen antagonism in endometrial cancer cells and tamoxifen-resistant breast cancer cells. Mol Cancer Ther 4:1239-1249.

49. Cai L, Mu LN, Lu H, Lu QY, You NC, et al. (2006) Dietary selenium intake and genetic polymorphisms of the GSTP1 and p53 genes on the risk of esophageal squamous cell carcinoma. Cancer Epidemiol Biomarkers Prev 15: 294-300.

50. Gao R, Zhao L, Liu X, Rowan BG, Wabitsch M, et al. (2012) Methylseleninic acid is a novel suppressor of aromatase expression. J Endocrinol 212: 199-205.

51. Wu M, Kang MM, Schoene NW, Cheng WH (2010) Selenium compounds activate early barriers of tumorigenesis. J Biol Chem 285: 12055-12062.

52. Wu M, Wu RT, Wang TT, Cheng WH (2011) Role for p53 in selenium-induced senescence. J Agric Food Chem 59: 11882-11887.

53. Wang L, Hu H, Wang Z, Xiong H, Cheng Y, et al. (2014) Methylseleninic acid suppresses pancreatic cancer growth involving multiple pathways. Nutr Cancer 66: 295-307.

54. Hagemann-Jensen M, Uhlenbrock F, Kehlet S, Andresen L, et al. (2014) The selenium metabolite methylselenol regulates the expression of ligands that trigger immune activation through the lymphocyte receptor NKG2D. J Biol Chem 289: 31576-31590.

55. Gromer S, Gross JH (2002) Methylseleninate is a substrate rather than an inhibitor of mammalian thioredoxin reductase. Implications for the antitumor effects of selenium. J Biol Chem 277: 9701-9706.

56. Gundimeda U, Schiffman JE, Chhabra D, Wong J, Wu A, et al. (2008) Locally generated methylseleninic acid induces specific inactivation of protein kinase C isoenzymes: relevance to selenium-induced apoptosis in prostate cancer cells. J Biol Chem 283: 34519-34531.

57. Gundimeda U, Schiffman JE, Gottlieb SN, Roth BI, Gopalakrishna R, et al. (2009) Negation of the cancer-preventive actions of selenium by over-expression of protein kinase Cepsilon and selenoprotein thioredoxin reductase. Carcinogenesis 30: 1553-1561.

58. Jiang W, Jiang C, Pei H, Wang L, Zhang J, et al. (2009) In vivo molecular mediators of cancer growth suppression and apoptosis by selenium in mammary and prostate models: lack of involvement of gadd genes. Mol Cancer Ther 8: 682-691.

59. Zhang J, Wang L, Anderson LB, Witthuhn B, Xu Y, et al. (2010) Proteomic profiling of potential molecular targets of methyl-selenium compounds in the transgenic adenocarcinoma of mouse prostate model. Cancer Prev Res (Phila) 3: 994-1006.

60. Ip C, Thompson HJ, Zhu Z, Ganther HE (2000) In vitro and in vivo studies of methylseleninic acid: evidence that a monomethylated selenium metabolite is critical for cancer chemoprevention. Cancer Res 60: 2882-2886.

61. Ip C, Hayes C (1989) Tissue selenium levels in selenium-supplemented rats and their relevance in mammary cancer protection. Carcinogenesis 10: 921-925.

62. Yan L, DeMars LC (2012) Dietary supplementation with methylseleninic acid, but not selenomethionine, reduces spontaneous metastasis of Lewis lung carcinoma in mice. Int J Cancer 131: 1260-1266.

63. Cao S, Durrani FA, Rustum YM (2004) Selective modulation of the therapeutic efficacy of anticancer drugs by selenium containing compounds against human tumor xenografts. Clin Cancer Res 10: 2561-2569.

64. Azrak RG, Yu J, Pendyala L, Smith PF, Cao S, et al. (2005) Irinotecan pharmacokinetic and pharmacogenomic alterations induced by methylselenocysteine in human head and neck xenograft tumors. Mol Cancer Ther 4: 843-854.

65. Azrak RG, Cao S, Pendyala L, Durrani FA, Fakih M, et al. (2007) Efficacy of increasing the therapeutic index of irinotecan, plasma and tissue selenium concentrations is methylselenocysteine dose dependent. Biochemical pharmacology 73: 1280-1287.

66. Azrak RG, Cao S, Durrani FA, Toth K, Bhattacharya A, et al. (2011) Augmented therapeutic efficacy of irinotecan is associated with enhanced drug accumulation. Cancer Lett 311: 219-229.

67. Hu H, Li GX, Wang L, Watts J, Combs GF Jr, et al. (2008) Methylseleninic acid enhances taxane drug efficacy against human prostate cancer and down-regulates antiapoptotic proteins Bcl-XL and survivin. Clin Cancer Res 14: 1150-1158.

68. Qi Y, Fu X, Xiong Z, Zhang H, Hill SM, et al. (2012) Methylseleninic acid enhances paclitaxel efficacy for the treatment of triple-negative breast cancer. PLoS One 7: e31539.

69. Li Z, Carrier L, Belame A, Thiyagarajah A, Salvo VA, et al. (2009) Combination of methylselenocysteine with tamoxifen inhibits MCF-7 breast cancer xenografts in nude mice through elevated apoptosis and reduced angiogenesis. Breast Cancer Res Treat 118: 33-43.

70. Zhan Y, Cao B, Qi Y, Liu S, Zhang Q, et al. (2013) Methylselenol prodrug enhances MDV3100 efficacy for treatment of castration-resistant prostate cancer. International journal of cancer Journal international du cancer 133: 2225-2233.

71. Li J, Sun K, Ni L, Wang X, Wang D, et al. (2012) Sodium selenosulfate at an innocuous dose markedly prevents cisplatin-induced gastrointestinal toxicity. Toxicology and applied pharmacology 258: 376-383.

72. Hu H, Jiang C, Ip C, Rustum YM, Lü J (2005) Methylseleninic acid potentiates apoptosis induced by chemotherapeutic drugs in androgen-independent prostate cancer cells. Clin Cancer Res 11: 2379-2388.

73. Yin S, Dong Y, Li J, Fan L, Wang L, et al. (2012) Methylseleninic acid potentiates multiple types of cancer cells to ABT-737-induced apoptosis by targeting Mcl-1 and Bad. Apoptosis 17: 388-399.

74. Azrak RG, Frank CL, Ling X, Slocum HK, Li F, et al. (2006) The mechanism of methylselenocysteine and docetaxel synergistic activity in prostate cancer cells. Mol Cancer Ther 5: 2540-2548.

75. Li Z, Carrier L, Rowan BG (2008) Methylseleninic acid synergizes with tamoxifen to induce caspase-mediated apoptosis in breast cancer cells. Mol Cancer Ther 7: 3056-3063.

76. Yamaguchi K, Uzzo RG, Pimkina J, Makhov P, Golovine K, et al. (2005) Methylseleninic acid sensitizes prostate cancer cells to TRAIL-mediated apoptosis. Oncogene 24: 5868-5877.

77. Bhattacharya A, Seshadri M, Oven SD, Toth K, Vaughan MM, et al. (2008) Tumor vascular maturation and improved drug delivery induced by methylselenocysteine leads to therapeutic synergy with anticancer drugs. Clin Cancer Res 14: 3926-3932.

78. Chintala S, Toth K, Cao S, Durrani FA, Vaughan MM, et al. (2010) Se-methylselenocysteine sensitizes hypoxic tumor cells to irinotecan by targeting hypoxia-inducible factor 1alpha. Cancer chemotherapy and pharmacology 66: 899-911.

79. Cao S, Durrani FA, Rustum YM, Yu YE (2012) Ugt1a is required for the protective effect of selenium against irinotecan-induced toxicity. Cancer Chemother Pharmacol 69: 1107-1111.

80. Fakih MG, Pendyala L, Smith PF, Creaven PJ, Reid ME, et al. (2006) A phase I and pharmacokinetic study of fixed-dose selenomethionine and irinotecan in solid tumors. Clin Cancer Res 12: 1237-1244.

81. Clark LC, Combs GF, Jr., Turnbull BW, Slate EH, Chalker DK, et al. (1996) Effects of selenium supplementation for cancer prevention in patients with carcinoma of the skin. A randomized controlled trial. Nutritional Prevention of Cancer Study Group. JAMA: the journal of the American Medical Association 276: 1957-1963.

82. Corcoran NM, Hovens CM, Michael M, Rosenthal MA, Costello AJ, et al. (2010) Open-label, phase I dose-escalation study of sodium selenate, a novel activator of PP2A, in patients with castration-resistant prostate cancer. Br J Cancer 103: 462-468.

83. Johnson WD, Morrissey RL, Kapetanovic I, Crowell JA, McCormick DL, et al. (2008) Subchronic oral toxicity studies of Se-methylselenocysteine, an organoselenium compound for breast cancer prevention. Food and chemical toxicology: an international journal published for the British Industrial Biological Research Association 46: 1068-1078.

84. Marshall JR, Ip C, Romano K, Fetterly G, Fakih M, et al. (2011) Methyl selenocysteine: single-dose pharmacokinetics in men. Cancer Prev Res (Phila) 4: 1938-1944.

85. Zhang J, Wang L, Li G, Anderson LB, Xu Y, et al. (2011) Mouse prostate proteomes are differentially altered by supranutritional intake of four selenium compounds. Nutr Cancer 63: 778-789.

18

Iodine, Thiocyanate and the Thyroid

Chandra Amar K*

Department of Physiology, University of Calcutta, University College of Science & Technology, Kolkata, India

Introduction

Thiocyanate is a ubiquitous metabolite in man and animals consuming plants containing cyanogenic glycosides and thioglycosides (glucionates) while iodine is present in the earth crust since its origin and is an essential constituent of thyroid hormone requires in trace amount. Iodine is essential for thyroid hormone synthesis while thiocyanate prevents the synthesis of thyroid hormone. As a result the physiological rather functional status of thyroid is very much dependent on the balance between these ions because of their similar ionic volume and charges and competition at different steps in thyroid hormone biosynthesis. Both iodine and thiocyanate enter in the body / thyroid gland through food and water. Thiocyanate in relatively higher concentration regulate the uptake, efflux, organification of iodide, thyroid peroxidase activity and biosynthesis of thyroid hormone. In addition the retaining capacity of iodide in the thyroid gland and body also depends on thiocyanate concentration or in other words the excretion of iodine is related with thiocyanate concentration. In the semi-arid region of earth, the consumption of cyanogenic food (thiocyanate precursor) is relatively high and many regions are environmentally iodine deficient therefore the people are at the risk of iodine deficiency disorders (IDD). The pregnant and lactating women and the women of childbearing age group are the most vulnerable group of IDD because the neuronal development of the fetus and neonate are greatly affected even in mid to moderate iodine deficiency. This article reviews the sources of thiocyanate and iodine in food and thyroid gland physiology in relation to thiocyanate and iodine based on experimental and epidemiological evidences.

From available literature along with our observations. thyroid gland morphology, iodide uptake, iodide influx, iodide organification, activity of thyroid peroxidase, thyroid hormone synthesis and the excretion of iodine in relation to thiocyanate concentration including thiocyanate metabolism have been discussed based on experimental and epidemiological evidences from available literature along with our observations.

In the semi-arid region of earth, the consumption of cyanogenic food is the cause for the development of goiter and associated iodine deficiency disorders (IDD). The pregnant and lactating women and the women of childbearing age group are the most vulnerable group for IDD because the neuronal development of the fetus and neonate are greatly affected even in mid to moderate iodine deficiency.

General Consideration

In thyroid gland iodine is an indispensable constituent for the synthesis of the thyroid hormone, thyroxine (T4) and triiodothyronine (T3) which are essential for normal growth, physical and mental development in man and animals. The most familiar effect of iodine deficiency is goitre (enlargement of thyroid gland) with a number of physiological disorders on the foetus, neonate, the child, adolescent and the adult in the whole population collectively termed as iodine deficiency disorders (IDD). The role of iodine deficiency as an environmental determination in the development of endemic goitre is established. However many agents in the environment interfere with thyroid gland morphology and function acting directly on the gland or indirectly by altering the regulatory mechanism of thyroid gland. The uptake and utilization of iodine, by the thyroid gland is impaired by the pseudo halide thiocyanate (SCN⁻). Thiocyanate is formed from cyanogenic substances. It is metabolized in thyroid gland. The role of thiocyanate ion in the homeostasis of thyroid is a provocative issue where IDD persists inspite of adequate iodine intake and consumption of cyanogenic plant food is relatively high. The article reviews the physiology of the thyroid gland in relation to iodine and thiocyanate metabolism.

Bioavailability of Iodine and Thiocyanate

Iodine

There is a cycle of iodine in nature. Most iodine is present in oceans. It was present during the primordial development of earth, but large amounts were carried by wind, rivers and floods into the sea. Iodine occurs in the deeper layers of the soil and is found in oil-well effluents. Water from deep wells can provide major source of iodine. In general, the older and explored soil surface the more likely it is to be leached of iodine [1].

The dietary source of iodine is the food crops grown in the region and drinking water. Meat, fish and dairy product are also the main source of iodine. In sea fish and seaweeds contain high amounts of iodine. Supplementations of iodine through salt, water, bread are the additional sources of iodine specially in iodine deficient area.

Thiocyanate

Cyanide in trace amount is almost ubiquitous in plant kingdom and occurs mainly in the form of cyanogenic glucosides and glucosinolates (thioglucosides); both are nitrogen containing secondary metabolites share a number of common features. They derive biogenetically from amino acids and occur as glycosides which are stored in vacuoles. They function as prefabricated defense compounds that are activated by the action of a β-glucosidase in case of emergency, releasing the deterent: toxic cyanide from cyanogens or isothiocyanates from glucosinolates [2].

When the cyanogenic plants are wounded by herbivores and other organisms, the cellular compartments are broken down and the cyanogenic glucosides come in contact with an active β-glucosidase having broad specificity, which hydrolyses them to yield 2-hydroxynitrile (cyanohydrin) that is further cleaved into the corresponding aldehyde or ketone and HCN by a hydroxynitrile lyase.

*Corresponding author: Department of Physiology, University of Calcutta, University College of Science & Technology, 92,A.P.C. Road, Kolkata, 700009, India, E-mail: physiology.ac@gmail.com

HCN is highly toxic for animals and microorganism due to its inhibition on enzymes cytochrome oxidases (respiratory chain) and its binding to other enzymes containing heavy metal ions. The lethal dose of HCN in man is 0.5-3.5 mg/kg after oral administration and death of animals or man reported after the consumption of plants with cyanogenic glycosides, whose concentrations can be upto 500 mg HCN/100 g seeds. Normally 50-100 mg HCN/100g seeds and 30-200 mg/100 g leaves have been reported [3].

Animals can rapidly detoxify small amounts of HCN by rhodanese. A number of herbivores can tolerate HCN at rest in lower concentrations [4]. Cyanogens are active and potent chemical defense compounds. HCN is toxin for plants which synthesize them. To prevent autotoxicity, a detoxification pathway exists - HCN combines with L-cysteine to yield 3-cyanoalanine by β-cyanoalanine synthase, cyanoalanine is hydrolyzed by β-cyanoalanine hydrolase to L-aspargine. β-cyanoalanine synthase occurs in all plants but likely to be more in strongly cyanogenic species [2] shown in (Figure 1).

Glucosinolate

Glucosinolates are similar to cyanogens in many respects, but they contain sulphur as an additional atom. Under hydrolysis, glucosinolates liberate D-glucose, sulphate and an unstable aglycone, which may form isothiocyanate (common name mustard oil) as main product under certain conditions, or a thiocyanate, a nitrile or cyano-epithioalkane.

All plants which sequester glucosinolates also possess thioglucoside glucohydrolases (commonly known as myrosinase) that can hydrolyze glucosinolates to D-glucose and an aglycone, spontaneously rearranging to isothiocyanate. These hydrolases are stored in the cell wall, in endoplasmic reticulum, Golgi vesicles and mitochondria.

When the tissues are wounded or disintegrated, the enzyme and its substrate come together liberating the pungent and repellant isothiocyanate. Depending on the environmental condition, enzymes and other compounds, present, the aglycone can rearrange to isothiocyanates as the most common product, or to nitriles, thiocyanates or cyano-epithioalkanes or oxazolidine-2-thiones (Figure 2).

A number of isothiocyanates are liophilic, volatile with a pungent smell and taste, while others are not volatile and pungent smelling, but have otherwise similar properties. Isothiocyanates can penetrate

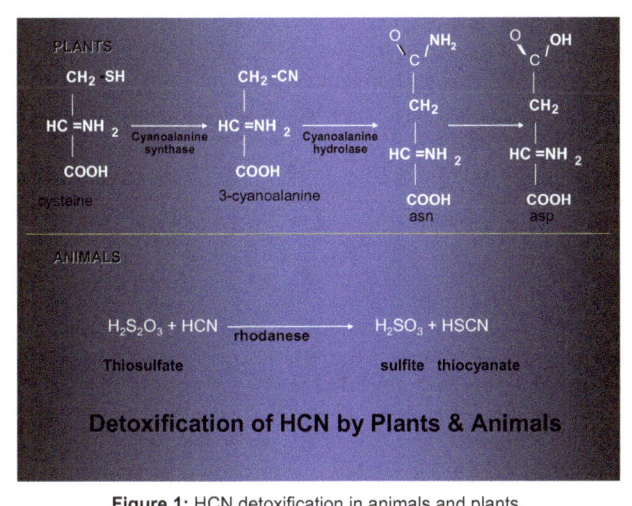

Figure 1: HCN detoxification in animals and plants.

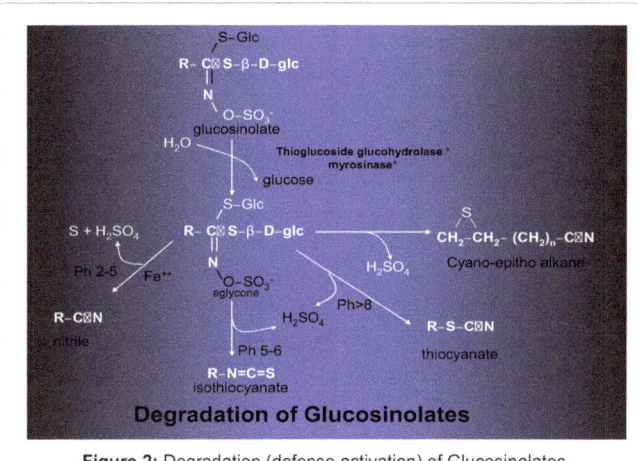

Figure 2: Degradation (defense activation) of Glucosinolates.

through biomembranes and they have many physiological actions.

Glucosinolates are thus considered as preformed defense chemicals which are activated during emergency. They have a wide range of activities and important specially in plant-harbivore but also in plant-plant and plant-microbe interactions.

Thyroid Physiology

Thyroid morphology/histology

The morphological profile of thyroid cells can be altered by dietary iodine. A low iodine diet causes distinctive functional alteration in thyroid cells. Some of the effects are direct result of iodine deficiency and the others are the secondary by elevated serum TSH level. In contrast high doses of iodine cause various responses depending on the dose of iodine given, the duration of the experiment and the route of administration [5].

Feeding of thiocyanate in rats at relatively high dose showed increased weight and abnormal histology of the thyroid. The histological features of the thyroid of animals from iodine non-supplemented thiocyanate added groups (-KI+SCN) indicated hypo functioning of the thyroid with a marked decrease in colloid containing follicles and significant proliferation of new follicles with indistinct lumen (hyperplasia) in contrast to the iodine supplemented control animals. The thyroid of rats deprived of KI (-KI) also showed a decreased in mature follicles and mild follicular hyperplasia. Colloid content of the follicles was however unaltered [6].

Cruciferous plants viz., cabbage, cauliflower, mustard (seeds and leaves), turnip, radish, brussel sprout, sprouts of Brassica family, bamboo shoot and cassava from non-Brassica family constitute a major portion of human diet contain naturally occurring goitrogenic substances or thiocyanate precursors (glucosinolates and cyanogenic glucoside). Extreme differences in the goitrogen content of these plants belong to same family and same taxonomy owing to their genetic and ecological backgrounds have also been reported [7]. Besides, the goitrogenic / anti-thyroid potential of the plant foods not only depend on their relative concentrations of the goitrogenic constituents as found in fresh plants but as also on their processing as foods [8]. The histological status of thyroid after prolonged feeding of cyanogenic plant foods e.g., fresh and cooked radish, turnip, cassava, bamboo shoot etc. by replacing 1/3 portion of the diet with and without iodine supplementation was investigated [9]. The thyroid follicles were lined by cuboidal cells with distinct nucleus showing hypertrophy and hyperplasia filled with less homogeneous colloid; some follicles were invaded by epithelial cell. Increase in the number of comparatively small follicles was one of the characteristic features. On the contrary, in the control rat, thyroid follicles were almost equal in size, lined by follicular cells filled with colloid. Alterations were found in the thyroid structure between the fresh and cooked cyanogenic plant fed rats. Variation in the number and size of follicular cells and colloid content was observed in KI- supplemented and non- supplemented plant fed group of rats. In addition, colloid stained more with eosin in the experimental group (-KI) as compared to control and KI- supplemented (+KI) group of rat for the variation of concentration of iodine [10,11].

Consumption of excess cyanogenic plants in relation to iodine is considered as an etiological factor for the persistence of iodine deficiency disorders in many regions. Moreover, in spite of salt iodization, residual goiter still persists [12-14].

Therefore moderate intake of iodine could be sufficient to meet the requirement but may not ensure normal thyroid in the presence of goitrogens like thiocyanate that come through cyanogenic plant which contributes a major portion of human diet of the people living in semi-arid region of the world.

Iodide uptake

Thiocyanate has been considered as a possible cause of thyroid disorders because it inhibits iodide transport [15-17]. The effect of thiocyanate on iodide transport in different TSH concentrations were studied in porcine thyroid cultured cells and found that SCN concentration >10 μmol/ L inhibited iodide uptake in a dose response manner regardless of TSH concentration. It has also been reported that follicles without preincubation and with 24hr preincubation by thiocyanate showed identical inhibition [18].

cAMP production and Na$^+$K$^+$ - ATPase activity

cAMP production and Na$^+$K$^+$- ATPase activity were measured in thyroid follicular cells to investigate the mechanism of inhibition of iodide uptake by thiocyanate. The presence of 200μmol/L thiocyanate for 24hr did not inhibit TSH mediated cAMP production in the cultured thyroid follicular activities of Na$^+$K$^+$- ATPase in the control and the thiocyanate group were almost same [18].

All these results indicate that inhibition of iodide uptake by thiocyanate is independent of TSH concentration and that thiocyanate does not affect cAMP generation or Na$^+$K$^+$- ATPase activity. Then the question arises how thiocyanate inhibits iodide transport. [19] have described thyroid iodide translocator, a Na dependent iodide transport protein different from Na$^+$K$^+$- ATPase, in the phospholipids vesicle of plasma membrane; and speculated that thiocyanate inhibits the system [17]. Their model is also convenient to explain competitive inhibition of iodide transport as thiocyanate and iodide are common substrates for the iodide transporting protein. Competitive inhibition is important to understand the action of thiocyanate *in vivo* because iodine deficiency may facilitate action of thiocyanate or an excessive iodine intake may diminish the action of thiocyanate in thyroid gland.

Metabolism of thiocyanate in thyroid

The concentration of thiocyanate in thyroid is fairly constant. There is no concentration gradient for thiocyanate between the thyroid and serum, the ratio (T/S) varying from 0.29 - 0.34.Thiocyanate ion is metabolized by the thyroid of rat. Sulphate is the major sulfur product; iodine is a potent inhibitor of the metabolism of thiocyanate. On the contrary there is a maximal inhibition of the concentration of iodide

by the thyroid at time when the serum level of thiocyanate ranged from 180 – 286 μmol/ml. It would appear that there is narrow ranged between the level of thiocyanate in the serum of rat and the level at which there is an inhibition of the concentration of iodide by the thyroid. Thus the role thiocyanate ion if any in the homeostasis of thyroid was found important [20].

Monovalent anions with a molecular size corresponding to that of iodine viz. SCN are concentrated in the thyroid and inhibits the normal metabolism of iodine [21]. Thiocyanate not only interferes with the uptake of iodide but also on the iodination of thyroglobulin. Thiocyanate is therefore, a potent antithyroid substance and may cause hypothyroidism at high concentrations [22]. However, short term administration of thiocyanate, serum levels of thiocyanate < 18mg/L did not suppress thyroid function. Because thiocyanate is largely exerted through kidney and can therefore, be accumulated in the body, results from short – and long term – experiments are however, not fully comparable [22].

Iodide efflux

Thiocyanate has been reported to increase iodide efflux [23] and in vivo model thiocyanate is more potent for iodide efflux than for inhibition of iodide transport. In culture thyroid follicles thiocyanate at 10μmol/L or greater increased iodide efflux from the thyroid follicles. The degrees of iodide efflux by 10μmol/L and 100μmol/L thiocyanate were almost the same. Even the increment of iodide efflux was minor at 200μmol/L in comparison with that of 10μmol/L thiocyanate [18].

Iodide organification

Thiocyanate decreases iodine organification in a dose response manner. The decrease in iodine organification occurred in parallel to the decrease in iodide uptake. To study whether thiocyanate has an independent inhibitory action on iodine organification, thyroid follicles were incubated with the mixture of Na ^{125}I and NaI for 2 hrs to load iodide; then 50 μmol/L thiocyanate was added. After the addition of thiocyanate, iodide uptake becomes plateau and iodine organification decreased significantly indicating that thiocyanate inhibits iodine organification independent of iodide uptake [18].

Thyroid peroxidase (TPO)

Cyanogenic constituents affect hormone synthesis in thyroid gland either by inhibiting iodide uptake or interfering the activity of thyroid peroxidase (TPO) i.e., by inhibiting the organification of iodide (I$^-$ leads to I$_2$) or iodination of tyrosine in thyroglobulin followed by coupling reaction [24-28]. The goitrogen content of a number of cyanogenic plant foods of Indian origin and their *in vitro* anti thyroid activity in raw, boiled and cooked extract s with and without extra iodine have been studied by Chandra et al, (2004). The relative anti TPO potency of the studied plants and PTU equivalence was also determined by estimating the amount of plant food or PTU capable of producing 50% inhibition (IC$_{50}$) of TPO activity. The IC$_{50}$ was highest in bamboo shoot, followed by cassava, mustard, cauliflower, radish, turnip and cabbage. This observation was confirmed by PTU equivalence of the studied plants

After the feeding of the cyanogenic plants in experimental animals for a prolonged period, the TPO activity of thyroid of the treated animals was reduced markedly [29-42]. As mentioned cyanogenic glucosides are readily converted into active goitrogenic agent thiocyanate by glucosidases and sulphur transferase enzymes present in the plant or in the animal tissue. Thiocyanate or thiocyanate like compounds primarily inhibit iodide concentrating mechanism of the thyroid, however at high concentration thiocyanate (SCN) inhibits the incorporation of iodide into thyroglobulin by competing with iodide at the thyroid peroxidase level [43] and forming insoluble iodinated thyroglobulin in thyroid [44]. High concentration of thiocyanate is also responsible for inhibition of TPO catalyzed oxidation (I leads to I_2) [28] while glucosinolates undergo a rearrangement to form isothiocyanate derivatives [26]. Isothiocyanate reacts spontaneously with amino groups to form thiourea that interferes in thyroid gland with organification of iodide and formation of thyroid hormone and this action cannot be antagonized by the iodide [43].

T3/T_4 synthesis

At low doses, thiocyanate was shown to inhibit the uptake of iodide; in addition it also affects the organic binding there by influence in the thyroxine synthesis. The latter effect of thiocyanate cannot be counteracted by excess iodide. Further, thiocyanate causes depression in protein bound thyroxine levels with concomitant increase in free thyroxine levels [45]. The reduced total circulating thyroxine levels could be a consequence of reduced thyroxine synthesis, depression in protein bound thyroxine levels and the utilization of free thyroxine levels by the peripheral tissues. Feeding of cyanogenic foods viz., bamboo shoot [39-41], radish (*Raphanus sativus Linn*) [34-36], cassava (*Manihot esculata crantz*) [34-36], maize (*Zea mays Linn*), cabbage, cauliflower, mastered etc. decreased the serum total T_3 and T_4 levels significantly. As mentioned, reduced TPO activity may be responsible for decreasing thyroid hormone levels because it regulates the synthesis of thyroid hormone.

Iodine/ thiocyanate ratio

The studies in Zaire have shown that cassava a staple diet in the region has definite antithyroid action in man and animals, resulting in the development of endemic goiter and cretinism. This action is due to the endogenous release of thiocyanate (SCN) from linamarin, a cyanogenic glucoside contained in cassava despite the fact that the cassava is consumed a large scale within tropics, however goiter and cretinism are not found in all population, where staple food is cassava. One possible explanation for the lack of goitrogenic action of cassava in some populations may be that they have a high iodine intake [46].

The development of goiter is critically related to the balance between dietary supplies of iodine and SCN. Under normal conditions, the urinary excretion of iodine (UEI) and thiocyanate (UESCN) or UEI/ UESCN or I/SCN is higher than 7. Endemic goiter develops when it reaches a critical threshold about 3 and becomes hyperendemic, complicated by endemic cretinism when it is lower than 2. The validity of this ratio as an index of the risk of development of goiter has been demonstrated by comparative studies conducted in different regions of Zaire [46].

In Manipur and Tripura of north- east India and Siddhartha nagar in the foot hills of Himalayas, universal salt iodization is in progress and the people consume adequate iodine, they also consume cyanogenic plant foods regularly in relatively considerable amount. Goiter is prevalent in the areas as mentioned and the UIE is almost adequate. In India, mean urinary thiocyanate level from non-endemic population is 0.504 ± 0.19 mg/dl [14]; the SCN levels in all those areas is much more. Therefore the contribution of SCN in the persistence of residual goiter during post salt iodization phase may not be ruled out. However the validity of I/SCN as mentioned (i.e., below 7) is not universal. This is consistent with earlier studies / report [8]; I/SCN ratio was a useful

indicator in the epidemiological studies in Zaire that elucidated the goitrogenic effect of SCN from cassava consumption [46]. However the proposed use of a defined threshold of 3 for this ratio for prediction of goiter frequency has several limitations. First it requires that the ratio is not clearly defined. It has been used as both the mean of individual I/ SCN ratio, and as the ratio between mean I/ mean SCN. As there ratios are mathematically different, they yield different results. Secondly, the distribution of individual I/SCN ratio is much skewed and that if any summary statistics is to be used the median and mode are preferable to the mean. A third limitation with the use of this ratio is that very high thiocyanate load will yield serum levels that exceed the kidney threshold. Urinary excretion of SCN is therefore not linearly related to the serum levels that exert the effect on the thyroid. Finally the often pronounced seasonal variation of cyanide exposure from cassava can result in 10 to 15 fold variations of SCN and this must be considered when estimating goitrogenic effect [47].

In the semi-arid region where the agricultural production of cyanogenic plant food and consumption of thiocyanate are more, the balance between the dietary supplies of iodine (I) and thiocyanate (SCN) play important role in the etiopathogenesis of endemic goiter and associated disorders but for the prediction of this ratio is yet to be determined.

Excretion of Iodine and Thiocyanate

The concentration of iodine in urine is the most widely used as biochemical marker of nutritional iodine deficiency as most of the body's iodine is excreted in the urine, usually over 90%. For surveys it is to collect 40-50 samples from an area and express the iodine as a concentration (μg/dl urine). A median urinary iodine concentration of 10 μg/dl in an area indicates no iodine deficiency [48].

Ingeston of the Brassica vegetables in human causes a rise of thiocyanate ion in blood followed by its appearance in urine. The thiocyanate level was found to drop as soon as the eating of the plants was discontinued [49]. As mentioned the urinary excretion of SCN (after a very high thiocyanate level) is not linearly related to the serum levels that exert the effect on the thyroid [50,51].

Inspite of adequate iodine nutritional status, endemic goiter is prevalent in many regions because the urinary iodine does not always truly reflect the iodine nutritional status in an environment where consumption of food containing thiocyanate precursors is relatively high [31-33]. Excess thiocyanate thus not only inhibit the iodine concentrating mechanism by inhibiting unidirectional clearance iodide from the thyroid gland but also the iodine retaining capacity of thyroid and body is also dependent on the consumption pattern of cyanogenic plant food [34-36].

Closing Remarks

In the semi-arid region, the cyanogenic plant food is grown and commonly consumed by the people and thus regular exposure of thiocyanate or its precursor is relatively high. It is also higher in cigarette smokers. When the dietary supplies of iodine and thiocyanate reach a critical point, endemic goiter and associated iodine disorders develops. On the other hand, iodine enters in the body through food and water but its availabilities vary on the geographical location. Therefore dietary supplies of iodine and thiocyanate vary from region to region depending on the availability and consumption patterns. The intake of iodine in relation to SCN and vice versa is a determinant for the causation of thyroid disorders viz. iodine deficiency disorders (IDD).

• Iodide itself is goitrogenic when it is presented in excessive in serum. Indiscriminate consumption of iodide salt regularly in environmental iodine sufficient region may be a risk factor for the development of autoimmune thyroid disorders, thyroid carcinoma, iodine- induced hypo and hyper thyroidism in long run. Conversely, intake of high thiocyanate is also goitrogenic if the intake of iodine is not satisfactory.

• Thus the question arises what should the 'adequate' or 'optimum' level of iodine? Will this remain at uniform level all over the country irrespective of its geographical distribution of iodine and consumption pattern of dietary goitrogens as cyanogenic plant foods.

• Experimental observations revealed that thiocyanate feeding inhibits iodine absorption by the mammary gland as well as by the thyroid. Such an effect on mammary gland conserves the iodine for the lactating animals but lowers iodine content milk for his young. Therefore lactating mothers ingesting thiocyanate ion could possibly cause goiter in her young affecting the development of foetus.

• Mild and moderate iodine deficiency due to thiocyanate overload associated with iodine deficiency affects intelligence, fine motor skills, problem solving capacity etc of the children and thus evaluation of their brain damage is important.

References

1. Hetzel BS (1989) The biology of iodine. In: Story of Iodine Deficiency. ed. B.S. Hetzel Oxford University Press, Delhi 21-35.

2. Conn EE (1981) Secondary Plant Products. In The Biochemistry of Plants, ed. P.K. tumpf, E.E. Conn 7: 279-501.

3. Teuscher E, Lindequist U (1994) Biogene Gifts, Fisher Verlag, Stuttgart, New York.

4. Seigler DS (1991) The Chemical Participants. In Herbivores – Their Interactions with Secondary Plant Metabolites. ed. G.A. Rosenthal, M.R. Berenbaum. Academic Press, New York 1: 35-37.

5. Krupp PP, Lee KP (1988) The effects of dietary iodine on thyroid ultrastructure. Tissue Cell 20: 79-88.

6. Lakshmy R, Rao PS, Sesikeran B, Suryaprakash P (1995) Iodine metabolism in response to goitrogen induced altered thyroid status under conditions of moderate and high intake of iodine.Horm Metab Res 27: 450-454.

7. Sundaresan S, Nambisian B, Easwari A (1987) Bitterness in cassava in relation to cyanoglucoside content. Indian J Agri Sci 57: 37-40.

8. Peterson S, Legue F, Tylleskar T, Kpizingui E, Rosling, et al. (1995) Improved cassava-processing can help reduce iodine deficiency disorders in the Central African Republic. Nutr Res 15: 803-12.

9. Chandra A K, Ghosh D, Mukhopadhyay S, Tripathy S (2006) Effect of cassava (Manihot esculenta Crantz) on thyroid status under conditions of varying iodine intake in rats. African J Traditional Complementary and Alterrnative Medicines 3: 87-99.

10. Sharpless GR, Pearsons J, Prato GS (1939) Production of goitre in rats with raw and with treated soyabean flour. J Nutr 17: 545-55.

11. Gaitan E, Cooksey RC, Legan J, Cruse JM, Lindsay RH, et al. (1993) Antithyroid and goitrogenic effects of coal-water extracts from iodine-sufficient goiter areas.Thyroid 3: 49-53.

12. Hennt P, Bourdoux P, Lagasse R, Thilly C, Putzeys G, et al. (1982) Epidemiology of goitre and malnutrition and dietary supplies of iodine, thiocyanate and proteins in Bas Zaire, Kivu and Ubangi, In Nutritional factors involved in the goitrogenic actions of cassava. ed. F. Delange, F.B. Iteke, A.M. Ermans. IDRC-184C, Ottawa, Canada 25-33.

13. Chandra AK, Ray I (2002) Evaluation of the effectiveness of salt iodization status in Tripura, north east India.Indian J Med Res 115: 22-27.

14. Marwaha RK, Tandon N, Gupta N, Karak AK, Verma K, et al. (2003) Residual goitre in the postiodization phase: iodine status, thiocyanate exposure and autoimmunity.Clin Endocrinol (Oxf) 59: 672-681.

15. Weiss SJ, Philp NJ, Grollman EF (1984) Iodide transport in a continuous line of cultured cells from rat thyroid.Endocrinology 114: 1090-1098.

16. Wolff J (1964) Transport of Iodide and Other Anions in The Thyroid Gland. Physiol Rev 44: 45-90.

17. Saito K, Yamamoto K, Nagayama I, Nemura J, Kuzuya T, et al. (1989) Effect of internally loaded iodide, thiocyanate and perchlorate on sodium dependant iodide uptake by phospholipids vesicles reconstituted with thyroid plasma membrane: iodide counterflow mediated by the iodide transport carrier. J. Biochem. 105:790-793.

18. Fukayama H, Nasu M, Murakami S, Sugawara M (1992) Examination of antithyroid effects of smoking products in cultured thyroid follicles: only thiocyanate is a potent antithyroid agent.Acta Endocrinol (Copenh) 127: 520-525.

19. Saito K, Yamamoto K, Takai T, Yoshida S (1984) Characteristics of the thyroid iodide translocator and of iodide-accumulating phospholipid vesicles. Endocrinology 114: 868-872.

20. Maloof F, Soodak M (1959) The inhibition of the metabolism of thiocyanate in the thyroid of the rat.Endocrinology 65: 106-113.

21. Green WL (1978) Mechanism of action of antithyroid compounds. In The Thyroid. ed. Werner, S.C., Ingbar S.H. 4th ed. New York. Harper & Row Publishers, NY 41-45.

22. Dahlberg PA, Bergmark A, Björck L, Bruce A, Hambraeus L, et al. (1984) Intake of thiocyanate by way of milk and its possible effect on thyroid function.Am J Clin Nutr 39: 416-420.

23. Scranton JR, Nissen WM, Halmi NS (1969) The kinetics of the inhibition of thyroidal iodide accumulation by thiocyanate: a reexamination.Endocrinology 85: 603-607.

24. Taurog A (1970) Thyroid peroxidase and thyroxine biosynthesis.Recent Prog Horm Res 26: 189-247.

25. Gaitan E (1990) Goitrogens in food and water.Annu Rev Nutr 10: 21-39.

26. Van Etten CH (1969) Goitrogens. In: Liener IE, eds. Toxic constituents of plant foodstuffs. New York: Academic Press 103-142.

27. Stoewsand GS (1995) Bioactive organosulfur phytochemicals in Brassica oleracea vegetables--a review.Food Chem Toxicol 33: 537-543.

28. Virion A, Deme D, Pommier J, Nunez J (1980) Opposite effects of thiocyanate on tyrosine iodination and thyroid hormone synthesis.Eur J Biochem 112: 1-7.

29. Chandra AK, Bhattarcharjee A, Malik T, Ghosh S (2009) Etiological Factors for the Persistence of endemic Goiter in selected areas of Siddharthanagar District in eastern Uttar Pradesh. J of Pediatric Endocrinology & Metabolism 22: 317-325.

30. Chandra A K, Ghosh D, and Tripathy S (2009) Effect of maize (Zea mays) on thyroid status under conditions of varying iodine intake in rats. J Endocrinol Reprod 13: 17- 26.

31. Chandra AK, Bhattacharjee A, Malik T, Ghosh S (2008) Goiter prevalence and iodine nutritional status of school children in a sub-Himalayan Tarai region of eastern Uttar Pradesh.Indian Pediatr 45: 469-474.

32. Chandra AK, Singh LH, Debnath A, Tripathy S, Khanam J (2008) Dietary supplies of iodine & thiocyanate in the aetiology of endemic goitre in Imphal East district of Manipur, north east India.Indian J Med Res 128: 601-605.

33. Chandra AK, Debnath A, Tripathy S (2008) Iodine nutritional status among school children in selected areas of Howrah District in West Bengal, India.J Trop Pediatr 54: 54-57.

34. Chandra AK, Mukhopadhyay S, Ghosh D, Tripathy S (2006) Effect of radish (Raphanus sativus Linn.) on thyroid status under conditions of varying iodine intake in rats.Indian J Exp Biol 44: 653-661.

35. Chandra AK, Tripathy S, Ghosh D, Debnath A, Mukhopadhyay S (2006) Goitre prevalence and the state of iodine nutrition in the sundarban delta of north 24-parganas in West Benegal.Asia Pac J Clin Nutr 15: 357-361.

36. Chandra AK, Singh LH, Tripathy S, Debnath A, Khanam J (2006) Iodine nutritional status of children in North East India.Indian J Pediatr 73: 795-798.

37. Chandra AK, Tripathy S, Ghosh D, Debnath A, Mukhopadhyay S (2005) Iodine nutritional status & prevalence of goitre in Sundarban delta of South 24-Parganas, West Bengal.Indian J Med Res 122: 419-424.

38. Chandra A K, Lahari D and Mukhopadhyay S (2005) Goitrogen content of cyanogenic plant foods of Indian origin. J Food Sc. & Tech 42: 212-218.

39. Chandra AK, Tripathy S, Lahari D, Mukhopadhyay S (2004) Iodine nutritional status of school children in a rural area of Howrah district in the Gangetic West Bengal.Indian J Physiol Pharmacol 48: 219-224.

40. Chandra AK, Mukhopadhyay S, Lahari D, Tripathy S (2004) Goitrogenic content of Indian cyanogenic plant foods & their in vitro anti-thyroidal activity. Indian J Med Res 119: 180-185.

41. Chandra AK, Ghosh D, Mukhopadhyay S, Tripathy S (2004) Effect of bamboo shoot, Bambusa arundinacea (Retz.) Willd. on thyroid status under conditions of varying iodine intake in rats.Indian J Exp Biol 42: 781-786.

42. Chandra AK, Ray I (2001) Dietary supplies of iodine and thiocyanate in the etiology of endemic goiter in Tripura.Indian J Pediatr 68: 399-404.

43. Ermans AM, Bourdoux P (1989) Antithyroid sulfurated compounds. In: Gaitan E, editor. Environmental goitrogens. Boca Raton, FL : CRC Press, 15-31.

44. van Middlesworth L (1985) Thiocyanate feeding with low iodine diet causes chronic iodine retention in thyroids of mice.Endocrinology 116: 665-670.

45. Langer P (1971) Extrathyroidal effect of thiocyanate and propylthiouracil: the depression of the protein-bound iodine level in intact and thyroidectomized rats.J Endocrinol 50: 367-372.

46. Delange F, Bourdoux P, Colinet E, Courtois P (1980) Nutritional factors involved in the goitrogenic action of cassava. In Cassava toxicity in thyroid: research and public health issues. ed. F.Delange, R. Ahluwalia. IDRC-207e, Ottawa, 148: 17-34.

47. Casadei E, Cliff J, Neves J (1990) Surveillance of urinary thiocyanate concentration after epidemic spastic paraparesis in Mozambique.J Trop Med Hyg 93: 257-261.

48. Indicators for tackling progress in IDD elimination (1994) In IDD Newsletter 10: 37-41.

49. Michajlovskij N, Langer P (1958) Studies on relation between thiocyanate formation and goitrogenic properties of foods. In Preformed thiocyanate contents of some foods (Studien uber Benziehungen Zwischen Rhodanbildung und Kropfbildender Eigenschaft Von Nahrungstteln. In Gehalt einiger Nahrungs Mittel an prafornierten Rhodanid). Hoppe Seyless. Z. Physiol. Chem. 312: 26-30.

50. Conn EE (1980) In Secondary Plant Products. Encyclopedia of Plant Physiology ed. E.A. Bell, B.V. Charlwood 8: 461-92.

51. Ruf J, Carayon P (2006) Structural and functional aspects of thyroid peroxidase. Arch Biochem Biophys 445: 269-277.

19

Morphology of the Small Intestine of Albino Wistar Rats Following Long Term Administration of Nevirapine

Umoren EB* and Osim EE

Department of Physiology, College of Medical Sciences, University of Calabar, Calabar, Nigeria

Abstract

Background: Nevirapine (NVP) is an antiretroviral medication that prevents human immunodeficiency virus (HIV) cells from multiplying in the blood. This study was undertaken to ascertain whether NVP administration affects intestinal morphology using albino Wistar rats.

Materials and methods: Sixty adult albino Wistar rats were used for the study. Rats in the control group (n=30) were fed normal rodent chow, while the NVP group (n=30) were fed by gavage NVP (0.4 mg/kg body weight) twice daily (7:00 am and 6:00 pm) in addition to normal rodent chow for 12 weeks. All animals were allowed free access to clean drinking water. Morphological examination of tissues (duodenum, jejunum and ileum) was done.

Results: Gross morphology of the duodenum in the NVP-treated group showed hypertrophy of the Bruner's glands within the sub-mucosa as compared to control where the tissues appeared intact. Gross morphology of the jejunum in the NVP-treated group showed hyperplasia of mucosal cells and mild desquamation of epithelia, when compared to control the tissues appeared intact. Gross morphology of ileum in the NVP-treated group showed reductions in the density of Payer's patches and diffused areas of necrosis of mucosal epithelium when compared to control where tissues appeared intact.

Conclusion: From the result of the study, long term administration of NVP may cause disorganization of the morphology of small intestine in albino Wistar rats.

Keywords: Nevirapine; Duodenum, Jejunum; Ileum

Abbreviations: ARV: Antiretroviral; H&E: Haematoxylin and eosin; HAART: Highly Active Antiretroviral Therapy; HIV: Human Immunodeficiency Virus; HIV-1: Human Immunodeficiency Virus-Type 1; NNRTI: Non-nuceosidereverse Transcriptase Inhibitor; NVP: Nevirapine

Introduction

Nevirapine (NVP) is an antiretroviral (ARV) medication that prevents human immunodeficiency virus (HIV) cells from multiplying in the blood. NVP binds directly to reverse transcriptase and blocks the RNA-dependent and DNA-dependent polymerase activities by causing a disruption of the enzyme's catalytic site (Bertram 2004). Widespread use of highly active antiretroviral therapy (HAART) has led to dramatic reductions in morbidity and mortality among individuals infected with the HIV-1 [1,2]. It is now clear that long term remission of HIV-1 disease can be achieved using various combinations of ARV agents, which suppress plasma viral loads to less than the limit of quantification of the most sensitive commercially available assays [3,4]. The clinical and immunological stabilization of HIV disease that is possible thanks to the availability of a broad spectrum of ARV compounds has its caveats in adherence, resistance and toxicity problems [5,6]. When HIV disease is associated with a viral hepatitis, other pharmacological treatments are needed concurrently and if substance abuse is still present (including intake of alcohol, heroin and methadone), the risk of increased drug-drug interaction and end-organ toxicity is increased significantly especially because of the central role of liver tissue in drug metabolism [6,7]. NVP like many other ARV agents have side effect and toxicities which affect the gastrointestinal system [8,9].

Epithelial tissue consists of a flat sheet of closely adhering cells; one or more cells thick, with the upper surface usually exposed to the environment or to an internal space in the body [10]. Epithelium covers the body surface, lines body cavities, forms the external and internal linings of many organs, and constitutes most gland tissue. Since the extracellular material is so thin, there is therefore a possibility that NVP a protease inhibitor also, an anti-inflammatory drug [11] will affect the morphology of the small intestine. Since there is paucity of information regarding the effect of NVP on intestinal tissues, this study was therefore set out to examine possible effect of NVP administration on morphology of the small intestine using albino Wistar rats as a model.

Materials and Methods

NVP was obtained from Strides Arcolab Ltd., Bangalore, India

Experimental animals

Sixty albino Wistar rats of initial body weight between 50-125 g were used for this study. They were obtained from the animal house of Physiology Department, University of Calabar, Nigeria. They were kept in improvised plastic metabolic cages with wire net covers. The ethics for the use of experimental animals were strictly adhered to. They were maintained in the animal facility of the Physiology Department University of Calabar.

*Corresponding author: Elizabeth B Umoren, Department of Physiology College of Medical Sciences, University of Calabar, Calabar 540001, Nigeria, E-mail: lizzyumoren@yahoo.com

Experimental protocol

Thirty albino Wistar rats used for this study were randomly assigned into three groups of ten rats each; each group was further subdivided into two groups. Each group had control (n=5) and NVP-treated group (n=10). Group one was used to study the effect of NVP administration on the duodenum, group two was used to study the effect of NVP administration on the jejunum; while group three was used to study the effect of NVP administration on the ileum. Rats in all the three groups were fed ad libitum for twelve weeks and were kept free from drought at room temperature (28 ± 2oC and 12 hours light/dark cycles) throughout the feeding period, after which the samples were collected for analyses. The test group received oral administration of NVP (0.4 mg/kg body weight) once daily for 2 weeks after which the dosage was doubled by administering the drug twice daily (07:00 h and 18:00 h). The dosage of NVP administration was calculated based on the animal weight (50 g body weight) equivalence to adult human (60 kg). In this study, the dosing regimen was well tolerated.

Histopathological grading

This was done using an electron microscope. The three segments of the small intestine (duodenum, jejunum and ileum) from the three groups of NVP-treated rats were examined and the result was compared to their control respectively.

Morphological examination of tissues (duodenum, jejunum and ileum)

The preparation for microscopic examination was done according to the method of Wallington et al. [12] as used by Igiri et al. [13]. Rats were anaesthetized by inhalation of chloroform and were then decapitated. The small intestine was removed and placed in cold normal saline. The intestine was slit open and carefully rinsed in normal saline. The tissue blocks from the small intestine were fixed for 24 hours in Bouin' fluid after which they were dehydrated accordingly in ascending grades of ethanol one hour each i.e. 70%, 95% and absolute ethanol. The tissues were then cleared in two changes of xylene one hour each, thereafter, were infiltrated in molten paraffin wax at oven temperature of 58oC, and finally, embedded in pure paraffin wax and thin sections cut at 5 microns. Sections were floated on water bath and picked on albuminized slides and incubated for 6 hours at 37oC. Furthermore, sections were stained with haematoxylin and eosin (H&E) for 15 minutes. The sections were de-wax in xylene and taken through absolute ethanol, 95% and 70% rinsed in water, stained in haematoxylin for 15 minutes and rinsed in water. Sections were differentiated briefly in 1% acid alcohol, blued in running tap water for 30 minutes, counter stained in 1% aqueous eosin for 2 minutes, dehydrated in alcohol clear in xylene and mounted with DPX. The sections were then viewed under the microscope and photomicrographs taken.

Results

Effect of long term administration of NVP on the duodenumGross morphology of the duodenum among the rats in the control group showed normal intestinal mucosa, sub mucosa and muscularisexterna (Figure 1a and 1b). However, gross morphology of the duodenum among the rats in the NVP-treated group revealed hypertrophy of Brunner's glands within the sub-mucosa. The muscularisexterna appeared distorted (Figure 2a and 2b).

Effect of long term administration of NVP on the jejunum

Gross morphology of the jejunum among the rats in the

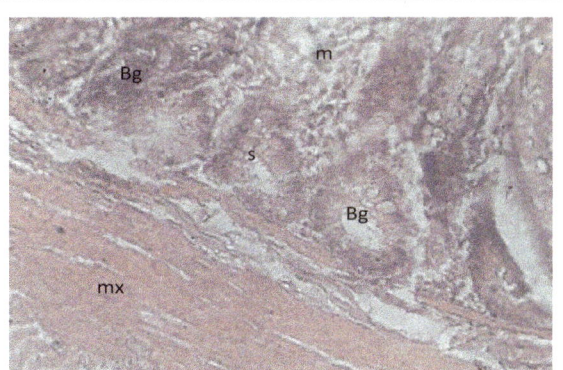

Figure 1a: Photomicrograph of duodenum of the control group. Showing intestinal mucosa (m), sub mucosa (s) and muscularis externa (mx).Within the sub mucosa are the Brunner's glands (Bg). Magnification x 25.

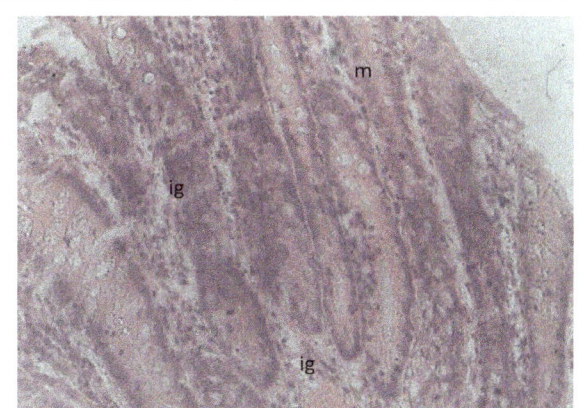

Figure 1b: Photomicrograph of the Jejunum of the control group. Showing the mucosa (m), submucosa (s) and muscularis externa (mx) appear normal. Magnification x 25.

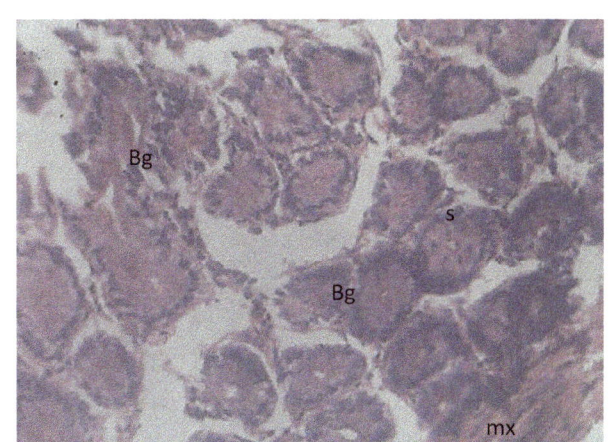

Figure 2a: Photomicrograph of duodenum of the NVP-treated group. Showing hypertrophy of the Brunner's glands (Bg) within the submucosa (S). Mx = muscularis externa. Magnification x 25.

control group showed normal intestinal mucosa, sub-mucosa and muscularisexterna (Figure 3a and 3b). However, gross morphology of the jejunum among the rats in the NVP-treated group revealed mucosal hyperplasia within the core of villi and mild desquamation of epithelia (Figure 4a and 4b).

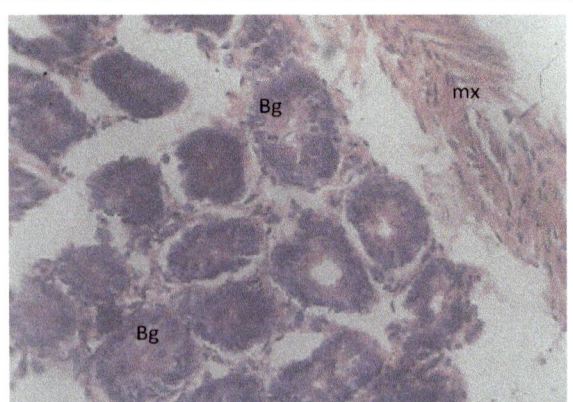

Figure 2b: Photomicrograph of duodenum of the NVP-treated group. Showing hypertrophy of Brunner's glands (Bg). Mx = muscularis externa. Magnification x 25.

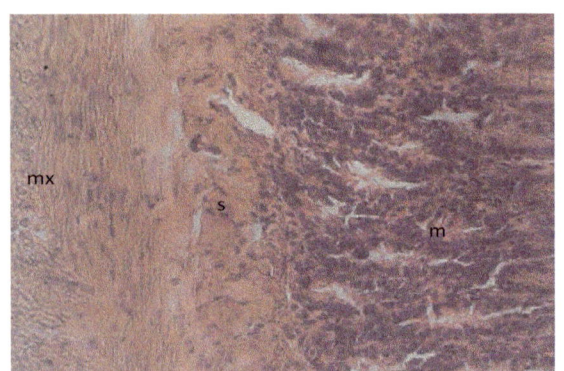

Figure 3a: Photomicrograph of the Jejunum of the control group. Showing the mucosa (m), submucosa (s) and muscularis externa (mx) appear normal. Magnification x 25.

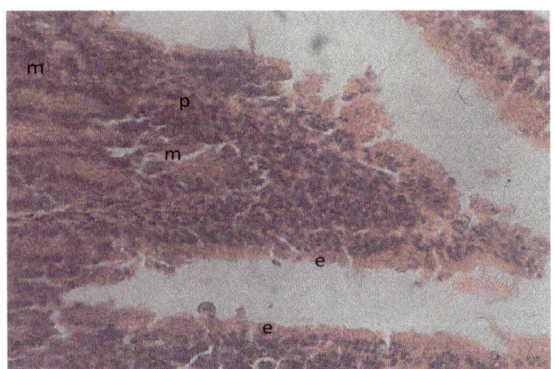

Figure 3b: Photomicrograph of jejunum of control group. Showing mucosa of the jejunum seen to be thrown into folds, with its core made of lamina propia (p) and the submucosal (s) tissue carrying blood vessels within. Magnification x 25.

Effect of long term administration of NVP on the ileum

Gross morphology of the ileum among the rats in the control group showed normal mucosa, within which was seen the Payer's patches limited externally by the sub mucosa and muscularisexterna (Figure 5). However, gross morphology of the ileum among the rats in the NVP-treated group revealed reductions in density of the Payer's patches and diffused areas of necrosis of mucosal epithelium (Figure 6).

Discussion

Effects of long term administration of NVP given through oral gavage on morphology of the small intestine of albino Wistar rats were studied. The results obtained from morphological examination revealed

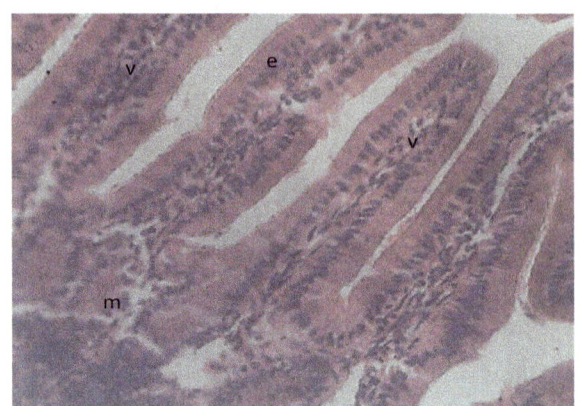

Figure 4a: Photomirogaph of jejunum of NVP-treated group. Showing mucosa (m) of jejunum with a continuum in the epithelium (e) which is composed of simple columnar cells. V= villi. Magnification x 25.

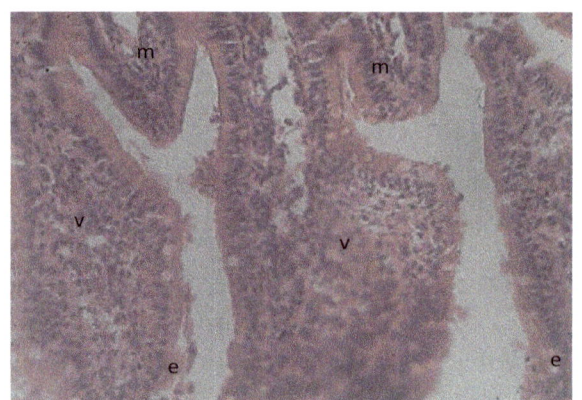

Figure 4b: Photomicrograph of jejunum of NVP-treated group. The mucosa (m) of jejunum in this treated group showed hyperplasia of cells within the core of villi and mild desquamation of epithelia (e). Magnification x 25.

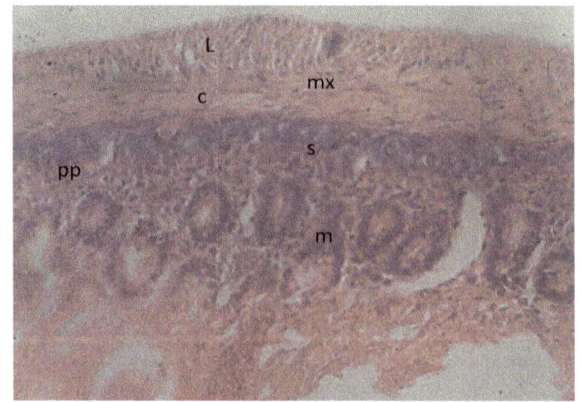

Figure 5: Photomicrograph of the ileum of control group. Showing the mucosa within which are seen the Payer's patches (PP), limited externally by the submucosa (s) and the muscularis externa (mx). L=longitudinal, C=circular layers of the muscularis externa. Magnification x 25.

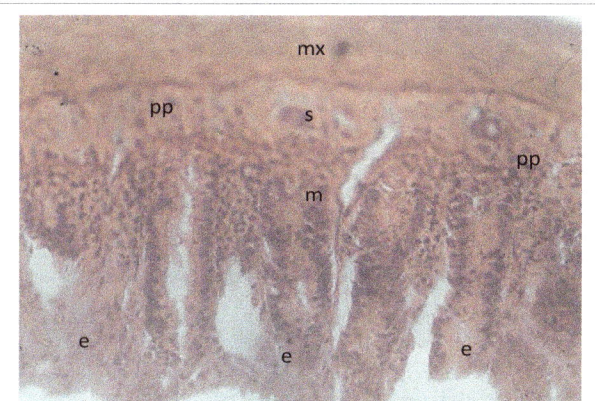

Figure 6: Photomicrograph of Ileum of NVP-treated group. Showing reduction in density of the Payer's patches (pp) and diffused areas of necrosis of mucosal epithelium (e). The submucosa (s) and muscularis externa (mx) appeared normal. Magnification x 25.

that the duodenum, jejunum and ileum of NVP-treated rats had hypertrophy of the Bruner's glands within the sub mucosa; hyperplasia of the mucosal cells and mild desquamation of the epithelia; reductions in density of the Payer's patches with diffused areas of necrosis of the mucosal epithelium, respectively, when compared to control groups of rat, the different segments of the intestinal tissues appeared normal.

Although, there is paucity of information with regards to the effect of NVP administration on the morphology of small intestine, there are series of reports as regards the toxicity of NVP a non-nucleoside reverse transcriptase inhibitor (NNRTI) on the liver, mitochondria, muscle and bone [14-17] had earlier reported that a direct or immune-mediated hepatic involvement seemed to be caused by NNRTIs, while [18-20] reported that the administration of nucleoside analogues acts via mitochondrial abnormalities prompting hepatosteatosis, lactic acidosis, and muscle and bone toxicity. Den Brinker et al. [21] reported that protease inhibitors seemed to be the main cause of glucose and lipid abnormalities.

The duodenum has prominent duodenal (Brunner) glands in the sub mucosa. They secrete an abundance of bicarbonate-rich mucus, which neutralizes stomach acid and shields the mucosa from its corrosive effects [10]. Unarguably, the mucosa can be damaged via a number of substances including prostaglandin inhibitors and other anti-inflammatory drugs [22]. It could be that NVP a protease inhibitor and also an anti-inflammatory drug, may be acting as an inhibitor of prostaglandins-which could confer protection on the intestinal mucosa. Further work on the effect of NVP on prostaglandins would substantiate this study.

Umoren et al. [8] had earlier reported intestinal motility/transit stimulating actions of NVP in albino Wistar rats. Disruption and erosion of the intestine of rats fed NVP exposed the muscle coat of intestine to various yaso-active agents causing contraction. Tissue and erosion degeneration can cause leakage of electrolytes such as sodium, potassium and hydrogen ions into the muscle coat layer of the intestine leading to amplification of the electrical activity of intestine [23]. This can result in increased intestinal motility and transit [24] had reported increased intestinal transit in NVP-treated HIV patients. Also, Deborah et al. [9] had reported gastrointestinal manifestations with protease inhibitor and NVP treatment to include diarrhea. These findings may be due to tissue erosion and degeneration caused by NVP administration, since damage to the cyto-architecture of the

small intestine results in the leakage of various ions, thus, affecting certain ion channels. Opening of calcium-sodium ion channels enhances calcium ion entry which causes contraction of smooth muscle cells [25]. Therefore, long term NVP administration may cause derangement of intestinal tissue leading to increased intestinal motility, contraction and transit [8]; these mechanisms can damage the intestinal mucosa. The circular folds of the intestine promote more thorough mixing and nutrient absorption. The core of the villus has a few smooth muscle cells that contract periodically. This enhances the mixing of chime in the intestinal lumen. Each absorptive cell of a villus has a fuzzy brush border that increases the absorptive surface area of the small intestine and contains brush border enzymes [10]. From the result of our laboratory studies [26] the NVP-treated rats had decreased nutrients (glucose + protein) absorption as compared to the control group. This could be a pointer to the fact that the intestinal tissues had been compromised. On the floor of the small intestine, between the bases of the villi, there are numerous pores that open into intestinal crypts which consist of absorptive and goblet cells like those of the villi Saladin [10]. Also, from the result of our laboratory studies (Umoren et al. [12]; unpublished results), the crypt height and crypt depths in the NVP-treated rats were significantly reduced respectively, when compared to their controls with normal crypt depth and crypt height. This also points to a possible intestinal mucosal damage caused by NVP administration, which could probably result in the abnormal (decreased) nutrients absorption.

In conclusion, the above results suggest that NVP administration may cause intestinal tissue erosion and degeneration in albino Wistar rat.

Limitations of the Study

The sample size (sixty rats) used in the study was small. Also, the choice of dose for the animal treatment though small was based on the weight equivalence of rat (50 g B/W) to adult physiological man (60 kg).

Acknowledgement

The financial assistance of Prof. Usua EJ is gratefully acknowledged Thanks to Dr Nana of Department of Anatomy uncial, Nigeria who interpreted the histological slides.

References

1. Carpenter CC, Cooper DA, Fischl MA, Gatell JM, Gazzard BG, et al. (2000) Antiretroviral therapy in adults: updated recommendations of the International AIDS Society-USA Panel. JAMA 283: 381-390.

2. Hogg RS, Heath KV, Yip B, Craib KJ, O'Shaughnessy MV, et al. (1998) Improved survival among HIV-infected individuals following initiation of antiretroviral therapy. JAMA 279: 450-454.

3. Raboud JM, Montaner JS, Conway B, Rae S, Reiss P, et al. (1998) Suppression of plasma viral load below 20 copies/ml is required to achieve a long-term response to therapy. AIDS 12: 1619-1624.

4. Bartlett J, DeMasi R, Quinn J, Moxham C, Rousseau F (2001) Overview of the effectiveness of triple combination therapy in antiretroviral-naive HIV-1 infected adults. AIDS 15: 1369-1377.

5. Ensoli F, Sirianni MC (2002) HIV/HCV co-infection: clinical and therapeutic challenges. AIDS 16: 1419-1420.

6. Bruno R, Sacchi P, Puoti M, Soriano V, Filice G (2002) HCV chronic hepatitis in patients with HIV: clinical management issues. Am J Gastroenterol 97: 1598-1606.

7. Kresina TF, Flexner CW, Sinclair J, Correia MA, Stapleton JT, et al. (2002) Alcohol use and HIV pharmacotherapy. AIDS Res Hum Retroviruses 18: 757-770.

8. Umoren EB, Obembe AO, Osim EE (2013) Ulcerogenic and intestinal motility/transit stimulating actions of nevirapine in albino Wistar rats. J Physiol Biochem 69: 547-557.

9. Deborah JE, Marriott, Jeffrey JP (2005) Gastrointesinal manifestations: in Immunology/HIV/Infectious Diseases. Clinical Services Unit, St. Vincent's Hospital, Sydney, NSW.

10. Saladin KS (2004) Anatomy & Physiology: the unity of form and function (3rd edn) McGraw-Hill companies, Inc., 1221 Avenue of the Americas, New York.

11. Smith ME, Morton DG (2001) The digestive system. Harcourt Publishers London 183-186.

12. Carleton HM, Drury RAS, Wallington SA (1980) Carleton's Histological techniques (5thed) CH 11:199-200. London University Press.

13. Igiri AO, Ibegbu AO, OsimEE (1994) The morphological and histological changes in the small intestinal induced by chronic consumption of palm oil diets   in rats. Trop J Appl Sci 3: 144-153.

14. Cattelan AM, Erne E, Salatino A, Trevenzoli M, Carretta G, et al. (1999) Severe hepatic failure related to nevirapine treatment. Clin Infect Dis 29: 455-456.

15. Martínez E, Blanco JL, Arnaiz JA, Pérez-Cuevas JB, Mocroft A, et al. (2001) Hepatotoxicity in HIV-1-infected patients receiving nevirapine-containing antiretroviral therapy. AIDS 15: 1261-1268.

16. Piliero PJ, Purdy B (2001) Nevirapine-induced hepatitis: a case series and review of the literature. AIDS Read 11: 379-382.

17. Sulkowski MS, Thomas DL, Mehta SH, Chaisson RE, Moore RD (2002) Hepatotoxicity associated with nevirapine or efavirenz-containing antiretroviral therapy: role of hepatitis C and B infections. Hepatology 35: 182-189.

18. Sulkowski MS, Thomas DL, Chaisson RE, Moore RD (2000) Hepatotoxicity associated with antiretroviral therapy in adults infected with human immunodeficiency virus and the role of hepatitis C or B virus infection. JAMA 283: 74-80.

19. Ensoli F, Sirianni MC (2002) HIV/HCV co-infection: clinical and therapeutic challenges. AIDS 16: 1419-1420.

20. Bruno R, Sacchi P, Filice G (2002) Mitochondrial toxicity in HIV-HCV co-infection: It depends on the choice of antiretroviral drugs? Hepatology 35: 500-501.

21. den Brinker M, Wit FW, Wertheim-van Dillen PM, Jurriaans S, Weel J, et al. (2000) Hepatitis B and C virus co-infection and the risk for hepatotoxicity of highly active antiretroviral therapy in HIV-1 infection. AIDS 14: 2895-2902.

22. Wallace JL (2008) Prostaglandins, NSAIDs, and gastric mucosal protection: why doesn't the stomach digest itself? Physiol Rev 88: 1547-1565.

23. Ladipo JK, Bradshaw LA, Halter S, Richards WO (2003) Changes in intestinal electrical activity during ischaemia correlate to pathology. West Afr J Med 22: 1-4.

24. Mavukani MP (2009) Maternal and fetal outcomes of pregnant women on antiretroviral (ARV) therapy at Dr George Mukhari Hospital: a case-controlled clinical study. PhD Dissertation, University of Limpopo (Medunsa campus).

25. Guyton AC, Hall JE (2006) Contration and excitation of smooth muscles. In: textbook of medical physiology(11thedn), Elsevier Saunders. Philadelphia 92-99.

26. Bertram GK (2004) Basic & Clinical Pharmacology (9thedn) International edition By McGraw. Hill Companies Appleton & Lang; Lange Medical Publications. Singapore 816-817.

20

Neuroprotection of Sesamin against Cerebral Ischemia *In-Vivo* and N-Methyl-D-Aspartate-Induced Apoptosis *In-Vitro*

Hong-liang Guo[1,2†], Jiao Tian[3†,] Xin-shang Wang[1†], Zhen Tian[1], Xu-bo Li[1], Le Yang[1], Ming-gao Zhao[1*] and Shui-bing Liu[1*]

[1]*Department of Pharmacology, School of Pharmacy, Fourth Military Medical University, Xi'an, Shaanxi 710032, China*
[2]*Department of Pharmacy, Fifth Hospital of PLA, Yin chuan, Ning xia 750004, China*
[3]*Department of Pediatrics, Tangdu Hospital, Fourth Military Medical University, Xi'an, Shaanxi 710038, China*
[†]*These authors contributed equally to this work.*

Abstract

Sesamin, a major lignan found in sesame oil, is widely used in traditional Chinese medicine for its bioactivities. However, the information on the neuroprotective effects of sesamin against ischemia- or glutamate-induced excitotoxic injury is limited. This study aimed to investigate the neuroprotective effects of sesamin against focal cerebral ischemia in vivo and N-methyl-d-aspartate (NMDA)-induced neurotoxicity in vitro. Sesamin (43.2 mg/kg) attenuated cerebral ischemic injury in mice induced by 2 h of middle cerebral artery occlusion and reperfusion. Furthermore, treatment with 0.1 µM sesamin significantly decreased the number of apoptotic neuronal cells in cultured neurons after exposure to 200 µM NMDA. Western blot and calcium imaging results indicated that sesamin protected neurons against excitotoxicity by restoring the balance of apoptotic proteins and inhibiting calcium overload in cultured neurons after exposure to NMDA. Our findings provide a new insight into the development of natural anti-excitotoxicity agents.

Keywords: Sesamin; Apoptosis; Neuroprotection; N-methyl-D-aspartate; Calcium

Introduction

Glutamate is the major excitatory neurotransmitter in the central nervous system (CNS) [1]. However, excessive glutamate is associated with numerous neurological disorders including stroke, traumatic brain injury [2,3], multiple sclerosis, Huntington's disease, Parkinson's disease and Alzheimer's disease [4]. Excessive glutamate can over activate glutamate receptors and result in high calcium ion (Ca^{2+}) influx, which activates a number of enzymes that damage cell structures such as the cell membrane, cytoskeleton components and DNA. This Ca^{2+} influx is thought to contribute to Ca^{2+}-mediated excitotoxic neuronal cell death in the processes of the abovementioned diseases [5]. N-methyl-D-aspartate (NMDA) receptors, a type of ionotropic glutamate receptors, perform a crucial function in mediating glutamate excitotoxicity because of its high calcium permeability [6]. NMDA receptors are permeable to Na^+, K^+, and Ca^{2+} ions, among which excess Ca^{2+} ions is linearly correlated with NMDA-mediated neuronal cell death triggered by intracellular Ca^{2+}-dependent cascades [7].

Apoptosis is a process of programmed cell death, which is a cascade produced by several apoptosis-regulatory genes [8]. Caspase-3, a member of the caspase family, determines the incidence of apoptosis. The members of the Bcl-2 family such as Bcl-2 and Bax proteins are the most prominent factors in the mitochondria-mediated apoptotic pathway [3,9]. Studies have shown the powerful properties of various natural polyphenols against neuronal exitotoxicity induced by NMDA [10,11]. Sesamin (a typical lignan with β-linkage) and sesamolin (a compound with a phenyl group with an acetaloxygen bridge) are two major lignans in sesame seeds and oil (Figure 1A), which are also found in several medicinal herbs, such as Acanthopanax senticosus. Sesamin is recognized to have various pharmacological effects, such as hypocholesterolemia, anti-hypertension, anti-inflammation, and protective effects against neurotoxicity, hypoxic and oxidative damage [12-15]. The neuroprotective effects of sesamin have been investigated in models of MCAO [15,16]. However, the underlying neuroprotective mechanisms of sesamin are not well known.

The present study was designed to investigate whether sesamin has neuroprotective effects against focal cerebral ischemia in vivo and NMDA -induced neurotoxicity in vitro. The treatment with sesamin was found to produce significant protection against the excitotoxicity triggered by NMDA and against a cerebral ischemic injury induced by a 2 h MCAO and reperfusion.

Materials and Methods

Chemicals and reagents

Sesamin (purity >98 %) was purchased from Shanghai Pure One Biotechnology (Shanghai, China). NMDA, Glycine, poly-L-lysine, propidiumiodide (PI), 3-(4,5-dimethylthiazol-2-yl)-2,5-diphenyltetrazoliumbromide (MTT), 2'-(4-Hydroxyphenyl)-5-(4-methyl-1-piperazinyl)-2,5'-bi-1H-benzimidazde, trihydrochloride (Hoechst33258), and β-actin antibody were purchased from Sigma (St. Louis, MO, USA). Anti-Bax, anti-Bcl-2, and anti-pro-caspase-3 antibodies were purchased from Santa Cruz (Santa Cruz, CA, USA). LDH Cytotoxicity Assay Kit was purchased from Beyotime (Beyotime, China). All secondary antibodies conjugated with horseradish peroxidase (HRP) were purchased from Santa Cruz (Santa Cruz, CA, USA). All of the other chemicals and reagents were standard.

*Corresponding author: Dr. Shui-bing Liu, , Department of Pharmacology, School of Pharmacy, Fourth Military Medical University, Xi'an 710032, China, E-mail: liushb@fmmu.edu.cn

Dr. Ming-gao Zhao, Department of Pharmacology, School of Pharmacy, Fourth Military Medical University, Xi'an 710032, China, E-mail: minggao@fmmu.edu.cn

Middle cerebral artery occlusion (MCAO).

Experiments were conducted in accordance with the Animal Care and Use Committee of the Fourth Military Medical University. C57BL/6J male mice (20 ~ 25 g) were provided by the Experimental Animal Center of the Fourth Military Medical University. They were housed with food and water available ad libitum in colony room at controlled temperature (25 ± 2°C), humidity (45 ~ 55 %) and 12:12 h light–dark cycle. To investigate the neuroprotective effects of sesamin on cerebral ischemia, MCAO mouse model was employed in this study [17]. In brief, mice were anesthetized with chloral hydrate (300 mg/kg) and a longitudinal incision of 10 ± 2 mm was made along the midline of the ventral cervical part. The right common carotid artery, internal carotid artery (ICA), and external carotid artery (ECA) were exposed and carefully isolated. A nylon mono filament (20 mm length and 0.2 mm diameter) was inserted from the lumen of the ECA to that of the right ICA to occlude the origin of the right middle cerebral artery (MCA). After 120 min, the nylon monofilament was removed to restore blood flow. Temperature was maintained at 37 ± 0.5°C throughout the surgery. All surgical procedures were performed under an operating stereomicroscope. Mice were randomly divided into three groups: (1) sham operated group, (2) MCAO group (120 min of MCAO followed by 24 h of reperfusion), and (3) sesamin + MCAO group. The mice in sham operated group were subjected to surgery and exposed the right ICA and the right ECA but did not suffer MCAO. The mice of MCAO and sesamin + MCAO groups were treated with saline or sesamin (43.2 mg/kg) (16) respectively by intragastric administration. Saline or drugs was fed once daily for seven consecutive days before the experiment. MCAO was carried out 30 min after the last drug administration.

Neurological Scoring and Infarct Size Measurement

The neurobehavioral evaluation and infarct volume assessment were performed 24 h after reperfusion in each group. Neurological scores were assessed on a scale: 0, no neurological deficit; 1, failure to extend left forepaw fully; 2, circling to the left; 3, inability to bear weight on the left; 4, no spontaneous walking with depressed level of consciousness [18].

After neurological evaluation, half of the mice (n=6) were killed and the brains were removed and cooled in iced saline for 10 min. Infarct volumes were measured as described previously [19]. Briefly, brains were cut into 1-mm-thick coronal sections and stained with 2% 2,3,5-triphenyltetrazolium chloride (TTC) for 30 min at 37°C followed by overnight immersion in 4% formalin. The infarct tissue remained unstained (white) and normal tissue was stained (red). The brain slices were photographed using a digital camera. White areas were defined as infarct and were measured using image analysis software (Adobe Photoshop CS3 for Windows). The infarct volume was calculated by measuring the unstained area in each slice, multiplying it by slice thickness (1 mm), and then summing all six slices.

Nissl staining

After neurological evaluation, another half of mice (n=6) were perfused with cold 4% paraformaldehyde in 0.01 M PBS (pH 7.4). Brain containing dorsal hippocampal and the prefrontal cortex area were cut into frozen coronal sections (30 μm) by using a Leica CM1950 and then stained with 0.1% cresylviolet for 40 min. The images were captured with light microscope (Olympus BX60). Six sections from each animal were selected for Nissl staining. Data were expressed according to the formula: intact neurons (%)=number of healthy neurons/number of total neurons × 100.

Primary mouse cortical neuronal culture

Embryos (E16 ~ 17, C57BL/6J mice for both genders) were employed in this experiment. The Animal Care and Use Committee of the Fourth Military Medical University approved all of the animal protocols used. Prefrontal cortex neurons were cultured as described previously [20]. Briefly, the prefrontal cortex was dissected, minced, and trypsinized at 37°C for 10 min using 0.25% trypsin (Invitrogen, Carlsbad, CA). Neurons seeded at a density of 2×10^4 cells/well in 96-well plate, 2×10^5 cells/well in 24-well plate containing glass coverslips (Fisher Scientific) and 1×10^6 cells/well in 6-well plate respectively for different treatments. All plates were pre-coated with 50 μg/ml poly-L-lysine (Sigma) in water. The cultures were incubated at 37°C in 95% air/5% carbon dioxide with 95% humidity. The cells were characterized by immunohistochemistry staining for anti-MAP2 antibody, revealing that this culture procedure yielded more than 95% neurons. Cultures were used for experiments on the day 7 in vitro (DIV 7). The culture medium was removed, and cells were washed with Mg^{2+}-free extracellular solution (ECS) containing (in mM): NaCl: 140, KCl: 3, CaCl: 22, HEPES: 10, glucose: 10, adjusted to pH 7.2 ~ 7.3 with NaOH and osmotic pressure 290 ± 5 with sucrose. Then the cortex neurons were exposed for 60 min to ECS supplemented with 200 μM NMDA (Sigma, St. Louis, MO, USA) and 20 μM glycine (Sigma). The cells were washed three times and returned to the original culture medium for 24 h. Sesamin was added into culture medium 24 h prior to addition of NMDA and were present throughout whole experiment.

Cell viability analysis

Neuronal cell viability was determined by MTT assay as previously described [21] with some modifications. Briefly, neurons were used on day 7 (DIV 7). MTT was dissolved in neurobasal medium and added to each well for incubation at 37°C for 4 h at a final concentration of 0.5 mg/ml. Then the medium was replaced by 150 μl dimethyl sulfoxide (DMSO). The optical density (OD) was read on a Universal Microplate Reader (Elx800, Bio-TEK instruments Inc., USA) at 570 nm (630 nm as a reference). Cell viability was expressed as a percentage of control value.

LDH assay

The LDH activity assay was performed with the LDH Cytotoxicity Assay Kit (Beyotime, China). LDH, a stable cytosolic enzyme, is released upon cell lysis. It was measured with a 30 min coupled enzymatic assay in culture supernatants, which resulted in the conversion of a tetrazolium salt into a red formazan product. The amount of color formed was proportional to the degree of damage to the cell membranes [22]. Absorbance data was collected using a Universal Microplate Reader (Elx800, Bio-TEK instruments Inc., USA) at 490 nm. LDH leakage was expressed according to the formula: LDH release (%)=(experimental LDH release-blank LDH release)/(maximum LDH release-blank LDH release) × 100.

Hoechst/PI double staining

Cell death was detected by Hoechst 33258 and PI double fluorescent staining as described previously [23] with some modifications. Neurons were cultured onto the cover slides in the 24-well plates at a density of 2×10^5 cells/well. Neurons were pretreated with sesamin (0.1 μM) for 24 h. Subsequently, they were subjected to excitotoxic injury with 200 μM NMDA and 20 μM glycine for 60 min. After that, the neurons were returned to the original culture medium including sesamin for 24 h. The cells were washed with ECS for three times, stained with PI (10 μg/ml) and Hoechst 33258 (10 μg/ml) for 15 min, and then fixed by 4 % paraformaldehyde for 10 min. Cells were observed under a fluorescence microscope (Olympus BX61, Japan). The Hoechst and PI dye were excited at 340 and 620 nm respectively. For each well, three visual fields were selected randomly.

Calcium imaging

Calcium imaging was performed as previously described [24,25]. Neurons were cultured in 3.5 cm plates at density 3×10^5 cells. The plate is made especially for laser scanning microscope. Cultured neurons were used on day 9, and then were washed twice using Mg^{2+}-free extracellular solution (ECS). The neurons were incubated with 2.5 μM fluo-3/AM at 37°C for 30 min, then washed twice and returned to the original culture medium for additional 20 min. Prior to NMDA treatment, the dye-loaded cells were scanned for 1 min to obtain a basal level of intracellular Ca^{2+} image by using a confocal laser scanning microscope (Olympus, Japan). NMDA (200 μM) was applied to the cultures, and an equal amount of ECS was added as a control. Sesamin was added to the culture medium for 24 h before the NMDA treatments and presented in the whole experiment process. The change of Ca^{2+} concentration was measured by the fluorescence ratio of the fluo-3/AM loaded neurons for another 4 min. The results expressed as the changes compared to the basal level.

Western blot

Western blot analysis was performed as previously described [26]. Protein samples (30 μg) were separated by 9 % SDS-polyacrylamide gel and electrotransferred onto PVDF membranes (Invitrogen). The membranes were blocked by 5% fat-free milk at room temperature for 2 h and incubated with anti-Bcl-2 antibody (1:1000), anti-Bax antibody (1:1000), anti-pro-caspase-3 antibody (1:500), and with β-actin (1:10000) at 4°C for overnight. After three washes with PBST, membranes were further incubated with HRP-conjugated secondary antibodies for 1 ~ 2 h and followed by three PBST washes. The target protein bands were visualized by an ECL chemiluminescence system (Bio-Rad, Hercules, CA).

Statistical analysis

Results were expressed as the mean ± SEM. Data were evaluated using independent samples test between two groups or one-way analysis of variance (ANOVA) for post hoc comparisons among multiple groups (SPSS 13.0). Data that passed the homogeneity test were analyzed by the one-way ANOVA Least Significant Difference (LSD) test. Data that did not pass the homogeneity test were analyzed by the one-way ANOVA Dunnett's T3 test. In all cases, p<0.05 was considered statistically significant.

Results

Attenuation of ischemia injury by sesamin

The neuroprotective effect of sesamin against ischemia-reperfusion injury was evaluated via neurological scoring, infarct size measurement, and Nissl staining. MCAO resulted in large infarct size (F (2, 15) =360.6, P<0.01, one-way ANOVA, Dunnett T3 test; Figure 1B and 1C) and high neurological deficit score (F (2, 15) =92.5, P<0.01, one-way ANOVA, Dunnett T3 test; Figure 1D). Sesamin (43.2 mg/kg) significantly decreased the infarct volume (F (2, 15) =360.6, P<0.01, one-way ANOVA, Dunnett T3 test; Figure 1B and 1C) and neurological deficit score (F (2, 15) =92.5, P<0.01, one-way ANOVA, Dunnett T3 test; Figure 1A and 1D) as compared with those of MCAO group. The Nissl staining showed that neuronal damage was obvious in the hippocampus CA1 region and prefrontal cortex

after MCAO (Figure 2A). The injured neurons showed shrunken cell bodies accompanied by shrunken and pyknotic nuclei. As shown in Figure 2B and 2C, the number of healthy neurons was reduced to 12.6 ± 1.0% in the hippocampus (F (2, 9) =908.3, P<0.01, one-way ANOVA, LSD test; Figure 2B) and 9.3 ± 0.8% in the prefrontal cortex (F (2, 9) =427.8, P<0.01, one-way ANOVA, LSD test; Figure 2C) in MCAO group, respectively. However, sesamin (43.2 mg/kg) markedly rescued the damaged neurons (hippocampus: F (2, 9) =908.3, P<0.01, one-way ANOVA, LSD test; prefrontal cortex: F (2, 9) =427.8, P<0.01, one-way ANOVA, LSD test; Figure 2B and 2C).

Sesamin protected neurons against NMDA-induced cell death.

To further evaluate the neuroprotective effects of sesamin, primary cortical neuron culture was performed and the neuroprotection of sesamin was detected by MTT assay in vitro. Cultured cortical neurons (DIV 7) were pretreated with sesamin for 24 h and then treated with NMDA for 60 min. The cells were returned to the original culture medium, which contains sesamin, for another 24 h (Figure 3A, top). Exposure to NMDA (200 μM) for 60 min markedly induced cell injury (F (6, 35) =11.6, P<0.01, one-way ANOVA, LSD test; Figure 3A, bottom). Treatment with sesamin (0.1-1 μM) significantly protected neurons against NMDA injury (F (6, 35) =11.6, P<0.01 and P<0.05, one-way ANOVA, LSD test). However, the higher concentration of sesamin (10 μM) failed to protect the neurons against NMDA exposure. Sesamin (0.1 μM) alone did not affect cell viability.

To further demonstrate the neuroprotection of sesamin, the amount of LDH release was measured using the LDH assay. NMDA caused a significant amount of LDH release (F (4, 25) =38.8, P<0.01, one-way ANOVA, Dunnett T3 test; Figure 3B), and sesamin (0.1 μM) completely protected the cells from cell damage (F(4, 25) = 38.8, P < 0.01, one-way

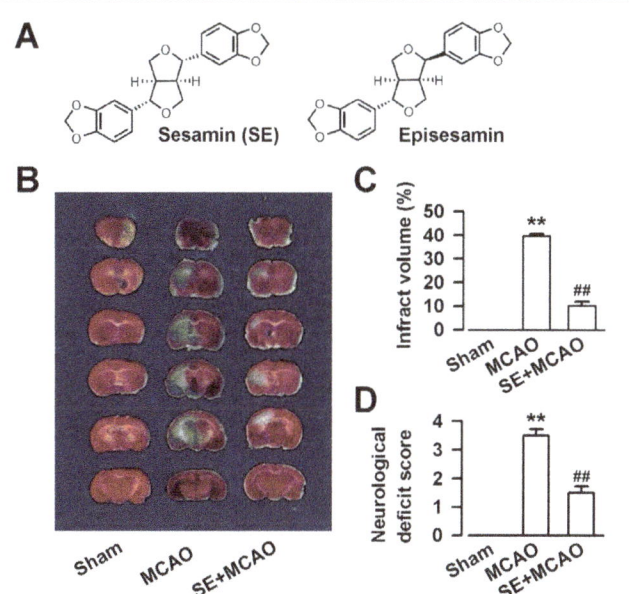

Figure 1: Neuroprotective effects of sesamin on ischemia injury after MCAO in mice.

(A) Structure of sesamin and episesamin. (B) Infarct areas were visualized by TTC staining of coronal brain sections (1 mm thick) from mice subjected to sham or MCAO. Non-ischemic region is in red and the infarct region appears in white. (C) The infarct volume percentage of the mice was measured 24 h after MCAO. (D) The quantification of neurological scores was performed 24 h after MCAO. n=6, ** p<0.01 compared with Sham group; ## p<0.01 compared with MCAO group. SE: sesamin.

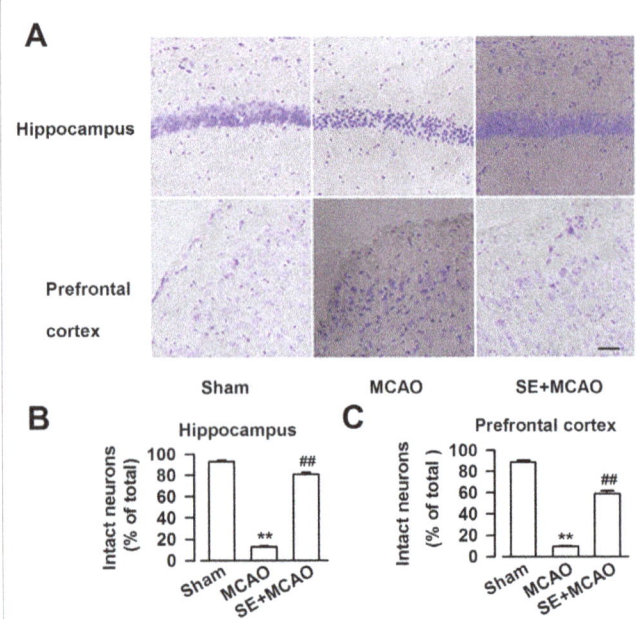

Figure 2: Nissl staining showing the effects of sesamin. (A) Morphological evaluation in the hippocampus and prefrontal cortex 24 h after MCAO in sham-, MCAO-, and SE + MCAO-treated groups. Scale bar=20 μm. (B–C) The percentage of healthy neurons in hippocampus (B) and prefrontal cortex (C) in sham-, MCAO-, and SE + MCAO-treated groups. n=4, ** $p < 0.01$ compared with sham group; ## $p < 0.01$ compared with MCAO alone. SE: sesamin.

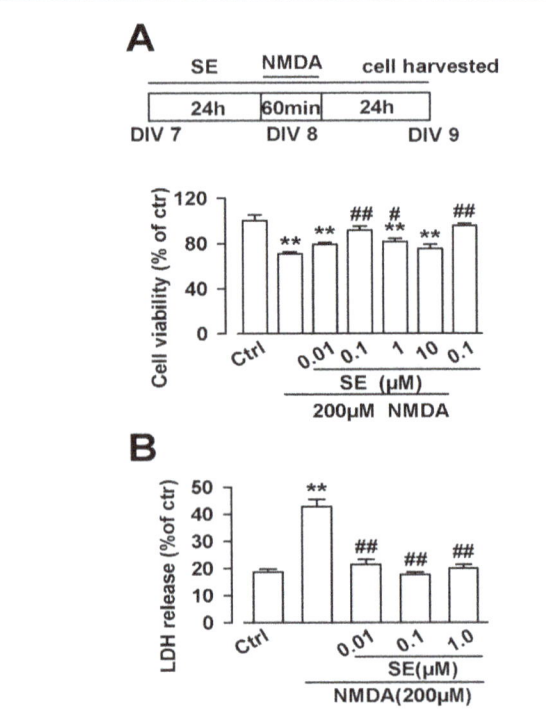

Figure 3: Effects of sesamin on cell viability upon NMDA injury. (A) Cultured cortical neurons (DIV 7) were pretreated with sesamin for 24 h and then with NMDA for 60 min. The cells were returned to the original culture medium with sesamin for 24 h, and the cell viability (DIV 9) was assessed by MTT assay (top). Effects of sesamin on the cell viability in cultured cortical neurons after exposure to NMDA (bottom). (B) Percentage of LDH release (DIV 9) was determined using LDH analysis. n=6, ** $p < 0.01$ compared with control; # $p < 0.05$, ## $p < 0.01$ compared with NMDA alone. SE: sesamin.

ANOVA, Dunnett T3 test; Figure 3B). The results were consistent with the data from MTT assay.

Hoechst 33258 and PI double staining were carried out to further determine the neuroprotective effects of sesamin. The results suggested that 8.1 ± 1.4 % cells in the control group and 43.4 ± 4.7 % cells in NMDA group underwent cell apoptosis or death (F (2, 9) =32.3, P<0.01, one-way ANOVA, LSD test; Figure4A and 4B). However, 0.1 μM sesamin markedly attenuated the excitotoxicity induced by NMDA in cultured cortical neurons (F (2, 9) =32.3, P<0.01, one-way ANOVA, LSD test; Figure4A and 4B).

Sesamin reduced the NMDA-evoked Ca²⁺ increase in cortical neurons

The calcium concentration in the control neuron was stable as shown by the unchanged fluorescence intensity during the whole detection process (Figure 5A and 5B). NMDA (200 μM) treatment produced a persistent elevation of Ca²⁺ level in cultured neurons (Figure 5A and 5C). However, treatment with sesamin (0.1 μM) reduced the NMDA-evoked increase of Ca²⁺ concentration as shown by decreased fluorescence intensity (T=8.0, p<0.01, independent samples test; Figure 5A and 5C).

Effects of sesamin on the expression of apoptosis-related proteins

Whether the protection of sesamin was associated with the changes in the expression of apoptosis-related proteins was determined. As shown in Figure 6, NMDA treatment down-regulated the Bcl-2 expression (F (2, 9) =17.0, P<0.01, one-way ANOVA, LSD test; Figure 6A and 6B), up-regulated the Bax expression (F (2, 9) =28.5, P<0.01, one-way ANOVA, LSD test; Figure 6A and 6C), and thus increased the Bax/Bcl-2 ratio (F (2, 9) =124.9, P<0.01, one-way ANOVA, LSD test; Figure 6D). However, 0.1 μM sesamin showed anti-apoptotic activity with increasing Bcl-2 expression (F (2, 9) =17.0, P<0.01, one-way ANOVA, LSD test; Figure 6A and 6B), decreasing Bax expression (F (2, 9) =28.5, P<0.01, one-way ANOVA, LSD test; Figure 6A and 6C), and decreasing Bax/Bcl-2 ratio (F (2, 9) =124.9, P<0.01, one-way ANOVA, LSD test; Figure 6D). Caspase-3 is known to have a crucial function in the apoptotic process. Pro-caspase-3 is an inactive precursor of caspase-3 and cleaves into active caspase-3, thereby causing Bcl-2 dialysis [27]. Subsequently, changes in the pro-caspase-3 expression were observed. Cultures treated with NMDA resulted in the decrease of pro-caspase-3 (F (2, 9) =12.1, P<0.01, one-way ANOVA, LSD test; Figure 6A and 6E). Sesamin (0.1 μM) significantly increased the levels of pro-caspase-3 (F (2, 9) =12.1, P<0.05, one-way ANOVA, LSD test; Figure 6A and 6E).

Discussion

Sesamin produces effective neuroprotection against cerebral ischemia [15]. Sesamin has been reported to rescue neuronal PC12 cells from apoptosis and death induced by the MPP+ activation of microglia cells [28], protect neuronal PC12 cells from high-glucose-induced oxidation and apoptosis [29], and protect neurons against hypoxic neuronal injury [30]. Sesamin is also a free radical scavenger, which has been proven to exhibit prominent antioxidant and free radical scavenging properties [31-33]. In the present study, a mouse model of transient focal cerebral ischemia induced by a 2 h MCAO and 24 h reperfusion was used to evaluate the neuroprotective effects of sesamin. Previous studies have reported that MCAO damages the structure of the neurons and other cells that support the neurons [20,34] and decreases neurological function [20]. Our results suggested that sesamin

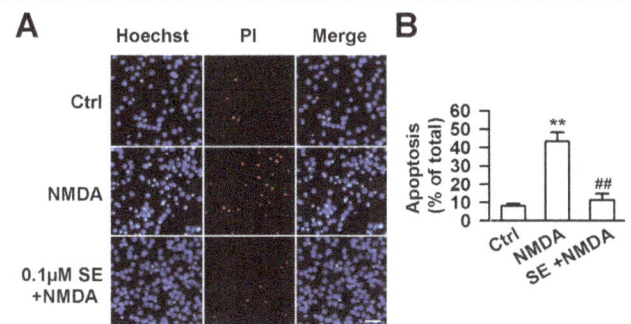

Figure 4: Hoechst 33258 and PI double staining in cultured cortical neurons.

Representative fluorescence images were obtained after Hoechst 33258 and PI double staining in the control, NMDA-, and 0.1 μM SE + NMDA-treated groups. Scale bar=20 μm. (B) The percentage of apoptotic neurons in control, NMDA-, and 0.1 μM SE + NMDA-treated groups. n=4, $**p<0.01$ compared with control; $##$ $p<0.01$ compared with NMDA alone. SE: sesamin.

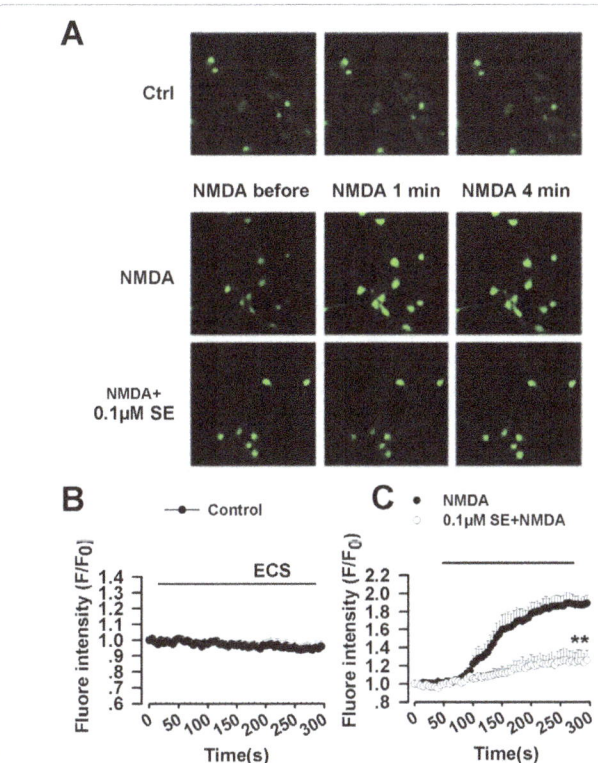

Figure 5: Effects of sesamin on intracellular calcium clearance in cultured cortical neurons.

(A) Cultured neurons were loaded with fluo-3, and then the fluorescence images were obtained before and after ECS or NMDA treatment. (B) The fluorescence intensity of ECS-perfused neurons was normalized, and the values represent the means ± SEM in three separate experiments. (C) The fluorescence intensities of the neurons in NMDA-treated (black dots) and NMDA + 0.1 μM sesamin-treated (empty dots) groups were detected and normalized according to the fluorescence intensity of the control. n=3. SE: sesamin.

reduces the infract volume in the brain of MCAO mice and improves the neurological deficit score. Meanwhile, the abnormal neuronal morphology in prefrontal cortex and hippocampus is ameliorated.

Glutamate is the main excitatory neurotransmitter in the CNS. High glutamate concentration induces excitotoxicity, which injures neuronal cells under in vitro and in vivo conditions [35]. NMDA receptor is a type of ionotropic glutamate receptor that regulates cell survival in vivo as well as in vitro. Over-stimulation of NMDA receptors leads to neuronal excitotoxicity because the subsequent influx of free Ca^{2+} results in the overload of intracellular Ca^{2+}, which has a vital function in NMDA-induced neuronal cell apoptosis [36]. Calcium influx activates a number of enzymes that damage cell structures such as the membrane, components of the cytoskeleton, and DNA. Many studies have shown that Ca^{2+} overload triggers several downstream lethal reactions, including cGMP elevation, NOS activation, and glutamate release [37,38]. In this study, the results of the MTT assay, LDH assay, Hoechst 33258 and PI double staining, and Fluo-3/AM fluorescent intensity test show that NMDA induces neuronal injury, which is consistent with previous reports [9,22]. Sesamin reduces neuronal apoptosis and inhibits the elevation of intracellular Ca2+ triggered by NMDA. These effects may be involved in the neuroprotection of sesamin against excitotoxicity.

A number of proteins influence and guide the apoptotic progression of mitochondrial pathway. The family of Bcl-2 proteins contains both the pro-apoptotic molecule Bax and the anti-apoptotic molecules Bcl-2 and Bcl-XL [39]. Their functions on cell survival in various stimuli including cytotoxic injury and oxidative stress have been well studied. The balance between Bcl-2 and Bax plays critical roles in regulating of cell death or survival [40]. The increase in the Bax/Bcl-2 protein ratio has been shown to be responsible for excitotoxic apoptosis and death mediated by NMDA in neurons [41]. The activations of initiator caspase-9 and the effector caspase-3 are very important in the apoptosis pathway. Caspase-3 activation is associated with stroke-induced apoptotic neuronal cell death [42,43]. Pro-caspase-3 is an inactive form of active caspase-3 and a major physiologic target of caspase-8 and -9 [44]. Our study showed that sesamin (0.1 μM) significantly increases the expression of Bcl-2 protein, decreases the Bax expression, and restores the increasing ratio of Bax/Bcl-2 induced by NMDA. The high level of pro-caspase-3 is related with high survival rate in cells [45]. The level of pro-caspase-3 is obviously decreased after NMDA exposure in cultured neurons, suggesting the activation of pro-caspase-3 to caspase-3. However, sesamin (0.1 μM) markedly restores the level of pro-caspase-3. A study demonstrates that sesamin can diminish iNOS and COX-2 protein expressions and significantly restore the SOD activity and protein expression levels in the acute hepatic injury rats [46]. Furthermore, sesamin treatment also significantly reduces inflammatory and oxidative stress markers including Iba1, Nox-2, and Cox-2 [15].

There are limitations of the present study. First, different protocols were used for the in vivo and in vitro experiments. Sesamin was used for seven days before the MCAO in vivo experiment, which is the standard protocol for in vivo studies. For the in vitro study, the cells were exposed to sesamin both before and after NMDA administration. The concentration of the drugs (sesamin in the present study) was speculated to decrease gradually in vivo. Actually, the pharmacokinetics of sesamin was not detected. Therefore, whether the pretreatment or post-treatment with sesamin was associated with neuroprotection could not be discriminated in the present study. More experiments need to be performed to reveal the best time window for sesamin treatment. Furthermore, there are a sex-dependent response to excitotoxicity, oxygen-glucose deprivation and nutrient deprivation in neurons in vitro [47]. Therefore, mixing male and female neurons in the present cultures may not be adequate, as differences in the ratio between male/female neurons could result in a different response to the treatments.

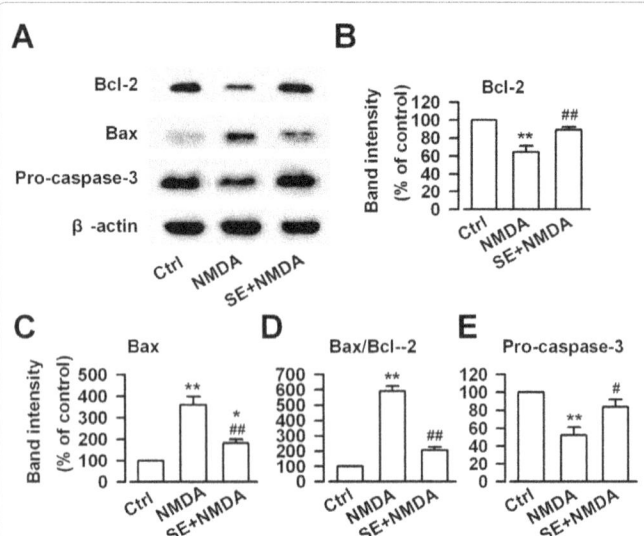

Figure 6: Effects of sesamin on Bcl-2, Bax, and pro-caspase-3 protein expression.

(A) Representative Western blot for Bcl-2, Bax, and pro-caspase-3 expression in the control, NMDA-, and SE + NMDA-treated cultured cortical neurons. (B) Sesamin (0.1 μM) evidently reversed the decreased Bcl-2 expression after exposure to NMDA in cultured cortical neurons. (C–D) Sesamin (0.1 μM) markedly reversed the increased Bax expression (C) and Bax/Bcl-2 ratio (D) after exposure to NMDA in cultured cortical neurons. (E) Sesamin (0.1 μM) significantly blocked the effect of NMDA on the pro-caspase-3 expression in cultured cortical neurons. * $p < 0.05$, ** $p < 0.01$ compared with control; # $p < 0.05$, ## $p < 0.01$ compared with NMDA alone. n=4. SE: sesamin.

In summary, the current study investigated the neuroprotective effects of sesamin on focal cerebral ischemia in vivo and against NMDA-induced cell apoptosis in vitro. This effect is partially attributed to anti-apoptotic activities. However, more experiments are necessary to elucidate the underlying mechanisms for the neuroprotective effect of sesamin.

Acknowledgement

This work was supported by NSF of China No.31470052, 31271126, and the Program for Elite Talents in University 4138C4IA75.

References

1. Choi DW (1988) Glutamate neurotoxicity and diseases of the nervous system. Neuron 1: 623-634.

2. Soundarapandian MM, Zhong X, Peng L, Wu D, Lu Y (2007) Role of K (ATP) channels in protection against neuronal excitatory insults. J Neurochem 103: 1721-1729.

3. D'Orsi B, Kilbride SM, Chen G, Perez Alvarez S, Bonner HP, et al. (2015) Bax regulates neuronal Ca²⁺ homeostasis. J Neurosci 35: 1706-1722.

4. Gonzalez J, Jurado-Coronel JC, Ávila MF, Sabogal A, Capani F, et al. (2015) NMDARs in neurological diseases: A potential therapeutic target. Int J Neurosci 125: 315-327.

5. Bano D, Young KW, Guerin CJ, Lefeuvre R, Rothwell NJ, et al. (2005) Cleavage of the plasma membrane Na⁺/Ca²⁺ exchanger in excitotoxicity. Cell 120: 275-285.

6. Brittain MK, Brustovetsky T, Brittain JM, Khanna R, Cummins TR, et al. (2012) Ifenprodil, a NR2B-selective antagonist of NMDA receptor, inhibits reverse Na⁺/Ca²⁺ exchanger in neurons. Neuropharmacology 63: 974-982.

7. Pankratov Y, Lalo U (2014) Calcium permeability of ligand-gated Ca²⁺ channels. Eur J Pharmacol 739: 60-73.

8. Elmore S (2007) Apoptosis: a review of programmed cell death. Toxicol Pathol 35: 495-516.

9. Tian Z, Liu SB, Wang YC, Li XQ, Zheng LH, et al. (2013) Neuroprotective effects of formononetin against NMDA-induced apoptosis in cortical neurons. Phytother Res 27: 1770-1775.

10. Campos-Esparza MR, Sánchez-Gómez MV, Matute C (2009) Molecular mechanisms of neuroprotection by two natural antioxidant polyphenols. Cell Calcium 45: 358-368.

11. Chang-Mu C, Jen-Kun L, Shing-Hwa L, Shoei-Yn LS (2010) Characterization of neurotoxic effects of NMDA and the novel neuroprotection by phytopolyphenols in mice. Behav Neurosci 124: 541-553.

12. Jeng KC, Hou RC, Wang JC, Ping LI (2005) Sesamin inhibits lipopolysaccharide-induced cytokine production by suppression of p38 mitogen-activated protein kinase and nuclear factor-kappaB. Immunol Lett 97: 101-106.

13. Lee CC, Chen PR, Lin S, Tsai SC, Wang BW, et al. (2004) Sesamin induces nitric oxide and decreases endothelin-1 production in HUVECs: possible implications for its antihypertensive effect. J Hypertens 22: 2329-2338.

14. Hou RC, Huang HM, Tzen JT, Jeng KC (2003) Protective effects of sesamin and sesamolin on hypoxic neuronal and PC12 cells. J Neurosci Res 74: 123-133.

15. Ahmad S, Elsherbiny NM, Haque R, Khan MB, Ishrat T, et al. (2014) Sesamin attenuates neurotoxicity in mouse model of ischemic brain stroke. Neurotoxicology 45: 100-110.

16. Khan MM, Ishrat T, Ahmad A, Hoda MN, Khan MB, et al. (2010) Sesamin attenuates behavioral, biochemical and histological alterations induced by reversible middle cerebral artery occlusion in the rats. Chem Biol Interact 183: 255-263.

17. Zhang K, Li YJ, Yang Q, Gerile O, Yang L, et al. (2013) Neuroprotective effects of oxymatrine against excitotoxicity partially through down-regulation of NR2B-containing NMDA receptors. Phytomedicine 20: 343-350.

18. Longa EZ, Weinstein PR, Carlson S, Cummins R (1989) Reversible middle cerebral artery occlusion without craniectomy in rats. Stroke 20: 84-91.

19. Han D, Zhang S, Fan B, Wen LL, Sun M, et al. (2014) Ischemic post conditioning protects the neurovascular unit after focal cerebral ischemia/reperfusion injury. J Mol Neurosci 53: 50-58.

20. Liu SB, Zhang N, Guo YY, Zhao R, Shi TY, et al. (2012) G-protein-coupled receptor 30 mediates rapid neuroprotective effects of estrogen via depression of NR2B-containing NMDA receptors. J Neurosci 32: 4887-4900.

21. Yang L, Li XB, Yang Q, Zhang K, Zhang N, et al. (2013) The neuroprotective effect of praeruptorin C against NMDA-induced apoptosis through down-regulating of GluN2B-containing NMDA receptors. Toxicol In Vitro 27: 908-914.

22. Penugonda S, Mare S, Goldstein G, Banks WA, Ercal N (2005) Effects of N-acetylcysteine amide (NACA), a novel thiol antioxidant against glutamate-induced cytotoxicity in neuronal cell line PC12. Brain Res 1056: 132-138.

23. Shen H, Yuan Y, Ding F, Liu J, Gu X, et al. (2008) The protective effects of Achyranthes bidentata polypeptides against NMDA-induced cell apoptosis in cultured hippocampal neurons through differential modulation of NR2A- and NR2B-containing NMDA receptors. Brain Res Bull 77: 274-281.

24. Li YJ, Yang Q, Zhang K, Guo YY, Li XB, et al. (2013) Cytisine confers neuronal protection against excitotoxic injury by down-regulating GluN2B-containing NMDA receptors. Neurotoxicology 34: 219-225.

25. Nishimura Y, Yamaguchi JY, Kanada A, Horimoto K, Kanemaru K, et al. (2006) Increase in intracellular Cd(2+) concentration of rat cerebellar granule neurons incubated with cadmium chloride: Cadmium cytotoxicity under external Ca(2+)-free condition. Toxicol in vitro 20: 211-216.

26. Liu SB, Han J, Zhang N, Tian Z, Li XB, et al. (2011) Neuroprotective effects of oestrogen against oxidative toxicity through activation of G-protein-coupled receptor 30 receptor. Clin Exp Pharmacol Physiol 38: 577-585.

27. Kirsch DG, Doseff A, Chau BN, Lim DS, de Souza-Pinto NC, et al. (1999) Caspase-3-dependent cleavage of Bcl-2 promotes release of cytochrome c. J Biol Chem 274: 21155-21161.

28. Bournival J, Plouffe M, Renaud J, Provencher C, Martinoli MG (2012) Quercetin and sesamin protect dopaminergic cells from MPP+-induced neuroinflammation in a microglial (N9)-neuronal (PC12) coculture system. Oxid Med Cell Longev 2012: 921941.

29. Bournival J, Francoeur MA, Renaud J, Martinoli MG (2012) Quercetin and sesamin protect neuronal PC12 cells from high-glucose-induced oxidation, nitrosative stress, and apoptosis. Rejuvenation Res 15: 322-333.

30. Hou CW, Chen YL, Chuang SH, Wang JS, Jeng KC (2014) Protective effect of a sesamin derivative, 3-bis (3-methoxybenzyl) butane-1, 4-diol on ischemic and hypoxic neuronal injury. J Biomed Sci 21: 15.

31. Fujikawa T, Kanada N, Shimada A, Ogata M, Suzuki I, et al. (2005) Effect of sesamin in Acanthopanax senticosus HARMS on behavioral dysfunction in rotenone-induced parkinsonian rats. Biol Pharm Bull 28: 169-172.

32. Kiso Y (2004) Antioxidative roles of sesamin, a functional lignan in sesame seed, and its effect on lipid- and alcohol-metabolism in the liver: A DNA microarray study. Biofactors 21: 191-196.

33. Wu WH, Kang YP, Wang NH, Jou HJ, Wang TA (2006) Sesame ingestion affects sex hormones, antioxidant status, and blood lipids in postmenopausal women. J Nutr 136: 1270-1275.

34. Mabuchi T, Lucero J, Feng A, Koziol JA, del Zoppo GJ (2005) Focal cerebral ischemia preferentially affects neurons distant from their neighboring micro vessels. J Cereb Blood Flow Metab 25: 257-266.

35. Hardingham GE, Bading H (2003) The Yin and Yang of NMDA receptor signalling. Trends Neurosci 26: 81-89.

36. Sibarov DA, Bolshakov AE, Abushik PA, Krivoi II, Antonov SM (2012) Na$^+$, K$^+$-ATPase functionally interacts with the plasma membrane Na$^+$, Ca^{2+} exchanger to prevent Ca^{2+} overload and neuronal apoptosis in excitotoxic stress. J Pharmacol Exp Ther 343: 596-607.

37. Mei JM, Chi WM, Trump BF, Eccles CU (1996) Involvement of nitric oxide in the deregulation of cytosolic calcium in cerebellar neurons during combined glucose-oxygen deprivation. Mol Chem Neuropathol 27: 155-166.

38. Baltrons MA, Saadoun S, Agulló L, García A (1997) Regulation by calcium of the nitric oxide/cyclic GMP system in cerebellar granule cells and astroglia in culture. J Neurosci Res 49: 333-341.

39. Adams JM, Cory S (1998) The Bcl-2 protein family: arbiters of cell survival. Science 281: 1322-1326.

40. Chang HJ, Yoon G, Park JS, Kim MH, Baek MK, et al. (2007) Induction of apoptosis by the licochalcone E in endothelial cells via modulation of NF-kappaB and Bcl-2 Family. Biol Pharm Bull 30: 2290-2293.

41. Gu B, Nakamichi N, Zhang WS, Nakamura Y, Kambe Y, et al. (2009) Possible protection by notoginsenoside R1 against glutamate neurotoxicity mediated by N-methyl-D-aspartate receptors composed of an NR1/NR2B subunit assembly. J Neurosci Res 87: 2145-2156.

42. Fuentes-Prior P, Salvesen GS (2004) The protein structures that shape caspase activity, specificity, activation and inhibition. Biochem J 384: 201-232.

43. Ji X, Luo Y, Ling F, Stetler RA, Lan J, et al. (2007) Mild hypothermia diminishes oxidative DNA damage and pro-death signaling events after cerebral ischemia: a mechanism for neuroprotection. Front Biosci 12: 1737-1747.

44. Stennicke HR, Jürgensmeier JM, Shin H, Deveraux Q, Wolf BB, et al. (1998) Pro-caspase-3 is a major physiologic target of caspase-8. J Biol Chem 273: 27084-27090.

45. Putt KS, Chen GW, Pearson JM, Sandhorst JS, Hoagland MS, et al. (2006) Small-molecule activation of procaspase-3 to caspase-3 as a personalized anticancer strategy. Nat Chem Biol 2: 543-550.

46. Chiang HM, Chang H, Yao PW, Chen YS, Jeng KC, et al. (2014) Sesamin reduces acute hepatic injury induced by lead coupled with lipopolysaccharide. J Chin Med Assoc 77: 227-233.

47. Manole MD, Tehranian-DePasquale R, Du L, Bayir H, Kochanek PM, et al. (2011) Unmasking sex-based disparity in neuronal metabolism. Curr Pharm Des 17: 3854-3860.

21

Novel Targeted Therapy for Advanced Gastric Cancer

Hui-yan Luo[1,2] and Rui-hua Xu[1]*

[1]Department of Medical Oncology, Sun Yat-Sen University Cancer Center, State Key Laboratory of Oncology in Southern China, Guangzhou 510060, People's Republic of China
[2]Department of Biomedical Engineering, School of Engineering, Sun Yat-sen University, Guangzhou, Guangdong 510006, People's Republic of China

Abstract

Despite its decreasing incidence in western countries, the care of gastric cancer remains a concern. As gastric cancer is often diagnosed at an advanced stage, the prognosis of patients with advanced disease remains dismal. Recent trials in advanced gastric cancer have been focused on targeted therapies. Agents targeting EGFR1 and HER2 have been widely tested. The addition of trastuzumab to cisplatin/fluoropyrimidine-based combination chemotherapy significantly improved survival in patients with HER2 positive advanced gastric cancer, which is now the new standard of care by recent ToGA trial. Other agents targeting VEGF, the PI3K–Akt–mTOR pathway, and other biological pathways have also been investigated in clinical trials, but showed little impact on the survival of patients. This review will focus on the recent progress in targeted agents for the treatment of AGC and summarize the current clinical evidence and ongoing trials supporting the use of targeted agents in the treatment of patients with AGC.

Keywords: Targeted therapy; Advanced gastric cancer; Novel; HER2; VEGF

Introduction

Gastric cancer (GC) is the fifth most common cancer in the world and is the third-leading cause of cancer death. There were nearly one million new cases worldwide in 2012 (631,000 men, 320,000 women) with approximately 723,000 deaths (469,000 men, 254,000 women) [1]. Over 70% of new cases and deaths occurred in developing countries, with the highest incidence in Eastern Asia, especially in Japan and China [2]. According to the 2012 Chinese cancer registry annual report, gastric cancer had become the third most common cancer and the second leading cause of cancer related death in China [3].

The survival of patients with gastric cancer is substantially worse than that of patients with most other solid malignancies, and the only treatment that offers a potential cure is complete resection of the tumor. However, in most of countries, the majority of patients is diagnosed at advanced stages and has a poor prognosis. Despite the improvement of surgical techniques and the recent availability of new chemotherapy regimens, outcome of the patients with advanced disease is usually poor, the median overall survival (OS) is approximately 7 to 11 months, and the median progression-free survival (PFS) is 6 to 7 months [4-6]. These results suggested that even the most widely accepted regimens, such as fluoropyrimidine and/or platinum based chemotherapy regimens, have not been able to achieve satisfactory survival. Thus, there is an urgent need to develop more efficient therapies.

During the past few decades, remarkable progress in tumor biology has led to the development of new agents that target critical aspects of oncogenic pathways. Recent trials in advanced gastric cancer have been focused on targeted therapies, the agents including: targeting the membrane HER2 and EGFR membrane receptors, as well as antiangiogenic drugs targeting VEGF. A number of small trials have also appeared in the literature, exploring the inhibition of the Akt–mTOR pathway (Figure 1). However, only HER2-targeting drugs have been proven efficacy so far. This review will focus on the recent progress in targeted agents for the treatment of AGC and summarize the current clinical evidence and ongoing trials supporting the use of targeted agents in the treatment of patients with AGC.

Targeting HER2 in Advanced Gastric Cancer

Among HER family members, such as human epidermal growth factor receptor (EGFR, also referred to as HER1), HER2, HER3 and HER4, HER2 has become the focus of investigations in GC. HER2 overexpression is observed in 10%–38% of gastric cancer tumor samples, and it is more frequent in intestinal type compared with that in diffuse type GC and in cancers of the gastroesophageal junction (GEJC) compared with that in cancers located elsewhere in the stomach [7-9].

Trastuzumab

Trastuzumab is a humanized recombinant monoclonal antibody that selectively binds to the extracellular domain of HER-2, thereby blocking its downstream signaling. Up to now, trastuzumab is the first and only targeted agent for gastric cancer approved by both the U.S [10] and European [11] authorities.

Trastuzumab has been evaluated in ToGA study. A major breakthrough was achieved in the care of advanced gastric cancer since the results of the ToGA trial were published [12]. This was a large multicenter, randomized, controlled phase III clinical study, exploring the benefit of trastuzumab in addition to chemotherapy, in HER2 overexpression advanced cancer of the stomach or gastroesophageal junction. In this trial, a total of 3665 patients were screened for HER2 overexpression, leading to the randomization of 298 and 296 HER2-positive (IHC 3+ or FISH-positive) patients in the chemotherapy (capecitabine or 5-fluorouracil plus cisplatin) plus trastuzumab or chemotherapy alone arms, respectively. Importantly, cross-over to the trastuzumab-containing arm was not allowed for patients progressing in the reference arm. The addition of trastuzumab to chemotherapy led to a significantly longer OS duration, 13.8 months versus 11.1 months (p =0.0046), significantly longer PFS interval, 6.7 months versus 5.5

*Corresponding author: Rui-hua Xu, M.D. Ph.D., Department of Medical Oncology, Sun Yat-Sen University Cancer Center, 651 Dong Feng Road East, Guangzhou 510060, People's Republic of China,
E-mail: xurh@mail.sysu.edu.cn

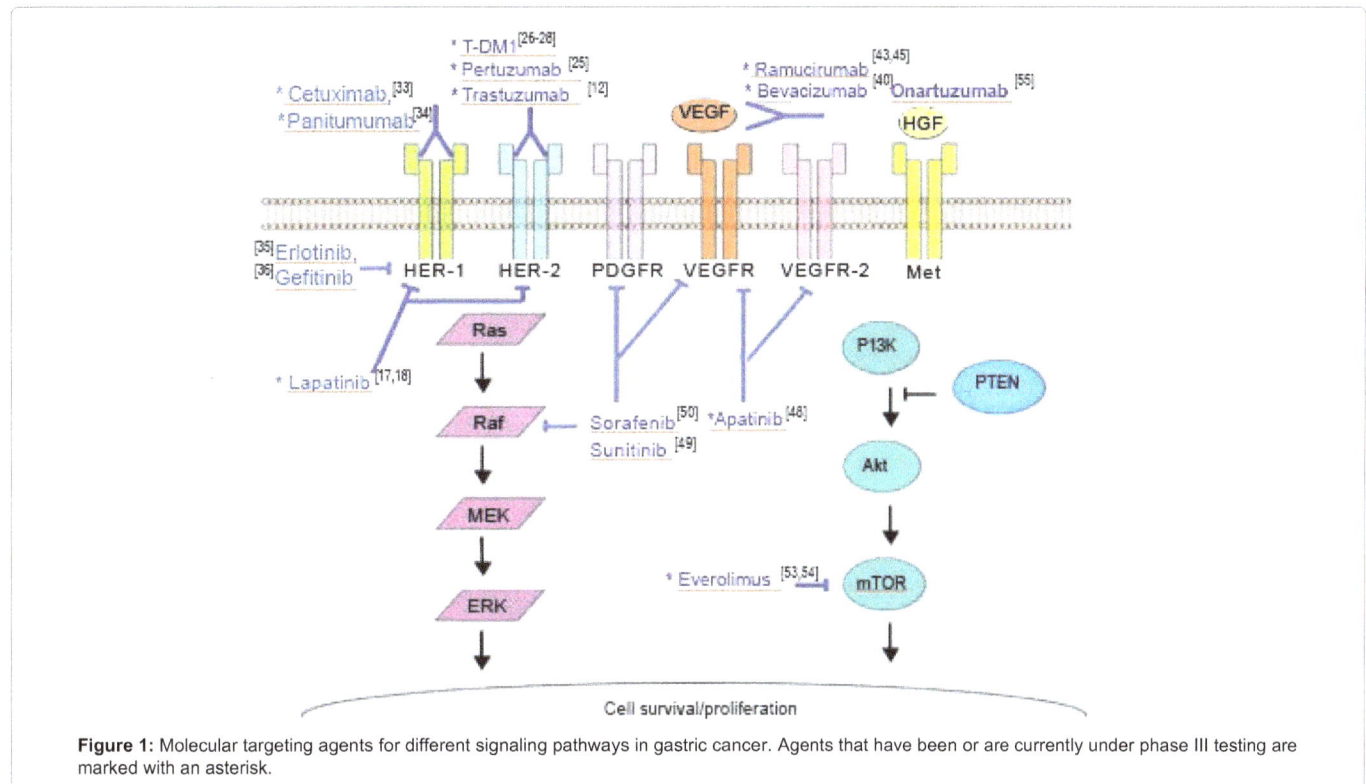

Figure 1: Molecular targeting agents for different signaling pathways in gastric cancer. Agents that have been or are currently under phase III testing are marked with an asterisk.

months (p<0.0002), and significantly higher overall response rate (ORR), 47% versus 35% (p<0017). The greatest benefit was seen in patients with higher levels of HER-2 expression, with either an IHC score of 3 or 2 plus FISH positivity; the OS time of those patients reached 16 months. Adverse effects were comparable between the two treatment groups. Moreover, the addition of trastuzumab did not affect quality of life. Based on the findings of this trial, trastuzumab, in combination with cisplatin–fluoropyrimidine chemotherapy has been approved by US FDA and European Medicines Agency as first-line therapy in HER2 positive GC and GEJC.

However, the OS gain was shorter than expected by comparison with breast cancer studies, and the GC patients who achieved an initial therapeutic response to trastuzumab eventually exhibited disease progression within 7 months. Those findings suggested that a significant proportion of patients with HER2-positive GC either do not satisfactorily respond to trastuzumab or develop an acquired resistance to this antibody.

Lapatinib

Lapatinib is a dual inhibitor of the tyrosine kinase domains of HER-1 and HER-2 based on its interference with adenosine triphosphate binding. Lapatinib has been proven efficacy and approved in HER2-positive breast cancer [13]. With regard to GC, several preclinical studies demonstrated the anti-proliferative effects of lapatinib [14], in addition to the synergic action of lapatinib with trastuzumab [15] or with other chemotherapeutic agents, such as 5-fluorouracil, cisplatin, oxaliplatin and paclitaxel, and irinotecan [14]. However, a phase II study of lapatinib in combination with chemotherapy as first-line treatment achieved only a 9% response rate, with a median OS of 4.8 months [16]. Subsequently, the TYTAN trials, investigated weekly paclitaxel plus or minus lapatinib in second-line therapy in HER2 positive GC. It failed to demonstrate any OS and PFS benefit in the

ITT population, but statistically significant improvements in OS and PFS were observed in patients with HER2-positive IHC3 + tumors and in Chinese patients [17]. The LOGiC phase III trial investigated capecitabine and oxaliplatin plus or minus lapatinib in first-line therapy in advanced or metastatic HER2 + upper GI tract (UGIT) adenocarcinomas, the results were reported in 2013 ASCO meeting and demonstrated a non-significant prolongation (1.7 months) of OS with the addition of lapatinib [18].

The limited efficacy of trastuzumab in the ToGA trial [12] and the unsatisfactory results of the TYTAN [17] and LOGiC trials [18] mentioned above suggest that the presence of drug resistance mechanisms or alternative pathways of escape from HER2 targeted therapy. To improve the treatment results of targeting HER2 in HER2-positive GC patients, there is an urgent need to elucidate the mechanisms underlying the alterations in tumor cell sensitivity to anti-HER2 therapy and to establish rational strategies to overcome this phenomenon.

Pertuzumab

Pertuzumab is a recombinant, humanized immunoglobulin IgG 1k monoclonal antibody, which targets HER2, a transmembrane glycoprotiein with intrinsic tyrosine kinase activity. It is the first one in a new class of targeted cancer treatment called HER2 dimerization inhibitors. Pertuzumab prevents HER2 from dimerizing with other ligand-activated HER receptors, most notably HER3 [19,20]. Like trastuzumab, pertuzumab can also stimulate antibody-dependent, cell-mediated cytotoxicity (ADCC). Because pertuzumab and trastuzumab bind to different HER2 epitopes and have complementary mechanisms of action, these two agents, when given together, provide a more comprehensive blockade of HER2 signaling and result in greater antitumor activity than either agent alone in HER2-positive tumor models [21,22]. Its efficacy and safety in combination with trastuzumab in HER2-positive metastatic breast cancer patients has been demonstrated in some phase III clinical trials [23,24].

In gastric cancer, an ongoing randomized phase IIa study (Study BP27836, JOSHUA) is being conducted in patients with inoperable or metastatic HER2 positive adenocarcinoma of GC or GEJC. This study has shown activity and safety of pertuzumab combined with cisplatin and capecitabine in patients with HER2-positive metastatic gastric cancer. Now a double-blind, placebo- controlled, randomized phase III study (Study BO25114, JACOB) is being conducted to compare overall survival (OS) in patients with HER2-positive AGC or GEJC treated with pertuzumab in addition to trastuzumab plus fluoropyrimidine and cisplatin (TFP) versus patients treated with placebo in addition to TFP. The primary objective is OS, the secondary objectives include PFS, ORR, quality of life and safety. The result of this study is worth expecting [25].

T-DM1

Trastuzumab-DM1 (T-DM1) is a novel anti-HER2 antibody-drug conjugate (ADC) in development for treatment of patients with HER2-positive cancer. T-DM1 combines the HER2-targeting properties of trastuzumab with intracellular delivery of DM1, a highly potent derivative of the antimicrotubule agent maytansine [26-28]. DM1 binds to tubulin and inhibits microtubule assembly with greater potency than vincristine or vinblastine. In T-DM1, trastuzumab and DM1 are covalently linked via the thioether linker (N-maleimidomethyl) cyclohexane-1-carboxylate (MCC).

T-DM1 has now demonstrated significant therapeutic effects in some phase III trials and may set a new standard for anticancer therapy as a drug with minimal toxicity and significant efficacy in previously treated HER2 overexpressing breast cancer patients. A trial (NCT01641939) is now ongoing to examine the efficacy and safety of T-DM1 compared with standard taxane therapy in patients with HER2-positive gastric cancer in second line setting. In this study, patients will be randomized to one of the three groups, 3.6 mg/kg T-DM1 every 3 weeks, 2.4 mg/kg T-DM1 every week, or standard taxane therapy for at least 12 weeks. The primary endpoint of the study was OS. If this study can achieve a positive result, it will provide a more effective strategy to improve the survival of patients on the current basis of trastuzumab treatment. .

Targeting EGFR (HER1) in Advanced Gastric Cancer

The EGFR is overexpressed in about 25% of gastric cancer and has been associated with more aggressive phenotype and poorer survival, which suggests that EGFR may be a rational therapeutic target [29]. Interestingly, and in contrast to colorectal cancer findings, where KRAS mutations occur in approximately 40% of patients and predict for lack of anti-EGFR efficacy, KRAS mutations are less common in gastric cancer, as these are only found in 3–13% of cases [30-32]. Similarly, no correlation was found between the KRAS genotype and response to treatment in gastric cancer, although further data may be needed to ascertain these findings [32]. Anti-EGFR mAbs and TKIs are currently undergoing clinical trials for GC patients.

Cetuximab

Cetuximab is a chimeric (mouse/human) mAb targeting to EGFR. Cetuximab is already approved for use in metastatic colorectal cancer and head and neck cancer. In several phase II trials of gastric cancer, cetuximab has shown some promising results when combined with various chemotherapeutic agents in first-line settings. The

phase III trial (EXPAND) [33] assessed the efficacy of cetuximab in combination with cisplatin and capecitabine as a first-line treatment for patients with advanced GC or GEJC. 904 patients in 24 countries were randomized to receive capecitabine and cisplatin, or the same combination plus cetuximab. The primary study end point is PFS, and secondary objectives include OS, quality of life and safety. The results are disappointing. This study has failed to meet its primary end point, the addition of cetuximab did not extend PFS, compared with chemotherapy alone (4.4 months in cetuximab plus chemotherapy group vs. 5.6 months in chemotherapy alone group, p=0.3158).

Panitumumab

Panitumumab is a fully humanized IgG2 mAb targeting EGFR, and which has been approved in metastatic, wild-type KRAS genotype colorectal cancer patients, in combination with chemotherapy. In gastric cancer, a phase II–III trial (the REAL-3 trial) was designed to assess the combination of panitumumab with the standard epirubicin, oxaliplatin and cisplatin (EOC). However, the survival in the panitumumab arm was inferior to that in the chemotherapy-alone arm (PFS, 6.0 months vs. 7.4 months, p = 0.068; OS, 8.8 months vs. 11.3 months, p = 0.013) [34].

The EGFR tyrosine kinase inhibitors (TKIs) gefitinib and erlotinib were evaluated in phase II trials but produced disappointing results as monotherapy for AGC [35,36]. Accordingly, there is no plan to move forward with anti-EGFR mAbs in further clinical investigation of AGC.

The clinical results of anti-EGFR agents might suggest that the role of EGFR pathway and the value of anti-EGFR therapy in GC need more evaluation and the concrete strategy including appropriate target patients population, combination and sequence with chemotherapy agents also need further investigation.

Targeting the VEGF–VEGF Receptor Pathway

Bevacizumab

VEGF is a key factor to the development of tumor angiogenesis and its blockade has been extensively studied in a variety of solid tumors. Hence bevacizumab, an anti-VEGF monoclonal antibody, has been approved in colororectal, kidney, lung and breast cancer. Several phase II trials combining bevacizumab with different chemotherapeutic agents were conducted on treatment-naive or pretreated patients with AGC or GEJC, demonstrating results which were initially promising [37-39]. A Phase II trial of bevacizumab 15 mg/kg at day 1 plus cisplatin 30 mg/m^2 and irinotecan 65 mg/m^2, both at day 1 and day 8, every 3 weeks, was administered in 47 advanced gastric or gastroeosophageal junction cancer patients, showing a promising 65% overall response rate and a median time to progression of 8.3 months. The tolerance was well [37]. In another report, bevacizumab 7.5 mg/kg was combined with docetaxel 70 mg/m^2 and oxaliplatin 75 mg/m^2 every 2 weeks, showing a 42% response rate in 38 advanced gastric cancer patients, with a median PFS of 6.6 months [38]. On the basis of results from these phase II studies, a large prospective phase III randomized, double-blind, contrast study (AVAGAST) was conducted internationally [40]. In this study, 774 advanced gastric or gastroeosophageal junction cancer patients were randomized to receive cisplatin and capecitabine with or without bevacizumab. Although the study did not reach its primary endpoint of OS (12.1 vs 10.1 months; p = 0.1002), the ORR was significantly better in the bevacizumab arm (46% versus 37%; p =.0315) and the PFS interval was significantly longer (6.7 vs. 5.3 months; HR: 0.8; p = 0.003). Interestingly, there was a discrepancy between OS HRs according to the geographical regions. Survival was longer in patients in pan-America with the addition of bevacizumab, but not in Asians or Europeans despite the better prognosis of the latter. That might be related to a higher rate of further treatment as 66, 31 and 21% of patients received a second-line therapy in Asia, Europe and pan-America, respectively. Suffice it to say, it seems inappropriate to incorporate bevacizumab in the treatment algorithm of AGC patients now.

Ramucirumab

Vascular endothelial growth-factor receptor (VEGFR)-2 and the VEGF A, C, and D ligands are known mediators of angiogenesis. VEGFR-2 is an important mediator in the VEGF pathway [41,42].

Ramucirumab is a fully human monoclonal antibody (IgG1) that binds the extracellular domain of VEGFR-2 and blocks VEGF ligands binding, shutting down VEGF signaling and inhibiting the growth of new blood vessels that feed the tumor. Ramucirumab is being tested in several phase III clinical trials for the treatment of metastatic gastric adenocarcinoma [43], non-small cell lung cancer [44] , among other types of cancer.

REGARD [43] is a global, randomized, double-blinded, placebo-controlled phase III study of ramucirumab and best supportive care (BSC) compared to placebo and BSC as treatment in patients with locally advanced or metastatic gastric cancer including gastroesophageal junction adenocarcinoma following progression after initial fluoropyrimidine or platinum-containing chemotherapy. In total, 355 patients were randomized in 29 countries. The primary endpoint was overall survival and the secondary endpoint was progression-free survival. Results demonstrated that ramucirumab (8 mg/kg by infusion every two weeks) plus best supportive care (BSC), as compared to placebo plus BSC, increased the median overall survival of patients with advanced gastric cancer by 37 percent (median overall survival of 5.2 months [95% CI 4.4, 5.7] vs. 3.8 months [95% CI 2.8, 4.7] for placebo, P=0.047, hazard ratio 0.78 [95% CI 0.60, 0.998]). Additionally, ramucirumab significantly improved progression-free survival, demonstrating a 62 percent increase in median progression-free survival (2.1 months [95% CI 1.5, 2.7] vs. 1.3 months [95% CI 1.3, 1.4] for placebo, P < 0.001, hazard ratio 0.48 [95% CI 0.38, 0.62]).

It is the first phase III trial to show improved overall survival and progression-free survival with a biologic agent in advanced gastric cancer after prior chemotherapy. Based on results of REGARD, on April 21, 2014, the U.S. Food and Drug Administration (FDA) has approved ramucirumab as a single-agent treatment for patients with advanced or metastatic gastric cancer or gastroesophageal junction (GEJ) adenocarcinoma with disease progression on or after prior fluoropyrimidine- or platinum-containing chemotherapy. This approval represents a meaningful advance for patients and gives them an important new second-line treatment option.

Similar to REGARD study, in RAINBOW study, ramucirumab adds to an efficacy of chemotherapy also improved overall survival in second-line gastric cancer.

RAINBOW [45] study is a global, phase III, randomized, double-blind study of ramucirumab plus paclitaxel versus placebo plus paclitaxel in the treatment of metastatic gastric adenocarcinoma following disease progression on first-line platinum- and fluoropyrimidine-containing combination therapy. Patients with gastric or gastroesophageal junction cancer who experienced disease progression during or within 4 months of first-line therapy with a platinum agent and a fluoropyrimidine were randomly assigned to 1 of 2 treatment regimens. All 665 patients

received paclitaxel 80 mg/m² on days 1, 8, and 15 of every 4-week cycle until disease progression, unacceptable toxicities, or death. They were also randomly assigned to receive intravenous ramucirumab 8 mg/kg every 2 weeks or placebo. The ramucirumab and paclitaxel combination was associated with better OS (9.6 vs. 7.4 months, HR, 0.87, 95% CI, 0.678 - 0.962; P = .0169) and PFS (4.4 vs. 2.8 months; HR, 0.635; 95% CI, 0.536 - 0.752; P <.0001) than monotherapy. Patients treated with the combination also had a significantly better median TTP (5.5 vs. 3.0 months; P <.0001) and a better objective response rate (28% vs. 16%; P =.0001). This largest gastric cancer second-line trial clearly demonstrated that an effective second-line therapy can improve survival of patients with metastatic advanced gastric cancer. This is the only study to date to demonstrate a 2-month improvement in survival in this setting, and with a relatively high 28% response rate for the combination therapy.

The results of the RAINBOW trial, combined with findings from REGARD trial of ramucirumab monotherapy, support the routine use of second-line therapy in patients with advanced gastric cancers who can tolerate the regimens. It also seemed that the targeting VEGFR agents might be more rational in the second-line therapy of AGC rather than in the first-line therapy.

Targeting VEGFR and PDGFR in Advanced Gastric Cancer

Apatinib

Apatinib (YN968D1) is a small-molecular TKI agent that highly and selectively inhibits the VEGFR-2 [46]. In a randomized, three-arm, double-blind, phase II trial of apatinib as a third-line treatment in patients with metastatic gastric cancer, 141 patients were randomized to receive apatinib (850 mg, qd), apatinib (425 mg bid) or placebo [47]. The study was reported during the 2011 ASCO Annual Meeting, and the results were as follows: median PFS, 3.4 months vs. 3.4 months vs. 1.4 months; median OS, 4.8 months vs. 4.3 months vs. 2.5 months. Common AEs included hypertension and hand-foot syndrome. Based on this result, a randomized, double blinded, placebo controlled, multicenter phase III study in a third-line setting in AGC is currently being conducted in China, the preliminary results were reported during the 2014 ASCO Annual Meeting [48]. Totally 273 patients were randomized to apatinib 850 mg qd p.o. or placebo and were treated until disease progression, intolerable toxicity or withdrawal of consent. The primary endpoint is OS. Median OS was 6.5 months with apatinib vs. 4.7 months with placebo (HR, 0.709; 95% CI, 0.537-0.937; P = .0149). Median PFS was 2.6 vs. 1.8months (HR, 0.444; 95% CI, 0.331-0.78; p < .0001). The AE including hypertension, proteinuria, hand-foot syndrome, bleeding, cardiac and liver toxicities, but all were manageable and reversible. Apatinib is the first small molecule targeting VEGFR to show a survival benefit in AGC, which made it as a new treatment option for AGC patients who failed to second line of chemotherapy.

Sunitinib & Sorafenib

Sunitinib is an orally available tyrosine kinase inhibitor that is approved in kidney cancer and gastrointestinal stromal tumors, which targets VEGFR1–3, PDGFR, RET and KIT. In gastric cancer, sunitinib was investigated in patients as second line treatment in a Phase II study that enrolled 78 patients with advanced gastric cancer. At a dose of 50 mg/day for 4 weeks every 6 weeks, disease control was obtained in 34.7% of patients (partial response: 2.6%; stable disease: 32.1%). The median PFS was 2.3 months and median OS was 6.8 months respectively. Adverse events were unremarkable at 50mg dosing (fatigue, neutropenia, nausea, diarrhea and stomatitis) [49]. These data suggested that single-agent sunitinib has little clinical interest as salvage therapy for chemotherapy-refractory AGC patients. At this time, there is no plan to move forward with sunitinib in further clinical investigations of GC.

Other tyrosine kinase inhibitors, such as the multikinase inhibitor sorafenib, similar to sunitinib in activity, are studied in Phase I and Phase II trials for gastric cancer. A phase II study of sorafenib combined with docetaxel and cisplatin as a treatment for chemo-naive metastatic or local advanced unresectable GC or GEJC patients was recently reported [50]. The study enrolled 44 patients who received sorafenib 400 mg bid, in combination with docetaxel 75 mg/m² day 1 and cisplatin 75 mg/m² on day 1 in a 3 weeks cycle. The ORR was 41 %, the median PFS was 5.8 months, and the median OS was 13.6 months. The authors concluded that sorafenib, combined with docetaxel and cisplatin, was effective and tolerable as a treatment for GC or GEJC. However, the results of this study did not show superiority over historical data from the cisplatin and docetaxel combination chemotherapy, thereby unlikely to be further clinical development of sorafenib in GC.

Other Targets in Advanced Gastric Cancer

Everolimus

mTOR is a key regulator of cell growth and proliferation, cellular metabolism, and angiogenesis, belonging to the PI3K–Akt–mTOR signaling pathway. The mTOR pathway has been shown to be frequently activated in a variety of human cancers, including gastric cancer [51]. Inhibitors of the PI3K–Akt–mTOR pathway have been developed at multiple levels, such as PI3K–Akt inhibitors and mTOR inhibitors. Among these drugs, everolimus (RAD001) has been investigated in advanced gastric cancer, as preclinical data suggested that the drug reduced peritoneal dissemination of a gastric cancer cell line in a mouse model [52]. In a multicenter phase II trial using everolimus as salvage therapy for pretreated AGC patients, the disease control rate was 55%, and the median PFS were 2.7 months. At a median follow-up duration of 9.6 months, the median OS was 10.1 months and good tolerability was observed [53]. Based on this provocative result, a phase III randomized trial, GRANITE-1 study was conducted to compare everolimus with placebo plus best supportive care in patients with progressive disease after one or two prior lines of chemotherapy [54]. A total of 656 patients from 23 countries were enrolled; 439 were randomized to everolimus, 217 to placebo. Median OS was 5.39 months with everolimus vs. 4.34 months with placebo (HR, 0.90; 95% CI, 0.75-1.08; P = 0.1244). Median PFS was 1.68 vs. 1.41 months (HR, 0.66; 95% CI, 0.56-0.78; p < 0.0001). Compared with BSC, everolimus did not significantly improve overall survival for advanced gastric cancer that progressed after one or two lines of previous systemic chemotherapy.

Onartuzumab

c-Met is a proto-oncogene encoding a membrane tyrosine kinase receptor – hepatocyte growth factor receptor (HGFR). HGFR plays an important role in tumor development through activation of key oncogenic pathways, angiogenesis, and tumor metastasis [55]. In gastric cancer patients, over-expression and amplification of c-Met often indicates poor prognosis [56–58]. c-Met inhibitors include monoclonal antibodies and small molecules that inhibit the enzymatic activity of the c-Met TK. Onartuzumab is a humanized monoclonal antibody directed against HGFR. A randomized, multicenter, double-blind, placebo-controlled, phase III study evaluating the efficacy and

safety of onartuzumab combined with mFOLFOX6 in patients with metastatic Her2-negative, c-Met positive gastroesophageal cancer is now ongoing (ClinicalTrials.gov Identifier: NCT01662869).

Pembrolizumab

Pembrolizumab is a highly selective, humanized IgG4/kappa isotype monoclonal antibody designed to block the interaction between PD-1 and its ligands, PD-L1 and PD-L2, thus reactivating the immune system to eradicate the host tumor. PD-1 is a negative co-stimulatory receptor expressed primarily on activated T cells. Binding of PD-1 to its ligands inhibits effector T-cell function. Expression of PD-L1 on tumor cells and macrophages can suppress immune surveillance and permit neoplastic growth. Pembrolizumab is able to achieve a dual blockade (PD-L1 and PD-L2) and shows no cytotoxic (ADCC/CDC) activity. The drug demonstrated a clinical activity in multiple tumor types, and recently became the first PD-1 inhibitor approved by the FDA when it was granted marketing approval for advanced melanoma.

The phase Ib study (Clinicaltrials.gov:NCT01848834) presented at ESMO 2014 assessed the safety, tolerability, and antitumor activity of pembrolizumab in gastric cancer patients [59]. Using a prototype IHC assay, PD-L1 expression was assessed in archival tumor samples from patients with recurrent/metastatic adenocarcinoma of the stomach or gastroesophageal junction. Eligible patients with PD-L1 staining in stroma or ≥ 1% of tumor cells were enrolled and treated with pembrolizumab 10 mg/kg every 2 weeks for up to 24 months or until complete response, disease progression, or unacceptable toxicity. Enrollment was designed to include an equal number of patients from Asia Pacific (AP) and the rest of the world (ROW). Of the 39 patients enrolled, 19 were from AP and 20 from ROW. AP patients were more likely to have received two or more therapies than ROW (79% vs. 55%). At a median follow-up of approximately 6 months, the ORR was 31% (31.6% in AP and 30% in ROW). Responses were ongoing for 6/6 Asia Pacific patients and 5/6 patients from the rest of world (median response duration not reached; range 8 + to 20 + weeks). Evidence of an association between PD-L1 expression and PFS (p = 0.032) and ORR (p = 0.071) was observed. The most common treatment-related adverse effects were hypothyroidism and fatigue. The author concluded that pembrolizumab was generally well tolerated and provided antitumor activity in patients with advanced gastric cancer that expressed PD-L1. These findings supported the potential of the PD-L1 pathway in gastric cancer and further development of pembrolizumab as a treatment option for patients with advanced gastric cancer. On the basis of the antitumor activity observed in this trial, a phase II study in advanced gastric cancer (KEYNOTE-059) is expected to begin enrollment in early of 2015.

Future Perspective

Targeted therapies have showed promise for improving the current grim prognosis of advanced gastric cancer. Contemporary targeted cancer therapy has progressed rapidly over the past decade. The ToGA trial has marked the beginning of a new era in AGC treatment. The addition of trastuzumab to combination chemotherapy is now considered a standard first-line treatment for HER2 positive advanced GC patients. However, this benefit is limited to only approximately 20% of AGC patients (HER2-positive), and sooner or later it will be development of resistance.

Unfortunately, up to now, no similar encouraging results was obtained in other targeting agents except ToGA trial, we still have a long way to go. EGFR-targeted therapy has not been successful in

Target	Agent	Trail	Regiment	N	Results
First-line					
VEGF	Bevacizumab	AVAGAST	XP+ Bevacizumab	774	Negative
EGFR	Panitumumab	REAL-3	EOC+ Panitumumab	553	Negative
EGFR	Cetuximab	EXPAND	CP+ Cetuximab	904	Negative
HER2	Trastuzumb	ToGA	XP+Trastuzumb	584	Positive
HER2	Lapatinib	LOGiC	Capox+ Lapatinib	545	Negative
HER2	Pertuzumab	JACOB	XP+Trastuzumb+ Pertuzumab	780	Ongoing
HGF/c-MET	Rilotumumab	RILOMET-1	ECX+ Rilotumumab	450	Ongoing
HGF/c-MET	Onartuzumab	MetGastric	FOLFOX+ Onartuzumab	800	Ongoing
Second-line					
VEGFR2	Ramucirumab	REGARD	BSC+ Ramucirumab	355	Positive
VEGFR2	Ramucirumab	RAINBOW	Paclitaxol+ Ramucirumab	665	Positive
HER2	Lapatinib	TyTAN	Paclitaxol+ Lapatinib	261	Negative
mTOR	Everolimus	GRANITE-1	BSC+ Everolimus	656	Negative
mTOR	Everolimus	AIO-STO-0111	Paclitaxol+ Everolimus	480	Ongoing
HER2	T-DM1	GATSBY	Paclitaxol vs T-DM1	412	Ongoing
PARP	Olaparib	GOLD	Paclitaxol + Olaparib	500	Ongoing

Table 1: Phase III studies of targeted agents in AGC

gastric cancer to date. Antiangiogenic treatment in gastric cancer is now focused on ramucirumab, which was recently approved by the US FDA for the treatment of advanced gastric cancer or gastroesophageal junction adenocarcinoma with disease progression after prior platinum and fluoropyrimidine chemotherapy. Anti-HGF therapy is potentially effective in gastric cancer, but we have to wait for the results of Phase III trials. Another potentially interesting target is the modulation of immune checkpoints, such as PD-1 and PD-L1. The PD-1 inhibitor pembrolizumab has demonstrated promise in patients with gastric cancer. The development of drugs against stem cell characteristics will probably become another important new approach. A randomized phase III study (BRIGHTER) has now been started in which BBI608, is being investigated as second-line therapy in gastric/gastroesophageal junction cancer [60].

Targeted therapies are beginning to change the course of gastric cancer. However, at present, little is known about the outcome of gastric cancer patients after targeted therapies. Molecular heterogeneity, a defining feature of gastric tumors, is driven by mutations and other genetic alterations. As other malignacies, the signal pathways involving in the carcinogenesis and development of gastric cancer are interactive and complex. The further researches of the signal pathways network will help us understand better about the molecular mechanism of gastric cancer and figure out potential therapy targets.

The key goals of future studies in the research field of GC treatment should include the development of better combination for validated targets, more new effective agents for novel targets, and the detection of novel predictive molecular markers to identify better and optimal treatment modalities for metastatic gastric cancer. A number of phase III clinical trials are ongoing (Table 1). These novel agents, once verified and validated, may become the next 'gold standard' and, if combined with reliable biomarkers for resistance and response prediction, may ultimately introduce a new era of personalized medicine.

References

1. Jemal A, Bray F, Center MM, Ferlay J, Ward E, et al. (2011) Global cancer statistics. CA Cancer J Clin 61: 69-90.

2. Cancer Fact Sheet (2012) Globocan: Cancer estimated incidence, mortality and prevalence worldwide in 2012.

3. Hao J, Chen WQ (2012) Chinese cancer registry annual report. Beijing: Military Medical Science Press.

4. Cunningham D, Starling N, Rao S, Iveson T, Nicolson M, et al. (2008) Capecitabine and oxaliplatin for advanced esophagogastric cancer. N Engl J Med 358: 36-46.

5. Van Cutsem E, Moiseyenko VM, Tjulandin S, Majlis A, Constenla M, et al. (2006) Phase III study of docetaxel and cisplatin plus fluorouracil compared with cisplatin and fluorouracil as first-line therapy for advanced gastric cancer: a report of the V325 Study Group. J Clin Oncol 24: 4991-4997.

6. Wagner AD, Grothe W, Haerting J, Kleber G, Grothey A, et al. (2006) Chemotherapy in advanced gastric cancer: a systematic review and meta-analysis based on aggregate data. J Clin Oncol 24: 2903-2909.

7. Yano T, Doi T, Ohtsu A, Boku N, Hashizume K, et al. (2006) Comparison of HER2 gene amplification assessed by fluorescence in situ hybridization and HER2 protein expression assessed by immunohistochemistry in gastric cancer. Oncol Rep 15: 65-71.

8. Lordick F, Bang YJ, Kang YK (2007) HER2- positive advanced gastric cancer: Similar HER2- positivity levels to broast cancer [abstract 3541]. Eur J Cancer 5: 271.

9. Gravalos C, Màrquez A, García-Carbonero R (2007) Correlation between HER2/neu overexpression/amplification and clinicopathological parameters in advanced gastric cancer patients: A prospective study 2007 [abstract 189]. Presented at the 2007 American Society of Clinical Oncology Gastrointestinal Cancers Symposium, Orlando, FL.

10. U.S. Food and Drug Administration (2011) Herceptin (trastuzumab).

11. European Medicines Agency (2011) Herceptin.

12. Bang YJ, Van Cutsem E, Feyereislova A, Chung HC, Shen L, et al. (2010) Trastuzumab in combination with chemotherapy versus chemotherapy alone for treatment of HER2-positive advanced gastric or gastro-oesophageal junction cancer (ToGA): a phase 3, open-label, randomised controlled trial. Lancet 376: 687-697.

13. Frampton JE (2009) Lapatinib: a review of its use in the treatment of HER2-overexpressing, trastuzumab-refractory, advanced or metastatic breast cancer. Drugs 69: 2125-2148.

14. Kim JW, Kim HP, Im SA, Kang S, Hur HS, et al. (2008) The growth inhibitory effect of lapatinib, a dual inhibitor of EGFR and HER2 tyrosine kinase, in gastric cancer cell lines. Cancer Lett 272: 296-306.

15. Wainberg ZA, Anghel A, Desai AJ, Ayala R, Luo T, et al. (2010) Lapatinib, a dual EGFR and HER2 kinase inhibitor, selectively inhibits HER2-amplified human gastric cancer cells and is synergistic with trastuzumab in vitro and in vivo. Clin Cancer Res 16: 1509-1519.

16. Iqbal S, Goldman B, Fenoglio-Preiser CM, Lenz HJ, Zhang W, et al. (2011)

Southwest Oncology Group study S0413: a phase II trial of lapatinib (GW572016) as first-line therapy in patients with advanced or metastatic gastric cancer. Ann Oncol 22: 2610-2615.

17. Satoh T, Xu RH, Chung HC, Sun GP, Doi T, et al. (2014) Lapatinib plus paclitaxel versus paclitaxel alone in the second-line treatment of HER2-amplified advanced gastric cancer in Asian populations: TyTAN--a randomized, phase III study. J Clin Oncol 32: 2039-2049.

18. Hecht JR, Bang YJ, Qin S, Chung HC, Xu JM, et al. (2013) Lapatinib in combination with capecitabine plus oxaliplatin (CapeOx) in HER2_ positive advanced or metastatic gastric, esophageal, or gastroesophageal adenocarcinoma (AC): The TRIO_013/LOGiC Trial. J Clin Oncol Suppl 31: LBA4001.

19. Agus DB, Akita RW, Fox WD, Lewis GD, Higgins B, et al. (2002) Targeting ligand-activated ErbB2 signaling inhibits breast and prostate tumor growth. Cancer Cell 2: 127-137.

20. Baselga J, Swain SM (2009) Novel anticancer targets: revisiting ERBB2 and discovering ERBB3. Nat Rev Cancer 9: 463-475.

21. Scheuer W, Friess T, Burtscher H, Bossenmaier B, Endl J, et al. (2009) Strongly enhanced antitumor activity of trastuzumab and pertuzumab combination treatment on HER2-positive human xenograft tumor models. Cancer Res 69: 9330-9336.

22. Lee-Hoeflich ST, Crocker L, Yao E, Pham T, Munroe X, et al. (2008) A central role for HER3 in HER2-amplified breast cancer: implications for targeted therapy. Cancer Res 68: 5878-5887.

23. Baselga J, Gelmon KA, Verma S, Wardley A, Conte P, et al. (2010) Phase II trial of pertuzumab and trastuzumab in patients with human epidermal growth factor receptor 2-positive metastatic breast cancer that progressed during prior trastuzumab therapy. J Clin Oncol 28: 1138-1144.

24. Cortés J, Fumoleau P, Bianchi GV, Petrella TM, Gelmon K, et al. (2012) Pertuzumab monotherapy after trastuzumab-based treatment and subsequent reintroduction of trastuzumab: activity and tolerability in patients with advanced human epidermal growth factor receptor 2-positive breast cancer. J Clin Oncol 30: 1594-1600.

25. Tabernero J, Hoff PM, Shen L, Ohtsu A, Eng-Wong J, et al. (2013) Pertuzumab (P) with trastuzumab (T) and chemotherapy (CTX) in patients (pts) with HER2-positive metastatic gastric or gastroesophageal junction (GEJ) cancer: An international phase III study (JACOB). J Clin Oncol suppl 31: TPS4150.

26. Remillard S, Rebhun LI, Howie GA, Kupchan SM (1975) Antimitotic activity of the potent tumor inhibitor maytansine. Science 189: 1002-1005.

27. Cassady JM, Chan KK, Floss HG, Leistner E (2004) Recent developments in the maytansinoid antitumor agents. Chem Pharm Bull (Tokyo) 52: 1-26.

28. Widdison WC, Wilhelm SD, Cavanagh EE, Whiteman KR, Leece BA, et al. (2006) Semisynthetic maytansine analogues for the targeted treatment of cancer. J Med Chem 49: 4392-4408.

29. Kitagawa Y, Ueda M, Ando N, Ozawa S, Shimizu N, et al. (1996) Further evidence for prognostic significance of epidermal growth factor receptor gene amplification in patients with esophageal squamous cell carcinoma. Clin Cancer Res 2: 909-914.

30. Pinto C, Di Fabio F, Barone C, Siena S, Falcone A, et al. (2009) Phase II study of cetuximab in combination with cisplatin and docetaxel in patients with untreated advanced gastric or gastro-oesophageal junction adenocarcinoma (DOCETUX study). Br J Cancer 101: 1261-1268.

31. Lordick F, Luber B, Lorenzen S, Hegewisch-Becker S, Folprecht G, et al. (2010) Cetuximab plus oxaliplatin/leucovorin/5-fluorouracil in first-line metastatic gastric cancer: a Phase II study of the Arbeitsgemeinschaft Internistische Onkologie (AIO). Br J Cancer 102: 500–505.

32. Park SR, Kook MC, Choi IJ, Kim CG, Lee JY, et al. (2010) Predictive factors for the efficacy of cetuximab plus chemotherapy as salvage therapy in metastatic gastric cancer patients. Cancer Chemother Pharmacol 65: 579-587.

33. Lordick F, Kang YK, Chung HC, Salman P, Oh SC, et al. (2013) Capecitabine and cisplatin with or without cetuximab for patients with previously untreated advanced gastric cancer (EXPAND): a randomised, open-label phase 3 trial. Lancet Oncol 14: 490-499.

34. Waddell TS, Chau I, Barbachano Y, de Castro DG, Wotherspoon A, et al. (2012) A random-ized multicenter trial of epirubicin, oxaliplatin, and capecitabine (EOC) plus panitumumab in advanced esophagogastric cancer (REAL3) . J Clin Oncol 30: LBA4000.

35. Dragovich T, McCoy S, Fenoglio-Preiser CM, Wang J, Benedetti JK, et al. (2006) Phase II trial of erlotinib in gastroesophageal junction and gastric adenocarcinomas: SWOG 0127. J Clin Oncol 24: 4922-4927.

36. Adelstein DJ, Rybicki L, Carrol MA (2005) Phase II trial of gefitinib for recurrent or metastatic esophageal or gastroesophageal junction (GEJ) cancer. Proc Am Soc Clin Oncol 23: A4054.

37. Shah MA, Ramanathan RK, Ilson DH, Levnor A, D'Adamo D, et al. (2006) Multicenter phase II study of irinotecan, cisplatin, and bevacizumab in patients with metastatic gastric or gastroesophageal junction adenocarcinoma. J Clin Oncol 24: 5201-5206.

38. Shah MA, Jhawer M, Ilson DH, Lefkowitz RA, Robinson E, et al. (2011) Phase II study of modified docetaxel, cisplatin, and fluorouracil with bevacizumab in patients with metastatic gastroesophageal adenocarcinoma. J Clin Oncol 29: 868-874.

39. El-Rayes BF, Zalupski M, Bekai-Saab T, Heilbrun LK, Hammad N, et al. (2010) A phase II study of bevacizumab, oxaliplatin, and docetaxel in locally advanced and metastatic gastric and gastroesophageal junction cancers. Ann Oncol 21: 1999-2004.

40. Ohtsu A, Shah MA, Van Cutsem E, Rha SY, Sawaki A, et al. (2011) Bevacizumab in combination with chemotherapy as first-line therapy in advanced gastric cancer: a randomized, double-blind, placebo-controlled phase III study. J Clin Oncol 29: 3968-3976.

41. Shibuya M (2008) Vascular endothelial growth factor-dependent and -independent regulation of angiogenesis. BMB Rep 41: 278-286.

42. Spratlin J (2011) Ramucirumab (IMC-1121B): Monoclonal antibody inhibition of vascular endothelial growth factor receptor-2. Curr Oncol Rep 13: 97-102.

43. Fuchs CS, Tomasek J, Yong CJ, Dumitru F, Passalacqua R, et.al. (2014) Ramucirumab monotherapy for previously treated advanced gastric or gastro-oesophageal junction adenocarcinoma (REGARD): an international, randomised, multicentre, placebo-controlled, phase 3 trial. Lancet 383: 31-39.

44. NCT01168973 (2010) Study of Chemotherapy and Ramucirumab Versus (vs.) Chemotherapy Alone in Second Line Non-Small Cell Lung Cancer Participants Who Received Prior First Line Platinum Based Chemotherapy.

45. Wilke H, Cutsem EV, Oh SC, Bodoky G, Shimada Y et al. (2014) RAINBOW: A global, phase III, randomized, double-blind study of ramucirumab plus paclitaxel versus placebo plus paclitaxel in the treatment of metastatic gastroesophageal junction (GEJ) and gastric adenocarcinoma following disease progression on first-line platinum- and fluoropyrimidine-containing combination therapy rainbow IMCL CP12-0922 (I4T-IE-JVBE). J Clin Oncol 32: suppl 3; abstr LBA7.

46. Tian S, Quan H, Xie C, Guo H, Lü F, et al. (2011) YN968D1 is a novel and selective inhibitor of vascular endothelial growth factor receptor-2 tyrosine kinase with potent activity in vitro and in vivo. Cancer Sci 102: 1374-1380.

47. Li J, Qin S, Xu J, Guo WJ, Xiong JP, et al. (2011) A randomized, double-blind, multicenter, phase II, three-arm, placebo control study of apatinib as third-line treatment in patients with metastatic gastric carcinoma. J Clin Oncol 29:4019.

48. Li J, Qin S, Xu J (2014) Phase III study of Apatinib in metastatic gastric cancer. J Clin Oncol: abstract 4003.

49. Bang YJ, Kang YK, Kang WK, Boku N, Chung HC, et al. (2011) Phase II study of sunitinib as second-line treatment for advanced gastric cancer. Invest New Drugs 29: 1449-1458.

50. Sun W, Powell M, O'Dwyer PJ, Catalano P, Ansari RH, et al. (2010) Phase II study of sorafenib in combination with docetaxel and cisplatin in the treatment of metastatic or advanced gastric and gastroesophageal junction adenocarcinoma: ECOG 5203. J Clin Oncol 28: 2947-2951.

51. Martín ME, Pérez MI, Redondo C, Alvarez MI, Salinas M, et al. (2000) 4E binding protein 1 expression is inversely correlated to the progression of gastrointestinal cancers. Int J Biochem Cell Biol 32: 633-642.

52. Cejka D, Preusser M, Woehrer A, Sieghart W, Strommer S, et al. (2008) Everolimus (RAD001) and anti-angiogenic cyclophosphamide show long-term control of gastric cancer growth in vivo. Cancer Biol Ther 7: 1377-1385.

53. Doi T, Muro K, Boku N, Yamada Y, Nishina T, et al. (2010) Multicenter phase II study of everolimus in patients with previously treated metastatic gastric cancer. J Clin Oncol 28: 1904-1910.

54. Van Cutsem E, Yeh KH, Bang YJ, Shen L, Ajani JA, et al. (2012) Phase III trial of everolimus (EVE) in previously treated patients with advanced gastric cancer (AGC): GRANITE-1. J Clin Oncol (Suppl 4):LBA3.

55. Appleman LJ (2011) MET signaling pathway: a rational target for cancer therapy. J Clin Oncol 29: 4837-4838.

56. Lee J, Seo JW, Jun HJ, Ki CS, Park SH, et al. (2011) Impact of MET amplification on gastric cancer: possible roles as a novel prognostic marker and a potential therapeutic target. Oncol Rep 25: 1517-1524.

57. Graziano F, Galluccio N, Lorenzini P, Ruzzo A, Canestrari E, et al. (2011) Genetic activation of the MET pathway and prognosis of patients with high-risk, radically resected gastric cancer. J Clin Oncol 29: 4789-4795.

58. Lennerz JK, Kwak EL, Ackerman A, Michael M, Fox SB, et al. (2011) MET amplification identifies a small and aggressive subgroup of esophagogastric adenocarcinoma with evidence of responsiveness to crizotinib. J Clin Oncol 29: 4803-4810.

59. Muro K, Bang Y, Shankaran V, Geva R, Catenacci DVT, et al. (2014) LBA15 - A phase 1b study of pembrolizumab (Pembro; MK-3475) in patients (Pts) with advanced gastric cancer. Program and abstracts of the European Society for Medical Oncology Congress, Madrid, Spain.

60. A study of BBI608 plus weekly paclitaxel to treat gastric and gastro-esophageal junction cancer (BRIGHTER) (2014) ClinicalTrials.gov Identifier: NCT02178956, Sponsor: Boston Biomedical, Inc.

22

Pharmacological Effects of Ethanol Extract of Artemisia Herba Alba in Streptozotocin-induced Type 1 Diabetes Mellitus in Rats

Heba MI Abdallah[1]*, Rehab F Abdel-Rahman[1], Gehad A Abdel Jaleel[1], Heba AM Abd El-Kader[2], Salma A El-Marasy[1], Eman R Zaki[3], Samir AE Bashandy[1], Mahmoud S Arbid[1] and Abdel Razik H Farrag[4]

[1]Department of Pharmacology, National Research Centre, Cairo, Egypt
[2]Department of Cell Biology, National Research Centre, Cairo, Egypt
[3]Department of Molecular Biology, National Research Centre, Cairo, Egypt
[4]Department of Pathology, National Research Centre, Cairo, Egypt

Abstract

Background: Diabetes mellitus has been treated orally with herbal remedies based on folk medicine since ancient times. The current study investigates the protective effect of Artemisia herba alba (Ah) against experimentally-induced type 1 diabetes mellitus and its complications.

Methods: Diabetes was induced in adult male Wister rats by administration of (Streptozotocin; STZ) at a dose of 52.5 mg/kg, i.p. Animals with diabetes were treated with either Ah ethanolic extract or gliclazide (10mg/kg, p.o.) for 14 days. Biochemical analysis was done such as glucose, insulin, homocysteine, lipid profile (cholesterol, triglyceride), liver function tests (T.bilirubin, AST and ALT), kidney function tests (BUN, sr. creatinine) and oxidative stress biomarkers. In addition, pancreas, liver, kidney, heart and aorta tissues were dissected out for pathological examination. Immuno histochemical study was done on pancreatic tissues for determination of insulin and glucagon immune reactivities. Liver tissues were also separated for genetic analysis.

Results: Oral administration of Ah ethanolic extract at a concentration of 400, 200and 100 mg/kg daily for 14 days results in decreased fasting blood glucose and homocysteine levels as well as enhancement of plasma insulin level as compared with STZ-treated rats. The extract improved lipid profile, liver and kidney function tests. It also increased hepatic and renal contents of GSH, diminished lipid peroxidation, and inhibited pathological alterations induced in the different organs. Treatment with Ah extract increased insulin expression while decreased glucagon immunoreactivity and DNA band polymorphism.

Conclusion: Thus, our results show that Ah possesses a promising antihyperglycemic effect that is comparable with gliclazide.

Keywords: Medicinal plants; Diabetes; Streptozotocin; Rats

Introduction

Diabetes mellitus (DM) is a worldwide endocrine disorder that impairs many physiological functions of the body.Type1 DM is primarily characterized by high blood glucose levels (hyperglycemia) induced by insulin insufficiency [1] due to inherited and/or acquired deficiency in production of insulin by the pancreas. Complications affecting eyes, kidneys, nerves and arteries are produced under the clinical settings of diabetes due to persistent hyperglycemia [2]. Current drugs for treatment of DM are associated with many side effects including obesity, osteoporosis sodium retention, hypoglycemia, and lactic acidosis [3,4]. The beneficial role of medicinal plants in the treatment of DM has been evolved due to their lower cost and lack of serious side effects. Thus, the traditional medicine has been extensively studied for its several therapeutic effects [5-7].

Artemisia herba-alba (Ah) "Shih-balady" is one of the plants that grown in Sinai, the most impressive vegetational regions of Egypt. It is a greyish-white perennial dwarf shrub, with small flowers. It is commonly grown in the central and southern wadis [8]. The plant has been used in folk medicine since ancient times as vermifuge, tonic, diuretic, skin troubles, emmenagogue, stomachic, intestinal, cholagogue, depurative and anthelmintic due to presence of volatile oils [9]. The plant is used also as digestive and analgesic against the rheumatic pains. Herbal tea from this species has been used antibacterial, antispasmodic, and hemostatic agents [10]. It has been used in Moroccan folk medicine to treat arterial hypertension and/or diabetes [11]. Recent studies have reported that aqueous extract of Ah showed hypoglycemic activity

in treated animals [12]. Administration of the extract also caused a reduction of serum lipids [13].

The chemical composition of Ah was previously studied. Several structural types of sesquiterpene lactones were found in the aerial parts of Ah. Eudesmanolides followed by germacranolides seem to be the most abundant types of lactones found in this species [14]. Flavonoids were detected in Ah ranging from common flavone and flavonol glycosides to more unusual highly methylated flavonoids such as Hispidulin and Cirsilineol which possess an anti-proliferative activity against multiple types of cancer cells [15]. In studies of the leaves and stems of Ah collected from Sinai, a total of eight flavonoids O- and C-glycoside were isolated and identified [16]. During a survey for antiulcerogenic principles of Ah, eight polyphenolics and related constituents were isolated. These included chlorogenic acid, 4, 5-O-dicaffeoylquinic acid,

*Corresponding author: Heba Mohammed Ibrahim Abdallah, Department of Pharmacology, National Research Centre, Cairo, Egypt,
E-mail: heba21_5@yahoo.com

isofraxidin 7-O-D-glucopyranoside, 4-O-D-glucopyranosylcaffeic acid, rutin, schaftoside, isoschaftoside, and vicenin-2 [17].

The current research was carried out to assess the hypoglycemic effect of the ethanol extract of Ah aerial parts in STZ model of type1 DM in rats. In addition, the protective effects of the extract on the other complications of diabetes were investigated.

Material and Methods

Plant material

Artemisia herba-alba (Ah) belongs to family Asteraceae. The dried aerial parts of the plant were purchased from the Egyptian markets and were grinded by electric grinder.

Preparation of plant extract

The plant powder was soaked in 70% ethyl alcohol for about 3 days, filtered using filter paper and the filtrate was concentrated under vacuum using the rotating evaporator (Rotavap), then percolated several times till exhaustion. The yielded ethanolic extract of Ah (55gm out of 200gm dried powder) was ready for both toxicological and pharmacological studies.

Toxicological studies (Determination of LD50)

The LD50 was determined as described by [18]. 1/10, 1/20 and 1/40 of the maximum dose (4 gm/kg b.wt.) that did not cause mortalities nor toxic symptoms in rats for the plant extract were chosen to be used for the biological investigation throughout the study.

Animals and chemicals

Sixty male Wister rats weighing 250-300g were used. The animals were obtained from the animal house colony of the National Research Center and housed in the animal facility of the pharmacology department, National Research Center. The animals were housed in a conditioned atmosphere (22°C ± 2, 50-60% humidity and 12h dark and light cycles) and kept on a standard diet pellets (El-Nasr, Abu Zaabal, Egypt) contained not less than 20% protein, 5% fibre, 3.5% fat, 6.5% ash and a vitamin mixture. They received water ad libitum. The experiments were carried out according to the national regulations of animal welfare and Institutional Animal Ethical Committee (IAEC).

Streptozotocin (STZ) was obtained from Sigma Chemical Company (U.S.A.). Gliclazide (standard antidiabetic drug) was purchased from SERVIER subsidiary SERDIA Pharmaceuticals (Canada) in tablet form and ground using a mortar. The powder was dissolved in distilled water and orally administered at a dose of 10 mg/kg body weight per day for the experimental period of 14 days. The dose of gliclazide was based on previous studies [19].

Phytochemical study

Determination of total phenolic content (TPC): Total concentration of phenolic compounds in the extracts was determined using a series of gallic acid standard solutions (2.5- 25 µg/ml) as described by [20] but with some modifications. Each extract solution (0.1ml) was mixed with 2ml of a 2% (w/v) sodium carbonate solution and vortexed vigorously. The same procedure was also applied to the standard solutions of gallic acid. After 8 min, 0.1 ml of Folin Ciocalteau's phenol reagent was added and each mixture was vortexed again. The absorbance at 765 nm of each mixture was measured, after incubation for 2 hrs at room temperature.

Determination of total flavonoid content (TFC): Total concentration of flavonoid compounds in extracts was determined using a series of standard rutin solutions (2.5-50 µg / ml) as described in the aluminum chloride colorimetric method. A known volume of each extract solution was mixed with 5% sodium nitrite solution, vortexed vigorously, then 10% aluminum chloride solution was added and vortexed again. After 6 min, 4.3% of sodium hydroxide solution was added, followed by addition of water, shaken, and left to stand for 15 min before determination. The sample solution without coloration was used as reference solution and the colour was read at 510 nm wavelength [21].

Induction of diabetes and Animal grouping

Type 1 DM was induced by a single i.p. injection of a freshly prepared solution of STZ (52.5 mg/kg body weight) in 0.1 M citrate buffer (pH 4.3) after a fasting period of 24 h [22]. On the third day of STZ injection, diabetes in surviving rats was confirmed by measuring the glucose level of blood obtained from the tail vein. Rats with a plasma glucose level of 180 mg/dl or greater and exhibited polyuria were accepted as diabetic and included in this study.

After induction of diabetes, rats were divided into six equal groups (ten rats per group). Group I (control negative group) comprises rats that receive 1 ml saline. Group II (control positive) comprises rats that receive streptozotocin (STZ) as mentioned above. Group III comprises rats that receive STZ and gliclazide (standard antidiabetic drug). Groups IV, V and VI comprise rats that receive STZ and oral administration of the Ah extract at the three selected doses. Treatment with either the standard drug or Ahextract was started 3 days after STZ injection and lasted for 14 days. Blood Samples will be drawn from the tail veins of fasted rats for recording fasting blood glucose (FBG) each group on days 3 (beginning of diabetes induction) and 17 (last day of the experiment, after treatment) of the study. Blood glucose was measured using glucose kit (Stanbio Laboratory, USA) according to Trinder [23].

Sampling and processing

At the end of the experiment, animals were anaesthetized by ether and blood samples were collected via the retro-orbital venous plexus and left for 20min to allow clotting. Serum samples were obtained by centrifugation at 3000 rpm for 10 min using the cooling centrifuge (Sigma and laborzentrifugen, 2k15, Germany). It was used for biochemical measurements. Animals were sacrificed by cervical dislocation. Kidney and liver tissues were dissected out and washed with ice-cold saline. Tissues were homogenized in saline solution and stored at -80°C.

Biochemical analysis: The collected sera were used for determination of insulin hormone level was evaluated by the enzymatic immunoassay method according to Eastham [24]. Homocystiene was estimated using a microplate enzyme immunoassay (Glory Science Co., USA).Serum triglycerides level was determined according to Fossati and Lorenzo [25] and total Cholesterol was evaluated according to Abell et al. [26]. Total bilirubin was estimated colorimetrically according to the method of Walter and Gerade [27]. AST and ALT were determined according to the method of Reitman and Frankel [28].

Antioxidant activity: The concentration of reduced glutathione (GSH) and lipid peroxides were estimated in liver and kidney tissue homogenates. GSH was estimated by the method of Ellman [29]. Lipid peroxides were assayed using thiobarbituric acid reactive substances (TBARS) method according to Ohkawa et al. [30].

Histopathological examination: After blood samples were obtained,the histopathological samples (pancreas, liver, Kidney, heart and aorta) were excised and fixed in 10% buffered neutral formalin. The paraffin sections were taken at 5 μm thickness processed in alcohol-xylene series and was stained with alum hematoxylin and eosin. The sections were examined microscopically for histopathology changes.

Immunocytochemistry staining: The pancreas was removed immediately and placed in 10% formalin in phosphate-buffered saline (PBS), pH 7.4, for 18 hrs before paraffin embedding. Tissues were routinely processed through a graded series of alcohols, cleared in xylol and embedded in paraffin. 5μm thick sections were obtained and processed for immunohistochemical staining for immunocytochemical localization of glucagon and insulin. Immunohistochemical staining was carried out by the peroxidase linked avidin-biotin complex (ABC) method as in the instruction manual provided with the kit (Mouse extravidin peroxidase staining kit Stock No EXTRA-2, Sigma, USA) [31].

Molecular analysis: The genomic DNA was isolated from liver tissue of mice using phenol/chloroform extraction and precipitation method. The concentrations of the extracted DNAs were measured at 260 nm as described by John et al. [32].

RAPD-PCR analysis: Primer screening for RAPD analysis was performed using six commercially available decamer random primers (Operon, Almeda, CA, USA). Four out of six primers amplified clear and reproducible bands, the other two primers amplified monomorphic bands : OPA02 (5'-TGCCGAGCTG-3'), OPA03(5'-AGTCAGCCAC-3'),OPA05 (5'-AGGGGTCTTG-3'), OPB13 (5'- TTCCCCCGCT-3'). The PCR protocol for RAPD analysis was followed as described by Williams et al. [33].

Results

Phytochemical investigation showed that 70% ethanolic extract of Artemisia herba alba contains high content of total phenolics (248.6 ± 20.4) mg gallic acid/g dry extract and flavonoids (62.15 ± 5.8) mg rutin/g dry extract. Results are represented as the mean values of three replicates of the same sample ±SE. Statistical analysis was performed using one way analysis of variance.

Biochemical analysis

FBG and insulin levels of groups are shown in Table 1. In the STZ (control positive) group, a significant increase in FBG level was observed on days 3 (start of treatment) and 17 (end of the experiment) as compared to the control negative (normal) group. Treatment with Ah extract significantly decreased the elevated FBG levels as compared to the control positive group at the end of the experiment. The extract at doses 400, 200, 100mg/kg exhibited % change in FBG: 65, 64.9 and 69%, respectively before and after treatment. This anti-hyperglycemic effect was comparable to that of the standard drug, gliclazide (71% changes in FBG). STZ induced a significant decrease in serum insulin level reached 64% of normal group. Treatment of diabetic rats with Ah for 14 days normalized serum insulin level as compared to STZ-treated group. Homocysteine level showed significant decreased in diabetic rats group compared to normal control. Ah extract administration increased the level of homocysteine significantly (Figure 1).

STZ-induced diabetic rats showed non-significant increase in the level of serum t. cholesterol as compared to the negative control. However, gliclazide therapy significantly decreased serum cholesterol by 31% as compared to STZ-treated group. Similarly, Ah extract at doses of 400, 200 and100mg/kg showed a significant decrease in serum

cholesterol level by 43.2, 42.8 and 34.7% as compared to STZ-treated group. This positive impact is, however, more pronounced in the rats treated with 100 mg/kg body weight extract. Treatment with both the standard gliclazide and Ah extract reduced t. cholesterol level below the normal value. A significant increase in serum triglycerides level was shown in diabetic rats, with an increase of 33.5% compared to the negative control group. Gliclazide treatment significantly decreased serum triglycerides level by 23.2% as compared to STZ-treated group. Treatment with Ah extract significantly reduced serum triglycerides level below the normal value. It showed a decrease of 39.5, 39.2 and 34.4% compared to STZ-positive control group (Table 2).

As shown in Table 2, serum activities of ALT and AST enzymes were significantly increased in STZ-treated group reached 129.5 and 119.1%, respectively as compared to the normal group. Treatment with Ah extract decreased ALT and AST activities as compared to the control positive group. Doses of 400, 200 and100 mg/kg of the plant extract recorded a decrease in ALT serum activity of 31.4, 31.4 and 34.7%, respectively compared to STZ-treated group. The same doses showed a decrease in AST serum activity of 11.2, 12.1 and 13% compared to

Treatment	Fasting Blood glucose (mg/dl)			Insulin
	Before	After	% change	(μ IU/ml)
Normal control	98.2 ± 4.0ᵃ	99.5 ± 5.9ᵃ	-1.3	4.52 ± 0.13ᵃ
STZ control	385.0 ± 15.5˙	333.2 ± 16.6˙	13.5	2.90 ± 0.04˙
Standard (gliclazide)	382.5 ± 24.9˙	109.7 ± 8.9ᵃ	71.3	4.27 ± 0.31ᵃ
Ah extract (400mg/kg)	347.5 ± 20.1˙	121.7 ± 8.4ᵃ	65.0	4.74 ± 0.37ᵃ
Ah extract (200mg/kg)	320.0 ± 26.4˙	112.2 ± 7.1ᵃ	64.9	4.81 ± 0.12ᵃ
Ah extract (100mg/kg)	365.0 ± 19.4˙	113.1 ± 6.0ᵃ	69	4.75 ± 0.14ᵃ

All groups except normal were injected STZ (52.5mg/kg, once), s.c. Treatment started 3 days after STZ injection. Blood glucose was measured twice; after 3days of STZ injection (before treatment) and at the end of the experiment (after treatment). Each value represents the mean glucose level or insulin level (mg/dl) ± SEM (n=10). *Significantly different from control negative (saline) at P<0.05, ᵃ significantly different from control positive (STZ) at P<0.05. Statistical analysis was carried out using one-way ANOVA test followed by Tukey post hoc test.

Table 1: Effect of 70% ethanolic extract of Ah on blood glucose level before (induction) and after treatment (end of experiment) and serum insulin level in rats:

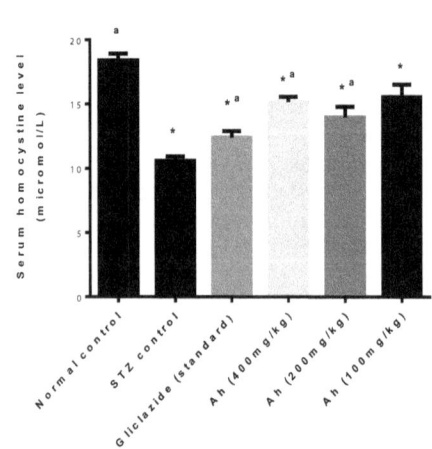

Figure 1: Effect of 70% ethanolic extract of Ah on serum homocysteine level. All groups except normal were injected STZ (52.5mg/kg, once), s.c. Treatment with gliclazide or Artemisia herba alba (Ah) started 3days after STZ injection. Each value represents the mean homocysteine level (mg/dl) ± SEM (n=8). *Significantly different from normal control (saline) at P<0.05, ᵃ significantly different from control positive (STZ) at P<0.05. Statistical analysis was carried out using one-way ANOVA test followed by Tukey post hoc test.

Treatment	T.bilirubin mg/dl	ALT U/L	AST U/L	BUN mg/dl	S. creatinine mg/dl	Cholesterol mg/dl	Triglycerides mg/dl
Control negative (normal)	1.91 ± 0.07	37.3 ±0.6[a]	107.1 ± 2.1[a]	14.7 ± 0.7[a]	0.57 ± 0.03[a]	83.7 ± 2.8	86.0 ± 2.6[a]
Control positive (STZ)	2.23± 0.11	48.3 ±1.1*	127.5 ± 1.1*	23.8 ± 2.2*	1.29 ± 0.02*	93.8 ± 4.6	114.8 ± 6.9*
Standard (gliclazide)	1.60 ± 0.06[a]	31.9 ±3.0[a]	110.7 ± 3.5[a]	18.1 ± 1.8[a]	0.86 ± 0.03	63.8 ± 4.2*[a]	88.1 ± 1.9[a]
Ah extract (400mg/kg)	1.59 ± 0.07[a]	33.1 ±1.2[a]	113.1 ± 3.8[a]	13.8 ± 0.5[a]	0.69 ± 0.01[a]	53.3 ± 2.5*[a]	69.4 ± 2.1*[a]
Ah extract (200mg/kg)	1.63 ± 0.10[a]	33.1 ±1.6[a]	112.0 ± 2.1[a]	13.5 ± 0.7[a]	0.75 ± 0.05[a]	53.1 ± 3.0*[a]	69.8 ± 3.7*[a]
Ah extract (100mg/kg)	1.54 ± 0.14[a]	31.5 ±1.0[a]	110.4 ± 2.8[a]	14.5 ± 0.8[a]	0.74 ± 0.16[a]	61.2 ± 4.6*[a]	75.3 ± 3.6[a]

All groups except normal were injected STZ (52.5mg/kg, once), s.c. Treatment with gliclazide or Artemisia herba alba (Ah) started three days after STZ injection. Each value represents the mean ± SEM (n=8). *Significantly different from control negative (saline) at P<0.05, [a] significantly different from control positive (STZ) at P<0.05. Statistical analysis was carried out using one-way ANOVA test followed by Tukey post hoc test.

Table 2: Effect of 70% ethanolic extract of Ah on selected biochemical parameters:

	Liver		Kidney	
	GSH (µmol/g tissue)	MDA (nmol/g tissue)	GSH (µmol/g tissue)	MDA (nmol/g tissue)
Normal (saline)	6.98 ± 0.12[a]	155.3 ± 8.8[a]	4.60 ± 0.03[a]	192 ± 13.6[a]
STZ control	4.32 ± 0.09*	474.6 ± 25.0*	3.39 ± 0.03*	390.9 ± 14.7*
Gliclazide (10mg/kg)	5.98 ± 0.05*[a]	247.8 ± 17.6*[a]	4.33 ± 0.40[a]	216.7 ± 7.3[a]
Ah extract (400mg/kg)	6.25 ± 0.03*[a]	262.4 ± 8.5*[a]	4.28 ± 0.06[a]	225.0 ± 11.6[a]
Ah extract (200mg/kg)	6.23 ± 0.05*[a]	204.4 ± 4.4[a]	4.33 ± 0.01[a]	248.1 ± 16.5*[a]
Ah extract (100mg/kg)	6.45 ± 0.15*[a]	220.1 ± 15.2[a]	4.25 ± 0.05[a]	247.4 ± 10.5*[a]

herba alba (Ah) started 3days after STZ injection. Each value represents the mean GSH or MDA level (mg/dl) ± SEM (n=8). *Significantly different from normal control (saline) at P<0.05, [a] significantly different from control positive (STZ) at P<0.05. Statistical analysis was carried out using one-way ANOVA test followed by Tukey post hoc test.

All groups except normal were injected STZ (52.5mg/kg, once), s.c. Treatment with gliclazide or Artemisia

Table 3: Effect of 70% ethanolic extract of Ah on oxidative stress biomarkers:

STZ-treated group. The protective effect of the plant extract on liver enzymes was comparable to the standard drug, gliclazide (33.9% for ALT, 13% for AST).

Levels of BUN and sr.creatinine increased significantly in diabetic groups (23.8±2.2mg/dl and 1.29±0.02mg/dl for BUN and sr.creatinine vs 14.7±0.7mg/dl and 0.57±0.03mg/dl in normal rats). Gliclazide treatment recorded a 39% decrease in BUN level and 33% decrease in sr.creatinine level as compared to STZ-treated group. The ethanol extract of Ah improved the kidney function indices of diabetic rats by significantly reducing the concentrations of BUN and sr.creatinine. It showed a decrease of 42, 43 and 39% in BUN levels at the doses, 400, 200, 100mg/kg, respectively and 46.5, 41.9 and 42.6% in sr.creatinine level compared to STZ-treated group (Table 2).

Antioxidant activity

The results are summarized in Table 3. As shown, STZ injection increased hepatic and renal contents of TBARs and decreased their GSH contents as compared to the normal control group. On the other hand, Ah extract at doses of 400, 200 and100 mg/kg and gliclazide treatment decreased TBARs content by 44.7%, 56.9%, 53.6%, 47.8%; respectively in the liver tissue and by 42.4% , 36.5%,36.7%,44.6%; respectively in the kidney tissue as compared to STZ control group. All treatment groups increased GSH content that reached 144.7%, 144.2%, 149.3%, 138.4%; respectively in the liver tissue and 126.2%, 127.7%, 125.4%, 127.7%; respectively in the kidney tissue as compared to STZ control group.

Histopathological findings

Sections of the normal pancreas of rats showed the exocrine component of the pancreas that consisted of closely packed acini. The interlobular duct, surrounded with the supporting tissue. The endocrine tissue of the pancreas, islets of Langerhans, scattered throughout the exocrine tissue (Figure 2A).In case of pancreas of diabetic rats, histopathological examination showed the acinar cells around the islets does not look classical. The islets were largely occupied by a uniform eosinophilic material and few atrophic cells (Figure 2B). Pancreas of diabetic rats also showed congested blood vessel and inter acinar haemorrhage (Figure 2C). Diabetic rats treated with the standard anti-diabetic, gliclazide, showed normal acinar cells and islets which were present with a smaller volume as compared with control (Figure 2D). In some examination islets were present with a very scanty inflammatory cells infiltration (Figure 2E). Similarly, diabetic rats treated with Ah (400 mg/kg) showed normal acinar cells were seen to be normal. The islets were present with a large proportion of islet cells though smaller than control (Figure 2F). Treatment with Ah extract (200 mg/kg) showed relatively larger islets of Langerhans than the control one (Figure 2G), whereas, rats treated with Ah (100 mg/kg) showed smaller acinar cells and islets than normal control (Figure 2H).

Liver of normal rats showed a normal structure of the hepatic lobule. The central vein is surrounded by the hepatocytes with eosinophilic cytoplasm and distinct nuclei. The hepatic sinusoids are shown between the hepatocytes (Figure 3A). However, liver of diabetic rats showed inflammatory infiltration and periportal necrosis of the hepatocytes appeared around the portal area was also shown (Figure 3B). Focal necrosis of the hepatocytes and some pyknotic nuclei of the hepatocytes were also shown (Figure 3C). Rats treated with gliclazide, showed hepatic lobules appeared more or less like control (Figure 3D). In some rats, focal necrosis associated with inflammatory infiltration were seen (Figure 3E). Treatment with Ah extract (400, 200 and 100 mg/kg) showed the hepatocytes appeared more or less as the control (Figure 3. F-H; respectively).

Histological examination of sections of kidney of control rats showed normal structure of distal convoluted tubules that could be differentiated from the proximal convoluted tubules as having a larger

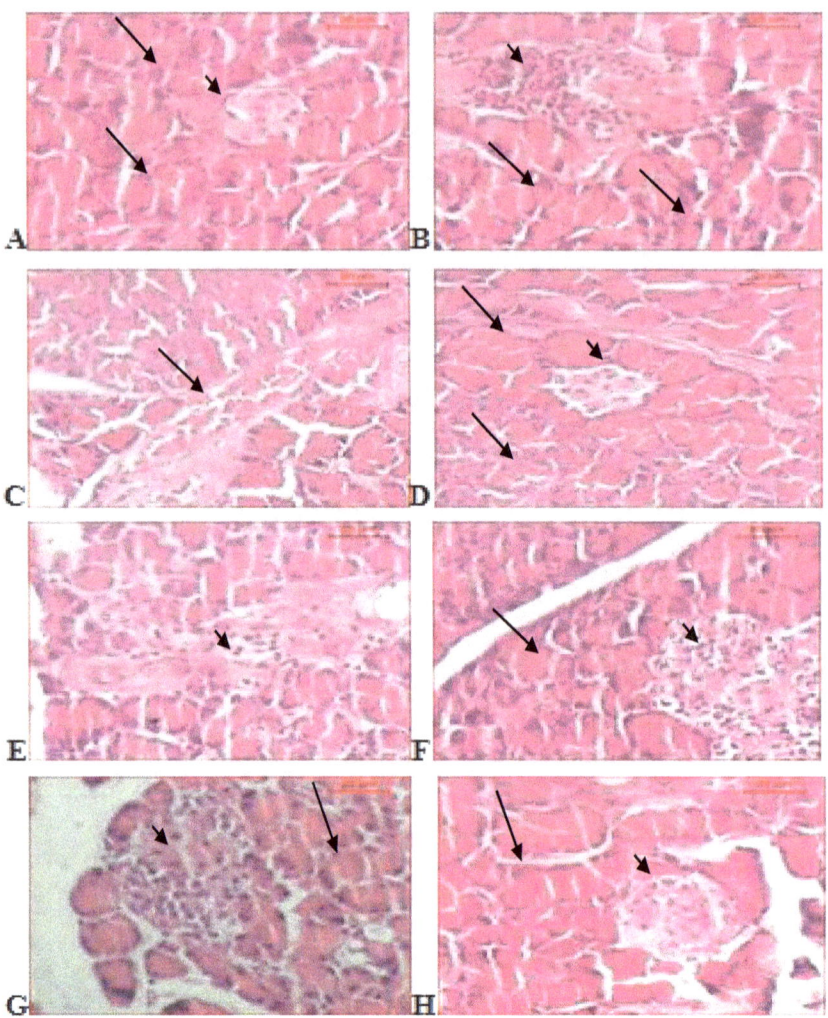

Figure 2: Sections of pancreas of A) control rat shows dense-staining acinar cells (arrows) and a light-staining islet of Langerhans (arrowhead) just right of the center of the field, **B):** a diabetic rat shows normal acinar cells (arrows). The islets are occupied by a uniform eosinophilic material (arrowhead), **C):** a diabetic rat shows congested blood vessel and inter acinar haemorrhage (arrow), **D):** a diabetic rat treated with the standard anti-diabetic, gliclazide, shows the acinar cells and islets are seen to be normal. The islets are present with a smaller volume (arrowhead) as compared with control, **E):** a diabetic rat treated with gliclazide shows the islets is present with a very scanty inflammatory cell infiltration (arrowhead), **F):** diabetic rat treated with *Artemisia* extract (400 mg/kg) shows acinar cells are seen to be normal (arrow). Islets are present with a large proportion of islet cells (arrowhead) as compared with control, **G):** a diabetic rat treated with *Artemisia* extract (200 mg/kg) shows islets of Langerhans that appeared relatively larger than the control one (arrowhead). Exocrine pancreas appeared more or less as control (arrow), **H):** a diabetic rat treated with *Artemisia* extract (100 mg/kg) shows acinar cells and islets are seen to be normal (arrow). Islets are present with a large proportion of islet cells though with a smaller volume as compared with control (arrowhead) **(H & E, Scale Bar: 20 µm)**

and well defined lumina, and glomerulus (Figure 4A). Sections of kidney of diabetic rat showed the development of necrosis of epithelial cells of some proximal tubules. Some cellular debris and hemorrhage in the dilated interstitial space were noticed (Figure 4B). In some rats, lobulation and hypercellularity of glomeruli and large interstitial hemorrhagic were shown (Figure 4C). Treatment with gliclazide showed normal structure of the renal corpuscles and renal tubules (Figure 4D). In some cases, lobulated glomeruli, partially degenerative glomeruli, and haemorrhagic areas were shown (Figure 4E). Ah treatment (400, 200,100 mg/kg), microscopic examination showed normal renal corpuscles and renal tubules (Figure 4 F-H; respectively).

Examination transverse section normal rat aorta showed the normal histological structure of the tunica intima, tunica media and tunica adventitia (Figure 5A).Diabetic rats aorta showed a significant atherosclerosis, vacuolation in the cells of the tunica media (Figures 5B,C). In diabetic rats treated with gliclazide, Ah extract (400,200,100 mg/kg) aorta showed the normal histological structure of the tunica intima, tunica media and tunica adventitia (Figure 5 D-G, respectively).

Immunohistochemical results

Glucagon immunoreactive cells were distributed normally in the marginal zone of the islets but some positive cells in the central zones as brown color (Figure 6). The diabetic rats show much more abundant and ubiquitous immunostaining for glucagon as compared with normal control. Treatment with gliclazide shows distribution of glucagon that appears more or less like normal. Similarly, Ah extract at the different doses shows reduction of glucagon staining but it did not reach to the normal control.

Figure 7 shows Insulin immunoreactive cells were detected with a high frequency in the central regions of the pancreatic islets of normal

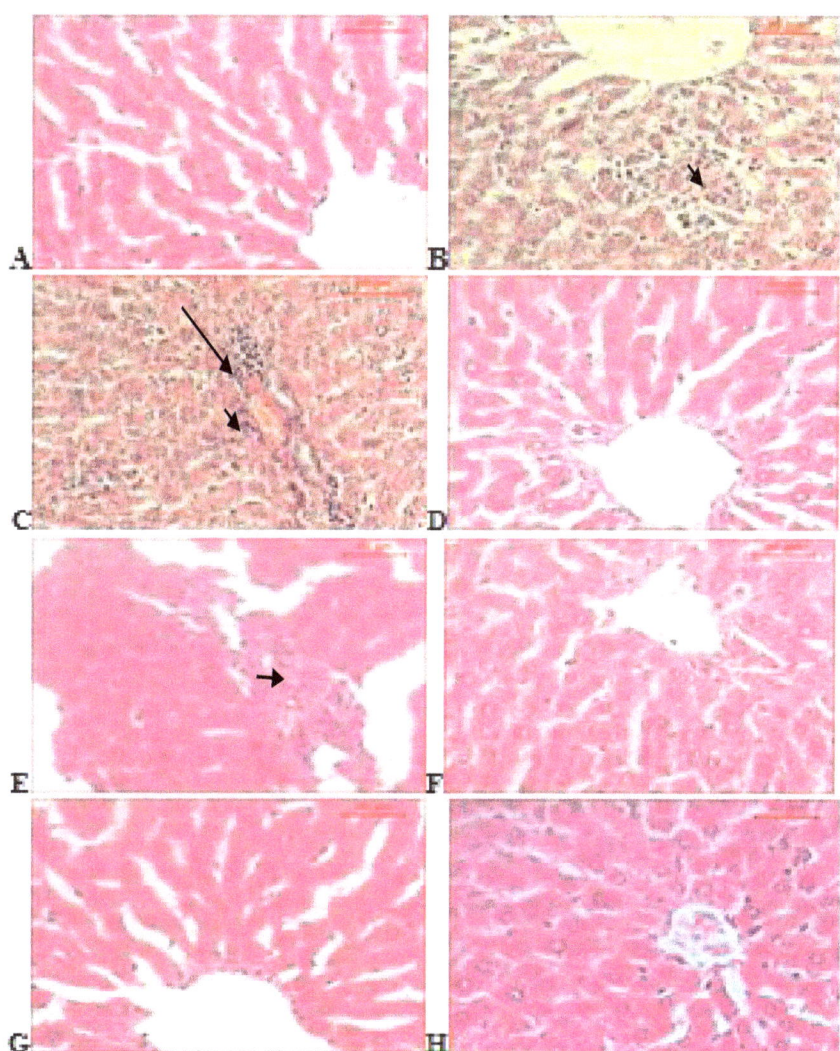

Figure 3. Sections of liver of A) control rat shows the architecture of a hepatic lobule, B): a diabetic rat shows focal necrosis of the hepatocytes. Some of the nuclei of the hepatocytes are pyknotic (arrowhead), C): a diabetic rat shows the periportal tract with dilated and congested vein (arrow) and periportal necrosis of the hepatocytes (arrowhead), **D**): diabetic rat treated with gliclazide shows hepatic lobule that appears more or less like control, **E**): a diabetic rat treated with the standard anti-diabetic, gliclazide, shows focal necrosis associated with inflammatory infiltration (arrowhead), **F**): a diabetic rat treated with *Artemisia* extract (400 mg/kg) shows the hepatocytes appear more or less as the control, G): a diabetic rat treated with *Artemisia* extract (200 mg/kg) shows the hepatocytes appear more or less as the control, H): a diabetic rat treated with *Artemisia* extract (100 mg/kg) shows the hepatocytes appear more or less as the control **(H & E, Scale Bar: 20 µm)**.

control rat appeared in brown color. No insulin positive cells were found in the peripheral regions or in the exocrine portions. On the other hand, the diabetic rat shows weaker immunostaining for insulin. However, diabetic rats treated by gliclazide or Ah extract appear with more dense insulin immunoreactivity as compared to the STZ-diabetic rats.

Molecular analysis

The results of RAPD analysis were determined by considering the bands which appeared in the control STZ sample as the criterion of the judgment. Polymorphism observed in RAPD profiles included disappearance of a normal control band and appearance of a new band. As illustrated in Table 4, four random primers generated a total of 12 bands in normal group. The molecular size of these bands ranged from 944 to 264 bp. The highest number of band appearance and disappearance was determined in control STZ group (25), the lowest

number was determined in Ah extract at doses 200 and 100 groups (20). The Percentage of polymorphic bands recorded in standard gliclazide group was (88%), percentages of polymorphic bands determined in Ah extract at doses400, 200 and 100 groups were (88%, 80% and 80%, respectively). Changes in RAPD profiles were significantly increased in control STZ group compared to normal group. The polymorphic bands percentages were decreased in the groups treated by standard gliclazide and Ah extract at all doses compared to Control STZ group.

On the other hand, the total number of bands generated by four primers in six groups was (121) with band sizes ranged from (1177-244pb) and the total number of polymorphic bands was (109). Primer OPA03 recorded the highest number of polymorphic bands with band size ranged (944-276) among the six groups while the lowest number of polymorphic bands was generated by primer OPA02 with band size ranged (539-265) (Figure 8)

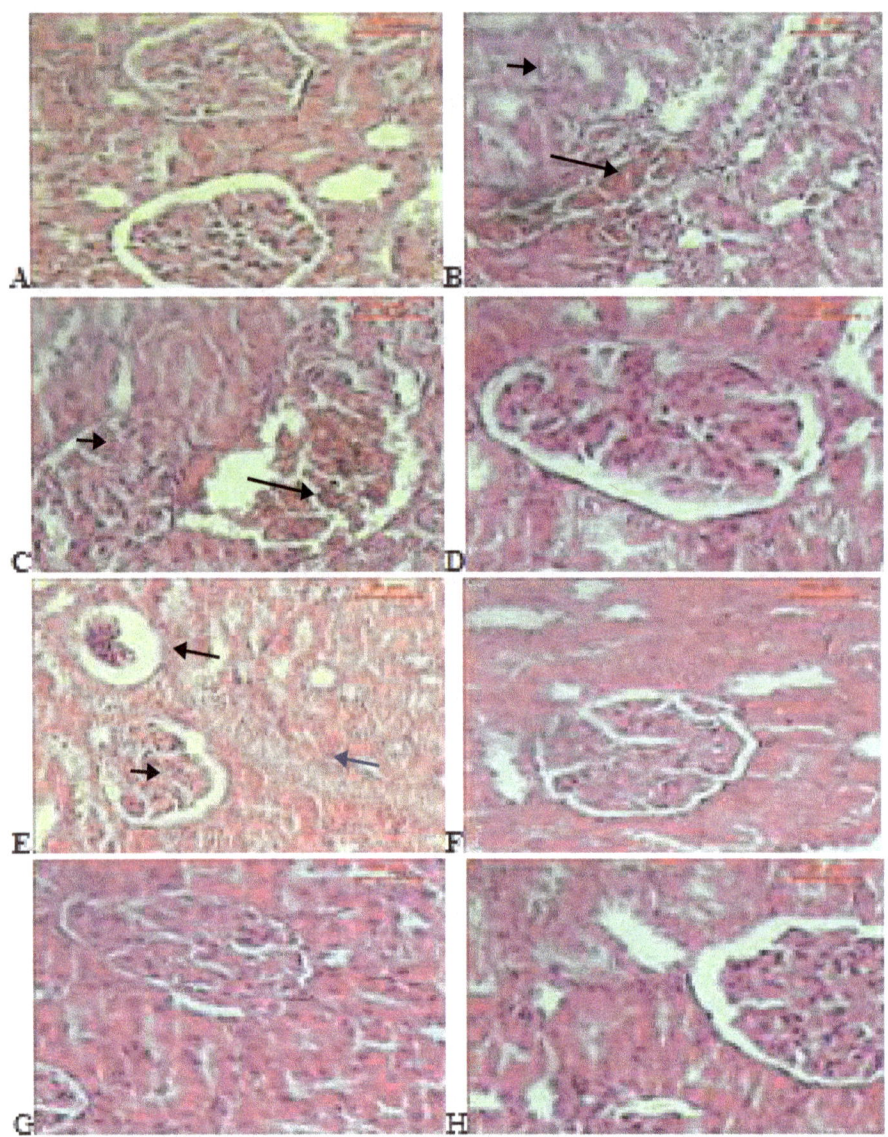

Figure 4. Sections of kidney of A): control rat shows normal structure of glomeruli and renal tubules, B): a diabetic rat shows the development of necrosis (arrowhead) of epithelial cells of some proximal tubules. Some cellular debris and hemorrhage in the dilated interstitial space (arrow), **C),** a diabetic rat shows lobulated and hypercellularity glomerulus (arrow). Large interstitial hemorrhagic is noticed (arrowhead), **D):** a diabetic rat kidney treated with the standard anti-diabetic, gliclazide, shows normal structure of the renal corpuscles and renal tubules, **E):** a diabetic rat treated with gliclazide shows the lobulated glomerulus (arrowhead), partially degenerative glomerulus (arrow), and haemorrhagic areas (blue arrow), **F):** a diabetic rat treated with *Artemisia* extract (400 mg/kg) show normal renal corpuscles and renal tubules, **G):** a diabetic rat treated with *Artemisia* extract (200 mg/kg) shows normal renal corpuscles and renal tubules, **H):** a diabetic rat treated with *Artemisia* extract (100 mg/kg) shows normal renal corpuscles and renal tubules **(H & E, Scale Bar: 20 µm)**.

Discussion

The present study investigates the different pharmacological effects of Ah ethanolic extract in rats with type 1 diabetes. STZ injection induced hyperglycemia and decreased serum insulin level. STZ-induced diabetes is widely used as type-1 like diabetic animal model to investigate hyperglycemia [34]. It has been reported that STZ induce an autoimmune process that results in the destruction of the Langerhans islets beta cells. Symptoms of diabetes type 1 are clearly seen in rats within 2-4 days following single intravenous or intraperitoneal injection of STZ [35, 36]. Ah extract lowered plasma glucose concurrently with an increase of plasma insulin in STZ-diabetic rats. Its hypoglycemic effect was comparable with that of the standard drug, gliclazide. Gliclazide is known to produce a hypoglycemic activity by pancreatic (stimulating insulin secretion by blocking K±channels in the pancreatic β cells) and extra pancreatic (increasing tissue uptake of glucose) mechanisms [37, 38]. Hence, it can be postulated that Ah extract produce similar effects as gliclazide. In addition, hypoglycemic effects of Ah could, possibly, be due to increased peripheral glucose utilization. Recently, Tastekin et al. [39] has concluded that Ah could reduce the absorption of glucose from the intestine and inhibit the absorption of glucose by the kidney tubules thus lowers blood glucose.

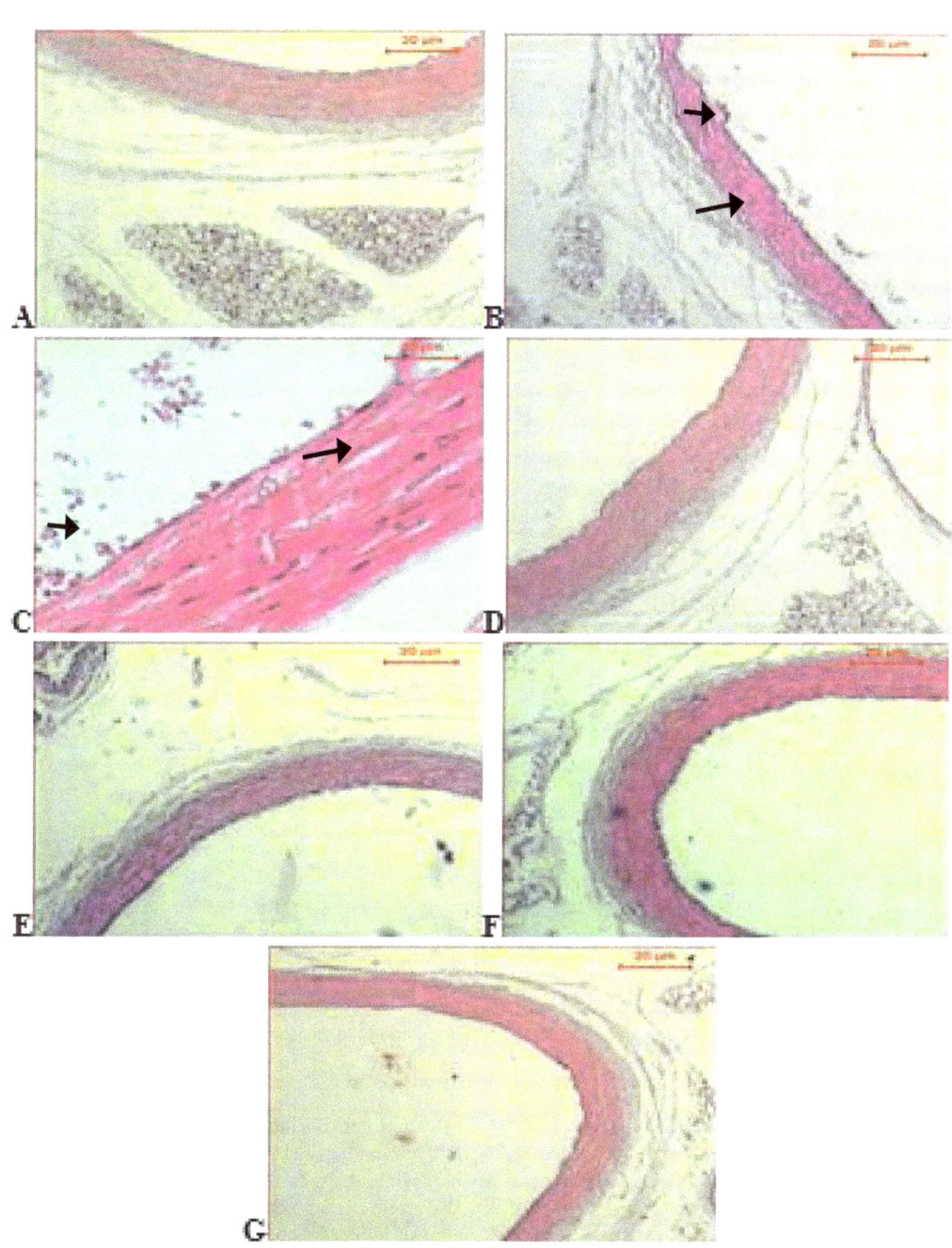

Figure 5. Transverse sections of aorta of rat **A)**: control shows the normal histological structure, **B)**: a diabetic rat shows a significant atherosclerosis (arrowhead), vacuolation in the cells of the tunica media (arrow), **C)**: Magnification of **(B)** shows a significant atherosclerosis (arrowhead), vacuolation in the cells of the tunica media (arrow), **D)**: a diabetic rat treated with gliclazide shows the normal histological structure of the tunica intima, tunica media and tunica adventitia, **E)**: a diabetic rat treated with *Artemisia* extract (400 mg/kg) shows the normal histological structure, **F)**: a diabetic rat treated with *Artemisia* extract (200 mg/kg) shows the normal histological structure, **G)**: a diabetic rat treated with *Artemisia* extract (100 mg/kg) shows the normal histological structure (H & E, Scale Bar: 20 μm).

Alterations in homocysteine metabolism have also been observed in diabetic patients. Elias and Eng [40] recorded that plasma homocysteine levels have been elevated in patients with diabetes. However, the plasma concentration of homocysteine in patients with diabetes is further confounded by the use of medication used to treat the disease and by the development of renal impairment. In the current study, STZ-treated rats presented decreased serum level of HCY and this reduction was normalized by Ah extract and gliclazide treatment. In agreement, Gursu et al., [41] found that homocysteine levels were reduced in STZ-induced diabetic rats. This reduction was normalized by insulin in a dose-dependent manner. HCY is converted to methionine by remethylation and cysteine by transsulfuration. Insulin administration reduced activities of transsulfuration and remethylation enzymes and hence prevented conversion of Hcy to methionine

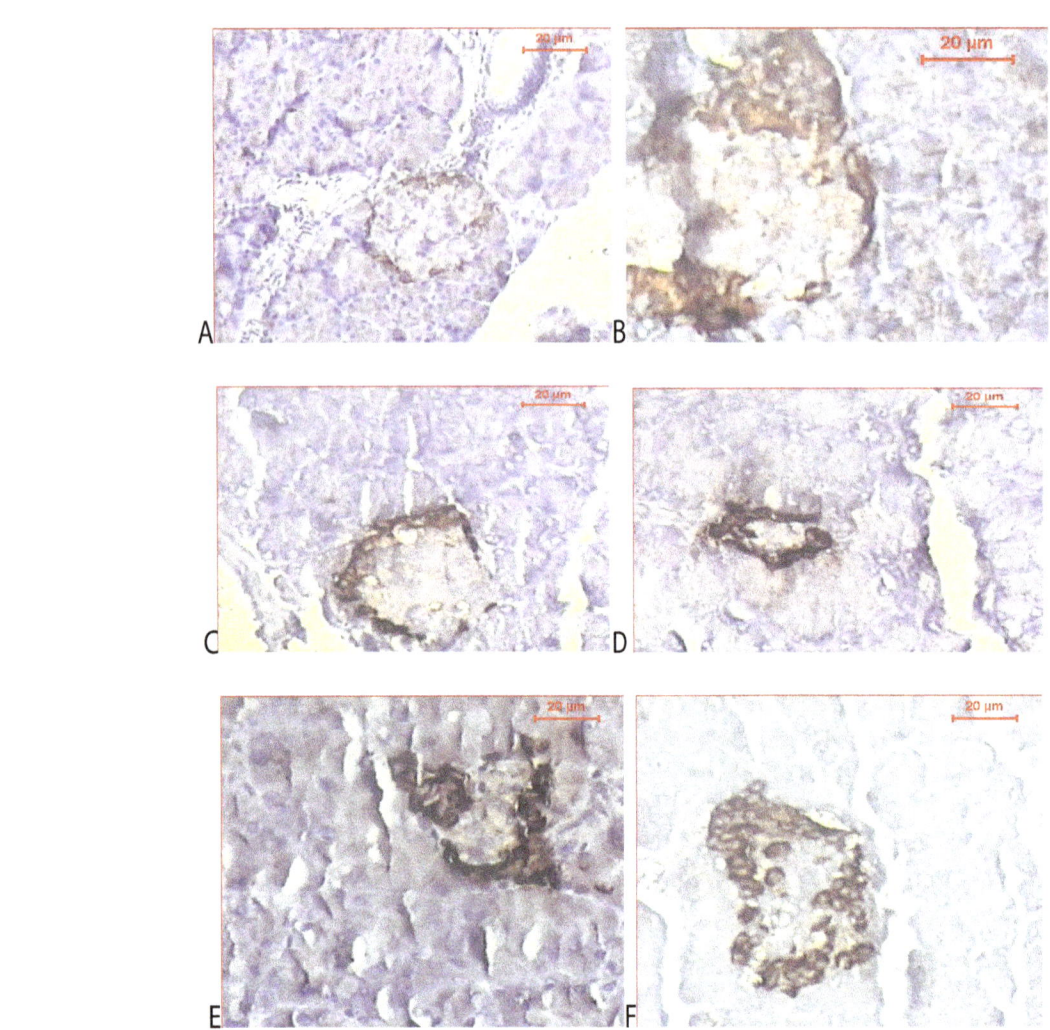

Figure 6. Immunohistochemical staining for glucagon antibody to identify the alpha cells in the islets of Langerhans of pancreas in **(A):** control rat **B):** a diabetic rat **C):** a diabetic rat treated with gliclazide **D):** a diabetic rat treated with Ah (400 mg/kg) **E): and F):** a diabetic rat treated with Ah (200 and 100mg/kg; respectively) (Immunoreactivity for insulin, Scale Bar: 20 μm).

and cysteine. Similarly, Jacobs and colleagues [42] observed a 30% reduction in plasma homocysteine in the diabetic rats. Given the above insulin results, it could be postulated that the treatment with Ah extract corrected HCY metabolism via increasing insulin level back to normal.

Diabetes is also associated with hyperlipidemia [43]. Serum lipids concentration is raised during diabetes due to increased mobilization of fatty acids from peripheral depots, since insulin inhibits the hormone sensitive lipase [44]. Excess fatty acids in the serum of diabetic rats are converted into phospholipids and cholesterol in the liver. These two substances along with excess triglycerides formed at the same time in the liver may be discharged into the blood in the form of lipoproteins [45]. In the present study, increased levels of serum triglycerides observed in STZ-induced diabetic rats were in accord with other studies [46, 47]. Administration of Ah at the three dose level normalized serum triglycerides and decreased serum cholesterol level even below the normal value. These results are in agreement with that of Abass [48] who found significant reductions were recorded in serum cholesterol upon treatment of normoglycemic rats with Ah aqueous

extract. It was concluded that this extract could present a good adjuvant to hyperlipidemia classical therapy compared to consuming the crude herb without any further modification like extraction. Mansi et al. [13] also reported that administration of Ah water extract (0.39 g/kg bwt) to alloxan-induced diabetic rats for 14 days showed considerable lowering of serum total cholesterol, triglycerides, LDL cholesterol, TC/HDL-C and an increase in HDL cholesterol.

In the current study, the significant increase in serum ALT and AST levels that was observed in STZ-induced diabetic rats represents liver damage compared to control rats. Serum enzyme activities can be used as useful biomarkers for monitoring the cytotoxicity of xenobiotics including STZ. Similar to our results, some earlier studies noted increases in serum ALT and AST activities in STZ-diabetic rats [49]. Significant reductions in serum activities of these enzymes were currently observed in A. Herba alba extract-treated groups. It is most likely that leakage of enzymes from tissues to serum was reduced after supplementation with this extract. It might have provided muscle integrity and ameliorated injuries of liver and heart tissues in diabetic

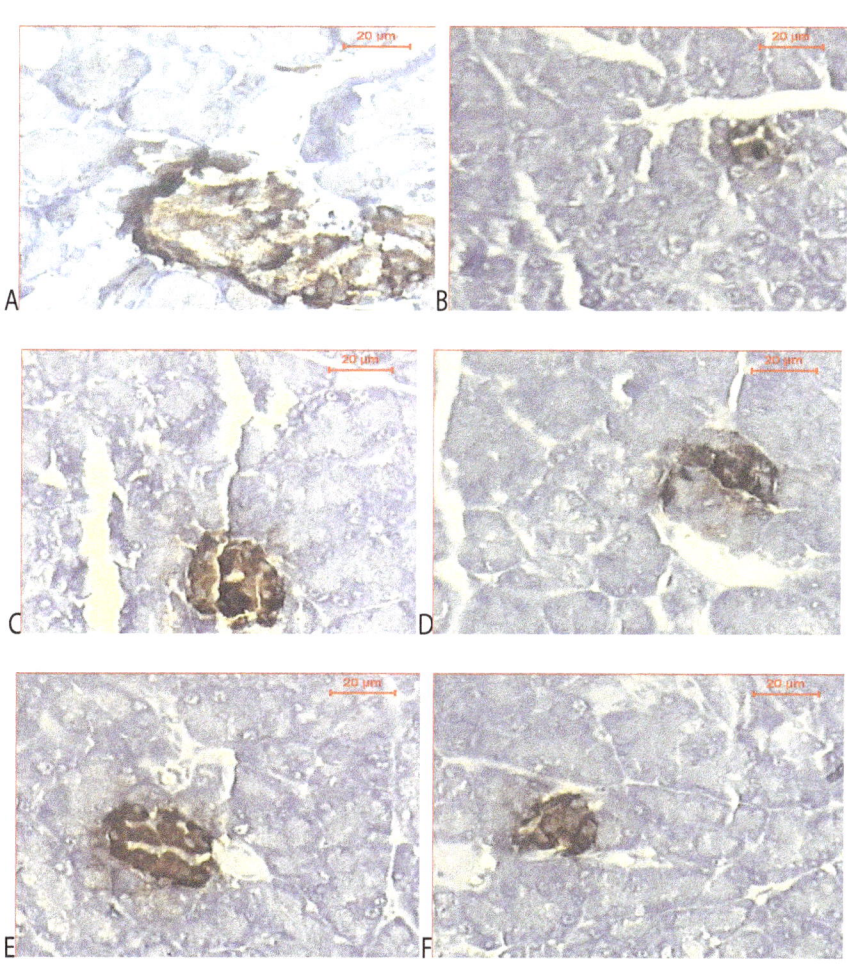

Figure 7. Immunohistochemical staining for insulin antibody to identify the beta cells in the islets of Langerhans of pancreas in **(A)**: control rat **(B)**: a diabetic rat **(C)**: a diabetic rat treated with gliclazide **D): and E): and F):** a diabetic rat treated with Ah (400,200,100mg/kg; respectively) (Immunoreactivity for insulin, Scale Bar: 20 μm).

rats. In accord with present results, Farhad et al. [50] demonstrated the reduction the complications of diabetes brought on liver after treatment with the hydro-alcoholic extract of Ah (200 and 300mg/kg bwt).

The present data revealed elevations in BUN and sr.creatinine in STZ-induced diabetic rats as expected. A similar effect was recorded previously [51]. Deficiency of insulin and consequent inability of glucose to reach the extrahepatic tissues stimulate gluconeogenesis as an alternative route of glucose supply [52]. This route is sustained by increased proteolysis which releases free glucogenic amino acids into the plasma that are deaminated in the liver with the consequence of increased urea in the blood. Creatinine is produced from creatine, a molecule of major importance for energy production in muscles. The kidneys maintain the blood creatinine in a normal range; hence, abnormally high levels of creatinine indicate impairment of renal function. [53]. In the current study, administration of ethanol extract of Ah produced a reduction in the levels of these metabolites, thereby conferring protection against impairment due to diabetes. It is worthy to mention that this herb showed better improvement of kidney function than the standard gliclazide.

Diabetes mellitus (hyperglycemia) is a metabolic disorder that results in excessive production of free radicals which leads to severe oxidative damage of cell components like lipids, proteins and DNA. In the present study, Ah extract showed strong antioxidant activity via enhancement of GSH concentration and inhibition of lipid peroxidation in hepatic and renal tissues. It has been documented that Ah plant contain wide variety of antioxidant molecules, such as phenolic acids, flavonoids and other natural antioxidants [54]. Additional studies have shown the antioxidant effect of Ah. The phenolic compounds have been reported to be significantly associated with the antioxidant activity of plant and food extracts [55]. It has been also found that Ah essential oils have some antioxidant abilities for preventing the linoleic oxidation and to reduce DPPH radicals [56].

The histopathological findings of STZ-treated rats further indicated the presence of pathological alterations in the pancreatic tissue as well as the other organs (liver, kidney, heart, aorta) revealing progression of diabetic complications. Treatment with Ah extract restored the morphological changes and began to recover the normal tissues histology. Hence, the pancreatic, hepatic, renal, cardiac and aortic lesions induced by STZ were significantly diminished by administration of Ah at lower to higher doses. The current Immunohistochemical results showed that the plant could reverse the catabolic features of

Primer	Normal Control	STZ Control		Gliclazide (Standard)		Ah ext (400mg/kg)		Ah ext (200mg/kg)		Ah ext (100mg/kg)	
		a	b	a	b	a	b	a	b	a	b
OPA02	3	2	2	3	3	2	2	2	3	1	2
OPA03	3	4	1	1	4	2	6	2	6	2	6
OPA05	3	5	1	1	5	1	5	0	4	0	4
OPB13	3	7	3	1	4	1	3	0	3	2	3
Total	12	18	7	6	16	6	16	4	16	5	15
a+b		25		22(88%)		22(88%)		20(80%)		20(80)	

a:appearance of new bands, b:disappearance of control bands , a+b: polymorphic bands.

Table 4: Changes of total bands in control, polymorphic bands and varied bands in samples:

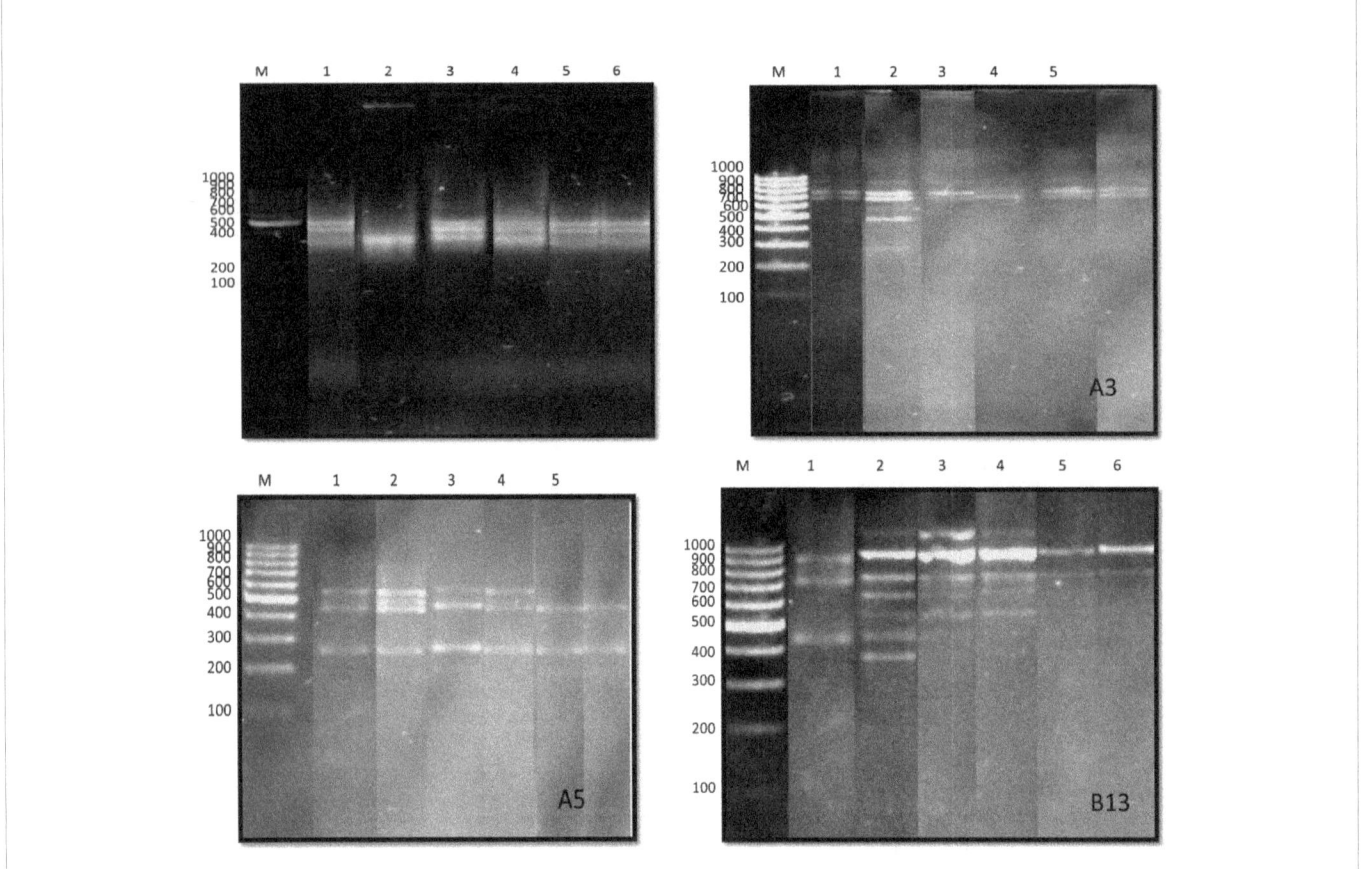

Figure 8: RAPD-PCR fingerprints generated by OPA02, OPA03, OPA05 and OPB13 primers for genomic DNA isolated mice and DNA fragmentation. *Lane M: ladder DNA (1000-100pb). Lane1 (normal control), Lane2 (STZ control), Lane3 (gliclazide), Lane4 (Ah, 400mg/kg) Lane 5 (Ah, 200mg/kg), Lane 6 (Ah, 100mg/kg).*

insulin deficiency, decrease the release of glucagon and increase that of insulin which may be via direct stimulation of glycolysis in peripheral tissues, increase glucose removal from blood or reduce glucose absorption from the gastrointestinal tract [57].

In the current study, STZ-induced diabetes caused DNA damage in rat liver, which was decreased in gliclazide and Ah extract treated groups as compared to diabetic one. This is in accordance with Iriadam et al. [58] who found that Ah possesses antidiabetic effects. Sliwinska et al. [59] found that gliclazide has antioxidant properties and diminished DNA damage induced by free radicals. Araki and Nishikawa [60] and Mckillop and Schrum [61] reported that oxidative stress is one of the main etiologies for complications of diabetes, which involves the formation of highly reactive OH and leads to severe oxidative damage of the cell's components like DNA. Therefore, the current study reveals

that besides having a beneficial effect on reducing oxidative stress in diabetic rats through the scavenging of free radicals, Ah extract may be used as protective agent against DNA damage.

Conclusion

Oral administration of ethanol extract of Ah for 14 days showed hypoglycemic activity in STZ-induced diabetes in Wistar rats. The findings indicated the beneficial effects of this herb in reducing hyperlipidemia accompanying diabetes. Other complications such as hepatic and renal impairment were also improved.

Additional investigations are warranted to study the active principles of Ah that are responsible for these pharmacological activities. Further studies are also needed to know more about the mechanisms of hypoglycemic action of this plant.

Acknowledgments

Authors acknowledge National Research Centre for funding this research and supplying materials, animals, and all necessary facilities to conduct this study with grant number 10010307. Authors also acknowledge Dr. Gihan Farag Mohammed Asaad, Pharmacology department, National Research Centre for her sincere help in performing the current experimental work.

References

1. Singh SK, Rai PK, Jaiswal D, Watal G (2008) Evidence-based Critical Evaluation of Glycemic Potential of Cynodon dactylon. Evid Based Complement Alternat Med 5: 415-420.

2. Tripathi BK, Srivastava AK (2006) Diabetes mellitus: complications and therapeutics. Med Sci Monit 12: RA130-147.

3. Stades AM, Heikens JT, Erkelens DW, Holleman F, Hoekstra JB (2004) Metformin and lactic acidosis: cause or coincidence? A review of case reports. J Intern Med 255: 179-187.

4. Chiang CK, Ho TI, Peng YS, Hsu SP, Pai MF, et al. (2007) Rosiglitazone in diabetes control in hemodialysis patients with and without viral hepatitis infection: effectiveness and side effects. Diabetes Care 30: 3-7.

5. Grover JK, Yadav S, Vats V (2002) Medicinal plants of India with anti-diabetic potential. J Ethnopharmacol 81: 81-100.

6. Jung M, Park M, Lee HC, Kang YH, Kang ES, et al. (2006) Antidiabetic agents from medicinal plants. Curr Med Chem 13: 1203-1218.

7. Balaraman AK, Singh J, Dash S, Maity TK (2010) Antihyperglycemic and hypolipidemic effects of Melothria maderaspatana and Coccinia indica in Streptozotocin induced diabetes in rats. Saudi Pharm J 18: 173-178.

8. Abou El-Hamd H, Mohamed AE, El-Sayed MA, Hegazy ME, Helaly SE, et al. (2010) Chemical Constituents and Biological Activities of Artemisia herba-alba .Rec Nat Prod 4: 11-25.

9. Di Stasi LC, Oliveira GP, Carvalhaes MA, Queiroz M Jr, Tien OS, et al. (2002) Medicinal plants popularly used in the Brazilian Tropical Atlantic Forest. Fitoterapia 73: 69-91.

10. Laid M, Hegazy M-E F, Ahmed AA (2009) Sesquiterpene lactones from Algerian Artemisia herba alba. Phytochemistry let 1: 85-88.

11. Tahraoui A, El-Hilaly J, Israili ZH, Lyoussi B (2007) Ethnopharmacological survey of plants used in the traditional treatment of hypertension and diabetes in south-eastern Morocco (Errachidia province). J Ethnopharmacol 110: 105-117.

12. Awad NE, Seida AA, El-Khayat Z, Shaffie N, Abd El-Aziz AM, et al. (2007) Hypoglycemic Activity of Artemisia herba-alba (Asso.) used in Egyptian Traditional Medicine as Hypoglycemic Remedy. Journal of Applied Pharmaceutical Science 3: 30-39.

13. Mansi K, Amneh M, Nasr H (2010) The hypolipidemic effects of Artemisia sieberi (A. herba-alba) in alloxan induced diabetic rats. Int J Pharm 3: 487-491.

14. Mohamed AHH, El-Sayed MA, Hegazy ME, Helaly SE, Esmail AM, et al (2010) Chemical constituents and biological activities of Artemisia herba-alba. Rec Nat Prod 4: 1-25.

15. He L, Wu Y, Wang LL, Wu Y (2011) Hispidulin a small flavonoid molecule, suppresses the angiogenesis and growth of human pancreatic cancer by targeting vascular endothelial growth factor receptor 2-mediated PI3K/Akt/mTOR signaling pathway. Cancer Sci 102: 219-225.

16. Saleh, NAM, El-Negoumy SI, Abou-Zaid MM (1987) Flavonoids of Artemisia judaica, A. monosperma and A. herba-alba. Phytochemistry 26: 3059-3064.

17. Kim T-H, Ito H, Hatano T, Taniguchi S, Khennouf S, et al. (2004) Chemical constituents of Artemisia herba-alba Asso. Nat Med 58: 165.

18. Behrens H, Karber S (1953) Determination of LD50. Archives for Experimental Pathology and Pharmacy 2: 177-1372.

19. Alberti KG, Johnson AB, Taylor R (2007) Beneficial effects of gliclazide on improving free radical status through its antioxidant properties. Human Diabetes and Metabolic Research Centre, University of Newcastle

20. Blois MS (1958) Antioxidant determinations by the use of a stable free radical. Nature 26: 1199-1200.

21. Hossain MM, Shaha SK, Aziz F (2009) Antioxidant potential study of some synthesized N-heterocycles. Bangladesh Med Res Counc Bull 35: 49-52.

22. Barrière DA, Rieusset J, Chanteranne D, Busserolles J, Chauvin MA, et al. (2012) Paclitaxel therapy potentiates cold hyperalgesia in streptozotocin-induced diabetic rats through enhanced mitochondrial reactive oxygen species production and TRPA1 sensitization. Pain 153: 553-561.

23. Veiga F, Fernandes C, Teixeira F (2000) Oral bioavailability and hypoglycaemic activity of tolbutamide/cyclodextrin inclusion complexes. Int J Pharm 202: 165-171.

24. Eastham RD (1985) Biochemical values in clinical medicine. 7th ed. Bristol, England John Wright & Sons Ltd.

25. Fossati P, Prencipe L (1982) Serum triglycerides determined colorimetrically with an enzyme that produces hydrogen peroxide. Clin Chem 28: 2077-2080.

26. ABEL LL, LEVY BB, BRODIE BB, KENDALL FE (1952) A simplified method for the estimation of total cholesterol in serum and demonstration of its specificity. J Biol Chem 195: 357-366.

27. Walter M, Gerade RW (1970) Bilirubin direct / total. Microchem J 15: 231.

28. REITMAN S, FRANKEL S (1957) A colorimetric method for the determination of serum glutamic oxalacetic and glutamic pyruvic transaminases. Am J Clin Pathol 28: 56-63.

29. ELLMAN GL (1959) Tissue sulfhydryl groups. Arch Biochem Biophys 82: 70-77.

30. Ohkawa H, Ohishi N, Yagi K (1979) Assay for lipid peroxides in animal tissues by thiobarbituric acid reaction. Anal Biochem 95: 351-358.

31. Hsu SM, Raine L, Fanger H (1981) Use of avidinÂ±biotin peroxidase complex (ABC) in immunoperoxidase techniques: a comparison between ABC and unlabelled antibody procedures. J Histochem Cytochem 29: 277-280.

32. John SW, Weitzner G, Rozen R, Scriver CR (1991) A rapid procedure for extracting genomic DNA from leukocytes. Nucleic Acids Res 19: 408.

33. Williams JG, Kubelik AR, Livak KJ, Rafalski JA, Tingey SV (1990) DNA polymorphisms amplified by arbitrary primers are useful as genetic markers. Nucleic Acids Res 18: 6531-6535.

34. Biswas M, Kar B, Bhattacharya S, Kumar RB, Ghosh AK, et al. (2011) Antihyperglycemic activity and antioxidant role of Terminalia arjuna leaf in streptozotocin-induced diabetic rats. Pharm Biol 49: 335-340.

35. Weiss RB (1982) Streptozocin: a review of its pharmacology, efficacy, and toxicity. Cancer Treat Rep 66: 427-438.

36. Elias D, Prigozin H, Polak N, Rapoport M, Lohse AW, et al. (1994) Autoimmune diabetes induced by the beta-cell toxin STZ. Immunity to the 60-kDa heat shock protein and to insulin. Diabetes 43: 992-998.

37. Campbell DB, Lavielle R, Nathan C (1991) The mode of action and clinical pharmacology of gliclazide: a review. Diabetes Res Clin Pract 14 Suppl 2: S21-36.

38. Wajchenberg BL, Santomauro AT, Porrelli RN (1993) Effect of a sulfonylurea (gliclazide) treatment on insulin sensitivity and glucose-mediated glucose disposal in patients with non-insulin-dependent diabetes mellitus (NIDDM). Diabetes Res Clin Pract 20: 147-154.

39. Tastekin D, Atasever M, Adiguzel G, Keles M, Tastekin A, et al. (2006) Hypoglycaemic Effect of Artemisia Herba Alba in Experimental Hyperglycaemic Rats. Bull Vet Inst Pulawy 50: 235-223.

40. Elias AN, Eng S (2005) Homocysteine concentrations in patients with diabetes mellitus--relationship to microvascular and macrovascular disease. Diabetes Obes Metab 7: 117-121.

41. Gursu MF, Baydas G, Cikim G, Canatan H (2002) Insulin increases homocysteine levels in a dose-dependent manner in diabetic rats. Arch Med Res 33: 305-307.

42. Jacobs RL, House JD, Brosnan ME, Brosnan JT (1998) Effects of streptozotocin-induced diabetes and of insulin treatment on homocysteine metabolism in the rat. Diabetes 47: 1967-1970.

43. de Sereday MS, Gonzalez C, Giorgini D, De Loredo L, Braguinsky J, et al. (2004) Prevalence of diabetes, obesity, hypertension and hyperlipidemia in the central area of Argentina. Diabetes Metab 30: 335-339.

44. Pushparaj P, Tan CH, Tan BK (2000) Effects of Averrhoa bilimbi leaf extract on blood glucose and lipids in streptozotocin-diabetic rats. J Ethnopharmacol 72: 69-76.

45. Bopanna KN, Kannan J, Sushma G (1997) Antidiabetic and antihyperlipaemic effects of neem seed kernel powder on alloxan diabetic rabbits. Indian J Pharmacol 29: 162-167.

46. Annida B, Stanely Mainzen Prince P (2004) Supplementation of fenugreek leaves lower lipid profile in streptozotocin-induced diabetic rats. J Med Food 7: 153-156.

47. Tunali S, Yanardag R (2006) Effect of vanadyl sulfate on the status of lipid parameters and on stomach and spleen tissues of streptozotocin-induced diabetic rats. Pharmacol Res 53: 271-277.

48. Abass OA (2012) Therapeutic Effect of Artemisia Herba- Alba Aqueous Extract. Iraqi J. Comm Med 4: 320-323.

49. Ozkol H, Tuluce Y, Dilsiz N, Koyuncu I (2013) Therapeutic potential of some plant extracts used in Turkish traditional medicine on streptozocin-induced type 1 diabetes mellitus in rats. J Membr Biol 246: 47-55.

50. Farhad K, Hossein KG, Shahla Z, Sara A, Mohammed F, et al. (2013) The effect of hydroalcoholic extract of Artemisia (Artemisia herba-alba) and markers of liver damage compared with metformin in streptozotocin-induced diabetic rats. Advances in Environmental Biology 6: 743.

51. GawroÅ„ska-Szklarz B, MusiaÅ‚ DH, Pawlik A, Paprota B (2003) Effect of experimental diabetes on pharmacokinetic parameters of lidocaine and MEGX in rats. Pol J Pharmacol 55: 619-624.

52. Robinson G, Johnston DE (1997) Mechanisms of Disease: An Introduction to Clinical Science, 1st edition, Cambridge University Press, Cambridge, Mass, USA.

53. Loeb S (1991) Clinical Laboratory Test: Values and Implication, Springhouse Corporation, Pa, USA.

54. Moufid A, Eddouks M (2012) Artemisia herba alba: a popular plant with potential medicinal properties. Pak J Biol Sci 15: 1152-1159.

55. Gupta S, Prakash J (2009) Studies on Indian green leafy vegetables for their antioxidant activity. Plant Foods Hum Nutr 64: 39-45.

56. Kadri A, Chobba IB, Zarai Z, BÃ©kir A, Gharsallah N, et al. (2011) Chemical constituents and antioxidant activity of the essential oil from aerial parts of Artemisia herba-alba grown in Tunisian semi-arid region. Afr J Biotechnol. 10: 2923-2929.

57. Marrif HI, Ali BH, Hassan KM (1995) Some pharmacological studies on Artemisia herba-alba (Asso.) in rabbits and mice. J Ethnopharmacol 49: 51-55.

58. Iriadam M, Musa D, GÃ¼mÃ¼ï¬,han H, Baba F (2006) Effects of two Turkish medicinal plants Artemisia herba-alba a n d Teucrium polium on blood glucose levels and other biochemical parameters in rabbits. Journal of Cell and Molecular Biology 5: 19-24.

59. Sliwinska A, Blasiak J, Kasznicki J, Drzewoski J (2008) In vitro effect of gliclazide on DNA damage and repair in patients with type 2 diabetes mellitus (T2DM). Chem Biol Interact 173: 159-165.

60. Araki E, Nishikawa T (2010) Oxidative stress: A cause and therapeutic target of diabetic complications. J Diabetes Investig 1: 90-96.

61. McKillop IH, Schrum LW (2005) Alcohol and liver cancer. Alcohol 35: 195-203.

23

Pharmacological Properties of Resveratrol. A Pre-Clinical and Clinical Review

Muñoz O[1,2]*, Muñoz R[3] and Bustamante S[2,4]

[1]Chemistry Department, Faculty of Science, University of Chile, Santiago, Chile
[2]Chilean Society of Phytotherapy (SOCHIFITO), Chile
[3]School of Medicine, University of Chile, Avda, Independencia 1027, Santiago, Chile
[4]Program of Molecular and Clinical Pharmacology, Faculty of Medicine, University of Chile, Avda, Independencia 1027, Santiago, Chile

Abstract

Resvertrol (Resv) is an extensively studied molecule – as of 2015 PubMed held more than 7100 publications on the subject. The First International Resveratrol Conference in 2010 found insufficient evidence to justify recommending chronic administration of Resv in humans, a finding in stark contrast with the claims of its therapeutic effects often made by the media, based on its supposed role in the beneficial properties of red wine and in the so-called French Paradox. However, pharmacological studies carried out on different formulations of Resv from 2010 onwards suggest that these recommendations should be reviewed.

Pharmacokinetic Resv is characterized by high inter-individual variability within pharmacokinetic parameters. Resv exhibits a rapid absorption rate, with extensive pre-systemic metabolism by human cytochrome P 450 and intestinal microbiota. Its metabolism leads mainly to conjugation products, the biological activity of which is still under discussion. It is also rapidly cleared by the kidneys. Finally, the estimated bioavailability of Resv is around 1% of orally-administered doses.

Clinical trials have shown that Resv seems to exert a therapeutic effect on endothelial dysfunction consistent with in vitro observations demonstrating that Resv stimulates the eNOS enzyme. Inflammatory markers and CRP reductions obtained from doses of Resv equal to or less than 20 mg/day are not observed in larger doses, which imply hermetic behavior. Resv has also been shown to reduce the atherogenic potential of LDL cholesterol by reducing oxidized LDL and ApoB levels, which would in turn reduce atherogenesis. Resv is a well-tolerated compound; short-term clinical trials have shown frequent gastrointestinal discomfort or spontaneously resolving diarrhea only with the administration of high doses.

Keywords: Resveratrol; Pharmacology; Cardiovascular

Introduction

Resveratrol (Resv) or 3,5,4'-stilbenotriol (Figure 1), is a secondary metabolite present in around 70 plant species, which was isolated for the first time in 1940 from white hellebore (*Veratrum grandiflorum*) root extract [1]. It is a phytoalexin, that is, a compound synthesized by plants in response to stress and infections. Structurally, it is a non-flavonoid polyphenol from the stilbene family present in a number of regularly consumed plant species such as berries, peanuts, and the epidermis of grapes, although its highest concentration is in *Polygonum cuspidatum* roots, a plant mentioned in traditional Chinese and Japanese pharmacopoeias [2], and currently used for commercial extraction. Even when biosynthesized in both its *cis* and *trans* forms, a wide consensus considers the *trans* form as more biologically active, besides being the most stable isomer [1,3].

Scientific interest in Resv grew significantly fifty years later, when work was published in *The Lancet* [4] on the low incidence of cardiovascular disease in the French population despite its high intake of saturated fats, possibly due to moderate and habitual consumption of red wine, which contains Resv among other polyphenols, a contradiction that soon became known as the so-called *French Paradox*. Later, it was shown that Resv had a preventive effect on the initiation, promotion and progression phases of *in vitro* and *in vivo* models of carcinogenesis [5]. While the *French Paradox* suggested the effectiveness of Resv at dietary concentrations by consuming food containing Resv, it was soon realized that the results in cancer research were in fact the reflection of an exponentially growing number of *in vitro* experiments that, at least in the first years, used concentrations far above those attainable *in vivo* [6,7]. Consequently, the initially high expectations arising from these experiments were soon tempered in the light of results from studies in animal models [8]. Different mechanisms have been proposed to explain the observed effects of Resv, especially in therapeutic areas as dissimilar as cancer [9], obesity, metabolic syndrome and diabetes [10], cardiovascular health [11] and neurodegenerative diseases [4,12-14].

This article reviews aspects regarding the pharmacokinetics and safety of resveratrol in animal and human models, and discusses evidence that could support its possible use as a therapeutic agent in cardiovascular health.

Pharmacokinetics

A range of assays have been carried out to determine whether Resv can reach the proposed sites of action after oral administration in humans, as the different pharmacokinetic stages may necessitate *in vivo* Resv concentrations that greatly differ from those used *in vitro*.

Absorption

Six healthy volunteers were administered ^{14}C-resveratrol in 25

*Corresponding author: Orlando Muñoz, Chemistry Department, Faculty of Science, University of Chile, Las Palmeras 3425, 7800003, Santiago, Chile, E-mail: omunoz@uchile.cl

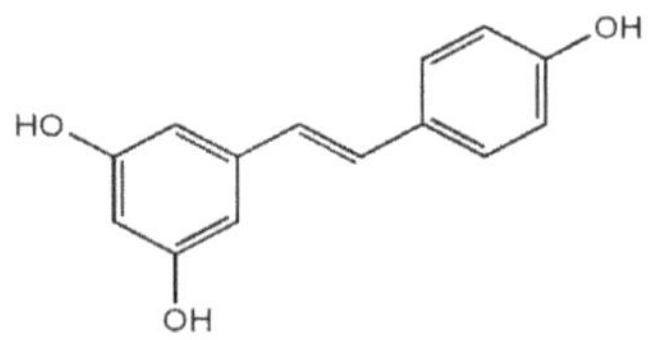

Figure 1: Chemical structure of *trans*-resveratrol (3,5,4'-stilbenotriol, MW: 228.5).

g oral doses [15]. Absorption was estimated to be equivalent to 70% of the dose, however, in plasma; Resv was only detected in quantities slightly above the detection limit (5 ng/ml). The majority of the dose was detected in urine, both for Resv and its three metabolites. In another study, 40 healthy volunteers were exposed to single oral doses of 0.5 g, 1.0 g, 2.5 g, or 5.0 g [16], and the time taken to establish the maximum plasma concentration (t_{max}) was estimated at between 0.83 and 1.5 h. This estimate was corroborated by a study administering *trans*-resveratrol in doses of 25, 50, 100 and 150 mg to eight healthy volunteers, in whom average t_{max} levels between 0.8 and 1.5 h were subsequently observed, depending on the dose received [17].

The passing mechanism for oral Resv would seem to be passive diffusion through the apical membrane of the enterocytes, which may be inferred from an *in vitro* study carried out on a monolayer of Caco-2 cells [18], consistent with its low water solubility estimated at less than 0.05 mg/ml [19]. Nonetheless, enterocytes express ATP-Binding Cassette (ABC) type transporters, which have been demonstrated to actively secrete Resv in the opposite direction, from the cytosol to the lumen, thus limiting the concentration of Resv passing into portal circulation.

After administering a single dose of 5.0 g of Resv to 10 healthy volunteers, its maximum plasma concentration (C_{max}) reached 539 ng/ml ± 384 ng/ml [16]. Another pharmacokinetic study administered chemically synthetized Resv *per os* to 10 healthy volunteers, with a daily dose per group of 0.5, 1.0, 2.5 and 5.0 g, for 29 days [20]. Its accumulated plasma concentration was determined between days 21 and 28, and showed an average C_{max} of 967 ng/ml. In order to increase Resv absorption, another study used micronized Resv (SRT501) and determined its pharmacokinetic parameters [21]. 5.0 g of SRT501 was administered daily for 14 days to six patients with rectal colon cancer and hepatic metastasis; the C_{max} after the single administration of SRT501 was 1942 ng/ml ± 1422 ng/ml, a value two to four times higher than the value reported for non-micronized forms [16, 20]. The average t_{max} was 2.8 h, far above that reported in other pharmacokinetic assays for Resv [16,17]. Considering the molecular weight of Resv (228.25), none of the pharmacokinetic studies *in vivo* in humans have shown plasma concentrations greater than 10 µM, far below the concentrations of up to 200 µM observed in *in vitro* studies.

It is widely accepted in pharmacology that the absorption and bioavailability stages of drugs administered by mouth can be modified by the presence of food and in certain cases it is decided to administer the drug on an empty stomach. Along these lines, one study administered *trans*-Resv to healthy volunteers in red wine in three different dietary conditions: while fasting (1920 µg of *trans*-Resv in 600 ml of red wine, n=5), after a standard meal (246 µg of *trans*-Resv in 300 ml of red wine, n=10) and after consuming a meal rich in fats (480 µg de *trans*-Resv in 600 ml of red wine, n=10). According to the authors of the study [22], *trans*-Resv bioavailability was not related with dietary status or lipid content, subsequently confirmed by another study in humans [23]. However, it should be noted that *trans*-Resv metabolites 3'- and

4'-glucuronate were detected, and that the pure compound was present only in trace amounts below the detection limit. Therefore, caution should be exercised with regards to the beneficial effects of dietary consumption of Resv [23], as the benefits associated with red wine consumption and its role in the *French Paradox*, are probably due to the total antioxidant content in red wine. The quantity of *trans*-resveratrol in red wine fluctuates from undetectable to 14.3 mg/l, with an average value of 1.9 ± 1.7 mg/l (8.2 ± 7.5 µM); however, the quantity of the *trans*- and *cis*-resveratrol-glucoside conjugate (*trans*- and *cis*-piceid) can be up to three times greater than Resv and, although it is absorbed in lower amounts than Resv, the Resv isomer can be produced by metabolization [24].

Metabolism

After oral administration, Resv undergoes intense metabolism by the bacterial flora in the human intestine [25]. Twelve healthy volunteers were orally administered a single dose of 0.5 mg/kg body weight of *trans*-Resv (Vineatrol, 7.7% *trans*-Resv and a range of stilbenes). In addition to the aforementioned dihydro-resveratrol metabolite [8], two new *trans*-Resv metabolites were reported due to bacterial metabolism, probably by the *Slackia equolifaciens* and *Adlercreutzia equolifaciens* strains of 3,4'-dihidroxi-*trans*-stilbeno and lunularin (3,4'dihidroxibibenzil). Bacterial metabolism was up to 62.7% of administered doses. On the other hand, the bacteria responsible for the dehydroxylation reactions have not been identified [25].

The most important metabolites arising from the human metabolism of Resv are created by phase II reactions. Mono- and di-glucuronide, mono- y di-sulfate and glucuronide sulfate metabolites have been described, of which Resv-3-O-sulfate is consistently identified as the most abundant [16,20,26]. The concentrations reached by these metabolites in plasma have been shown to be greater than those reached by pure *trans*-resv, exhibiting an AUC 20 [20] to 23 [16] times greater than those of the original molecule in the case of the majority metabolite. The intense metabolism of Resv explains why, despite its quick absorption, its bioavailability remains around 1% [8].

Based on *in vitro* experiments, it has been suggested that the metabolites are biologically active, as ubiquitous enzymes such as β-glucuronidase could convert these metabolites to the original Resv molecule either locally or systematically [3,27]. Sulfate metabolites [3] and dihydro-resveratrol [25] have also been shown to be active *in vivo*.

When plotting C_{max} using escalated doses from 25 to 5,000 mg, near linear behavior is seen in Resv plasma concentration, which would prove non-saturation of the metabolism [8]. However, some studies show that sulfate-conjugated Resv metabolites can be found in higher amounts as long as the highest doses of Resv are administered [16,28]. It should be noted that these results could indicate possible saturation of glucuronosyltransferase enzymes at high Resv doses, contrasting with observations of the sulfation route, as the latter present's non-competitive substrate inhibition [29]. Such saturation in Resv metabolism implies a change in the route from glucuronidation to sulfatation [30], which would explain the high amount of sulfate metabolites in reports of studies using high doses of dietary Resv [16,28].

In a clinical study, the metabolic interaction of Resv with the activity of enzymes from the CYP-P450 family and phase II detoxification enzymes was quantified in 40 healthy volunteers subjected to 1.0/g doses of Resv for four weeks [26]. Resv was shown to inhibit the phenotypical index of CYP3A4, CYP2D6 and CYP2C9 and was able to induce the phenotypical index of CYP1A2. On the other hand, in phase II enzymes, GST and UGT1A1 activity was minimally affected, although in volunteers with low base levels of enzyme activity, induction of GST-π was observed. Drugs such as caffeine, dextrometorphan, losartan and buspirone, could potentially increase dose-dependent adverse reactions or alter the efficacy of Resv co-administration [26].

Table 1 shows main resveratrol metabolites, metabolic route/agent, *in vivo* metabolite activity, and molecular structure.

Distribution

In vitro studies have determined that Resv is reversibly bonded to bovine serum albumin at a bonding constant of $2.52 \pm 0.50 \times 10^4 \, M^{-1}$, in addition to likely partial protein cleavage [31]. Resv metabolites, sulfates, disulfates and resveratrol-C/O-diglucoronide are non-covalently bonded to plasma proteins [28].

In dried colon tissues from 20 patients treated with Resv SRT501 in daily doses of 500 mg or 1,000 mg per 29 days, it was observed that non-conjugated Resv was distributed in greater concentrations to the colon tissue than to plasma [21]. In any case, this organ forms part of the administration route, which is also exposed to the entire non-absorbed fraction. The Resv concentrations in tissue from dried liver with metastasis and healthy liver in 5 of 6 patients were 4.81 nmol/g and 1.84 nmol/g, respectively [21]. In a preclinical study administering 100 Resv mg/kg body weight to 15 rats, tissue concentrations between 5 to 10 times greater than those found in liver, heart, lung, spleen and kidney tissue were detected in the stomach and the small intestine [32].

The estimated apparent distribution volume of Resv ranges from 16.07 liters for a 500 mg dose [20] to 66.99 liters for a dose ten times greater [17].

Excretion

Little information is available on the excretion of Resv. It is estimated that the total clearance of Resv ranges between 2.5 to 3.0 l/h (41.7 ml/min to 50 ml/min) [16,20]. The elimination half-life ($t_{\frac{1}{2}}$) has been calculated at 1.1 h after a dose of 100 mg Resv, while after 1.0 g/day administration for 21 days, the $t_{\frac{1}{2}}$ is 9.7 h [17]. Resv is eliminated relatively quickly and it has been reported that up to 77% of the dose is eliminated within the first four hours post-administration [33].

Resv plasma level curves consistently show a second peak after C_{max},

Source	Metabolization	Metabolite	Activity	Molecular structure
tra	bacterial flora	dihydro-resveratrol	Active	
		3,4'-dihydroxy-trans-stilbeno	Non active	
		3,4'-dihydroxybibenzyl (*lunularin*)	Non active	
	phase II glucuronosyl-transferase route	resveratrol-3-O-glucuronide	active	
	phase II sulfation route	resveratrol-3-O-sulfate	active	
		resveratrol-3,4'-disulfate	active	
	phase II mixed route	resveratrol-3-sulfate-4'-glucuronide	active	

Table 1: Main resveratrol metabolites and activity (see text).

which has been interpreted as proof of enterohepatic recirculation. Conjugated forms of Resv metabolites excreted via biliary routes may be metabolized by bacterial hydroxylase enzymes in the small intestine, facilitating their reabsorption [33], which has been demonstrated in animal models [34]. Fecal excretion is highly variable, between 0.3% and 23% of the administered dose, with an average of 12.7% ± 6.1% [15].

Chronopharmacology and variability

The pharmacokinetics of Resv show two interesting characteristics worth consideration, however, these require further study for corroboration. Firstly, the administration of Resv is circadian-dependent, as the AUC in a plasma level graph is larger after morning than after afternoon oral administration [17]. Consequently, Resv bioavailability would be higher if administered in the morning. Secondly, as mentioned, the pharmacokinetic parameters have high interindividual variability, with variance coefficients of around 40%, in which the impact of patient gender or age is insignificant, as shown in comparisons of groups of men and women, young and older people [35].

Cardiovascular therapeutic potential

Resv has hormetic effects, that is, it is active at low doses and less responsive or non-responsive at high doses. This characteristic has been observed in preclinical studies on Resv and at least six types of human cell tumors in the breast, prostate, leukemia, colon, uterus, and lung [36]. In another *in vitro* assay of ischemia-reperfusion in Sprague-Dawley rats that were administered Resv in escalated doses of 2.5 and 5.0 mg/kg body weight for 14 days, after which the size of the infarction and the cardiomyocyte apoptosis were compared [37]. In comparison with the control group, both the size of the infarction and the cardiomyocyte apoptosis recorded were significantly less for the 2.5 and 5.0 mg/kg dose of body weight, while these variables increased in comparison with the control in groups subject to doses above or equal to 25 mg/kg body weight.

Consequently, the choice of a therapeutic dose of Resv must additionally include this non-linear behavior in dose-effect curves. This is particularly true for clinical trials in humans which, nonetheless, have not always been included.

Table 2 shows a summary of clinical trials with Resv in humans to determine its efficacy in cardiovascular problems. These seven clinical trials included a total of 426 patients administered Resv in different formulations including nutraceuticals from *Vitis vinifera* extracts (with other compounds such as polyphenols and vitamins) and red wine. If only those administered solely Resv are counted, this number drops to 175 patients.

Clinical trials have focused on the efficacy of Resv in the primary prevention of cardiovascular events in sub-populations with different factors of CV risk, such as arterial hypertension, diabetes, dyslipidemia, active smoking, or a family history of early cardiovascular disease. Resv was administered concomitantly with each patient's base medication. The most dose of Resv administered was 270 mg per day [38], in the form of supplements for hypertense obese patients. The lowest dose of Resv is 0.74 mg daily in 272 ml of red wine [39]. The longest study of the administration of Resv to humans in a nutraceutical formulation has been for 12 months, at a dose equivalent to 8 mg/day [40].

The effect of Resv on endothelial function has been determined by ultrasound as the percentage variance of flow measured dilatation (FMD) in the brachial artery. In a study of 19 overweight patients and/or patients with elevated values of arterial pressure given single doses of a *Vitis vinifera* nutraceutical equivalent to 30, 90 y 270 mg of Resv, a significant increase in the FMD percentage was recorded in all dose groups in contrast with the control group [40], demonstrating linear behavior between the logarithm of the dose used and percentage FMD values. Two additional studies corroborated this finding. In 34 patients diagnosed with metabolic syndrome (see criteria in Table 1), a significant increase in the FMD percentage was observed after three months of administering 100 mg/day of Resv in a preparation that also included quercetin, vitamin D_3 and rice bran phytic acid controlled against a placebo [41]. Similar results were observed in a clinical trial with 40 patients who showed significant increases both in the FMD percentage and diastolic function of the left ventricle in groups given 10 mg Resv daily for three months [42, 43]. These results show that Resv supplementation improves endothelial function, and thus reduces cardiovascular risk. However, the results should be interpreted carefully, due to the fact that the base diameter of the brachial artery conditions the flow increase percentage, especially in patients with developing atherosclerotic injuries, which could bias the conclusions, therefore studies based on this index are not recommended for assigning cardiovascular risk in asymptomatic adults [44].

Given that atherogenesis is an inflammatory process, different serum markers have been used to determine inflammation in the system, such as clinically significant C reactive protein levels (CRP), due to their prognostic value in patients with acute coronary syndrome. In a one year study administering a *Vitis vinifera* nutraceutical equivalent to 8 mg/day of Resv, significant and clinically relevant drops were reported in CRP levels in both hypercholesterolemic and diabetic patients undergoing statin treatment [40]. Similar results were reported in a study administering a 20 mg Resv supplement and calcium fructoborate daily for two months to overweight patients with stable angina [45]. However, not all CRP reduction can be attributed to Resv, as it has been shown that pharmacotherapy with statins *per se* induces statistically significant reduction in CRP levels [46].

Conversely, in a clinical trial administering Resv daily for three months as a nutritional supplement (Longevinex˚) equivalent to 100 mg of Resv, no changes of any type were registered in CRP levels [41]. Given that lower doses of Resv did have an effect, the authors consider that this result was due to the hormetic behavior of Resv when acting on CRP levels.

The effect of Resv on plasminogen-1 activator inhibitor levels has also been determined in a 12 month clinical trial, reporting clinically and statistically significant reductions in groups given Resv in comparison with the placebo group [41]. Nonetheless, no change in pro-inflammatory interleukin IL-6 levels was recorded in this trial. Similar results were shown in a study comparing the effect of ethanol with the phenolic compounds of red wine on the expression of inflammation markers related with atherosclerosis due to cardiovascular disease [39]. The results suggest that the phenolic compounds of dealcoholized red wine can modify leukocyte adhesion molecules, whereas the ethanol and polyphenols present in red wine may modulate soluble inflammation mediators, however the effects cannot be attributed exclusively to Resv, as it is probable that the other polyphenol molecules present in red wine could be responsible for the effect observed [39].

Several clinical trials show that administering Resv does not modify plasma HDL- or LDL-cholesterol levels [41,45,47], classical markers in evaluating cardiovascular risk. Nonetheless in a six-month study

Number and health of subjects	Study characteristics	Form of administration	Dose, administration intervals and duration	Variables studied (outcomes)	Noteworthy results	Ref
40 subjects who have previously suffered heart attacks	Randomized, double blind, controlled by placebo	RESV Capsules	10 mg of pure RESV daily for 3 months	Endothelial function, measured by the Flow Mediated Dilatation technique (FMD), diastolic function of the left ventricle	Increased FMD and diastolic function of the left ventricle	26
19 overweight or obese subjects and/or with high values of untreated AP (up to 160 mmHg SAP or 100 mmHg DAP)	Randomized, double-blind, controlled by placebo, cross-over	ResVida™ capsules containing RESV	Three doses of 30, 90 or 270 mg RESV in an interval of one per week. Study of acute effects	Endothelial function, measured by FMD	Significant increase of FMD in all dose groups. A linear relationship is observed between this variable and the vulgar dose logarithm.	54
116 overweight subjects suffering from stable angina	Randomized, double blind, controlled by placebo, parallel arms	Capsules of pure RESV and RESV with Calcium Fructoborate (CFB)	20 mg daily for 60 days	Plasma levels of PCR-as, NT-proBNP, LDL, HDL and triglycerides. Quality of life (1)	Significant reductions in PCR-as levels in all groups; greater in those consuming only CFB. The group receiving RESV obtained better results in NT-proBNP, total cholesterol, triglyceridemia reductions; and also 50% reductions in weekly angina episodes	28
67 diabetic subjects or subjects with 3 or more risk factors (2)	Randomized, blind, controlled (with ingestion of an alcoholic beverage without polyphenols), cross-over	Red wine (RW) and alcohol-free red wine (AFRW) with 5.26 + 0.83 mg/L and 5.01 + 0.86 mg/L total RESV (5) and 2.92 + 0.36 mg/L and 2.73 + 0.23 mg/L t-RESV, respectively	272 mL daily (0.79 and 0.74 mg pure RESV for RW and AFRW respectively); for 28 days	Expression of soluble cellular adhesion molecules and in leukocytes; expression of pro-inflammatory citoquins	In groups consuming wine a reduction was observed in serum ICAM-1 and IL-6, concentrations and in the expression of T lymphocyte and monocyte adhesion in molecule membranes.	13
75 patients with diabetes or hypercholesterolemia, in treatment with statins, and one or more CV risk factors (4)	Randomized, triple blind, controlled with grape extract capsules without RESV and placebo, parallel arms	Stilvid® capsules containing 8 mg RESV and standardized grape extract	8 mg daily for 6 months	Lipid markers: triglyceridemia, total cholesterolemia, plasma HDL, LDL, non-HDL cholesterol, apolipoprotein B (ApoB) and oxidated LDL (LDLox) concentrations	Significant reduction of plasma LDLox and ApoB concentrations only in the group consuming capsules with RESV. The ApoB values for this group reached the optimums proposed by the Canadian Cardiovascular Society (<90 mg/dL)	45
75 patients with diabetes or hypercholesterolemia, in treatment with statins, and one or more than three CV risk factors (4)	Randomized, triple blind, controlled with grape extract capsules without RESV and placebo, parallel arms	Stilvid® capsules containing 8 mg of RESV and standardized grape extract	8 mg daily for 12 months	Inflammation markers: soluble ICAM-1, Interleukins 6, 10 and 18; TNF-a, HS-RCP y PAI-1	Significant reduction HS-RCP, TNF-a and PAI-1 only in the group consuming capsules containing RESV. Reductions of "marginal significance" of soluble ICAM-1 and absence of changes in IL-6	44
34 subjects diagnosed with Metabolic Syndrome (3)	Randomized, not blind, controlled, cross-over	Longevinex® Capsules containing pure RESV (100 mg), quercetin, vitamin D3 and rice bran phytic acid	100 mg daily for three months	Anthropometric measurements and indexes, arterial pressure, fasting glycemia, fasting insulinemia, HbA1c, plasma levels of HDL, LDL, IL-6 and HS-RCP. Entothelial function measured by FMD	Significant rise of FMD; no significant changes in any of the other study variables	20

(1) Operationalized as the classification of angina according to the Canadian Cardiovascular Society and number of angina episodes per week

(2) Smokers, hypertension, dyslipidemic, overweight or obese patients, or with a family history of premature coronary disease

(3) Abdominal obesity and 2 or more of the following: triglyceridemia >150 mg/dL, [HDL] <40 mg/dL, SAP >130 mmHg, DAP >85 mmHg or fasting glycemia >110 mg/dL

(4) Smokers, hypertensive or obese patients

(5) Includes isomer and piceid forms

HS-RCP High Sensitivity Reactive C Protein, NTproBNP N-terminal prohormone brain natriuretic peptide, SAP Systolic Arterial Pressure, DAP Diastolic Arterial Pressure

Table 2: Clinical trials with resveratrol to determine cardiovascular health issues as an outcome. In the first three trials (above the dotted line) pure resveratrol was administered. In the last four trials (below the dotted line) resveratrol was administered as part of a nutraceutical formulation.

administering a *Vitis vinifera* nutraceutical equivalent to 8 mg of Resv to patients with cardiovascular risk showed significant reductions both in oxidated LDL and Apolipoprotein B (ApoB) concentrations, although LDL or total-cholesterol were not modified [47]. This finding, still unverified in additional clinical studies, is interesting and relevant, as oxidation of these particles is a recognized progression factor of atherosclerotic lesions, given that it facilitates their precipitation. ApoB, has become known as a valuable prognostic marker of the capacity for interaction of apolipoprotein as a specific cellular receptor [48]. Figure 2 shows a flow chart that summarized *in vitro* and *in vivo* resveratrol mechanism of action.

Safety and Toxicity

Toxicity in animal models

The toxicity of Resv in different animal models has already been discussed *in extenso*, including its acute, subchronic and chronic toxicity [49].

The acute toxicity of a commercial product (resVida') containing pure 99% *trans*-Resv was examined in three classic tests: dermic irritation, ocular irritation and cutaneous sensitization. In the dermic irritation test, semi-occlusive resVida' dermic patches equivalent to 500 mg of Resv were applied to the flanks of New Zealand rabbits for four hours; no adverse reaction was observed for 72 hours post-administration [49].

For the ocular irritation test, resVida', equivalent to 100 mg of undiluted Resv, was administered to corneas of New Zealand rabbits, which exhibited slight to moderate redness that disappeared 72 hours later, without any other adverse effect [49].

The cutaneous sensitization test (local lymph node assay) consisted of topical administration of the assayed drug to the earlobes of the rabbits for three consecutive days. Resv at 6.25%, 12.5%, 25% weight/volume was used, and compared with a control group. Five days after

the study began, radio-marked thymidine was injected, and incubated for five hours, after which animals were culled to examine auricular lymph node cells. The calculated sensitization index was <3, below the threshold that characterizes a sensitizing substance [49].

Subchronic and chronic Resv toxicity has been tested in numerous animal models, such as Wistar and Sprague-Dawley rats [49-51], rabbits and dogs [52]. Crowell [50], administered Resv in 300, 1000 y 3000 mg/kg body weight doses for 28 days to Sprague-Dawley rats through a gastric tube. The toxic effects observed in the group that was administered 3000 mg/kg were severe, and generally attributed to a process of nephrotoxicity due to Resv. On the other hand, the group that was administered 1000 mg/kg manifested effects depending on the sex of the animals; the males had increased white cell count, while the females did experience blood count alterations, but gained significantly less weight during the study compared with the control group. The lower female body weight gain was attributed to dehydration and not reduction in food consumption. The group that was administered the smaller 300 mg/kg dose did not show toxicity or any other adverse effect.

Based on these results, a study of the same duration in Wistar rats [49] used doses of up to 500 mg/kg Resv incorporated into the standard diet. Although weight loss was not verified in any of the groups, variations in food consumption were observed, which the authors judged as irrelevant without providing more details. Alterations were also reported in partial thromboplastin time, with a shorter average partial thromboplastin time in the group that was administered 50 mg/kg, while it increased in the group administered 500 mg/kg. In contrast to what was observed regarding partial thromboplastin time, other animal studies did not reveal changes in coagulation parameters [51].

In a 13 week study incorporating doses of Resv of up to 750 mg/kg into the diet of rats, the group of Wisar rats that was administered the higher dose of Resv exhibited a range of sex-dependent alterations in biochemical markers; the males had increased plasma levels of inorganic

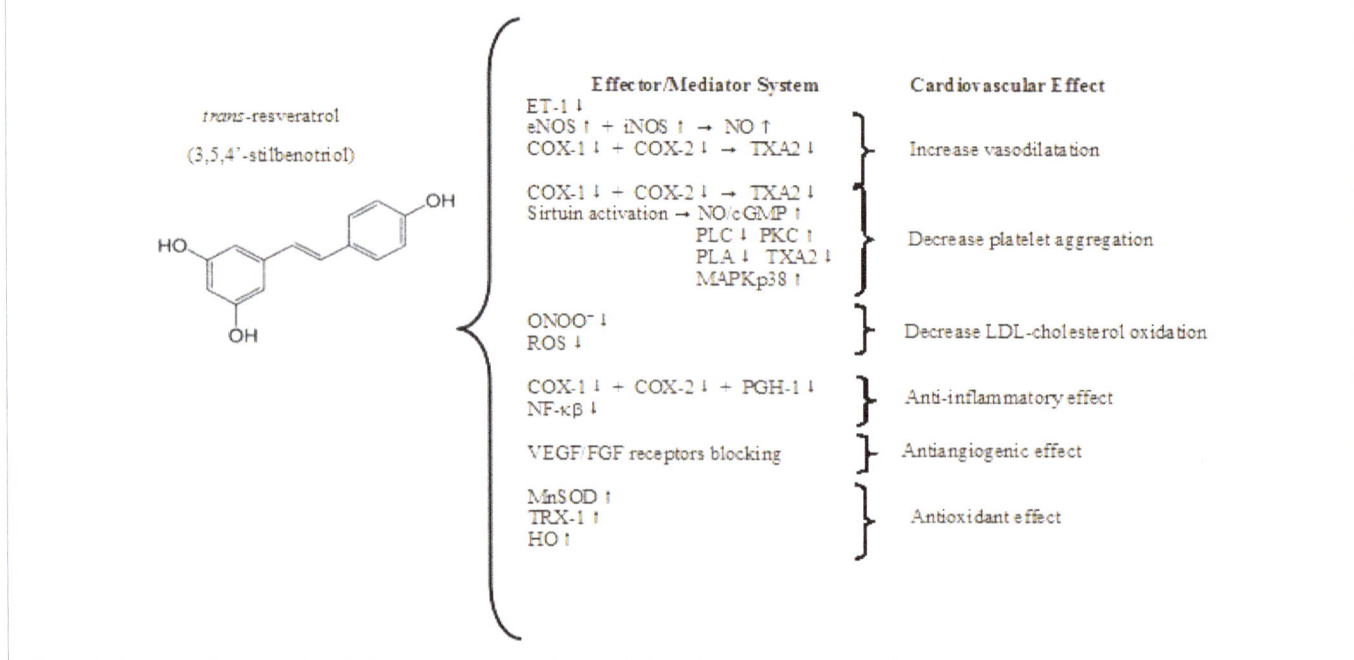

Figure 2: Summary of resveratrol mechanism of action proposed to explain its cardiovascular protection effect, derived from in vitro and in vivo experiments (see text) [36-48].

phosphate and albuminemia, and the latter was also observed in the groups of males administered even the lowest doses of 300 mg/kg [49]. The females exhibited only an increase in plasma alkaline phosphatase levels. As these findings did not follow a dose dependent pattern and as any macroscopic or hystopathological findings explaining them were also absent, they were judged to be toxicologically non-significant [49]. Other studies have not reported pathological changes in any organ within this dosage range of Resv [50].

In another toxicological study, Sprague-Dawley rats were administered Resv in doses of 200, 400 y 1000 mg/kg via gastric tube for 13 weeks. Even when a lower dose-dependent weight gain was observed in females in comparison with the control group, only the group administered the higher dose showed significantly lower body weight at the end of the study, without varying either group's food consumption [51]. In the group administered the highest dose increased average bilirubinemia was observed.

The administration of Resv to Beagle dogs over three months [51] led to lower body weight gain only in the higher dose group (1200 mg/kg), which was observed in both sexes and which may reflect lower dietary intake. At lower doses no adverse effects were observed. Dogs treated with Resv underwent cardiovascular monitoring, including ECG, but no alterations were detected throughout the range of the tested dose.

Another preclinical study was carried out to confirm the efficacy of Resv on the survival of mice consuming a diet rich in calories for more than 20 months [53]. Despite administering Resv in daily doses of up to 22.4 ± 0.4 mg/kg, no significant adverse effect was reported.

Adverse reactions and toxicity in human beings

A recent review addresses adverse reactions to Resv and Resv toxicity in human clinical trials [54] In these studies, Resv was used either in pure form or as part of nutraceutical formulations including polyphenols or other chemical compounds.

Tomé-Carneiro [40] carried out a 12-month clinical study divided into six-month phases. 25 healthy volunteers were administered capsules of a *Vitis vinifera* nutraceutical equivalent to 8 mg of Resv. Throughout the clinical trial, no adverse reactions or hypersensitivity were reported. Aminotransferase, thyroid hormone, albuminemia and creatininemia levels were determined, which did not reveal clinically or statistically significant evidence of changes.

Timmers [55] administered 150 mg of pure Resv to 11 obese subjects for 30 days. No alterations were observed in hematological, coagulation, general biochemical, or electrocardiographic parameters. However, statistically significant reductions were observed in plasma alanine-aminotransferase levels, white blood cell count and inflammatory parameters such as plasma IL-6 or TNF- concentrations in the treatment group. In contrast, another study carried out one year later with a 500 mg/day dose of Resv did not result in altered aminotransferase levels or inflammation factors [56]. The latter study, lasting only 28 days and involving 12 obese patients, was free of adverse events, except for the development of a generalized rash in one patient from the *vero* group during the first week of the clinical trial. The patient concerned subsequently left the study [56].

In a clinical study of 20 cancer patients, subjects were administered Resv in 500 or 1000 mg/day doses for 8 days before a colectomy [57]. In this short study, no adverse treatment-related events were observed, and both doses were well-tolerated.

Chow [26] administered 1000 mg/day of Resv to 24 healthy volunteers for 28 days, without reporting clinically significant alterations in biochemical or hematological parameters. Two volunteers prematurely abandoned the study, one due to a case of diarrhea after the first dose and the second due to the appearance of peri-menopausal symptoms – hot flushes – in a postmenopausal woman.

Coincidentally, in another study carried out on eight healthy volunteers who were administered 2 g/day doses of Resv daily for eight days [58], episodic diarrhea was reported in six of the eight volunteers undergoing treatment. Furthermore, a reaction of rash-type hypersensitivity was reported in one volunteer, which resolved spontaneously.

Howells [21] used a dose of 5 g/day of micronized Resv SRT501 in patients with hepatic metastasis. In five of the six patients undergoing treatment, episodes of light diarrhea were recorded; a second patient also presented nausea and anal pruritus, and a third developed symptoms of hypersensitivity.

A phase II clinical trial using micronized Resv SRT501 co-administered with bortezomib to patients with multiple refractory myelomas was terminated early as many patients developed chronic renal insufficiency during the assay [59]. The close causal relationship between multiple myeloma and deterioration of renal function prevents clearly associating these events with a toxic Resv effect.

The evidence would seem to show that adverse reactions to Resv in doses of less than 1,000 mg/day are scarce and mild, meaning that a cause-effect relationship cannot always be established. At higher doses, the most frequently reported adverse reactions are mild and spontaneously resolving diarrhea. Based on this data and the results of metabolic interactions with cytochrome P-450 complex enzymes at doses higher than 1,000 mg/day, it has been suggested that this dose is the upper limit for clinical trials [43,59].

Discussion

A large amount of information is available on Resv. A simple search for the keyword "resveratrol" in PubMed carried out in January 2015 delivered 7,130 results, with an exponential increase in publication of articles on this subject from 1999 to the present. This has led the scientific community to comment on recommendations of its use in humans. The recommendations proposed at the First International Resveratrol Conference, Resveratrol 2010, in Denmark, found insufficient evidence to justify recommending chronic administration of Resv in humans [43], in contrast to the therapeutic effects reported in commercial material and the media, based on the supposedly beneficial properties of red wine and as a potential explanation for the so-called *French Paradox* [60]. However, results from clinical assays carried out with different formulations of Resv from 2010 onwards suggest that these recommendations should be reviewed.

Pharmacokinetically, Resv is characterized as a rapidly absorbed compound, but which undergoes extensive pre-systemic metabolism by human cytochrome P-450 and intestinal microbiota [17,25,61]. Its metabolism mainly leads to conjugation products, the biological activity of which is still under discussion [28]. It is also rapidly cleared. All of this would explain the bioavailability estimated at around 1% of orally-administered doses [16,61]. Another distinctive feature of Resv is its high inter-individual variability in pharmacokinetic parameters [54].

Resv seems to exert a therapeutic effect on endothelial dysfunction that, although measured with a currently questioned technique [44], is consistent with the *in vitro* observation that Resv stimulates the endothelial nitric oxide synthase enzyme [11]. The inflammatory markers and CRP reductions obtained from doses of Resv equal to or less than 20 mg/day are not observed in larger doses, which could imply that the effects of Resv are hermetic [36]. On the other hand, Resv has been shown to reduce the atherogenic potential of LDL-cholesterol by reducing oxidized LDL and ApoB levels, which are important lipid markers for atherogenesis [47,48].

Analysis of the safety of Resv shows that it is well-tolerated. Short-term (29 days) human studies have shown frequent gastrointestinal discomfort or spontaneously resolving diarrhea only with the administration of high doses (2.5 g to 5 g per day). Only minor and inconsistent adverse effects have been observed in other short acute studies [60]. In animal models, toxic doses produce physiopathological processes in the kidney [40,49].

Conclusion

The published evidence suggests that Resv reduces cardiovascular risk, whether prophylactically or therapeutically. It reduces the incidence of arterial hypertension, heart failure and ischemic cardiac disease in different animal models. Similarly, there is sufficient evidence to suggest that Resv improves insulin sensitivity and reduces the plasma glycemia levels and obesity caused by high-fat diets in rodent models.

The data obtained from animal models is promising and justifies the need for more clinical trials in humans to show the cardiovascular therapeutic potential of Resv, whether administered in pure form or jointly with other formulated or nutraceutical natural compounds.

However it should be reiterated that the current published evidence is not sufficiently strong to recommend the chronic administration of Resv to human beings beyond doses able to be obtained from dietary sources. The administration of Resv in chronic doses, above the concentrations found in food should be considered experimental, until longer clinical trials can take place in humans to ensure the efficacy and safety of Resv.

Acknowledgements

The authors are grateful to the Dr. Tulio Nuñez (University of Chile) for his observations and suggestions.

References

1. Gambini J, López-Grueso R, Olaso-González G, Inglés M, Abdelazid K, et al. (2013) Resveratrol: distribution, properties and perspectives. Rev Esp Geriatr Gerontol 48: 79-88.

2. Aggarwal BB, Bhardwaj A, Aggarwal RS, Seeram NP, Shishodia S, et al. (2004) Role of resveratrol in prevention and therapy of cancer: Preclinical and clinical studies. Anticancer Res 24: 2783-2840.

3. Delmas D, Aires V, Limagne E, Dutartre P, Mazué F, et al. (2011) Transport, stability, and biological activity of resveratrol. Ann N Y Acad Sci 1215: 48-59.

4. Renaud S, de Lorgeril M (1992) Wine, alcohol, platelets, and the French paradox for coronary heart disease. Lancet 339: 1523-1526.

5. Jang M, Cai L, Udeani GO, Slowing KV, Thomas CF, et al. (1997) Cancer Chemopreventive Activity of Resveratrol, a Natural Product Derived from Grapes. Science 275: 218-220.

6. Baur JA, Sinclair DA (2006) Therapeutic potential of resveratrol: The in vivo evidence. Nat Rev Drug Discov 5: 493-506.

7. Tomé-Carneiro J, Larrosa M, González-Sarrías A, Tomás-Barberán FA, García-Conesa MT, et al. (2013) Resveratrol and clinical trials: The crossroad from in vitro studies to human evidence. Curr Pharm Des 19: 6064-6093.

8. Walle T (2011) Bioavailability of resveratrol. Ann N Y Acad Sci 1215: 9-15.

9. Shukla Y, Singh R (2011) Resveratrol and cellular mechanisms of cancer prevention. Ann N Y Acad Sci 1215: 1-8.

10. Szkudelski T, Szkudelska K (2011) Anti-diabetic effects of resveratrol. Ann N Y Acad Sci 1215: 34-39.

11. Petrovski G, Gurusamy N, Das DK (2011) Resveratrol in cardiovascular health and disease. Ann N Y Acad Sci 1215: 22-33.

12. Quincozes-Santos A, Gottfried C (2011) Resveratrol modulates astroglial functions: Neuroprotective hypothesis. Ann N Y Acad Sci 1215: 72-78.

13. Richard T, Pawlus AD, Iglésias ML, Pedrot E, Waffo-Teguo P, et al. (2011) Neuroprotective properties of resveratrol and derivatives. Ann N Y Acad Sci 1215: 103-108.

14. Singh N, Agrawal M, Doré S (2013) Neuroprotective properties and mechanisms of resveratrol in in vitro and in vivo experimental cerebral stroke models. ACS Chem Neurosci 4: 1151-1162.

15. Walle T, Hsieh F, DeLegge MH, Oatis JE Jr, Walle UK (2004) High absorption but very low bioavailability of oral resveratrol in humans. Drug Metab Dispos 32: 1377-1382.

16. Boocock DJ, Faust GE, Patel KR, Schinas AM, Brown VA, et al. (2007) Phase I dose escalation pharmacokinetic study in healthy volunteers of resveratrol, a potential cancer chemo-preventive agent. Cancer Epidemiol Biomarkers Prev 16: 1246-1252.

17. Almeida L, Vaz-da-Silva M, Falcão A, Soares E, Costa R, et al. (2009) Pharmacokinetic and safety profile of trans-resveratrol in a rising multiple-dose study in healthy volunteers. Mol Nutr Food Res 53 Suppl 1: S7-15.

18. Kaldas MI, Walle UK, Walle T (2003) Resveratrol transport and metabolism by human intestinal Caco-2 cells. J Pharm Pharmacol 55: 307-312.

19. Belguendouz L, Fremont L, Linard A (1997) Resveratrol inhibits metal ion-dependent and independent peroxidation of porcine low-density lipoproteins. Biochem Pharmacol 53: 1347-1355.

20. Brown VA, Patel KR, Viskaduraki M, Crowell JA, Perloff M, et al. (2010) Repeat dose study of the cancer chemopreventive agent resveratrol in healthy volunteers: Safety, pharmacokinetics, and effect on the insulin-like growth factor axis. Cancer Res 70: 9003-9011.

21. Howells LM, Berry DP, Elliott PJ, Jacobson EW, Hoffmann E, et al. (2011) Phase I randomized, double-blind pilot study of micronized resveratrol (SRT501) in patients with hepatic metastases-safety, pharmacokinetics, and pharmacodynamics. Cancer Prev Res (Phila) 4: 1419-1425.

22. Vitaglione P, Sforza S, Galaverna G, Ghidini C, Caporaso N, et al. (2005) Bioavailability of trans-resveratrol from red wine in humans. Mol Nutr Food Res 49: 495-504.

23. Vaz-da-Silva M, Loureiro AI, Falcao A, Nunes T, Rocha JF, et al. (2008) Effect of food on the pharmacokinetic profile of trans-resveratrol. Int J Clin Pharmacol Ther 46: 564-570.

24. Stervbo U, Vang O, Bonnesen C (2007) A review of the content of the putative chemo-preventive phytoalexin resveratrol in red wine. Food Chem 101: 449-457.

25. Bode LM, Bunzel D, Huch M, Cho GS, Ruhland D, et al. (2013) In vivo and in vitro metabolism of trans-resveratrol by human gut microbiota. Am J Clin Nutr 97: 295-309.

26. Chow HH, Garland LL, Hsu CH, Vining DR, Chew WM, et al. (2010) Resveratrol modulates drug- and carcinogen-metabolizing enzymes in a healthy volunteer study. Cancer Prev Res (Phila) 3: 1168-1175.

27. Wang LX, Heredia A, Song H, Zhang Z, Yu B, et al. (2004) Resveratrol glucuronides as the metabolites of resveratrol in humans: Characterization, synthesis, and anti-HIV activity. J Pharm Sci 93: 2448-2457.

28. Burkon A, Somoza V (2008) Quantification of free and protein-bound trans-resveratrol metabolites and identification of trans-resveratrol-C/O-conjugated diglucuronides - two novel resveratrol metabolites in human plasma. Mol Nutr Food Res 52: 549-557.

29. Maier-Salamon A, Hagenauer B, Wirth M, Gabor F, Szekeres T, et al. (2006) Increased transport of resveratrol across monolayers of the human intestinal Caco-2 cells is mediated by inhibition and saturation of metabolites. Pharmaceut Res 23: 2107-2115.

30. Kapetanovic IM, Muzzio M, Huang Z, Thompson TN, McCormick DL (2011) Pharmacokinetics, oral bioavailability, and metabolic profile of resveratrol and its dimethylether analog, pterostilbene, in rats. Cancer Chemother Pharmacol 68: 593-601.

31. Bourassa P, Kanakis CD, Tarantilis P, Pollissiou MG, Tajmir-Riahi HA (2010) Resveratrol, genistein, and curcumin bind bovine serum albumin. J Phys Chem B 114: 3348-3354.

32. Liang L, Liu X, Wang Q, Cheng S, Zhang S, et al. (2013) Pharmacokinetics, tissue distribution and excretion study of resveratrol and its prodrug 3,5,4'-tri-O-acetylresveratrol in rats. Phytomedicine 20: 558-563.

33. Patel KR, Scott E, Brown VA, Gescher AJ, Steward WP, et al. (2011) Clinical trials of resveratrol. Ann N Y Acad Sci 1215: 161-169.

34. Marier JF, Vachon P, Gritsas A, Zhang J, Moreau JP, et al. (2002) Metabolism and disposition of resveratrol in rats: extent of absorption, glucuronidation, and enterohepatic recirculation evidenced by a linked-rat model. J Pharmacol Exp Ther 302: 369-373.

35. Nunes T, Almeida L, Rocha JF, Falcão A, Fernandes-Lopes C, et al. (2009) Pharmacokinetics of trans-resveratrol following repeated administration in healthy elderly and young subjects. J Clin Pharmacol 49: 1477-1482.

36. Calabrese EJ, Mattson MP, Calabrese V (2010) Resveratrol commonly displays hormesis: Occurrence and biomedical significance. Hum Exp Toxicol 29: 980-1015.

37. Dudley J, Das S, Mukherjee S, Das DK (2009) Resveratrol, a unique phytoalexin present in red wine, delivers either survival signal or death signal to the ischemic myocardium depending on dose. J Nutr Biochem 20: 443-452.

38. Wong RH, Howe PR, Buckley JD, Coates AM, Kunz I, et al. (2011) Acute resveratrol supplementation improves flow-mediated dilatation in overweight/obese individuals with mildly elevated blood pressure. Nutr Metab Cardiovasc Dis 21: 851-856.

39. Chiva-Blanch G, Urpi-Sarda MLlorach R, Rotches-Ribalta M, Guillén M, Rosa Casas, et al. (2012) Differential effects of polyphenols and alcohol of red wine on the expression of adhesion molecules and inflammatory cytokines related to atherosclerosis: a randomized clinical trial. Am J Clin Nutr 95: 326-334.

40. Tomé-Carneiro J, Gonzálvez M, Larrosa M, Yáñez-Gascón MJ, García-Almagro FJ, et al. (2012) One-year consumption of a grape nutraceutical containing resveratrol improves the inflammatory and fibrinolytic status of patients in primary prevention of cardiovascular disease. Am J Cardiol 110: 356-363.

41. Fujitaka K, Otani H, Jo F, Jo H, Nomura E, et al. (2011) Modified resveratrol Longevinex improves endothelial function in adults with metabolic syndrome receiving standard treatment. Nutr Res 31. 842-047.

42. Magyar K, Halmosi R, Palfi A, Feher G, Czopf L, et al. (2012) Cardioprotection by resveratrol: A human clinical trial in patients with stable coronary artery disease. Clin Hemorheol Microcirc 50: 179-187.

43. Vang O (2013) What is new for resveratrol? Is a new set of recommendations necessary? Ann N Y Acad Sci 1290: 1-11.

44. Atkinson G, Batterham AM (2015) The clinical relevance of the percentage flow-mediated dilation index. Curr Hypertens Rep 17: 4.

45. Militaru C, Donoiu I, Craciun A, Scorei ID, Bulearca AM, et al. (2013) Oral resveratrol and calcium fructoborate supplementation in subjects with stable angina pectoris: effects on lipid profiles, inflammation markers, and quality of life. Nutrition 29: 178-183.

46. Zamani B, Saatlo BB, Naghavi-Behzad M, Taqizadeh-Jahed M, Alikhah H, et al. (2014) Effects of high versus low-dose atorvastatin on high sensitive C-reactive protein in acute coronary syndrome. Niger Med J 55: 490-494.

47. Tomé-Carneiro J, Gonzálvez M, Larrosa M, García-Almagro FJ, Avilés-Plaza F, et al. (2012) Consumption of a grape extract supplement containing resveratrol decreases oxidized LDL and ApoB in patients undergoing primary prevention of cardiovascular disease: A triple-blind, 6-month follow-up, placebo-controlled, randomized trial. Mol Nutr Food Res 56: 810-821.

48. Contois JH, Warnick GR, Sniderman AD (2011) Reliability of low-density lipoprotein cholesterol, non-high-density lipoprotein cholesterol, and apolipoprotein B measurement. J Clin Lipidol 5: 264-272.

49. Williams LD, Burdock GA, Edwards JA, Beck M, Bausch J (2009) Safety studies conducted on high-purity trans-resveratrol in experimental animals. Food Chem Toxicol 47: 2170-2182.

50. Crowell JA, Korytko PJ, Morrissey RL, Booth TD, Levine BS (2004) Resveratrol-associated renal toxicity. Toxicol Sci 82: 614-619.

51. Johnson WD, Morrissey RL, Usborne AL, Kapetanovic I, Crowell JA, et al. (2011) Subchronic oral toxicity and cardiovascular safety pharmacology studies of resveratrol, a naturally occurring polyphenol with cancer preventive activity. Food Chem Toxicol 49: 3319-3327.

52. Elliott PJ, Walpole S, Morelli L, Lambert PD, Lunsmann W, et al. (2009) Resveratrol/SRT501. Sirtuin SIRT1 activator, treatment of type 2 diabetes. Drugs Fut 34: 291-295.

53. Baur JA, Pearson KJ, Price NL, Jamieson HA, Lerin C, et al. (2006) Resveratrol improves health and survival of mice on a high-calorie diet. Nature 444: 337-342.

54. Cottart CH, Nivet-Antoine V, Beaudeux JL (2014) Review of recent data on the metabolism, biological effects, and toxicity of resveratrol in humans. Mol Nutr Food Res 58: 7-21.

55. Timmers S, Konings E, Bilet L, Houtkooper RH, van de Weijer T, et al. (2011) Calorie restriction-like effects of 30 days of resveratrol supplementation on energy metabolism and metabolic profile in obese humans. Cell Metab 14: 612-622.

56. Poulsen MM, Vestergaard PF, Clasen BF, Radko Y, Christensen LP, et al. (2013) High-dose resveratrol supplementation in obese men: an investigator-initiated, randomized, placebo-controlled clinical trial of substrate metabolism, insulin sensitivity, and body composition. Diabetes 62: 1186-1195.

57. Patel KR, Brown VA, Jones DJ, Britton RG, Hemingway D, et al. (2010) Clinical pharmacology of resveratrol and its metabolites in colorectal cancer patients. Cancer Res 70: 7392-7399.

58. la Porte C, Voduc N, Zhang G, Seguin I, Tardiff D, et al. (2010) Steady-State pharmacokinetics and tolerability of trans-resveratrol 2000 mg twice daily with food, quercetin and alcohol (ethanol) in healthy human subjects. Clin Pharmacokinet 49: 449-454.

59. Popat R, Plesner T, Davies F, Cook G, Cook M, et al. (2013) A phase 2 study of SRT501 (resveratrol) with bortezomib for patients with relapsed and or refractory multiple myeloma. Br J Haematol 160: 714-717.

60. Vang O, Ahmad N, Baile CA, Baur JA, Brown K, et al. (2011) What is new for an old molecule? Systematic review and recommendations on the use of resveratrol. PLoS One 6: e19881.

61. Rotches-Ribalta M, Andres-Lacueva C, Estruch R, Escribano E, Urpi-Sarda M (2012) Pharmacokinetics of resveratrol metabolic profile in healthy humans after moderate consumption of red wine and grape extract tablets. Pharmacol Res 66: 375-382.

24

Protective Effects of Cyclohexyl methyl dithiocarbamates Sodium Salts on Diclofenac Induced Reproductive Toxicity in Male Albino Rats

Adegbegi J Ademuyiwa[1*], Jose R Adeolu[1] and Adefegha S Adeniyi[2]

[1]Department of Science Laboratory Technology, Rufus Giwa Polytechnic, Owo, Ondo State, Nigeria
[2]Department of Biochemistry, Federal University of Technology, Akure, Ondo State, Nigeria

Abstract

The present study investigates the effect of cyclohexylmethyldithiocarbamates sodium salt (a synthetic compound) and vitamin E against diclofenac-induced blood and testes of experimental Wistar male albino rats. The study consists of six groups of six rats each. Group I (control) received corn oil (3 ml/kg b.w), Group II received diclofenac (100 mg/kg b.w), Group III rats were treated with diclofenac and cyclohexylmethyldithiocarbamates sodium salt (30 mg/kg b.w), Group IV was administered diclofenac and Vitamin E (30 mg/kg b.w), Group V was given cyclohexylmethyldithiocarbamates sodium salt (30 mg/kg b.w) only and Group VI received vitamin E only. The results showed a significant ($p<0.05$) decrease in the daily sperm production in the diclofenac only treated rats, diclofenac with Na (HxMedtc), diclofenac with vitamin E treated rats and Na (HxMedtc) treated rats but no significant ($p>0.05$) in the vitamin E only treated rats when compared with the control. There was a significant ($p<0.05$) decrease in the Testicular sperm number (TSN) in the diclofenac only treated rats, diclofenac with Vitamin E treated rats and vitamin E only treated rats and no significant ($p>0.05$) decrease in the diclofenac with Na (HxMedtc) treated rats and Na (HxMedtc) only treated rats when compared with the control. Also, there was a significant ($p<0.05$) decrease in TSN in the diclofenac with Na (HxMedtc) treated rats and diclofenac with vitamin E treated rats when compared with diclofenac only treated rats. And a decrease ($p<0.05$) in the daily sperm production (DSP) in the diclofenac only treated rats, and diclofenac with cyclohexylmethyldithiocarbamate sodium salt only treated rats when compared with the control.

Keywords: Cyclohexyl methyl dithiocarbamates sodium salt; Diclofenac; Albino rats; Vitamin E

Introduction

The testis is the organ responsible for the production of spermatozoa and hormones which are required for maintenance of secondary sexual functions [1]. Exogenous compounds such as drugs and other foreign substances may interfere with the synthesis, secretion, transport, binding, action or elimination of hormones responsible for the reproduction and other physiological functions of the body [2], thereby disrupting spermatogenesis. Exposure to varying concentrations of these endogenous compounds has also been reported to cause adverse effects on several organs and alter several defense mechanisms in both animal and human models [3].

Diclofenac, a 2-arylacetic acid, (marketed as Voltaren), is a non-steroidal anti-inflammatory drug (NSAID) taken to reduce inflammation and as an analgesic reducing pain in conditions such as arthritis or acute injury [4]. Recent evidence suggests that diclofenac metabolism involves the production of reactive oxygen species leading to oxidative stress and genomic DNA fragmentation [5,6]. Furthermore, there are indications that the mitochondrial inner membrane permeabilization and activity of caspases play a crucial role in the pathogenesis of diclofenac [7].

Furthermore, it has been reported that the extensive use of diclofenac increases the risk of acute myocardial infarction and several cases of severe local reactions associated with intramuscular injection of diclofenac have been reported [8]. Diclofenac was found to generate protein adducts in the livers of treated mice as well as in rat hepatocytes via protein acylation by the drug glucuronide [9]. *In vitro* experiments with cultured rat hepatocytes have shown, however, that the covalent binding of diclofenac is neither the only nor the major cause of acute cytotoxicity [10]. Moreover, previous work has suggested that diclofenac is cytotoxic to rat hepatocytes after cytochrome P-450 (CYP)-mediated metabolism [11].

Dithiocarbamates are the reduced forms of thiuram disulfides with strong complexing properties [11]. They exhibit very rich coordination chemistry with a large variety of transition metals and are used as vulcanizing (analytical agents) [12]. Thiuram disulfides (thiram), dithiocarbamate salts (nabam) or their complexes with iron (ferbam), manganese (maneb) and zinc (ziram, zineb, propineb, metiram) are well known as pesticides with an estimated annual global consumption of 25,000 – 35,000 metric tons [12].

Dithiocarbamates exert both antioxidant and pro-oxidant effects in cells [13]. Their antioxidant behaviour includes eliminating hydrogen peroxide and scavenging the superoxide radical, peroxynitrite and the hydroxyl radical [14] and lipid peroxidation products such as the peroxyl radical [13]. The reaction of dithiocarbamates with reactive oxygen and nitrogen species generates dithiocarbamate thiyl radicals which ultimately dimerize to form thiuram disulphides [13], the oxidized form of dithiocarbamates. The pro-oxidant consequences of dithiocarbamate action, including that of PDTC and diethyldithiocarbamate have recently been highlighted with respect to their effects on apoptosis [15]. However, there is limited information on the effects of dithiocarbamate sodium salts and diclofenac on reproductive system. The purpose of this study, therefore, is to investigate the effect of dithiocarbamate on diclofenac induced testicular damage in rats.

*Corresponding author: Adegbegi J Ademuyiwa, Department of Science Laboratory Technology, Rufus Giwa Polytechnic, Owo, Ondo State, Nigeria, E-mail: muyithegreat@yahoo.com

Materials and Methods

Materials

Chemicals and reagents: *N,N*-dibenzylamine (Boheringer), *N*-benzyl-*N*ethylamine (Aldrich), *N*-benzyl-*N*-isopropylamine (Boheringer), *N*-benzyl-*N*-methylamine (Aldrich), *N*-ethyl-*N*methylamine (Aldrich) and *N*-benzyl-2-phenethylamine (Boheringer).

Animal ethics

All of the animals received humane care according to the criteria outline in the Guide for the Care and the Use of Laboratory Animals prepared by the National Academy Science and published by the National Institute of Health (USA). The ethic regulations have been followed in accordance with national and institutional guidelines for the protection of animals' welfare during experiments. The experiment was carried out at the Drug Metabolism and Toxicology Laboratory, Department of Biochemistry, University of Ibadan, Oyo State, Nigeria.

Preparation of test compounds (Dithiocarbamates)

Synthesis of Cyclohexyldithiocarbamate salt: Thiophosgene, chlorothioformates and isothiocyanates were used in the synthesis of dithiocarbamates (DTCs) according to the method described by [12]. Amines were mixed with dithiocarbamate and sodium salts without any solvent and then maleic anhydride was slowly added to this mixture at room temperature. The combination produced dithiocarbamate derivatives of about 70% yields at room temperature. The product is stable even under reflux in toluene for 12 h.

Chemicals and reagents preparation

All chemicals were if an analytical grade and are supplied from sigma chemical co. USA. Distilled water was used in all biochemical assays.

Experimental Animals

Thirty-six (36) adults Laboratory breed male wistar albino rats weighing between 120-150 g were purchased from covenant Farm limited, Gbolasire, Iwo Road, Ibadan, and Oyo state. The animals were maintained under standardized environmental conditions in a well ventilated rat house in cages, in the departmental animal house at room temperature (22-28ºC), under controlled light cycle of 12 hrs light/ 12 hrs dark with free access to standard rat feed purchased from Ladokun Feeds Nig. Limited, Ibadan, Nigeria and water supplied *ad libitum*.

Experimental Design

The thirty-six rats used for the experiment were randomly assigned to six (6) groups at the end of acclimatization period. The animals in group 1 serve as control and received corn oil throughout the treatment period. Animals of groups 2, 3, 4, 5 and 6 received diclofenac only, diclofenac and Cyclohexylmethyldithiocarbamate sodium salt, Diclofenac and vitamin E, Cyclohexylmethyldithiocarbamate sodium salt only and vitamin E only respectively. The animals in the test group were pretreated with vitamin E (groups 5 and 6) and the test compound (groups 3 and 4) for one week. Appropriate dose dilutions were made with distilled water and corn oil for test compound and vitamin E respectively based on body weight (100 mg/kg) to provide for a total volume of 0.3 ml. Thus, 0.3 ml of dose dilution was similarly administered orally through gavage to each rat. All the surviving animals were sacrificed after 24 hrs of diclofenac.

Semen collection and characteristics

Daily feed intake and body weight were recorded weekly. Total sperm output calculated by multiplying semen ejaculate volume and semen concentration. Assessment of live and abnormal spermatozoa was performed using an eosin– nigrosine blue staining mixture [12]. The percentages of motile sperm were estimated by visual examination under low-power magnification (10×) using a phase-contrast microscope with heated stage. Total number of motile sperm calculated by multiplying percentage of motile sperm and total sperm outputs. Reaction time for the buck is calculated as the time needs for mounting a doe until complete ejaculation; it measured in seconds using a stopwatch. Initial hydrogen ion concentration (pH) of semen samples was determined immediately after collection using a pH cooperative paper (Universal indikator pH 0-14 Merck, Merck KgaA, 64271 Darmstadt, Germany). Packed sperm volume (PSV) was recorded. Total functional sperm fraction (TFSF) parameter was also calculated as (total sperm output × motility (%) × normal morphology (%) [16].

Blood collection and testosterone determination

Blood samples were collected from the ear vein of each buck every other week and placed immediately on ice in heparinized tubes. Plasma was collected from blood by centrifuged at 860 g for 20 min and stored at -60ºC. Testosterone concentration in plasma was measured by simple solid phase enzyme immunoassay utilizing horseradish peroxidase as a tracer (Equipar, via G. Ferrari, Saronno, Italy). Intra and interassay coefficient of variations were 3.9% and 6.2%, respectively. All rats were euthanized at the end of the experimental period (16 week). Weight of testis and epididymis was recorded.

Organ collection

The testes were collected, weighed and excised. Part of it was excised and stored in 50% formalin solution for Histology studies and the other was removed into ice-cold 0.25 M sucrose solution. It was then blotted with tissue paper and homogenized in ice-cold 0.25M sucrose solution (1:5 w/v) using Teflon homogenizer. This was kept frozen until required for the enzyme assay.

Statistical analysis

Results are presented as means ± SD. Effect of non-enzymatic antioxidants for different variables was analyzed by the analysis of variance (ANOVA). When the F–ratio was significant ($P < 0.05$), Tukey's Honestly significant difference was used to compare the treatment mean.

Results

Results show no significant decrease ($P < 0.05$) in the body weight of all animals administered with Diclofenac and cyclohexylmethyldithiocarbamates sodium salt (Na (HxMedtc)) as compared with control (Table 1).

Table 2 above is a significant ($p < 0.05$) decrease in the sperm motility and count in the diclofenac only treated rats, diclofenac with Na (HxMedtc) treated rats, diclofenac with Vitamin E treated rats, Na (HxMedtc) only treated rats and vitamin E only treated rats when compared with the control. There is also a significant decrease ($p < 0.05$) in the live/dead in the diclofenac with Na (HxMedtc) treated rats, diclofenac with Vitamin E treated rats, Na (HxMedtc) only treated rats when compared with the control. Also, no significant ($p > 0.05$) decrease in the number of dead/live diclofenac with vitamin E treated rats and diclofenac with Na (HxMedtc) treated rats, but there is a significant (p>0.05) in the sperm motility and sperm count in this treated rats when compared with the control. But there is no significant (p>0.05) decrease in the sperm motility, count and live/dead in the Na (HxMedtc) only treated rats, when compare with the diclofenac and Na (HxMedtc) treated rats. No significant (p>0.05) decrease in the sperm motility, live/dead and count in the vitamin E only treated rats when compared with vitamin E and diclofenac treated rats.

There was a significant (p<0.05) decrease in the daily sperm production in the diclofenac only treated rats, diclofenac with Na (HxMedtc), diclofenac with vitamin E treated rats and Na (HxMedtc) treated rats but no significant (p>0.05) in the vitamin E only treated rats when compared with the control. There is an increase (64%) inhibition in the diclofenac with Na (HxMedtc) treated rats when compared with the Na (HxMedtc) only treated rats against the control an increase (29%) inhibition in the daily sperm production in the diclofenac and vitamin E treated rats when compared with vitamin E only treated rats (Table 3).

There is a significant (p<0.05) decrease in the TSN in the diclofenac only treated rats, diclofenac with Vitamin E treated rats and vitamin E only treated rats and no significant (p>0.05) decrease in the diclofenac with Na (HxMedtc) treated rats and Na (HxMedtc) only treated rats when compared with the control. Also, there is a significant (p<0.05) decrease in Testicular sperm number (TSN) in the diclofenac with Na HxMedtc) treated rats and diclofenac with vitamin E treated rats when compared with diclofenac only treated rats (Table 4).

Discussion

Treatment with Diclofenac and Cyclohexylmethyldithiocarbamates Sodium Salts reduced testosterone levels, feed intake and body weight (BW) (Table 1). Moreover, previous studies also showed a decrease in these parameters in rabbits treated with cypermethrin [17,18]. Reported that the reduction of body weight of rabbits treated with carbofuran and glyphosate may be due to direct cytotoxic effect of the pesticides on somatic cells, and/or indirectly through the central nervous system which control feed and water intake and regulates the endocrine function. Also, the failure of different species exposed to environmental

toxicant to gain body weight may be due to the decrease in feed intake, malabsorption of nutrients from the gastrointestinal tract and impaired feed conversion efficiency [19]. The decline in the BW of treated rabbits with appeared as a result of lesser intake of feed Cyclohexyl methyl dithiocarbamates Sodium Salts and Diclofenac (Table 1).

Semen quality (Table 2) deteriorated following treatment with Cyclohexylmethyldithiocarbamates Sodium Salts and Diclofenac and these results are in agreement with the previous studies [20,21]. Exposure to Diclofenac caused sexual dysfunction in male rats [19]. The decline in ejaculate volume, sperm concentration, total sperm output, and packed sperm volume (PSV), and increased reaction time can be partly attributed to the Diclofenac-induced reduction in testosterone levels (Table 3). The effects of certain drugs on spermatogenesis may be mediated through their effects on hormonal balance.

Previous studies showed reduced semen quality in men occupationally exposed to various pesticides [22] and in animals [23]. Additionally, [24] found that treatment with cypermethrin caused reduction in the fertility of male rats. Also, the epididymal and testicular sperm counts as well as daily sperm production were significantly decreased and the number of implantation sites was significantly reduced in females mated with males that had ingested cypermethrin. The decrease in sperm packed volume of immobile sperms. Fructose synthesis and secretion by the accessory glands is dependent upon the secretion of testosterone by the testes [25,26] reported that generation of reactive oxygen species and peroxidation of sperm membranes could bring negative effects on motility, midpiece abnormalities and sperm-oocyte fusion [27]. Suggested that pesticide's disruption of reproductive processes might be in part due to adverse effects on sperm cell function. In general the effect of Diclofenac on sperm quality may be due to the decrease in plasma testosterone concentration and/or indirectly by reducing feed intake.

Vitamin E treatment

Treatment with vitamin E alone caused a slight significant (P<0.05) decrease in body weight and relative testes and epididymis weights (Table 1) [28] found that supplementation of vitamin E to California and New Zealand White rabbits increased body weight gain and improved feed efficiency compared to the control group. Our previous studies showed that vitamin E supplementation stimulated weight gain in rats and rabbits [29] which is in agreement with the present results. The beneficial effects of vitamin E noted in the present study can be attributed to the antioxidant effects of this vitamin; it is scavenger of oxygen-free radicals which are toxic byproducts of many metabolic processes [19,30,31]. Vitamin E protects critical cellular structures against damage caused by oxygen-free radicals and reactive products of lipid peroxidation. It has been reported that lipid peroxidation was prevented by vitamin E [29,30]. Vitamin E inhibits peroxidation of membrane lipids by scavenging lipid peroxyl radicals, as a consequence

Group	Initial weight (g)	Final weight (g)
Control	115 ± 5.48	116 ± 4.18
Diclofenac only	153 ± 5.16	132 ± 14.38
Diclofenac and Na(c-HxMedtc)	118 ± 11.69	116 ± 11.40
Diclofenac and Vitamin E	132 ± 4.08	107 ± 5.77
Na(c-HxMedtc) only	140 ± 0.00	135 ± 8.95
Vitamin E only	118 ± 11.69	116 ± 11.40

Values are expressed as means ± SEM of six independent experiments. Means in the same column not sharing the same letter(s) are significantly different (p < 0.05).
Table 1: Effects of administration on the initial and final body weight of experimental rats.

Treatment Group	Motility	Live/Dead	Count
Control	93.75 ± 2.50	98.00 ± 0.00	91.75 ± 7.67
Diclofenac only	76.00 ± 5.48*	93.5 ± 5.10	67.80 ± 4.44*
Diclofenac and Na(c-HxMedtc)	56.67 ± 5.77**	90.00 ± 5.00*	53.00 ± 2.65**
Diclofenac and Vitamin E	45.00 ± 7.07*	90.00 ± 5.00*	45.00 ± 4.58**
Na(c-HxMedtc) only	60.00 ± 8.94*	90.5 ± 5.24*	50.83 ± 7.00*
Vitamin E only	65.00 ± 5.77*	93.60 ± 3.51*	46.00 ± 2.65*

Values are expressed as means ± SEM of six independent experiments. Means in the same column not sharing the same letter(s) are significantly different (p < 0.05)
Table 2: Effect of cyclohexylmethyldithiocarbamates sodium salt , vitamin E, and Diclofenac on Spermatozoan of Albino rats

Group	Daily Sperm Production (10^6)
Control	4.83 ± 0.21
Diclofenac only	1.80 ± 0.24*
Diclofenac and Na(c-HxMedtc)	7.90 ± 0.94**
Diclofenac and Vitamin E	3.42 ± 0.62**
Na(c-HxMedtc) only	3.03 ± 0.35**
Vitamin E only	3.89 ± 0.49

Values are expressed as means ± SEM of six independent experiments. Means in the same column not sharing the same letter(s) are significantly different (p < 0.05).
Table 3: Effect of cyclohexylmethyldithiocarbamates sodium salt, vitamin E, and Diclofenac on daily sperm production of Albino rats

Group	Control	Diclofenac only	Diclofenac and Na (c-HxMedtc)	Diclofenac and Vitamin E	Na (c-HxMedtc) only	Vitamin E only
Tailess tail	0.83 ± 0.14	1.16 ± 0.14*	1.37 ± 0.20*	1.24 ± 0.25*	1.24 ± 0.25*	1.16 ± 0.14*
Headless tail	0.74 ± 0.01	1.24 ± 0.01*	1.13 ± 0.18**	0.83 ± 0.14*	0.92 ± 0.144	0.83 ± 0.14
Rudiment	0.66 ± 0.14	0.7 ± 0.01	0.75 ± 0.00**	0.5 ± 0.25	0.67 ± 0.14	0.67 ± 0.14
Bent tail	1.64 ± 0.12	2.24 ± 0.02*	2.47 ± 0.00**	2.66 ± 0.13**	2.57 ± 0.154**	2.42 ± 0.14*
Curved tail	1.73 ± 0.03	2.24 ± 0.02*	2.49 ± 0.02**	3.07 ± 0.60**	2.22 ± 0.03**	2.75 ± 0.00*
Bent mid-Pierce	1.63 ± 0.11	2.15 ± 0.25*	2.12 ± 0.19*	3.07 ± 0.16**	2.63 ± 0.15**	2.57** ± 0.13
Curved mid Pierce	1.48 ± 0.02	2.31 ± 0.11*	0.61 ± 0.16*	2.74 ± 0.02**	2.58 ± 0.14	2.67 ± 0.14*
Looped tail	0.40 ± 0.13	0.41 ± 0.14*	0.63 ± 0.18	0.5 ± 0.25	0.74 ± 0.01*	0.67 ± 0.14*
Total	9.11 ± 0.21	12.50 ± 0.51*	13.55 ± 0.60*	14.61 ± 0.31*	13.58 ± 0.36*	13.73 ± 0.03**

Values are expressed as means ± SEM of six independent experiments. Means in the same column not sharing the same letter (s) are significantly different (p < 0.05)

Table 4: Effect of cyclohexylmethyldithiocarbamates sodium salt, vitamin E, and Diclofenac on Testicular sperm number (TSN) of Albino rats

of which it is converted into a-tocopheroxyl radical. This radical is thought to be either recycled to a-tocopherol by interacting with soluble antioxidants, such as ascorbic acid, or irreversibly oxidized to a-tocopherylquinone. In fact, a-tocopherylquinone may act as a potent anticoagulant and as an antioxidant through its reduction to hydroquinone [31]. Also, [32] reported that the protective role of vitamin E against the toxicity of oxidants may be due to the quenching of hydroxyl radicals.

Similarly, [33] reported that vitamin E supplementation reduced ROS generation and protected spermatozoa from loss of motility [34] found that oral treatment with 200 mg vitamin E daily decreased reactive oxygen species significantly and increased fertilization rate of fertile normospermic human male after one month of treatment. Also, [35] reported that treatment with vitamin E decreased the formation of TBARS and improved semen quality of rabbits. In addition, in vitro study using rabbit sperm by [36] showed that vitamin E decreased TBARS and increased antioxidant enzymes (superoxide dismutase and catalase). They also reported that supplementation with vitamin E was more effective in improving sperm characteristics and in reducing the production of reactive oxygen species than Vitamin C [37] reported that in vivo experiments, seven weeks of oral vitamin E (1000 IU/d/ animal) administration in boar caused a significant fall in the level of seminal plasma TBARS from 2.2 to 1.2 nmol/ml and significantly increased the number of spermatozoa. Therefore, the improving effect of vitamin E on semen characteristics may be due to the reduction in lipid peroxidation potential. The ameliorating effect of vitamin E (Table 2) against the toxicity of lambda-cyhalothrin on semen quality may be due to their role as antioxidant through quenching 1O2 or free radical and reacting with peroxyl radicals [38].

From the present results, it can be concluded that concurrent administration of Cyclohexylmethyldithiocarbamates Sodium Salts and Vitamin E to Diclofenac-treated animals ameliorated the induced sperm quality damage, significantly improved the sperm parameters and reduced the induction of seminal plasma free radicals. This is consistent with a vital role of vitamin E in antioxidant systems that protect against Diclofenac damage, possibly by preventing oxidative damage to sperm.

The present study suggests therapeutic effects of Cyclohexylmethyldithiocarbamates Sodium Salts Vitamin E to minimize the reproductive toxicity of Diclofenac exposure.

References

1. Saradha B, Mathur PP (2006) Induction of oxidative stress by lindane in epididymis of adult male rats. Environ Toxicol Pharmacol 22: 90-96.

2. Mackey R, Eden J (1998) Phytoestrogens and the menopause. Climacteric 1: 302-308.

3. Richburg JH, Nañez A, Gao H (1999) Participation of the Fas-signaling system in the initiation of germ cell apoptosis in young rat testes after exposure to mono-(2-ethylhexyl) phthalate. Toxicol Appl Pharmacol 160: 271-278.

4. Sallmann AR (1986) The history of diclofenac. Am J Med 80: 29-33.

5. Hickey EJ, Raje RR, Reid VE, Gross SM, Ray SD (2001) Diclofenac induced in vivo nephrotoxicity may involve oxidative stress-mediated massive genomic DNA fragmentation and apoptotic cell death. Free Radic Biol Med 31: 139-152.

6. Inoue A, Muranaka S, Fujita H, Kanno T, Tamai H, et al. (2004) Molecular mechanism of diclofenac-induced apoptosis of promyelocytic leukemia: dependency on reactive oxygen species, Akt, Bid, cytochrome and caspase pathway. Free Radic Biol Med 37: 1290-1299.

7. Gómez-Lechón MJ, Ponsoda X, O'Connor E, Donato T, Castell JV, et al. (2003) Diclofenac induces apoptosis in hepatocytes by alteration of mitochondrial function and generation of ROS. Biochem Pharmacol 66: 2155-2167.

8. Pillans PI, O'Connor N (1995) Tissue necrosis and necrotizing fasciitis after intramuscular administration of diclofenac. Ann Pharmacother 29: 264-266.

9. Pumford NR, Myers TG, Davila JC, Highet RJ, Pohl LR (1993) Immunochemical detection of liver protein adducts of the nonsteroidal antiinflammatory drug diclofenac. Chem Res Toxicol 6: 147-150.

10. Kretz-Rommel A, Boelsterli UA (1993) Diclofenac covalent protein binding is dependent on acyl glucuronide formation and is inversely related to P450-mediated acute cell injury in cultured rat hepatocytes. Toxicol Appl Pharmacol 120: 155-161.

11. Schmitz G, Stauffert I, Sippel H, Lepper H, Estler CJ (1992) Toxicity of diclofenac to isolated hepatocytes. J Hepatol 14: 408-409.

12. Blom E (1950) A one-minute live-dead sperm stain by means of eosin–nigrosin. J Fertil Steril 1: 176–177.

13. Zanocco AL, Pavez R, Videla LA, Lissi EA (1989) Antioxidant capacity of diethyldithiocarbamate in a metal independent lipid peroxidative process. Free Radic Biol Med 7: 151-156.

14. Liu J, Shigenaga MK, Yan LJ, Mori A, Ames BN (1996) Antioxidant activity of diethyldithiocarbamate. Free Radic Res 24: 461-472.

15. Nobel CS, Burgess DH, Zhivotovsky B, Burkitt MJ, Orrenius S, et al. (1997) Mechanism of dithiocarbamate inhibition of apoptosis: thiol oxidation by dithiocarbamate disulfides directly inhibits processing of the caspase-3 proenzyme. Chem Res Toxicol 10: 636-643.

16. Correa JR, Zavos PM (1996) Preparation and recovery of frozen-thawed bovine spermatozoa via various sperm selection techniques employed in assisted reproductive technologies. Theriogenology 46: 1225–1232.

17. Ronconi L, MacCato C, Barreca D, Saini R, Zancato M, et al. (2005) Gold(III) dithiocarbamate derivatives of N-methylglycine: an experimental and theoretical investigation. Polyhedron 24: 521–531.

18. Yousef MI, Awad TI, Mohamed EH (2006) Deltamethrin-induced oxidative damage and biochemical alterations in rat and its attenuation by Vitamin E. Toxicology 227: 240-247.

19. Yousef MI, Salem MH, Ibrahim HZ, Helmi S, Seehy MA, et al. (1995) Toxic effects of carbofuran and glyphosate on semen characteristics in rabbits. J Environ Sci Health B 30: 513-534.

20. Ball LM, Chhabra RS (1981) Intestinal absorption of nutrients in rats treated

with 2,3,7,8-tetrachlorodibenzo-p-dioxin (TCDD). J Toxicol Environ Health 8: 629-638.

21. Ratnasooriya WD, Ratnayake SS, Jayatunga YN (2002) Effects of pyrethroid insecticide ICON (lambda cyhalothrin) on reproductive competence of male rats. Asian J Androl 4: 35-41.

22. Yousef MI, El-Morsy AM, Hassan MS (2005) Aluminium-induced deterioration in reproductive performance and seminal plasma biochemistry of male rabbits: protective role of ascorbic acid. Toxicology 215: 97-107.

23. Elbetieha A, Da'as SI, Khamas W, Darmani H (2001) Evaluation of the toxic potentials of cypermethrin pesticide on some reproductive and fertility parameters in the male rats. Arch Environ Contam Toxicol 41: 522-528.

24. Mann T (1964) Fructose, polylos, and organic acids. In: The Biochemistry of Semen and the Male Reproductive Tract. John Wiley and Sons Inc., New York, US 237–264.

25. Kim JG, Parthasarathy S (1998) Oxidation and the spermatozoa. Semin Reprod Endocrinol 16: 235-239.

26. Yousef MI, Bertheussen K, Ibrahim HZ, Helmi S, Seehy MA, et al. (1996) A sensitive sperm-motility test for the assessment of cytotoxic effect of pesticides. J Environ Sci Health B 31: 99-115.

27. Shetaewi MM (1998) Efficacy of dietary high levels of antioxidant Vitamins C and E for rabbits subjected to crowding stress. Egypt J Rabbit Sci 8: 95–112.

28. Yousef MI, El-Demerdash FM, Kamil KI, Elaswad FA (2006) Ameliorating effect of folic acid on chromium(VI)-induced changes in reproductive performance and seminal plasma biochemistry in male rabbits. Reprod Toxicol 21: 322-328.

29. Meydani M (1995) Vitamin E. Lancet 345: 170-175.

30. Arita M, Sato Y, Arai H, Inoue K (1998) Binding of alpha-tocopherylquinone, an oxidized form of alpha-tocopherol, to glutathione-S-transferase in the liver cytosol. FEBS Lett 436: 424-426.

31. Boldyrev AA, Bulygina ER, Volynskaia EA, Kurella EG, Tiulina OV (1995) [The effect of hydrogen peroxide and hypochlorite on brain Na,K-ATPase activity]. Biokhimiia 60: 1688-1696.

32. Hsu PC, Liu MY, Hsu CC, Chen LY, Guo YL (1998) Effects of vitamin E and/or C on reactive oxygen species-related lead toxicity in the rat sperm. Toxicology 128: 169-179.

33. Geva E, Bartoov B, Zabludovsky N, Lessing JB, Lerner-Geva L, et al. (1996) The effect of antioxidant treatment on human spermatozoa and fertilization rate in an in vitro fertilization program. Fertil Steril 66: 430-434.

34. Yousef MI, Bertheussen K, Ibrahim HZ, Helmi S, Seehy MA, et al. (1996) A sensitive sperm-motility test for the assessment of cytotoxic effect of pesticides. J Environ Sci Health B 31: 99-115.

35. Yousef MI, Salama AF (2009) Propolis protection from reproductive toxicity caused by aluminium chloride in male rats. Food Chem Toxicol 47: 1168-1175.

36. Brezezińska-Slebodzińska E, Slebodziński AB, Pietras B, Wieczorek G (1995) Antioxidant effect of vitamin E and glutathione on lipid peroxidation in boar semen plasma. Biol Trace Elem Res 47: 69-74.

37. El-Missiry MA, Shalaby F (2000) Role of beta-carotene in ameliorating the cadmium-induced oxidative stress in rat brain and testis. J Biochem Mol Toxicol 14: 238-243.

38. Makar AB, McMartin KE, Palese M, Tephly TR (1975) Formate assay in body fluids: application in methanol poisoning. Biochem Med 13: 117-126.

25

Research of New Molecules Able to Starve the Tumors by Molecular Docking's Method

Boucherit Hanane*, Chikhi Abdelouahab, Bensegueni Abderrahmane, Merzoug Amina, Hioual Khadidja Soulef and Mokrani El Hassen

Laboratory of Applied Biology and Health, Department of Biochemistry-Microbiology, Faculty of Natural And Life Sciences, Mentouri University, Constantine, Algeria

Abstract

In recent years, a promising new approach uses the anti-angiogenesis properties of certain molecules to try to block cancer by depriving tumors of nutrients and oxygen they need to grow. Endothelial cells, specialized in the development of new blood vessels, are the target of most anti-angiogenic strategies, Or methionine aminopeptidase (MetAp) type 2 is a member of a family of proteins that regulates the growth of these endothelial cells.

The molecular docking program, GOLD, was developed to assist in the development of molecules with therapeutic activity. It has been used to study the inhibition of 1QZY, human methionine aminopeptidase type 2, by bengamide derivatives, with the aim of discovering new anti-angiogenic drugs. The evaluation of the affinity of these molecules brought to light those presenting the best inhibitive effect. It is about the compound 16, the value of the score of which is 135.35.

Keywords: Tumor; Anti-angiogenesis; Methionine aminopeptidase; Docking; GOLD; RMSD

Introduction

Molecular docking techniques have shown great promise as a new tool in the discovery of novel small molecule drugs for targeting proteins, because of their speed, economy and increasing reliability [1].

In this context, methionine aminopeptidase (MetAp) is a dimetalloprotease that catalyzes the removal of N-terminal methionine in newly formed polypeptide chains. MetAps are found in both eukaryotic and prokaryotic cells, and two types of MetAps are recognized from amino acid sequence comparisons and structural studies: type 1 (MetAp-1) and type 2 (MetAp-2) [2].

The human MetAp2 isoform has been of considerable interest as a target for cancer chemotherapy, after the discovery that the antiangiogenic natural compound, fumagillin, is a covalent inhibitor selective for MetAP-2. On the basis of the antiangiogenic activity observed *in vitro*, a fumagillin analog TNP-470 has progressed to clinical trials; however, the compound has demonstrated dose limiting neurotoxicity. A second family of natural products, the bengamides, has recently been identified as inhibitors of both MetAp isoforms [3].

The purpose of this work is to test the reliability of the molecular docking program GOLD (Genetic Optimization for Ligand Docking), used in this study by determining the RMSD (root mean square deviation), then use this program to search for a new inhibitor of methionine aminopeptidase through similar of bengamide [4], with a degree of similarity up to 95% from the data bank PubChem.

Materials and Methods

Molecular docking

Docking is one of the commonly used computational methods in structure based drug design. Docking is the process of fitting of the ligand into the receptor. It not only gives an idea about how the ligand is going to bind with the receptors, but also about up to what extent conformational changes can be brought in the receptor structure. Docking comprises two distinct tasks, the first being the prediction of favorable binding geometries for a small molecule in the binding site of a target protein, and secondly, the estimation of the binding free energy of the complex so formed, also referred to as scoring.

Docking accuracy reflects an algorithm's ability to discover a conformation (pose) and alignment of a ligand relative to a cognate protein that is close to that experimentally observed, and to recognize the pose as correct. Scoring accuracy is the ability to correctly predict the rank order of binding affinities of ligands to a particular protein [5-7].

GOLD v 5.0.1 (2011)

GOLD [8] is one of the most successful docking program and widely used. It is based on three major parts:

A scoring function to rank different binding modes: The Goldscore function is a molecular mechanics–like function with four terms:

$$\text{GOLD Fitness} = Subtext + S\ vdw\_ext + S\ hb\_int + S\ vdw\_int$$

Where *Subtext* is the protein–ligand hydrogen-bond score and *Svdw_ext* is the protein-ligand van der Waals score. *Shb_int* is the contribution to the *Fitness* due to intramolecular hydrogen bonds in the ligand; *Svdw_int* is the contribution due to intramolecular strain in the ligand.

A mechanism for placing the ligand in the binding site: GOLD uses a unique method to do this, which is based on fitting points; it adds fitting points to hydrogen bonding groups on protein and ligand, and maps acceptor points on the ligand on donor points in the protein, and

*Corresponding author: Boucherit Hanane, Laboratory of Applied Biology and Health, Department of Biochemistry-Microbiology, Faculty of Natural And Life Sciences, Mentouri University, Constantine, Algeria, E-mail: Boucherithanane@hotmail.fr

vice versa. Additionally, GOLD generates hydrophobic fitting points in the protein cavity onto which ligand CH groups are mapped.

3. A *search algorithm* to explore possible binding modes; GOLD uses a genetic algorithm (GA).

Structure of the enzyme

Structure of the enzyme derived from the PDB "Protein Data Bank". The PDB (Protein Data Bank) is the single worldwide archive of structural data of biological macromolecules, established in Brookhaven National Laboratories (BNL) in 1971 [9]. It contains structural information of the macromolecules determined by X-ray crystallographic, NMR methods etc.

The 1QZY structure was chosen for this study, because it represents a compromise between good resolution (1.60), and the presence of an inhibitor (TDE).

Lipinski rule

Each drug must comply with several basic criteria, such as low cost of production, be soluble, stable, but must also conform to the schedules associated with its pharmacological properties of absorption, distribution, metabolism, excretion and toxicity (ADME/Tox) [10], which is based on the rule of five made by *Christopher Lipinski* [11]. The "rule of 5" states that: poor absorption or permeation is more likely when:

– There are more than 5 H-bond donors

– The MWT is over 500

– The Log P is over 5

– There are more than 10 H-bond acceptors

In addition, *Veber* has introduced two supplementary criteria to what is now commonly called "the rule of five". Surface area of the polar compound must be less than 140 Å and the number of rotatable bonds must be less than 15 [12].

Results and Discussion

The ability of molecular docking software GOLD

Program performance has been evaluated on 150 complexes available in the PDB. The docked binding mode is compared with the experimental binding mode, and a root-mean-square distance (RMSD) between the two is calculated (by GOLD); a prediction of a binding mode is considered successful if the RMSD is below a certain value (usually 2.0 Å) [5,8,13]. In the graph, the results are given in percent.

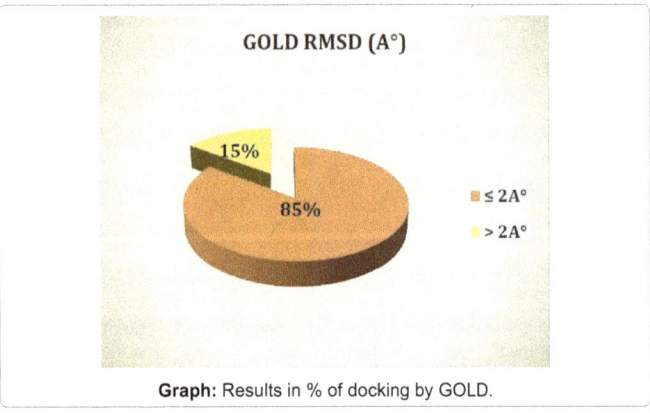

Graph: Results in % of docking by GOLD.

We notice from these results that the program GOLD reproduces well the experimental data. Indeed, 85% of RMSD values are less than 2 Å. It is clear from this graph that the RMSD values are consistent with the results of Abdelouahab C and Abderrahmane B [5], Vieth et al. [13] and Gabb et al. [14], showing that any program the docking is successful when the RMSD is less than 2 Å. This is also consistent with the results obtained by Zaheer-ul-Haq et al. [15], where six docking programs were used: FRED, GOLD, MOE, AutoDock, FlexX and Surflex-Dock, for a comparative study to determine their ability

N	Inhibitors	Fitness (score)
1	BENGAMIDE	115.28
2	CID_2322	109.94
3	CID_2323	115.06
4	CID_448235	112.71
5	CID_5353435	101.13
6	CID_638810	85.00
7	CID_6444155	113.15
8	CID_6476094	114.28
9	CID_6476095	114.02
10	CID_9975670	107.59
11	CID_10090681	99.27
12	CID_10316350	98.63
13	CID_11057452	96.50
14	CID_11245731	115.40
15	CID_11246226	116.79
16	**CID_11249087**	**135.35**
17	CID_11383607	114.47
18	CID_11639347	113.30
19	CID_11682243	103.99
20	CID_21637220	110.54
21	CID_24782418	118.73
22	CID_24782420	113.17
23	CID_24840580	94.27
24	CID_24840583	99.47
25	CID_44124768	110.89
26	CID_44124877	117.55
27	CID_44124881	111.65
28	CID_44125009	119.34
29	CID_44125012	114.49
30	CID_44125146	106.05
31	CID_44125148	105.36
32	CID_44125149	111.51
33	CID_44347653	108.49
34	CID_44347702	115.79
35	CID_44347715	109.43
36	CID_45027798	108.15
37	CID_46915399	115.60
38	CID_46915400	118.76
39	CID_46915538	109.65
40	CID_46915539	114.04
41	CID_46915540	97.08
42	CID_46936660	95.39
43	CID_53260818	99.07

Table 1: Results of the docking bengamide and its similar 95%.

to reproduce poses *via* the experimental RMSD. FRED was the best followed by Surflex-Dock and GOLD. In the same year [16] evaluated the performance of four programs: GOLD, AutoDock, Surflex-Dock and FRED by calculating the RMSD, the best results were obtained by GOLD and FRED. In addition, our results confirm the results obtained by Hioual et al. [17], where the program GOLD has been tested with the software FlexX; GOLD showed a large performance to reproduce the experimental tests with 64.05% of the RMSD values less than 2 Å. Thus, this software can be used to predict the interactions MetAP-inhibitors.

Docking bengamide derivatives

The docking by GOLD of the bengamide and its similar gave the following results, which are presented in the Table 1.

Of the 43 inhibitors tested the similar N° 16 (Table 1) forms the most stable complex protein-ligand, so it has the best inhibitory effect with fitness value of 135.35.

Lipinski rule

Before starting the study of interactions between the enzyme MetAP and the compound 16, it is necessary to evaluate the parameters for validation as an antibiotic (Table 2). These indices were calculated under the code "Molinspiration." It used to draw molecules and calculate molecular properties important (log P, polar surface, the number of donors and acceptors the hydrogen bond, ..., etc.) directly on a web page.

The results in Table 2 show that the molecule 16 used in this study responds to the rule of *Lipinski*.

Interaction MetAP-similar 16

To study the mode of interaction of different inhibitors with the active site of the human methionine aminopeptidase (MetAp- 2) by molecular docking, we used the latest version of the program GOLD

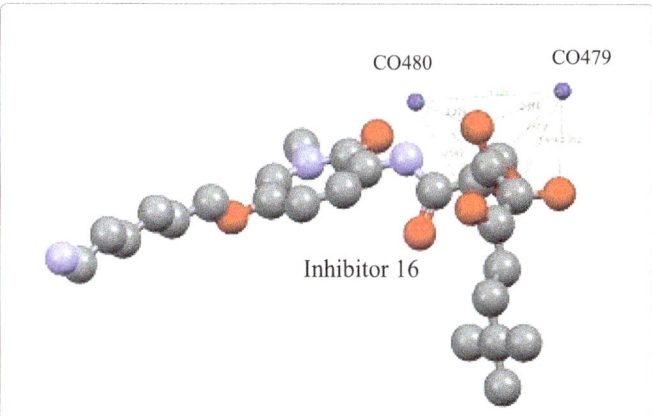

Figure 2: Representation of the interactions Van der Waals trained by the compound 16.

N	Residues involved	Atom of amino acid	Ligand atom	Distance Å
1	Asp251	O_{D2}	O_5	2.949
1	Asp262	O_{D2}	O_7	2.413
2	Glu364	O_{E1}	N_2	3.006
			O_4	2.851

Table 3: Hydrogen bonds.

N	Residues involved	Atom of amino acid	Ligand atom	Distance Å
4	CO479	-	O_4	2.218
		-	O_5	2.352
		-	C_8	2.613
			C_{12}	2.596
3	CO480	-	O_4	2.220
		-	O_7	2.668
		-	C_8	2.975

Table 4: Van der Waals interactions.

which can show the Van Der Waals contacts and the hydrogen bonds that are the most important among the weak links.

The Figure 1 shows that the inhibitor 16 penetrates well into the active site of the enzyme, forming 4 hydrogen bonds represented in the Table 3.

Note: We have neglected a few amino acids of some figures for clarity images. The ligand is represented "balls and sticks" of different colors, and amino acids in the active site of the enzyme are shown in "wireframe".

The compound 16 establishes several Van Der Waals interactions with metal ions. In the Table 4, we have summarized the different interactions (Figure 2).

The results obtained in our study are consistent with those found by other authors who have shown that bengamide derivatives are powerful inhibitors of methionine aminopeptidase [18,19].

Conclusion

The test by the RMSD allows us to conclude that GOLD is an

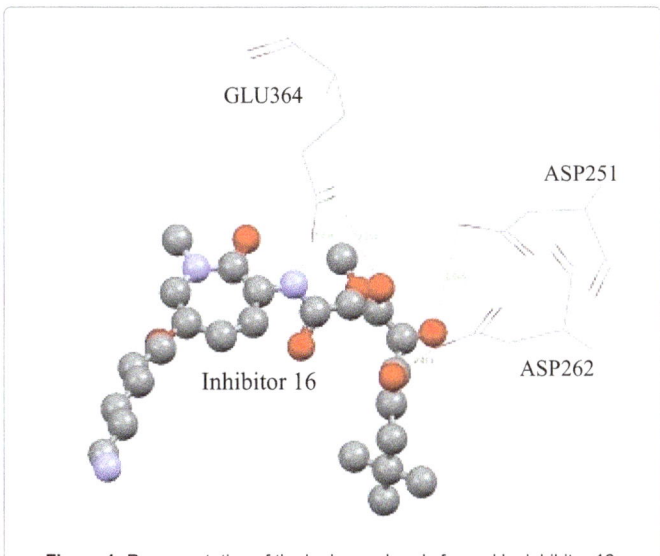

Figure 1: Representation of the hydrogen bonds formed by inhibitor 16.

Compound	Molecular weight (g/mol)	H Donors	H Acceptors	Log P	Flexible bonds
16	501.65658	5	8	0.8	15

Table 2: Lipinski rule.

excellent program for molecular docking, and seems well adapted to the study of this type of theoretical calculation. The docking results show that the compound 16 represents the best inhibitor to fight the tumors. An *in vitro* and *in vivo* experimental study will allow verifying later the theoretical results obtained *in silico*.

References

1. Ordog R, Grolmusz V (2008) Evaluating genetic algorithms in protein-ligand docking. LNBI 4983: 402-413.

2. Nonato MC, Widom J, Clardy J (2006) Human methionine aminopeptidase type 2 in complex with L- and D-methionine. Bioorg Med Chem Lett 16: 2580-2583.

3. Kim S, LaMontagne K, Sabio M, Sharma S, Versace RW, et al. (2004) Depletion of methionine aminopeptidase 2 does not alter cell response to fumagillin or bengamides. Cancer Res 64: 2984-2987.

4. Towbin H, Bair KW, DeCaprio JA, Eck MJ, Kim S, et al. (2003) Proteomics-based target identification. bengamides as a new class of methionine aminopeptidase inhibitors. J Biol Chem 278: 52964-52971.

5. Abdelouahab C and Abderrahmane B (2008) Comparative study of the efficiency of three protein-ligand docking programs. J Proteomics Bioinform 1: 161-165.

6. Ganguly S, Panigrahi N (2009) Docking studies of some novel 1-{2 (Diarylmethoxy) Ethyl]-2-Methyl-5 Nitroimidazole (DAMNI) analogs. Int J ChemTech Research 1: 974-984.

7. Wei BQ, Weaver LH, Ferrari AM, Matthews BW, Shoichet BK (2004) Testing a flexible-receptor docking algorithm in a model binding site. J Mol Biol 337: 1161-1182.

8. Verdonk ML, Cole JC, Hartshorn MJ, Murray CW, Taylor RD (2003) Improved protein–ligand docking using GOLD. Proteins 52 :609-623.

9. Berman HM (2008) The protein data bank:A historical perspective. Acta Crystallogr A 64: 88-95.

10. Miteva MA, Violas S, Montes M, Gomez D, Tuffery P, et al. (2006) FAF-Drugs: Free ADME/tox filtering of compound collections. Nucleic Acids Res 34: W738-W744.

11. Lipinski CA, Lombardo F, Dominy BW, Feeney PJ (2001) Experimental and computational approaches to estimate solubility and permeability in drug discovery and development settings. Adv Drug Deliv Rev 46: 3-26.

12. Veber DF, Johnson SR, Cheng HY, Smith BR, Ward KW, et al. (2002) Molecular properties that influence the oral bioavailability of drug candidates. J Med Chem 45: 2615-2623.

13. Vieth M, Hirst JD, Kolinski A, Brooks CL (1998) Assessing energy functions for flexible docking. J Comput Chem 19: 1612-1634.

14. Gabb HA, Jackson RM, Sternberg MJ (1997) Modelling protein docking using shape complementarity, electrostatics and biochemical information. J Mol Biol 272: 106-120.

15. Zaheer-ul-Haq, Halim SA, Uddin R, Madura JD (2010) Benchmarking docking and scoring protocol for the identification of potential acetyl cholinesterase inhibitors. J Mol Graph Model 28: 870-882.

16. Lape M, Elam C, Paula S (2010) Comparison of current docking tools for the simulation of inhibitor binding by the transmembrane domain of the sarco/endoplasmic reticulum calcium ATPase. Biophys Chem 150: 88-97.

17. Hioual KS, Chikhi A, Bensegueni A, Merzoug A, Boucherit H (2012) Comparative data on docking algorithms: Keeping the update in the field knowledge. Int J Applied Information Systems 2: 2249-0868.

18. Lu JP, Yuan XH, Yuan H, Wang WL, Wan B, et al. (2011) Inhibition of *Mycobacterium tuberculosis* methionine aminopeptidases by bengamide derivatives. ChemMedChem 6: 1041-1048.

19. Lu JP, Yuan XH, Ye QZ (2012) Structural analysis of inhibition of *Mycobacterium tuberculosis* methionine aminopeptidase by bengamide derivatives. Eur J Med Chem 47: 479-484.

26

Synthesis and Evaluation of Ornithine Decarboxylase Inhibitors with Oxime Moiety and MCF-7 Breast Cancer Cells

Hyunshun Shin[1]*, Heather Whitehead[1], Xian Zhou[2], Karl L Banta[3], Juliet V Spencer[3], Myung K Cho[4] and Sung-Kun Kim[4]

[1]Department of Chemistry and Biochemistry, McMurry University, McM station Box 158, Abilene, TX 79697, USA
[2]Department of Chemistry, University of Iowa, Iowa City, IA 52242-1294, USA
[3]Department of Biology, University of San Francisco, 2130 Fulton Street, San Francisco, CA 94117, USA
[4]Department of Chemistry and Biochemistry, Baylor University, Waco, TX 76798-7348, USA

Abstract

Cell proliferation can be regulated by small, aliphatic polyamines, and it is suggested that tumor tissues have significantly higher polyamine levels than surrounding tissues. The major biologically active polyamines present in mammalian cells are putrescine, spermidine, and spermine. The Ornithine Decarboxylase (ODC) catalyzes the decarboxylation of ornithine to produce putrescine which is aprecursor of polyamine synthesis. We report here the synthesis of 2-Amino-5-(Hydroxyimino) Pentanoic Acid (AHPA), based on the substrate of ODC, L-ornithine, derivatized with oxime functionality. In molecular docking studies, the E-isomer AHPA binds to ODC more favorably than does the Z-isomer. In addition, the growth of MCF-7 (Michigan Cancer Foundation–7) breast cancer cells in the presence of AHPA was significantly reduced. These results implicate that AHPA can be explored as a potential agent of cancer chemotherapy.

Keywords: Polyamine; Ornithine decarboxylase (ODC); Inhibitors of ODC; MCF-7 (Michigan Cancer Foundation–7)

Introduction

Cancer is the second most common cause of death for Americans and accounts for nearly 1 of every 4 deaths in the US [1,2]. An estimated 229,060 new cases of invasive breast cancer are expected to occur among women in the US during 2012; about 2,190 new cases are expected in men [1,2]. Cancer is a disease related to uncontrolled growth and spread of abnormal cells [2]. Targeting the polyamine pathway has been studied in possible therapeutic approaches [3]. One of the most promising areas for the development of novel anti-cancer therapeutics is polyamine biosynthesis [4,5]. The finding that inhibitors of polyamine biosynthesis can prevent, or at least limit cancer cell growth [6-9], together with the fact that polyamine concentrations are elevated in multiple cancer tissues [10-12], has made polyamine metabolism a promising target for cancer chemoprevention and therapy. The major biologically active polyamines present in mammalian cells are putrescine, spermidine, and spermine [3]. These molecules are synthesized in sequence starting from ornithine, which is derived from the amino acid arginine through the action of the enzyme arginase (Scheme 1). The first critical step is the synthesis of putrescine via the decarboxylation of ornithine, which is catalyzed by the enzyme Ornithine Decarboxylase (ODC) [13,14]. Subsequent steps involve the production of spermidine through the addition of Decarboxylated S-Adenosylmethionine (DAM) to the putrescine by spermidine synthase. A second DAM is then added to spermidine to produce spermine [15-17] (Scheme 1).

Difluoromethylornithine (DFMO), an inhibitor of the first enzyme in the mammalian polyamine biosynthetic pathway, ornithine decarboxylase, is approved for use in trypanosomiasis and has shown promise in the therapy of brain tumors [18]. DFMO was originally evaluated as an antitumor agent in the early 1980s, with limited success. Phase I studies suggested a dose of 2.25 g/m^2 every 6 h for patients with advanced solid tumors or lymphomas [19]. Phase II studies were carried out with melanoma patients including small cell lung carcinoma, colon cancer, and prostate cancer [20-22]. The drug was generally well tolerated, although significant but infrequent adverse effects including thrombocytopenia (a relative decrease of platelets in blood), transient hearing loss, and osmotic diarrhea were

noted. The results of these studies deterred continued evaluation of the drug as an antitumor agent. Although the ODC inhibitor may have significant effects on their respective target enzymes, only one inhibitor, R-Difluoromethylornithine (DFMO), has reached the market. DFMO was originally designed as an antitumor agent, but the drug was not effective enough to the further study of phase II trials. However, it has been shown to be an effective cure for infection caused by *Trypanosoma brucei gambiense*, which causes West African sleeping sickness [23,24].

Due to the limitation of use of DFMO, it is necessary to design new possible compounds that disturb the polyamine biosynthetic pathway. The oxime moiety is of great value in investigating binding affinities in arginine biosynthesis due to the geometrical isomers (E/Z) of the oxime functionality and biological activities [25]. The oxime moiety (-C=N-OH) is easily coordinated with metal ions or hydrogen bonds with conserved residues in active sites of various enzymes.

In this present study, we report the design and synthesis of 2-amino-5-(hydroxyimino) pentanoic acid (AHPA), 6, which contains an oxime functional group. The molecular docking study was conducted to extend Structure-Activity Relationship (SAR) studies based on AHPA with ODC (PDB code 2ON3). Although we synthesize the mixture of E and Z isomers of 2-Amino-5-(Hydroxyimino) Pentanoic Acid (AHPA), we can anticipate that the E isomer has a better binding affinity than the Z-isomer based on a molecular docking study. In

*Corresponding author: Hyunshun Shin, Department of Chemistry and Biochemistry, McMurry University, McM station Box 158, Abilene, TX 79697, USA, E-mail: shin.hyunshun@mcm.edu, hyunshun@yahoo.com

addition, the biological evaluation of AHPA with MCF-7 (Michigan Cancer Foundation–7) breast cancer cells was shown more potent when compared with DFMO *in vitro*. Our initial studies investigated the impact of AHPA on proliferation of human breast cancer cells, and the results indicate that inhibition of ODC greatly impairs the ability of these cells to replicate. Therefore, AHPA may have a considerable potential as a cancer chemopreventive and therapeutic agent.

Results and Discussion

Chemistry

We designed and synthesized a 2-amino-5-(hydroxyimino) pentanoic acid 6 (AHPA) inhibitor based on the modified substrate of ornithine decarboxylase with oxime functionality. The Compound 6 (APHA) was synthesized using the procedure described in scheme 2.

2-Amino-5-(hydroxyimino)pentanoic acid (AHPA), 6, was synthesized using L-glutamic acid derivative *(S)*-5-(*tert*-butoxy)-4- [(*tert*-butoxycarbonyl)amino]-5-oxopentanoic acid 1, as the starting material. Esterification of the compound 1 using methyl chloroformate by treatment with triethylamine and a catalytic amount of 4-dimethylaminopyridine (DMAP) in dry methylene chloride provided the ester derivative 2. Synthesis of di-*tert*-butyl dicarbonate (di-BOC) 3 was carried out by treatment with di-*tert*-butyl dicarbonate in the presence of DMAP in methylene chloride. The subsequent reduction of ester derivative 3 was performed with diisobutylaluminium hydride (DIBAL-H) in ether to provide the aldehyde 4 [26]. Oxime derivative 5 was prepared for hydroxylamine hydrochloride in methanol under reflux condition. Complete deprotection of the compound, 5 with trifluoroacetic acid (TFA) in methylene chloride yielded AHPA 6.

We have investigated the stabilities of geometric isomers in molecular modeling-docking studies to computationally evaluate the fit between the human and *Leishmania donovani* ODC (PDB code 2ON3) and the *E*- and *Z*-isomers of AHPA [27,28]. Calculated binding data are recorded in table 1. When *E*-AHPA is bound in an extended conformation, the oxime moiety can make hydrogen bonds with conserved enzyme residues, Lys 69, Arg154, and Glu274. When *Z*-AHPA is bound, the oxime moiety can make a hydrogen bond

with only one conserved residue, Asp364. Thus, the greater hydrogen bonding potential of the *E*-isomer of the oxime moiety suggests a stability preference for this isomer. Force-field based methods can predict the binding free energy of a protein-ligand complex by adding up individual contributions from different types of interactions. Programs for energetic analysis of receptor-ligand interaction based on force-field scoring functions and terms including van der Waals, electrostatics and hydrogen bonds can be available.

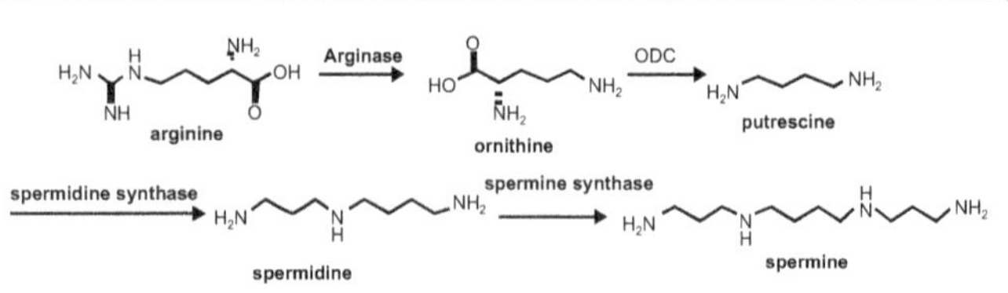

Interestingly, Autodock molecular modeling of the structure of human and *Leishmania donovani* ornithine decarboxylases14 (PDB code 2ON3) with geometric isomers (*E*/*Z*) of oxime ligands has shown that a high degree of affinity with *E* isomer rather than *Z* isomer (Table 1, Figure 1 and Figure 2).

To evaluate the impact of ODC inhibitors on cell proliferation, MCF-7 cancer cells were used. The cells were cultured in the presence or absence of varying doses of AHPA. As shown in figure 3, AHPA treatment significantly reduced cell proliferation. A seven point dilution series was performed, and even at the lowest concentration (0.391 mg/ml), AHPA was found to affect cell viability. At 24 hours post-treatment, the cells were viable and the level of ATP was roughly equivalent for cells under each experimental condition. By 48 hours post-treatment, there was no proliferation detected and viability of all cells that had been exposed to AHPA was decreasing. In contrast, the control cells exhibited healthy and robust proliferation, as evidenced by the increasing amounts of ATP detected. By 96 hours, cells that had been exposed to AHPA at any dose were dead. It thus appears that AHPA was a much more potent inhibitor of cell proliferation than comparable doses of DFMO (difluoromethylornithine), a well-known inhibitor of ornithine decarboxylase. Although there is a possibility that the reduction of cell proliferation by AHPA is due to the compound toxicity, the significant effect of AHPA on cell proliferation and the *in silico* analysis support the conclusion that the AHPA inhibit the cell proliferation by binding to ODC.

`MCF-7 breast cancer cells were cultured in the presence of absence of AHPA at the indicated time points. Cell viability and proliferation was measured via the Cell Titer Glo Assay, and results are expressed as relative light units.

As shown in figure 4, MCF-7 cell proliferation was not significantly affected by doses of DFMO lower than 3 mg/ml. At doses higher than 3 mg/ml DFMO, modest reduction of cell proliferation was observed. Proliferation of cells treated with AHPA was dramatically reduced by even the lowest doses of the compound. These results demonstrate that AHPA is a potent inhibitor of cell proliferation.

In conclusion, while exploring the design of new therapeutic inhibitors in arginine biosynthetic pathways, AHPA appears to be a potential cancer chemotherapeutic agent based on the observations of *in silico* docking and cell proliferation experiments. The docking studies have shown that geometric isomers of the ornithine-based

Scheme 1: Biosynthesis of Polyamines.

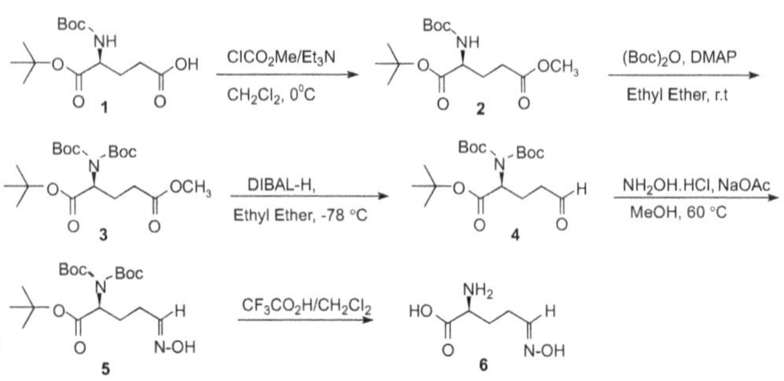

Scheme 2: BSynthesis of 2-amino-5-(hydroxyimino)pentanoic acid (AHPA).

Compound AHPA, 6	N_{tor}	ΔG_{AD4} (kcalmol)	RMSD (Å)	H-bonding interaction	H-bond distance (Å)
				HO...HN(Lys 69)	2.7
E-isomer *(trans)*	3	-7.92	2.347	HO...HN(Arg154)	1.9
				NH...OH(Glu274)	1.8
Z-isomer *(cis-)*	6	-5.51	0.485	OH...OC(Asp364)	1.9

Table 1: Comparison of the complex of *E*/*Z* isomers of 2-Amino-5-(Hydroxyimino) Pentanoic Acid (AHPA) with ODC (PDB code 2ON3) in molecular docking studies

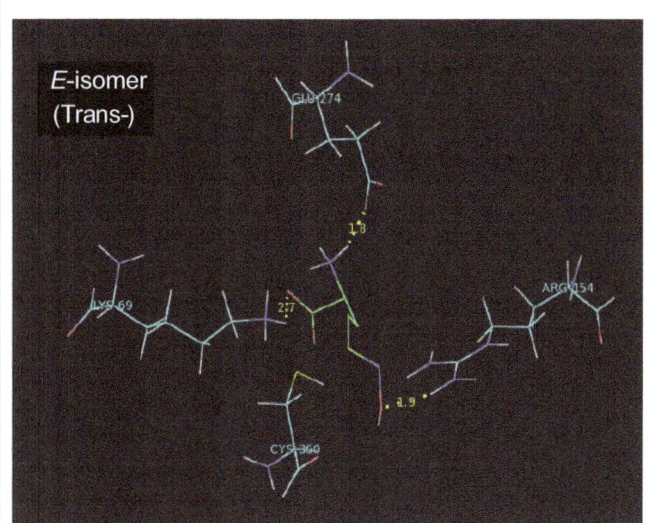

Figure 1: A schematic diagram showing the interactions of *E*-AHPA with neighboring groups within the active site of ODC (PDB code 2ON3)

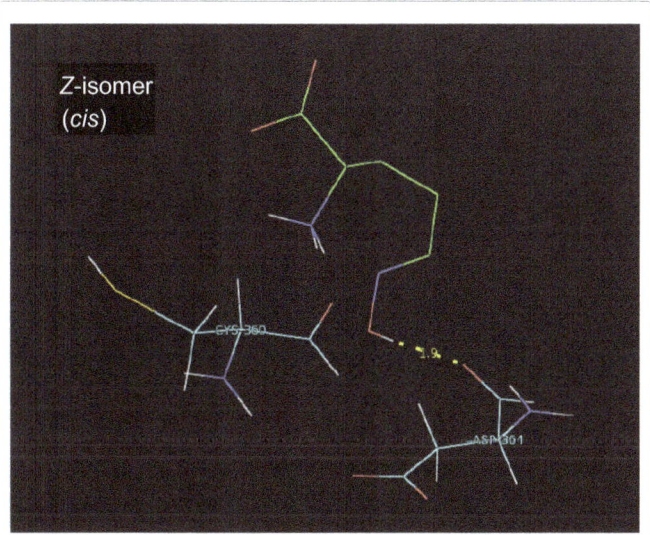

Figure 2: A schematic diagram showing the interactions of Z-AHPA with neighboring groups within the active site of ODC (PDB code 2ON3)

oxime AHPA play a significant biological role in blocking ODC activity. The predicted binding affinity of the *E*-isomer of AHPA is higher than that of its *Z*-isomer with ODC as calculated with AutoDock. Besides, AHPA significantly affects cell viability with MCF-7. It is, however, worth noting that the *in silico* and cell proliferation observations will not warrant the fact that the AHPA specifically binds to ODC. To assess this issue, more evidence by further investigations would conclusively support the binding specificity. Furthermore, exploring structure-activity relationships of additional AHPA analogues as well as determining their lowest effective doses would be considered as future studies.

Experimental section

Synthesis of an amino acid oxime analogue: Reactions requiring anhydrous conditions were carried out under a nitrogen atmosphere in oven-dried glassware, and solvents were freshly distilled. Diethyl ether and Tetrahydrofuran (THF) were distilled from sodium/benzophenone.

Dichloromethane and triethylamine were distilled from calcium hydride. All other reagents and solvents were used without further purification from commercial sources. Organic extracts were dried over anhydrous $MgSO_4$ or Na_2SO_4. Reactions were monitored by Thin-Layer Chromatography (TLC) with 0.25-mm E. Merck precoated silica gel plates and visualized with ninhydrin solution (0.1% ninhydrin in 95% *n*-butanol, 4.5% water, 0.5% glacial acetic acid) and $KMnO_4$ solution (3 g of $KMnO_4$, 20 g of K_2CO_3, 5 ml of 5% NaOH, and 300 ml of water). Flash column chromatography was carried out with E. Merck silica gel 60 (230-240 mesh ASTM). The 1H and 13C NMR spectra taken by Dr. Garner by were recorded on a Bruker AM-500 spectrometer. Chemical shifts were expressed in parts per million (ppm) and referenced to CDCl3, CD3OD, or DMSO-*d*6 at Baylor University. The general syntheses of *(S)-tert*-butyl 2- (bis(*tert*-butoxycarbonyl)amino)-5-(hydroxyimino)pentanoate 5 and *(S)*-2-amino-5-(hydroxyimino) pentanoic acid (AHPA) 6 are as follows.

Procedure

(S)-tert-butyl 2-(bis(*tert*-butoxycarbonyl)amino)-5-(hydroxyimino) pentanoate, 5

At room temperature to a solution of the appropriate aldehyde (1.0 g, 8.9 mmol) in methanol (5 ml) was added hydroxyamine hydrochloride (0.743 g, 0.107 mmol) followed by sodium acetate trihydrate (0.148 g,

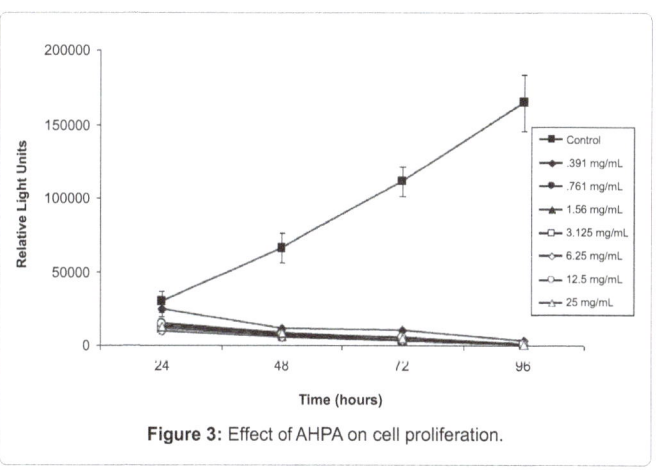

Figure 3: Effect of AHPA on cell proliferation.

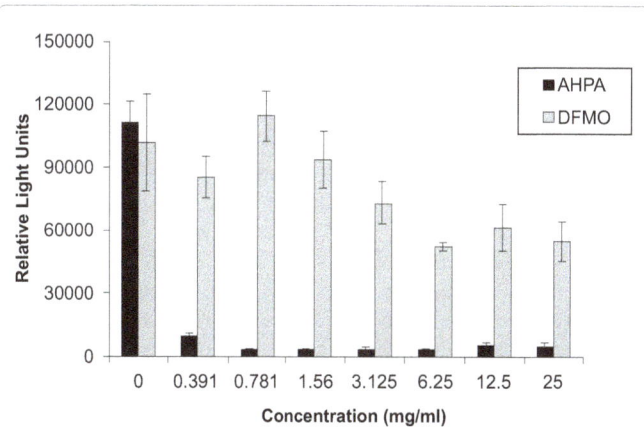

Figure 4: MCF-7 cells were cultured in the presence of DFMO or AHPA at the indicated concentrations and cell viability was measured at 72 hours using the Cell Titer Glo Assay. Results are representative of two separate experiments and error bars represent standard error

0.107 mmol) and methanol (10 ml). Enough methanol was then added to give a clear solution, and stirring at 60°C was refluxed for 3-4 hrs. The resulting solution was cooled to room temperature, diluted with water (10 ml), and extracted with ether (3×10 ml). The combined organic phases were washed with saturated sodium bicarbonate (2×10 ml) and brine and then dried over MgSO$_4$. The solvent was removed at reduced pressure, and the crude oximes was purified by column chromatography (1:9=ethylacetate:hexanes): clear oil. Yield (0.5 g 81.45%).

^{1}H NMR (CDCl3): δ 7.49-7.41 (t, 0.56H), 6.83-6.73 (s, 0.47H), 4.85-4.73 (m, 1H), 2.15-1.99 (m, 1H), 1.54-1.40 (m, 29H). IR (cm-1): 3550-2800, 1800-1700. MS (ES+) *(m/z)*: [M+Na] calcd for (C$_{19}$H$_{34}$N$_2$O$_7$Na) 425.2264, found 424.2245.

2-amino-5-(hydroxyimino)pentanoic acid (AHPA), 6: To a stirred solution of the compound 5 (0.425 g, 1.03 mmol) in CH$_2$Cl$_2$ (10 ml) was slowly added Trifluoroacetic Acid (TFA) (8 ml) at 0°C. The reaction mixture was stirred for 1-4 hrs and then allowed to equilibrate at room temperature until the end of the reaction. The solvent was removed on a rotary evaporator, and the crude residue was purified by silica gel chromatography to yield 6 (0.24 g, 87% yield).

^{1}H NMR (MeOD): δ 7.45-7.33 (m, 0.39H), 6.78-6.68(m, 0.29H), 4.08-3.90 (m, 1H), 2.25-1.95(m, 2H), δ1.38-1.20(m, 0.72H). IR (cm^{-1}): 3500-2100, 1800-1600.

MS (ES+) *(m/z)*: [M+H] calcd for (C$_5$H$_{11}$O$_3$N$_2$) 147.0770, found 147.0764.

Preparation of Target Protein Structure

The 3D structure of ODC (Ornithine Decarboxylase) from human and *Leishmania donovani* was obtained from the protein data bank (PDB code 2ON3). The X-ray crystal structure of the enzyme has been determined at 3.0 Å resolution [14]. All atom parameters were automatically created by AutoDockTools (ADT). Coordinates for the ODC (PDB code 2ON3) were processed in ADT by adding hydrogen atoms, assigning charges with the Gasteiger method, and merging the non-polar hydrogens. The 3D structure and active site residues of target protein were confirmed by PyMol [27].

Docking with Predefined Compounds

To increase the validity of potential inhibitor and docking studies, inhibitor candidates (geometric isomers (*E/Z*) of oxime ligands) were chosen as control dockings. We utilized the Dundee PRODRG28 server to generate a topological description of the both *E* and *Z* form. This server converted 2D compounds drawn by the JME editor to 3D coordinates in PDB format, adding hydrogen atoms. The 3D structures of the compounds, in the PDB format, were then docked with the (PDB code 2ON3) using AutoDock4.0 (http://autodock.scripps.edu). A grid map of 60Å×60Å×60Å points with 0.375Å grid spacing was centered on the active site and was calculated around the docking area by running AutoGrid. The Lamarckian genetic algorithm was used as the search method, and the docking parameters were set to 10 automated docking runs, as default setup, for a 150 population size with a 2,500,000 maximum number of energy evaluations for each docking experiment. The results showed the binding energies and hydrogen bonds' interactions between the ligands and (PDB code 2ON3), and the cluster analysis was performed based on Root Mean Square Deviation (RMSD).

Biological Assays

MCF-7 breast cancer cells were maintained in FK12/DMEM medium supplemented with 5% fetal bovine serum in a 37°C incubator with a humidified 5% CO$_2$ atmosphere. Cells were plated at 5×10^4 per well in white 96 well plates in the presence or absence of compound as indicated and each treatment was performed in triplicate. Cell growth was measured at the indicated time points using the Cell Titer Glo Kit (Promega, Madison, WI). Briefly, a luciferin substrate added to each well was converted to oxyluciferin in the presence of O$_2$ and ATP. The light produced was measured using a Veritas Microplate Luminometer (Turner Biosystems, Sunnyvale, CA) and the relative light units were proportional to the amount of ATP present, reflecting the number of viable cells in the well. DFMO was purchased from Sigma-Aldrich (St. Loius, MO).

Acknowledgment

We thank Professor Charles Garner for data analysis of 1H, 13C NMR supported by the NSF (Award #CHE-042802) and Dr. Alejandro Ramirez (High Resolution Mass Spectroscopy) at Baylor University. We acknowledge the Robert A. Welch Foundation to Department of Chemistry and Biochemistry at McMurry University and Lily Drake Cancer Research.

References

1. Estimated New Cancer Cases and Deaths by Sex for All Sites (2012) American Cancer Society. US.

2. Cancer Facts & Figures (2012) American Cancer Society. US.

3. Casero RA Jr, Woster PM (2009) Recent advances in the development of polyamine analogues as antitumor agents. J Med Chem 52: 4551-4573.

4. Bernacki RJ, Bergeron RJ, Porter CW (1992) Antitumor activity of N,N'-bis(ethyl) spermine homologues against human MALME-3 melanoma xenografts. Cancer Res. 52: 2424-2430.

5. Bernacki RJ, Oberman EJ, Seweryniak KE, Atwood A, Bergeron RJ, et al. (1995) Preclinical antitumor efficacy of the polyamine analogue N1, N11-diethylnorspermine administered by multiple injection or continuous infusion. Clin Cancer Res 1: 847-857.

6. McCloskey DE, Casero RA Jr, Woster PM, Davidson NE (1995) Induction of programmed cell death in human breast cancer cells by an unsymmetrically alkylated polyamine analogue. Cancer Res. 55: 3233–3236.

7. Mamont PS, Böhlen P, McCann PP, Bey P, Schuber F, et al. (1976) Alpha-methyl ornithine, a potent competitive inhibitor of ornithine decarboxylase, blocks proliferation of rat hepatoma cells in culture. Proc Natl Acad Sci U S A 73: 1626-1630.

8. Eskens FA, Greim GA, Van Zuylen C, Wolff I, Denis LJ, et al. (2000) Phase I and pharmacological study of weekly administration of the polyamine synthesis inhibitor SAM 486A (CGP 48 664) in patients with solid tumors. European Organization for Research and Treatment of Cancer Early Clinical Studies Group. Clin. Cancer Res. 6: 1736-1743.

9. Milovica V, Turchanowa L, Khomutov AR, Khomutov RM, Caspary WF, et al. (2001) Hydroxylamine-containing inhibitors of polyamine biosynthesis and impairment of colon cancer cell growth. Biochem. Pharmacol 61: 199-206.

10. Kingsnorth AN, Lumsden AB, Wallace HM (1984) Polyamines in colorectal cancer. Br J Surg 71: 791-794.

11. Löser C, Fölsch UR, Paprotny C, Creutzfeldt W (1990) Polyamines in colorectal cancer. Evaluation of polyamine concentrations in the colon tissue, serum, and urine of 50 patients with colorectal cancer. Cancer 65: 958-966.

12. Fogel-Petrovic M, Kramer DL, Vujcic S, Miller J, McManis JS, et al. (1997) Structural basis for differential induction of spermidine/spermine N1-acetyltransferase activity by novel spermine analogs. Mol Pharmacol 52: 69-74.

13. Cañizares F, Salinas J, de las Heras M, Diaz J, Tovar I, et al. (1999) Prognostic value of ornithine decarboxylase and polyamines in human breast cancer: correlation with clinicopathologic parameters. Clin Cancer Res 5: 2035-2041.

14. Dufe VT, Ingner D, Heby O, Khomutov AR, Persson L, et al. (2007) A structural insight into the inhibition of human and *Leishmania donovani* ornithine decarboxylases by 1-amino-oxy-3-aminopropane. Biochem J 405: 261-268.

15. Pegg AE (1988) Polyamine metabolism and its importance in neoplastic growth and a target for chemotherapy. Cancer Res 48: 759-774.

16. Casero RA Jr, Celano P, Ervin SJ, Porter CW, Bergeron RJ, et al. (1989) Differential induction of spermidine/spermine N1-acetyltransferase in human lung cancer cells by the bis(ethyl)polyamine analogues. Cancer Res 49: 3829-3833.

17. Heby O, Roberts SC, Ullman B (2003) Polyamine biosynthetic enzymes as drug targets in parasitic protozoa. Biochem Soc Trans 31: 415-419.

18. Levin VA, Hess KR, Choucair A, Flynn PJ, Jaeckle KA, et al. (2003) Phase III randomized study of postradiotherapy chemotherapy with combination alpha-difluoromethylornithine-PCV versus PCV for anaplastic gliomas. Clin Cancer Res 9: 981-990.

19. Abeloff MD, Slavik M, Luk GD, Griffin CA, Hermann J, et al. (1984) Phase I trial and pharmacokinetic studies of alpha-difluoromethylornithine--an inhibitor of polyamine biosynthesis. J Clin Oncol 2: 124-130.

20. Meyskens FL, Kingsley EM, Glattke T, Loescher L, Booth A (1986) A phase II study of alpha-difluoromethylornithine (DFMO) for the treatment of metastatic melanoma. Invest New Drugs 4: 257-262.

21. Abeloff MD, Rosen ST, Luk GD, Baylin SB, Zeltzman M, et al. (1986) Phase II trials of alpha-difluoromethylornithine, an inhibitor of polyamine synthesis, in advanced small cell lung cancer and colon cancer. Cancer Treat Rep 70: 843-845.

22. Herr HW, Warrel RP, Burchenal JH (1986) Phase I trial of alpha-difluoromethyl ornithine (DFMO) and methylglyoxal bis (guanylhydrazone) (MGBG) in patients with advanced prostatic cancer. Urology 28: 508-511.

23. Bacchi CJ, Garofalo J, Mockenhaupt D, McCann PP, Diekema KA (1983) In vivo effects of alpha-DL-difluoromethylornithine on the metabolism and morphology of Trypanosoma brucei brucei. Mol Biochem Parasitol 7: 209-225.

24. Bacchi CJ, Nathan HC, Livingston T, Valladares G, Saric M, et al. (1990) Differential susceptibility to DL-alpha-difluoromethylornithine in clinical isolates of Trypanosoma brucei rhodesiense. Antimicrob Agents Chemother 34: 1183-1188.

25. Ley JP, Bertram HJ (2001) Hydroxy- or methoxy-substituted benzaldoximes and benzaldehyde-O-alkyloximes as tyrosinase inhibitors. Bioorg Med Chem 9: 1879-1885.

26. Shin H, Cama E, Christianson DW (2004) Design of amino acid aldehydes as transition-state analogue inhibitors of arginase. J Am Chem Soc 126: 10278-10284.

27. DeLano WL (2002) The PyMOL molecular graphics system. DeLano Scientific, San Carlos, CA, USA.

28. Schüttelkopf AW, van Aalten DM (2004) PRODRG: a tool for high-throughput crystallography of protein-ligand complexes. Acta Crystallogr D Biol Crystallogr 60: 1355-1363.

Wound Healing and Anti-Ulcerogenic Activity of *Gardenia angustifolia* Extract in Rats

Omale James*, Abbah Okpachi Christopher, Ojogbane Eleojo Berikisu, David Ede Patience and Adah Gabriel Onuche

Faculty of Natural Sciences, Department of Biochemistry, Kogi State University, P.M.B. 1008, Anyigba, Kogi State, Nigeria

Abstract

Gardenia angustifolia is widely utilized in many parts of Nigeria to manage a wide range of ailments. As part of effort to elucidate its pharmacological activities and hence medicinal potential, wound healing and anti-ulcerogenic properties of the extract was evaluated using experimentally created wound and ulcers in albino rats. Wound healing properties was evaluated using excision wound model, while anti-ulcer activity was studied using ethanol induced ulcer model. Five groups of rats were experimentally wounded at the back area. An area of uniform wound of 7×7 mm using millimeter ruler was excised. The animal groups were topically treated with *Gardenia angustifolia* gel, wound dressed with leaf, fruit and root gel significantly healed earlier than those treated with paraffin base and povidone iodine (standard). In anti-ulcer studies, rats were orally administered with different doses of the root extract (100, 250 and 500 mg/kg body weight) and positive control group (Omeprazole, 8 mg/kg body weight) for five days. After induction of ulcer using 5 ml/kg body weight of ethanol, the stomach of the rats was opened, gastric volume and ulcer area were measured. The results indicated that *Gardenia angustifolia* root extract could prevent ulceration in rats in a dose dependent manner. The acute toxicity study revealed that the plant could be toxic at higher doses. Blood glucose reduction was dose and time dependent. From this study it is evident that *G. angustifolia* possess anti-ulcer properties and also wound dressed with the root, leaf and fruit gels significantly enhanced the acceleration of wound healing in rats.

Keywords: *Gardenia angustifolia*; Anti-ulcer; Wound healing; Albino rats; Omeprazole; Toxicity

Introduction

Wound is a breach in the normal tissue continuum, resulting in a variety of cellular and molecular sequelae. The basic principles of optimal wound healing which include minimizing tissue damage, debriding nonviable tissue, maximizing tissue perfusion and oxygenation, proper nutrition and moist wound healing environment have been recognized for many years [1].

A number of drugs ranging from simple non-expensive analgesics to complex and expensive chemotherapeutic agents administered in the management of wound affect healing either positively or negatively [2]. Aspirin, indomethacin, cytotoxic agents and immunosuppressant have been proved experimentally to affect healing negatively [3]. Wound is defined as the disruption of the cellular and anatomic discontinuity of a tissue and may be produced by chemical, physical, thermal, microbial or immunological insult to the tissue. Wound cause discomfort and are more proned to infection and other troublesome complications [4].

Peptic ulcer is a conglomerate of heterogeneous disorders, which manifests itself as a break in the lining of the gastrointestinal mucosa bathed by acid and or pepsin [5]. Mucosal injury may occur when noxious factors "overwhelm" an intact mucosal defense or when the mucosal defense is somehow in paired [6]. Although a number of anti-ulcer drugs such as H_2 receptors antagonists, proton pump inhibitors and cytoprotectants are available for ulceration all these drugs have side effects and limitations. Herbal medicine deals with plants and plant extracts in treating diseases. These medicines are considered safer because of the natural ingredients with no side effects [7]. These natural agents induce healing and regeneration of the tissue by multiple mechanisms, however, there is need for scientific validation, standardization and safety evaluation of plants of traditional medicine before they could be recommended for wound and ulcer treatment [8].

Gardenia angustifolia (*G. angustifolia*) is locally called *Ikaga* by the Igala people of Kogi State, Nigeria. *G. angustifolia* (*Rubiaceae*) is found in the tropical and subtropical regions of Africa and Southern Asia. Different parts of *G. angustifolia* are used in the management of many diseases traditionally including abdominal irritation, abortion abscesses, chicken pox, mental disorder, erectile dysfunction, cough, diabetes, etc. Inspite of being one of the well-known medicinal plants used in Nigerian traditional medicine, studies pertaining to the pharmacological properties of *G. angustifolia* are very rare. There is no scientific evidence available for wound healing and anti-ulcer activity of *G. angustifolia*; therefore, the present research was undertaken.

Materials and Methods

Plant material

The plant sample was collected from Abocho in Dekina Local Government Area of Kogi State, Nigeria during rainy season when the plant thrives well and produces fruit. Dirt was removed from the plant sample by rinsing properly in clean water. The sample was air-dried for three weeks and pulverized into powder form using mechanical hand blender and sieved.

Preparation of extract

Portions of the samples-600 g of the powdered root, 300 g of the leaf and 60 g of the powdered fruit were weighed out and soaked in containers containing 1200 ml, 800 ml and 200 ml of methanol

*Corresponding author: Omale James, Faculty of Natural Sciences, Department of Biochemistry, Kogi State University, P.M.B. 1008, Anyigba, Kogi State, Nigeria, E-mail: james.omale123@yahoo.com

respectively for 72 hours. The mixtures were then filtered under vacuum pressure and the filtrates were concentrated by evaporation using water bath at 60°C.

Animals

The animals selected for this study were albino rats of both sexes with average weight range between 130–220 g. They were obtained from Mr. Friday Titus Emmanuel who breeds them and housed in the departmental animal house during the experimental period in a standard environmental conditions. They were allowed free access to standard laboratory diet and drinking water without any form of restriction. This study was carried out in conformity with national and international laws and guidelines for care and use of laboratory animals in biomedical research; especially as promulgated and approved by United States Institute of Health (1985).

Ointment preparation for topical application

Methanol-free extract of *G. angustifolia* leaf, root and fruit gels were used for the preparation of the ointment for topical application [9]. A 50% (w/w) of extract ointments of *G. angustifolia* (leaf, root and fruit) were formulated using soft white paraffin base [10].

Excision wound model

Animals were anaesthetized with 0.3 ml of lindocane adrexyl (local an aesthetic) to prevent any movement of animals for at least two hours after administration and animals were left without being restrained [11].

The back of the animals were shaved and sterilized with 70% ethanol before 7×7 mm excision wound was created by a surgical blade from a predetermined shaved area on the back of each animal [12]. The experimental groups were topically applied with the extracts twice daily for consecutive 16 days. The group treated with povidone iodine drug served as a reference-standard. A progressive decrease in the wound area was periodically monitored. The wound contractions or closures were measured by a tracing paper on the wounded margin and calculated as percentage reduction in wounded area. The actual value was converted into percentage value taking the size of the wound at the time of wounding as 100%. The animals were divided into five groups of four animals per group.

Group 1: Control (wound treated with paraffin base).

Group 2: Standard (wound treated with povidone iodine).

Group 3: Wound treated with *G. angustifolia* root extract ointment.

Group 4: Wound treated with *G. angustifolia* leaf extract ointment.

Group 5: Wound treated with *G. angustifolia* fruit extract ointment.

Measurement of wound closure was taken the 4, 6, 8, 10 and 16th day post wound creation.

Acute toxicity

Seven groups (n=7) of albino rats of both sex were used in the acute toxicity of the root extract of *G. angustifolia*. Animals from all groups were fasted overnight and a safe dose of extract was determined through the acute oral toxicity test in rats at different doses up to 6000 mg/kg^{-1} was prepared by dissolving the extract in phosphate buffer saline (PBS). The extract was then administered (P.O.) with single dose (100, 200, 500, 1000, 2000, 5000 and 6000 mg/kg^{-1}) of the extract. The animals were observed for behavioral changes, any sign of toxicity and

mortality up to 48 hrs and their blood glucose level were measured after 12 and 24 hrs. Blood glucose measurement: The blood glucose level was determined according to the method described by [13].

Anti-ulcer activity study

Five groups (n=4) of albino rats were used to evaluate the anti-ulcerogenic activity of *G. angustifolia* methanol extract. Phosphate buffer saline (PBS), *G. angustifolia* methanol extract, Omeprazole and ethanol were administered to the group of animals per orally (P.O.). Group 1 received PBS (10 ml/kg^{-1}) for 4 days and on the 5th day received absolute ethanol (5 ml/kg^{-1}) and served as ulcer control. Group 2 was administered Omeprazole (8 ml/kg^{-1}) for 5 days and served as positive control. Group 3, 4 and 5 were respectively administered with 100, 250 and 500 ml/kg^{-1} of *G. angustifolia* methanol extract for 5 days. All groups were fasted for 24 hrs and again administered with the extract or drug at the respective dose. After 30 minutes of this treatment, animals of group 2-5 were administered with 5 ml/kg^{-1} ethanol to induce ulcer. After 15 minutes of ethanol administration, all the animals were sacrificed using anaesthetic ether. Gastric volume was measured by pylorus ligation approach [14].

Each animal's stomach was opened along the greater curvature and examined macroscopically for gastric erosions under a dissecting microscope (20x). The length and width (mm) of ulcer on the gastric mucosa were measured by plane glass square (10x10mm). The ulcer area (UA) was calculated. The percentage of protection (P%) availed the animals through various treatments which are calculated using the formula:

$$P\% = \frac{(\text{UA Ulcer Control} - \text{UA Treatment})}{\text{UA Ulcer Control}} \times \frac{100}{1}$$

Chemicals and reference drugs

All chemicals and reagents used in this investigation were of analytical grade and were obtained from BDH, Poole, England. Omeprazole and povidone iodine (reference drugs) were obtained from Kuzak Pharmacy in Anyigba, Kogi State, Nigeria. Omeprazole is an anti-ulcer drug which blocks the enzymes in the wall of the stomach from producing acid, the main culprit in peptic ulcer. By blocking the enzymes, the production of stomach acid is decreased, thus allowing the ulcer to heal [15].

Statistical analysis

All data were expressed as mean ± SEM. Statistical comparisons were performed using ANOVA. The level of significance was set at P<0.01.

Results

Wound healing

The topical application of *G. angustifolia* ointments increased the percentage of wound closure and this indicates rapid epithelization and collagenation. The administration of the extracts (root, leaf and fruit) accelerated the progression of wound healing. The root extract appears more potent than the leaf and fruit ointments (Table 1).

Acute toxicity evaluation

The result is as presented in table 2. Single dose (100, 200, 500, 1000, 2000, 5000 and 6000 mg/kg^{-1}) of *G. angustifolia* root methanol extract administered to albino rats elicited some behavioural characteristics in them. There were some physical signs of toxicity when doses up 500

Group/Treatment	Percentage Wound Contraction				
	4	6	8	10	16
1. Paraffin base	14.11 ± 0.35[a]	21.26 ± 0.05[a]	39.00 ± 6.97[a]	49.50 ± 7.67[a]	60.49 ± 6.77[a]
2. Povidone iodine	17.69 ± 7.27[a]	28.22 ± 0.42[a]	42.68 ± 11.37[a]	53.49 ± 7.09[a]	71.24 ± 0.36[a]
3. Root extract	21.24 ± 7.50[ab]	30.73 ± 7.76[ab]	48.53 ± 7.48[ab]	64.38 ± 8.19[ab]	87.36 ± 3.46[ab]
4. Leaf extract	17.50 ± 7.85[a]	28.39 ± 0.37[a]	46.07 ± 6.91[ab]	60.46 ± 7.12[ab]	81.81 ± 7.12[ab]
5. Fruit extract	21.07 ± 6.65[ab]	24.75 ± 6.98[a]	45.93 ± 7.11[a]	49.49 ± 8.34[a]	67.25 ± 6.74[ab]

Values are expressed as mean ± S.E. The mean values with the same superscript (ab) in the same column are significantly different (P<0.01). Values in the same column with (a) superscript are not significant (P<0.01) when compared with the reference standard.

Table 1: Effect of *G. angustifolia* extracts on wound closure.

Dosage (mg/kg) Time (hr)	100 2 4 6 8 12 24	200 2 4 6 8 12 24	500 2 4 6 8 12 24	1000 2 4 6 8 12 24	2000 2 4 6 8 12 24	5000 2 4 6 8 12 24	6000 2 4 6 8 12 24
Gross activity							
Respiration	- - - - - -	- - - - - -	- - - - - -	+ - - - - -	+ + - - - -	+ + - - - -	+ + +D
Writhing	- - - - - -	- - - - - -	- - - - - -	- - - - - -	- - - - - -	- - - - - -	- - -D
Tremors	- - - - - -	- - - - - -	- - - - - -	+ - - - - -	+ + - - - -	+ + - - - -	- - - D
Convulsion	- - - - - -	- - - - - -	- - - - - -	- - - - - -	- - - - - -	- - - - - -	- - - D
Salivation	- - - - - -	- - - - - -	- - - - - -	- - - - - -	- - - - - -	- - - - - -	- - - D
Diarrhea	- - - - - -	- - - - - -	- - - - - -	- - - - - -	- - - - - -	- - - - - -	- - + D
Mortality	- - - - - -	- - - - - -	- - - - - -	- - - - - -	- - - - - -	- - - - - -	- - - D
Hind limb paralysis	- - - - - -	- - - - - -	- - - - - -	- - - - - -	- - - - - -	- - - - - -	- - - D
Sedation	- - - - - -	- - - - - -	-- --- - -	+ + - - - -	+ + - - - -	+ + - - - -	- - -D
Skin irritation	- - - - - -	- - - - - -	- - - - - -	+ + + - - -	+ + - - - -	+ + - - - -	+ + -D
Eye irritation	- - - - - -	- - - - - -	- - - - - --	- - - - - -	- - - - - -	- - - - - -	- - -D
CNS depression	- - - - - -	- - - - - -	- - - - - --	- - - - - -	-- - - - -	--- - - -	+ + +D

+: Indicates that changes were observed; -: Indicates that there was no change; D: Indicates death.

Table 2: Changes in the animal's behavior after administration of *G. angustifolia* methanol root extracts.

mg/kg[-1] and above were administered. Death was recorded at 6000 mg/kg[-1] dose (Table 2). Fast respiration, mild tremor, sleepingness, and depression were observed. These observations showed that the oral LD_{50} of *G. angustifolia* is less than 6000 mg/kg[-1] in albino rats. The animals were able to overcome the effects after 7 days of post experiment.

Blood glucose

The plant extract elicits reduction in blood glucose and this is dose and time dependent as seen in table 3. This plant may be useful in the diabetic condition.

Anti-ulcerogenic activity study

As presented in table 4, *G. angustifolia* extract exhibited a dose-dependent protection from ethanol-induced ulceration. In comparison with the ulcer control group, *G. angustifolia* provided 48, 59 and 71% protection respectively at 100, 250 and 500 mg/kg[-1] dose. The reference standard, Omeprazole offered the highest protection at 8 mg/kg[-1] dose with 76.15% protection. The effect of 500 mg/kg[-1] dose of extract was quite comparable (71.37%) with the reference standard.

Discussion

The methanol extract of *G. angustifolia* was evaluated for wound healing activity using excision wound model in albino rats. The wound area measurement post wounding days (Table 1) showed that wound size of the test groups were reduced early as compared to control group. In addition to the reduction in wound size, the test group also showed a faster rate of healing. The order of increasing wound contraction of the various treatments is as follows:

Paraffin base ⟶ Fruit extract ointment ⟶ Povidone iodine ⟶ Leaf extract ointment ⟶ Root extracts ointment

The root extract showed the highest healing activity. Wound healing is a complex and dynamic process of restoring cellular structures and tissue layers in damaged tissues as closely as possible to its normal state.

Wound contracture is a process that occurs throughout the healing process, commencing in the fibroblastic stage whereby the area of the wound undergoes shrinkage. In maturation phase, the final phase of wound healing the wound undergoes contraction resulting in a smaller amount of apparent scar tissue.

Granulation tissue formed in the final part of the proliferative phase is primarily composed of fibroblasts, collagen, edema, and new small blood vessel [16]. In this study, it may be inferred that *G. angustifolia* ointments have the potential to satisfy all requirements of an ideal dressing material in that it provides an environment at the surface of the wound in which healing took place at the maximum rate consistent with the formation of granulation tissue with an acceptable cosmetic appearance and also provides a rationale for the use of *G. angustifolia* preparations in traditional system of medicine to promote wound healing.

Furthermore, it can be concluded that *G. angustifolia* extract has a beneficial effect as antiseptic and as an injury healing promoter. This effect may be explained by several mechanisms such as coating the wound, forming complexes with proteins of microorganism cell wall, chelating free radicals and reactive oxygen species, stimulating the contraction of the wound and increasing the formation of new capillaries and fibroblasts. Moreover, the extract did not produce any adverse effect on the wound surface and because of this it is possible to recommend its use in the treatment of skin wounds or ulcers.

Methanol extract of the root of *G. angustifolia* up to 5000 mg/kg[-1] did not cause any mortality in rats. All the doses below 5000 mg/kg[-1] did not produce any gross apparent effect on general motor activity; there was no convulsion, salivation, diarrhea and paralysis. Though there were mild signs of CNS depression at higher doses as well as sedation, respiration changes and slight tremor but all these signs faded as the time of exposure increased thus at 48 hrs after administration, the animals were near normal and well again (Table 2). Any substance that is not toxic at 5000 mg/kg[-1] is considered relatively safe [17].

Dosage (mg/kg⁻¹)	Blood Glucose (mg/dl) after 12 Hrs	Blood Glucose (mg/dl) after 24 Hrs
100	66	52
250	65	50
500	61	54
1000	60	46
2000	58	49
5000	54	48

Table 3: Effect of *G. angustifolia* on blood glucose level in rats.

Treatment	Dose (mg/kg⁻¹)	Gastric Volume (ML)	Ulcer Area (mm²)	Protection (%)
Ulcer control	0	2.98 ± 0.22ᵃ	753.33 ± 4.32ᵃ	0.00
Drug control (Omeprazole)	8	1.46 ± 0.12ᵇ	171.33 ± 8.62ᶜ	76.15
Treatment 1 (*G. angustifolia*)	100	1.63 ± 0.03ᶜ	379.33 ± 24.68ᵇ	47.59
Treatment 2 (*G. angustifolia*)	250	1.67 ± 0.10ᵇ	297.66 ± 23.16ᵈ	58.65
Treatment 3 (*G. angustifolia*)	500	1.55 ± 0.62ᶜ	191.67 ± 14.84ᵉ	71.37

Values are expressed as mean ± S.E. Values in a column followed by different letters are significantly different ($P<0.01$). Values in a column with an asterisk (*) are significantly different from ulcer control ($P<0.01$).

Table 4: Anti-ulcerogenic effect of *G. angustifolia* root methanol extract.

Ulcer has long been recognized as one of the most important gastrointestinal problem. Peptic ulcers are common disorder of the entire gastro-intestinal tract that occurs mainly in the stomach and the proximal duodenum [18]. With the ever growing interest in natural medicine, many plants have been screened and reported to be useful in treating and managing ulcer. *G. angustifolia* has been claimed to have several pharmacological properties. In spite of its use in the traditional medicine against various ailments, this plant has so far not been screened for anti-ulcer activity. This report on its anti-ulcer activity appears to be the first in literature. The results of the present study have shown that *G. angustifolia* root extract possess gastro-protective activity, as evidenced by its significant inhibition in the formation of ulcers induced by ethanol (Table 4).

Since ulcer is a multi-factorial disease, its treatment faces great difficulties due to the limited effectiveness and severe side effects of the currently available drugs [18]. Owing to the side effects of the available drugs and cost, many plant-derived natural products have been evaluated as therapeutics for the treatment of a variety of diseases, including the peptic ulcer [19].

As presented in table 4, the methanol extract of the root of *G. angustifolia* (100, 250 and 500 mg/kg⁻¹) and Omeprazole (8 mg/kg⁻¹) significantly inhibited ulcer formation in this model by 47.59, 58.65, 71.37 and 76.15% respectively. The reduction of the lesions seen with the methanol extract of *G. angustifolia* suggests that part of the protective mechanisms could involve mucosal defensive factors. Gastric mucosal damage caused by ethanol and related non-steroidal anti-inflammatory drugs result from the inhibition of prostaglandins synthesis via the arachidonic pathway [20]. Prostaglandins serve protective functions in the stomach by maintaining gastric microcirculation [20] and causing gastric secretion of bicarbonate and mucus [21]. Thus, the effect of the extract in this model suggests that it may possess cytoprotective action, probably by enhancing prostaglandin synthesis. The extract significantly ($P<0.01$) protected gastric mucosa against ethanol challenge.

Ethanol-induced gastric mucosal lesions, predominant in the glandular part of the stomach are cuased by the direct toxic action of ethanol, reduction of the secretion of bicarbonate and depletion of gastric wall mucus [22].

Conclusion

In conclusion, our results suggest that *G. angustifolia* methanol extract ointment possess wound healing activity and gastro-protective effect against acute ethanol-induced ulcer models in rats. In this regard, we suggest that natural gastro-protective agent in *G. angustifolia* may be effective as plant gastro-protector and thus may have some obvious therapeutic implications. This plant could be toxic at higher doses. Further work is needed in the area of biosafety, phytoconstituents and mechanisms of action of *G. angustifolia* in wound healing action.

Acknowledgment

We gratefully acknowledge the technical assistance of Mr. Friday T. Emmanuel and Olusegun Olupinyo in this work.

References

1. Pierce GF, Mustoe TA (1995) Pharmacologic enhancement of wound healing. Annu Rev Med 46: 467-481.

2. Prasad D, Rao CM (1995) Wound healing profiles of ketorolac, metronidazole and tinidazole administered post-surgically. Indian J Exp Biol 33: 845-847.

3. Rao CM, Ramesh KV, Bairy KL, Kulkarni DR (1991) A simple method to quantify maturation of wound collagen. Indian J Exp Biol 29: 156-158.

4. Meyer-Ingold W (1993) Wound therapy: growth factors as agents to promote healing. Trends Biotechnol 11: 387-392.

5. Wallace JL, McKnight W, Reuter BK, Vergnolle N (2000) NSAID-induced gastric damage in rats: requirement for inhibition of both cyclooxygenase 1 and 2. Gastroenterology 119: 706-714.

6. Laine L, Takeuchi K, Tarnawski A (2008) Gastric mucosal defense and cytoprotection: bench to bedside. Gastroenterology 135: 41-60.

7. Clouatre D, Rosenbaum M (1994) The diet and benefits of HCA. Keats Publishing, New York, USA.

8. Bennet RG (1988) Fundamentals of cutaneous surgery. St. Louis C.V. Mosby 78.

9. Yagi A, Hine MM, Nsyawa Y, Tateyama T, Fujioka K, et al. (1998) Tetrahydroantracene glucoside in calus tissue from Aloe barbadensis leaves. Phytochemistry 47:1267-1270.

10. Cooper SP (1987) Gunn's dispensing for pharmacentical sudent. In: Carter SL. (12thedn), C.B.S. Publisher and Distributors, New Delhi, India.

11. Rashed AN, Afifi FU, Disi AM (2003) Simple evaluation of the wound healing activity of a crude extract of *Portulaca oleracea* L. (growing in Jordan) in *Mus musculus* JVI-1. J Ethnopharmacol 88: 131-136.

12. Abu-Al-Basal M (2001) The incidence of some local medicinal plant extracts on skin wound healing activity: Evaluated by histological and ultra-structural studies. Ph.D. Thesis, University of Jordan, Amman, Jordan.

13. Obelis S, Sae H (2009) Fine test auto-coding premium blood glucose monitoring system. Infopia Co. Ltd. 431-716.

14. Kurasawa T, Chikaraishi Y, Naito A, Toyoda Y, Notsu Y (2005) Effect of *Humulus lupulus* on gastric secretion in a rat pylorus-ligated model. Biol Pharm Bull 28: 353-357.

15. Mohd Anur SFZ, Abdulla MA, Mohd Ali H, Suzita MN, Ismail S (2009) Anti-ulcerogenic activity of aqueous extract of *Ficus deltoidea* against ethanol-induced gastric mucosal injury in rats. Annals of Medicine and Healthcare Research 226-235.

16. Kumar R, Shenoy C, Patil MB (2006) Wound healing activity of *Hyptis suaveolens* (L.) Poit (Lamiaceae). International Journal of PharmTech Research 1: 737-744.

17. Lorke D (1983) A new approach to practical acute toxicity testing. Arch Toxicol 54: 275-287.

18. Mota KS, Dias GE, Pinto ME, Luiz-Ferreira A, Souza-Brito AR, et al. (2009) Flavonoids with gastroprotective activity. Molecules 14: 979-1012.

19. Musthaba M, Baboota S, Athar TM, Thajudeen KY, Ahmed S, et al. (2010) Patented herbal formulations and their therapeutic applications. Recent Pat Drug Deliv Formul 4: 231-244.

20. Vane JR (1971) Inhibition of prostaglandin synthesis as a mechanism of action for aspirin-like drugs. Nat New Biol 231: 232-235.

21. Garner A, Flemstrom G, Heylings JR (1979) Effects of antiinflammatory agents and prostaglandins on acid and bicarbonate secretions in the amphibian-isolated gastric mucosa. Gastroenterology 77: 451-457.

22. Marhuenda E, Martin MJ, De La Alarcon Lastra C (1993) Antiulcerogenic activity of aescine in different experimental models. Phytotherapy Research 7: 13-16.

28

The Role of Stroma in Tumour-Host Co-Existence: Some Perspectives in Stroma-Targeted Therapy of Cancer

Joseph Molnár[1], Ilona Mucsi[1], Helga Engi[1], Gabriela Spengler[1], Leonard Amaral[1,2], Attila Zalatnai[3], Qi Wang[4] and Ben Efraim Shlomo[5]

[1]Institute of Medical Microbiology and Immunobiology, University of Szeged, Szeged, Hungary
[2]Travel Medicine, Center for Malaria and other Tropical Diseases (CMDT), Institute of Hygiene and Tropical Medicine of Lisbon, Universidade Nove de Lisboa, Lisbon, Portugal
[3]Department of Pathology, University of Semmelweis, Budapest, Hungary
[4]Department of Respiratory Medicine, the Second Affiliated Hospital of Dalian Medical University, Dalian, China
[5]Department of Human Microbiology Sackler, Faculty of Medicine, Tel-Aviv –University, Tel Aviv, 62155, Israel

Abstract

Cancer grows at the expense of the host as a parasite or superparasite following the second law of thermodynamics (conservation of energy). When the cancer cell progresses via replication to the special state called "spheroid", a new phase begins with its intimate interaction and development of responses from the stroma which together assist in the formation of a full blown cancer. Among the processes involved are the development of blood vessels and lymphatic channels which are essential for maintenance and further growth of the cancer mass. In this way the condition of "parasitism" is completed with simultaneous suppression of the immune response of the host to the histoincompatability of the tumor mass. Stroma/parenchyma promotes cancer invasion by feeding cancer cells and inducing immune tolerance. The dynamic changes in composition of stroma and biological consequences as feeder of cancer cells and immune tolerance can give a perspective for rational drug design in anti-stromal therapy. There are differences between normal and cancer cells at subcellular level such as compartmentalzation and structure of cytoskeleton and energy distribution (that is low generally, but locally high in normal cells). In cancer cannibalism of normal cells, the growing cancer mass is a factor for progression and invasion.

Cancer cells have been shown to kill normal cells and the products of cell death used for progression of growth of the cancer cell. Serum and growth factors produced by tumor stroma also provide the needed nutrients and conditions for further tumor growth. Cancer cannot feed off other cancer cells and therefore grow poorly. Probably, although not yet proven, the inability of cancer to "parasitise" other cancer cell types is probably due to some kind of competition or interference. The tumor is in charge of its own development due to its induction proteinases, lipid mobilization factors and angiogenetic factors as well as its ability to negate immune responses of the host response to what is in essence a foreign body.

In our review co-existence of normal and cancer cells in tumor with the growth promoting factors, and the immune tolerance mediating factors produced in the stromal and cancer cells/tissues will be discussed with perspective of stroma targeted therapy.

Keywords: Development of a solid cancer; 2nd law of thermodynamics; Parasitic interaction between cancer and normal cells; Stroma cells; Interaction between stroma and cancer cells and immune responses; Therapeutic targets; existing compounds; Proteases; Immune regulators; Vascular and endothelial growth factors; Inhibition of signals between cancer and normal cells of surrounding and mestatic sites

Introduction

The clinical significance of cell cannibalism is well defined and described in a large number of publications [1,2]. The direction of process of cancer developmemt is defined as the tumor invades the normal tissue which never occurs in the reverse direction. This suggests that the cancer cell strives to achieve the lowest energy level possible. Therefore the first law of the development of a full blown cancer can be considered as the 2nd Thermodynamic principle [3] that explains, describes and drives the invading cancer into normal surrouding tissue.

From the normal living state, under particular conditions such as hypoxia, where ATP synthesis is decreased resulting in a switch to glycolytic pathways, cancer cells are selected from a fraction of the population [4]. Energetically, in the presence of electron transfer, by using high energy from respiration, the proliferating state is more stable than resting cells where a higher degree of protein stabilization occurs such as that needed for maintainance of the cytoskeleton of the cell. It

was proposed that tumor-promotion might be controlled or modulated by small electronic currents originating from reactive oxygen species and transported through the cytoskeletal microfilament network of the cancer cell [5].

Aerobic glycolysis is the main energy producing process in cancer cells [6]. Among many other aspects, recently the mitochondria have also been regarded as potential targets in the therapy of cancer. Several small molecules have been tested to restore their dysfunctional functions either by direct or indirect effects [7]. Because of poorly functioning mitochondria, the electron transfer component of the respiration cycle is inefficient; therefore, cancer cells have smaller Gibbs energy than

*Corresponding author: Joseph Molnar, Institute of Medical Microbiology and Immunobiology, University of Szeged, Szeged, Hungary, E-mail: molnar.jozsef@med.u-szeged.hu

healthy cells. This means, that these cancer cells exists in a metastable state [8] and are not able maintain normal cell structure. Therefore, the cytoskeleton system is collapsed and dielectric bilayers are formed as a lower grade of cellular structure with decreased electron conductivity. Consequently, to halt cancer growth, one has to evaluate the process of cancer cell development *in situ*, where the primary tumor is growing as well as that of the metastatic cell that is invading surrounding or distal tissues [9]. This affords one to suggest that the stroma is formed first during long term repeated oxidative stress, a process that is initially accompanied with inflammation due to an active immune response to the histo-incompatability antigens present on the surfce of the cancer cell. If the cancer cell evades the activity of killer T cells (Treg cells) by either secreting agents that reduce the response of the Treg cells or the immune system for whatever reason is ineffective (immunosuppresed states such as HIV/AIDS, pregnancy, transplatation therapy, etc.), the formed cancer cells have the opportunity to initiate tumor development. Because of the limited capacity of its electron transfer cycle, cancer cells are essentially starving cells that require glycolytically useful substrates. These substrates are obtained from the killing of normal cells by agents secreted by the cancer cell and the products yielded from dead normal cells "eaten" (phagocytosed) by the starving cancer cell which is digested by the cancer cells lysosomal system. This autophagic process of cannibalism keeps the cancer cell alive and thriving and is known as cytophagy, i.e., cannibalism of normal cells. This type of autophagocytosis results in a parasitic co-existence of tumor cells with normal cells and will determine the main pathway of interaction between the growing cancer tissue (tumor) and normal tissue where the cancer tissue gradually destroys normal tissues. This process obeys the scond law of thermodynamics-conservation of energy within a defined system.

The conduction of proteins and oxygen consumption are basically different in cancer and healthy tissues primarily due to the faulty mitochondrial structure. This difference bestows on the cancer cell an advantage over the normal cell that makes up the environment in which the cancer cell arose [10-12]. When cancer cells receive support from feeder fibroblasts for growth, they multiply independently from the ordered structure of tissue by forming a new agressive cell population that lives at the expense of normal tissue [8]. We have conducted a series of experiments that studied the specific coexistence between cancer and normal cells. Our aims were to analyse the various stages of tumor development with improving the opportunities of intervention for cancer therapy based upon the considerations of population biology and co-existance of normal and transformed cells or tissues. First of all, it should be noted that separate in vitro cultures which contain cancer cells and normal cells, repectively, when serum is omitted from the medium, the cancer cells survive for a longer period than do the normal cells [13]. When the culture contains a mixture of cancer cells and normal cells and serum is omitted, the cancer cells fluorish at the expense of dying normal cells [13]. These experiments clearly show that the cancer cells survive at the expense of the normal cells which when alive or dead, yield products that are ingested by the cancer cell.

As per the second law of thermodynamics, the developing cancer cell seeks a lower energy level for its stability. As this process continues, tremendous changes occur where the original status, including structure and function, can never be regained. In other words, the process leads to an irreversible state which progresses to lower energy levels. This lower energy state means that whereas the normal cell requires a much more stringent source of nutrients, the transformed cancer cell readily survives on cell debris, tissue fluid, fibroblasts and other connective tissue cells [14]. The limitation of avaliable nutrients does not affect the replication of the cancer cell as it does the normal cell. Whereas when insufficient nutrient is provided to the normal cell, receptors on the surface of the cell promote an inhibition of replication, the cancer cell, lacking these receptors, continues to replicate. The colonisation of surrounding tissue and organ just began from tumor spheroid state. 4) The Stroma Has a Role in the Invasion of Tumor Cells

Cancer cells invade normal tissue of an organ *via* different types of circulations, namely, the circulatory component that drains the site where the cancer cell exists and is not firmly attached to neighbouring cells or the lymphatic channels that provide similar drainage [15,16]. In the case of the circulatory system, the cancer cell may be taken to distal parts of the host's body. In the case of the lymphatic system, the cancer cell will reach the first lymphoid nodules where it is trapped, but continues to replicate. Therefore, different types of circulations specifically mediate the first steps of spreading and invasion into the surrounding tissues. The development of tumor stroma and the role of stress in tumor progression have been described in detail by several authors. There is a plethora of evidence that the tumor stroma differs significantly from that of the respective normal tissue. This is a very complex microenvironment, composed of connective tissue cells, blood vessels, lymphatics, nerves, smooth muscle elements, fat, lymphoid and macrophagic elements embedded in the extracellular matrix niche [17]. It is well established that there are dynamic and mutual interactions between the tumoral cells (e.g. tumor parenchyma) and the stroma, and recently, this concept provides the basis for novel treatment strategies by considering the opportunities given by the second law of thermodynamics [18]. The main components of tumor stroma are cancer cells, fibroblasts and immune cells. The biological role of stroma/parenchyma is feeding the cancer cells building a micro-environment for tumor and an interface between host healthy tissues and tumorous tissues [17].

The structure of the Extracelluar Matrix (ECM) or tumorous parenchyma may determine the degree of resistance the moving cell encounters. The malignant cells secreting various soluble factors that may remodel the ECM through collagen crosslinking, and tissue rigidity can potentially facilitate the directed cell migration. Tumoral chemotactic factors may trigger the monocyte → Tumor Associated Macrophage (TAM) transformation, and these cells are regarded as the major stromal cells responsible for the migration, invasion and metastasis formation. These cells are usually accumulated in the hypoxic areas of the cancer, and produce several pro-angiogenic factors [19]. In addition to TAM production, factors released from the tumor cells (interleukins, growth factors) stimulate TAMs to secrete Matrix Metalloproteases (MMPs) and other ECM degrading proteases which further enhance the invasiveness of the cancer cells [20,21]. Cancer cells can change their stroma by cell to cell contacts during tumor growth and are capable of modifying the invasiveness and metastasis formation of the tumor.

Another important cell population in the tumor stroma is the Cancer Associated Fibroblast (CAF) that is generated by transforming growth factor β1 (TGF-β1). They can produce a variety of cytokines, growth factors and ECM proteins in a paracrine manner that further alter the microenvironment of the cancer. CAFs, however, have a Janus-face, because they may promote tumor growth by enhancing angiogenesis and activating the endothelial cells, but they can also exert a tumor-suppressing effect [22]. Based on parenchyma protein production, the cancer associated fibroblast can determine the biophysical properties of the matrix favoring again the spreading of the cancer cell [23]. The main components and possible targets for intervention localised at the border (interfase) between "tumor –normal tissue" [24] are: 1. glycolysis [6], 2. lipid mobilization factor [25] and 3. proteolysis inducing factor at the microenvironment of the tumor-host interface [26].

The Stromal Cells as Possible Targets of Therapy

The stroma and parenchyma containing the various cells and ECM can be considered as a new therapeutic target having multiple sub-targets essential for tumor growth and the immunosuppressive property of the cancer cell. Several inhibitors of matrix metalloproteases needed for cancer growth, have been shown to inhibit tumor cell growth [20,21]. When therapeutic approach co-targets parenchymal, stromal cells, the ECM and cytokine elements, a good antitumor effect would be achieved. Experimental conditions provide the opportunity to exploit simultaneously more target interaction than targeting only a single cell or a single compartment interaction [27].

When the cancer cell is formed and the spheroid state develops gradually, the transformed cells will attract feeder cells, forming a new tissue structure, in which the polarity and place of cells are disturbed. Therefore, the tissue is disordered. The newly formed disordered tissue contains the tumor cells supported by the attracted stromal cells. The tumor cells are protected and fed by stroma and now have the possibility of invading the normal tissue, where tumor stroma functioning as a "Trojan horse".

The normal physiological activities of cells in the region of disordered tissue or an entire organ consisting of disordered tissue, will present gradients of electric potential that differ from normal ordered tissue. In a conventional sense, the movement of fluids that transport ions and other necessary materials to reaction sites in the disordered tissue, severely compromise colonization of normal tissue by cancer cells [9,15]. Others have demonstrated an additional pathway for energy exchange that permits reactions among distantly situated regions of the colonized tissue [28]. The living cells at the periphery of a tumor act as a "semipermeable" sieve or barrier between the surroundings and central necrosis in the tumor. This property may at first inspection not be quite obvious. The tumors consisting of cancer cells and stromal cells make the tissue firmer and denser than the surrounding normal tissues. This general firmness and greater density of the tumor serves to identify palpable cancers rather readily (breast and prostatic cancers are good examples). The sieve functions of various interstitial channels in tumors are increased compared to the surrounding normal tissue [15].

The development of stroma begins and is subsequently followed by invasion. Hence, the network of interstitial channels in a tumor potentially constitutes a relative barrier to interstitial flow, i.e., a "tumor barrier". On both sides of the tumor barrier, non-permeable bodies may be found. Many of these biological units may then be too large to pass through the intercellular spaces of an organized tissue. In this sense the intercellular sieve of a tumor acts as a barrier where material can be adsorbed or trapped by diffusion and closed electric transports [16]. What is the relationship of the electron deficiencies in cancer that result from less than adequate mitochondrial function? Various charge transfer cycles (CTC) of primary, secondary or tertiary nature exist in biological systems [28]. The electron deficiency is not a generalized deficiency, but a very specific one where one CTC cycle is not operating or is inactive [28]. Can a deficiency of one or more CTC cycles be exploited for inhibiting tumor growth? The answer is definitely no! They are responsible for tumor formation.

In general, we think that the direction of tumor growth and invasion of surrounding normal tissues is due to mechanism of auto-phagocytosis or cannibalism (self- and xeno-cannibalisms), defined as a superparasitism, is based on the 2nd law of thermodynamics [13,18,29]. Consequently, the application of well defined external force fields- may reverse the direction of tumor growth by the modification of the direction of some particular entropy flow therefore serving to modify parasitic interaction. Exposure of the "tumor-normal tissue area" to a physical force such as pulsed application of square wave electric potential, or, chemical (e.g. specific apoptosis inducers) may yield the desired modification of tumor growth. Blocking essential local energy producing mechanisms by the inhibition of anaerobic glycolysis, inhibition of the beta-oxidation of fatty acids as growth stimulators, blocking the alternative pathway of respiration branches by the application of SHAM (salicyl-hydroxamic acid) or, by biological intervention such as immunomodulation, can be promising ways to combat cancer.

Perspectives in immunology for stroma targeted therapy

The target of tumor killing activity of a low dose alkylating agent- an anticancer drug- was dissociated from its immunomodulating activity by treating mice bearing a tumor resistant to certain alkylating drugs. Induction of specific anti-tumor response by a low dose of alkylating drugs was due to expression of "latent anti-tumor" capability [30]. This fits the conception that "suppressed concomitant immunity" occurring in tumor-bearing animals can be activated. The immunomodulating activity of alkylating drugs was related to enhancement of T-cell functions by impairment of suppressor T-cell activity, enhancement of effector T-cell activity and increased production of cytokines at the tumor site. A low dose of anticancer agent had an immunomodulating effect in human cancer such as reduction of ConA-induced suppressor cell activity in melanoma, some improvement in addition to use of melanoma vaccine, and potentiation of DTH in cancer patients. The immunomodulating effect of alkylating drugs suggests that their use might be beneficial not only for killing tumor cells but also for promoting specific anti-tumor immune response [30].

The need to modify xenogenization of tumor cells *in vivo* to make the cancer cell more immunogenic and to raise an efficient protective immune response was studied in experimental models by the use of xenogenized human tumor cells for immunotherapy by using chemically and viral modified tumor cells [31]. Modified tumor cells were found partially effective as immunomodulating agents. Moreover, the mitogenic effects of agents on alveolar fibroblasts suggest a role for in fibrogenesis in support of cancer stroma, inasmuch as the supportive component of tumor stroma was reduced [32].

Some cancer vaccines that have been used in clinical trials which have resulted in partial beneficial therapeutic effects have not provided a full solution for rational use of thymic humoral factor as immunotherapy against cancer [33]. The use of cell free mediators for cancer immunotherapy in clinical trials suggests that much remains to be done in order to assure effective and reproducible therapeutic effectiveness of immunotherapy protocols for routine use in the treatment of human cancers [34]. Epstein Barr Virus (EBV) induces production of a suppressor factor in the supernatant of B-cell cultures [35]. BCG induces in the patient immune processes that target the early stages of a urinary bladder cancer. These findings above, collectively suggest that both T and B cells play important roles in the immune regulation and immune suppression by EBV [36].

Human melanoma cells secrete a factor that inhibits phytohemagglutinin induced T-cell proliferation and lipopolysaccharide induced B-cell proliferation. It is supposed that these factors have a role in protecting the melanoma tumor from attack by the immune system and reduce the antitumor responses of the host [37]. At any rate, antigen activated human macrophages have therapeutic activity against human tumor cells growing in mice [38]. The regulatory role of inflammatory mediators and their relationships with eicosanoids is a network that controls the expression of antitumor activity of the macrophages in cell to cell contact, and, because production of these anti-tumor factors can be shown in the medium containing the tumor and activated macrophage, these soluble factors as antitumor immunomodulators have potential for immunotherapy of human malignancies [39].

The stromal cells may regulate local immune responses by interacting cancer cells with the tumor-infiltrating T lymphocytes [40]. In addition, immune competent cells can mediate the cancer to accommodate, to adapt to the host and to avoid attack by host immune system. Stromal cells affect the immune response; create immune tolerance and barriers that avoid host immunity to the cancer cell. The tumor tolerizing mechanisms result in the inability of T-cells to destroy the tumor cells [41]. Suppression of T-cell activity is an important contributing factor by down regulation of MHC molecules, resulting in a decreased expression of HLA class I antigens [42], and the altered HLA class I phenotypes in human tumors is responsible for the immune suppression in cancer. Interestingly, the tumor cells do not only inhibit directly immune function, they kill infiltrating antigen specific T-lymphocytes [43,44]. However, these studies cannot be extrapolated to *in vivo* effects [45,31-38].

The tumor-shed soluble MHC class I homologues MICA and B are often produced by epithelial tumors resulting in the reduced responsiveness of tumor specific natural killer T cells [43,44]. In addition the tumor cells express T- cell stimulating antigens that are tolerated by the T-cells leading to insufficient antigen density [41,45,46].

Due to immune deficiencies in the host and immune tolerance of cancer cells, the tumor develops as a stealth object in the body by several mechanisms such as a tumor virus blocking the MHC1 antigen transport to the surface of the cells [47]. Consequently the cytotoxic immune response cannot eliminate the tumor cells. The production of a great variety of immunosuppressive factors involves complex mechanisms that contribute to the stealth behavior of cancer in the organism. Tumor gradually grows and invades the healthy tissues without early presentation of symptoms. Due to immunosuppression induced by human tumors, the tumor escapes immune surveillance and continues to grow [48].

Cancer cannibalism is an important mechanism of malignancy responsible for immunotolerance or resistance when metastatic tumor use cannibalism at low nutrient supply, The cannibal cells feed on sibling tumor cells and other cells under acidic environment that allow activation of lytic enzymes such as cathepsin B, and other factors as caveolin and actin-linker molecule ezrin. Various steps of cannibalisms may be explored and exploited for anti-stromal therapy [3,17,20,21,49]. From thermodynamic aspects the toxic effects of entropy flow from tumor to normal tissue plays an important role in the superparasitism, in the competitive exclusion between tumor and normal host cells where the possible targets are the proteolysis, extracellular matrix, various signal pathways, VEGF etc. [3,50]. Tumor gradually grows and invades the healthy tissues without early presentation of symptoms. Due to immunosuppression induced by human tumors, the tumor escapes immune surveillance and continues to grow [48].

As a by-product of oxidative phosphorylation Reactive Oxygen Species (ROS) are formed that may contribute to tumor initiation or progression [51]. Apart from damaging effects on nuclear and mitochondrial DNA, they are able to directly activate cell signaling such as MAP kinase, or phosphoinositide 3-kinase pathways [52], and they are implicated in the myc-induced tumorigenesis [53]. The hypoxia-inducible factor (HIF) seems to be a particularly important factor in the ROS-mediated tumorigenesis. HIF is known to mediate the upregulation of glycolytic genes and a global shift in cellular metabolism toward glycolysis, and the ROS stabilize and activate this factor under hypoxic conditions [54]. Therefore it is not surprising the targeting of mitochondrial ROS in cancer therapy is a novel approach. The tempting idea that large doses of antioxidants might interfere with the tumor development or progression proved to be inconsistent and controversial in human studies, still there are data about the ROS-mediated cell killing by different cytostatic drugs [55], or there is ongoing research to find selective anticancer compounds [56]. Similarly, targeted inhibition of HIF is also under investigation [57].

The redox-status in cancer stem cells is hardly understood. These cells are believed to be relatively radio-resistant and drug resistant because of low ROS-level and high concentration of scavenger molecules. Redox-modulating strategies could serve again new therapeutic approaches to overcome drug resistance. However, breaking their redox-adaptation has a Janus-face [58]. Nevertheless, some promising results are available indicating the selective killing effect of a thiol-depleting compound on leukemic stem cells without significant toxicity of normal hemopoetic cells [59].

Apparently the stroma has a key role in tumor development, consequently can be considered as possible target of therapy. There are opportunities in at least two different areas of therapy: a. focused on tumor stroma the modification cancer cell adhesion, proteolysis, extracellular matrix and various signal pathways as was suggested by Liotta et al. in 2002 [17]. Other opportunities are related to thermodynamics or physics. We had quantitively demonstrated that entropy production of rates of cancer cells is always higher than that of normal cells Molnar et al [60].When an electric field is applied to cells the entropy production rate of normal cells may exceed that of cancer cells [59]. The thermodynamical approaches as confirmed by calculations of the effects of external energy of electric field as the application of physical on the growth inhibition of cancer cells was a promising intervention as suggested by Luo et al. [29].

The electric effect of field was demonstrated recently *in vivo* where high electric fields induced the ablation of cancer in various metastatic tumors in mice and in clinical trials due to electric ablation in changes occurred in the tumor microenvironment. The induction of antitumor immunity was also involved in the complex effects of the pulsed electric forces [61].

Conclusion

Therapeutic opportunities that exploit various facets of cancer development, invasion, and the role that the stroma and its distinct composition of cell types play [17], are briefly summarized in Table 1. The *in situ* ablation of solid tumors by electric forces and effects on the tumor microenvironment and antitumor immunity has been discussed by others and suggestions for therapy well presented [61].

Due to the large number of distinct cancer cell types and subsequent departure from their appearance, functions, biochemical properties and energy and nutritional needs when they metastasize to different parts of the body that exhibit different stromal conditions, it is highly doubtful that any single form of therapy that specifically aims at one target, will

Target	Example agent	Comments
Adhesion	Vitaxin (anti-acfl3-mAb)	Cytostasis in patients, antitumor and anti-angiogenic in animal models
Proteolysis	Matrix metalloproteinase inhibitors	Cytostatic in patients
Extracellular matrix	Pirfenidone	Stromal fibrosis Suppresses stromal remodelling
	Squalamine	Selective to endothelial cells
Signal pathways	Anti-EGFR mAb (C225)	Active in animal models
	CAI (nonvoltage-gated Ca^{2+}-uptake inhibitor)	Active in combinations *in vitro*

Table 1: Examples for therapeutics targeting stroma-tumor interactions [17].

be effective against many cancer cell types. These differences may not be as limiting as one may think. Rather they may present the ability to selectively target the sensitive target of a distinct cancer cell type. This in turn may result in far less damage to normal cells as is the case with the "shot-gun approaches" of chemotherapy and radiotherapy in use today.

References

1. Alva AS, Gultekin SH, Baehrecke EH (2004) Autophagy in human tumors: cell survival or death? Cell Death Differ 11: 1046-1048.

2. Kojima S, Sekine H, Fukui I, Ohshima H (l998) Clinical significance of cannibalism in urinary cytology of bladder cancer. J Acta Cytologica 42: 1365-1369.

3. Molnar J, Varga ZG, Thornton-Benko E, Thornton B (2011) The second Law of Thermodynamics and Host–Tumor Relationships: Concepts and opportunities. Application of Thermodynamics to Biological and Material Science Edited by Tadashi Mizutani (ISBN 978-953-980-6).

4. Goldblatt H, Cameron G (1953) Induced malignancy in cells from rat myocardium subjected to intermittent anaerobiosis during long propagation in vitro. J Exp Med 97: 525-552.

5. Cavelier G (2000) Theory of malignant cell transformation by superoxide fate coupled with cytoskeletal electron-transport and electron-transfer. Med Hypotheses 54: 95-98.

6. WARBURG O (1956) On the origin of cancer cells. Science 123: 309-314.

7. Wang F, Ogasawara MA, Huang P (2010) Small mitochondria-targeting molecules as anti-cancer agents. Mol Aspects Med 31: 75-92.

8. Fröhlich H (1980) The biological effects of microwaves and related questions. Advances in Electronics and Electron Physics 53: 85.

9. Thornton BS (1984) Inversion of Raman spectra of living cells indicates dielectric structure related to energy control. Physics Letters 106: 198-202.

10. Chen N, Schoenbach KH, Kolb JF, James Swanson R, Garner AL, et al. (2004) Leukemic cell intracellular responses to nanosecond electric fields. Biochem Biophys Res Commun 317: 421-427.

11. Barsamian ST, Barsamian SP (1988) Dielectric investigation of murine cancer cells. J of Biological Physics 16: 25-30.

12. Yoo DS (2004) The dielectric properties of cancerous tissues in a nude mouse xenograft model. Bioelectromagnetics 25: 492-497.

13. Molnar J, Liao-fu L, Gyemant N, Mucsi I, Vezendi K, et al. (2007) Cancer growth is superparasitism in host: a Predator-Prey Relationship Acta Scientiarum Naturalium Universitas NeiMongol 38: 44-63.

14. Varro A, Holmberg C, Quante M, Steele I, Kumar J, et al. (2012) Release of TGFssig-h3 by gastric myofibroblasts slows tumor growth and is decreased with cancer progression. Carcinogenesis. [Epub ahead of print]

15. Nordenström BEW (1989) Biologically Closed Electric Circuits. Nordic Medical Publications: 122-124.

16. Nordenström BEW (1989) Biologically Closed Electric Circuits, Clinical, Experimental and Theoretical Evidence for an Additional Circulatory System. Nordic Medical Publications: 148.

17. Liotta LA, Kohn EC (2001) The microenvironment of the tumour-host interface. Nature 411: 375-379.

18. Molnar J, Thornton BS, Thornton-Benko E, Amaral L, Schelz Zs, et al. (2009) Thermodynamics and Electrobiologic properties for therapies to intervene in cancer progression, Current Cancer Therapy Reviews 5: 158-169.

19. Hockel M, Vaupel P (2001) Biological consequences of tumor hypoxia. Semin Oncol 28: 36-41.

20. Engi H, Gyémánt N, Ohkoshi M, Amaral L, Molnár J (2009) Modelling of tumor-host coexistence in vitro in the presence of serine protease inhibitors. *In vivo* 23: 711-716.

21. Ohkoshi M, Sasaki Y (2005) Antimetastatic activity of a synthetic serine protease inhibitor, FOY-305 (Foypan). *In vivo* 19: 133-136.

22. Rasanen K, Vaheri A (2010) Activation of fibroblasts in cancer stroma. Exp Cell Res 316: 2713-2722.

23. Ungefroren H, Sebens S, Seidl D, Lehnert H, Hass R (2011) Interaction of tumor cells with the microenvironment. Cell Commun Signal 9: 18.

24. Watchorn TM, Waddell I, Dowidar N, Ross JA (2001) Proteolysis-inducing factor regulates hepatic gene expression *via* the transcription factors NF-(kappa)B and STAT3. FASEB J 15: 562-564.

25. Islam-Ali BS, Tisdale MJ (2001) Effect of a tumour-produced lipid-mobilizing factor on protein synthesis and degradation. Br J Cancer 84: 1648-1655.

26. Tisdale MJ (2003) Pathogenesis of cancer cachexia. J Support Oncol 1: 159-168.

27. Zalatnai A (2006) Molecular aspects of stromal-parenchymal interactions in malignant neoplasms. Curr Mol Med 6: 685-693.

28. Guttmann F, Johnson C, Keyzer H, Molnar J (1997) Charge transfer complexes in biological systems, Marcel Dekker Inc., New York Basel Hong Kong 1997.

29. Liao-fu L, Molnar J, Ding H, Lv X, Spengler G (2006) Attempts to introduce thermodynamics in anticancer therapy using entropy production difference between cancer and normal cells. Acta Scientiarum Naturalium Universitatis Nei Mongol 37: 295-303.

30. Ben-Efraim S (2001) Immunomodulating anticancer alkylating drugs: targets and mechanisms of activity. Curr Drug Targets 2: 197-212.

31. Ben-Efraim S, Bizzini B, Relyveld EH (2000) Use of xenogenized (modified) tumor cells for treatment in experimental tumor and in human neoplasia. Biomed Pharmacother 54: 268-273.

32. Shahar I, Fireman E, Topilsky M, Grief J, Schwarz Y, et al. (1999) Effect of endothelin-1 on alpha-smooth muscle actin expression and on alveolar fibroblasts proliferation in interstitial lung diseases. Int J Immunopharmacol 21: 759-775.

33. Ben-Efraim S, Keisari Y, Ophir R, Pecht M, Trainin N, et al. (1999) Immunopotentiating and immunotherapeutic effects of thymic hormones and factors with special emphasis on thymic humoral factor THF-gamma2. Crit Rev Immunol 19: 261-284.

34. Ben-Efraim S (1999) One hundred years of cancer immunotherapy: a critical appraisal. Tumour Biol 20: 1-24.

35. Drucker I, Ben-Efraim S, Klajman A (1996) Secretion of suppressor factors by EBV infected B cell lines. Anticancer Res 16: 2857-2861.

36. Ben-Efraim S (1996) Cancer immunotherapy: hopes and pitfalls: a review. Anticancer Res 16: 3235-3240.

37. Giacomoni D, Ben-Efraim S, Najmabadi F, Dray S (1990) Inhibitors of lymphocyte activation secreted by human melanoma cell lines. Med Oncol Tumor Pharmacother 7: 273-280.

38. Ben-Efraim S, Tak C, Romijn JC, Fieren MJ, Bonta IL (1994) Therapeutical effect of activated human macrophages on a human tumor line growing in nude mice. Med Oncol 11: 7-12.

39. Bonta IL, Ben-Efraim S (1993) Involvement of inflammatory mediators in macrophage antitumor activity. J Leukoc Biol 54: 613-626.

40. Gorgun G, Anderson KC (2011) Intrinsic modulation of lymphocyte function by stromal cell network: advance in therapeutic targeting of cancer. Immunotherapy 3: 1253-1264.

41. Restifo NP (2001) Hierarchy, Tolerance and Dominance in the Antitumor T-cell Response. J Immunother 24: 193-194.

42. Garrido F, Ruiz-Cabello F, Cabrera T, Perez-Villar JJ, Lopez-Botet M, et al. (1997) Implications for immunosurveillance of altered HLA class I phenotypes in human tumors. Immunol Today 18: 89-95.

43. Bergmann-Leitner ES, Duncan EH, Leitner WW (2003) Identification and targeting of tumor escape mechanisms: a new hope for cancer therapy? Curr Pharm Des 9: 2009-2023.

44. M, O'Connel J, O'Sulivan GC, Brady C, Roche D, et al. (1998) The Fas counterattack *in vivo*: apoptotic depletion of tumor infiltrating lymphocytes associated wih Fas ligand expression by human esophageal carcinoma. J Immunology 160: 5669-5675.

45. Restifo NP (2000) Not so Fas: Re-evaluating the mechanisms of immune privilege and tumor escape. Nat Med 6: 493-495.

46. Groh V, Wu J, Yee C, Spies T (2002) Tumour-derived soluble MIC ligands impair expression of NKG2D and T-cell activation. Nature 419: 734-738.

47. Whiteside TL, Rabinowich H (1998) The role of Fas/FasL in immunosuppression induced by human tumors. Cancer Immunol Immunother 46: 175-184.

48. Garrido F, Algarra I (2001) MHC antigens and tumor escape from immune surveillance. Adv Cancer Res 83: 117-158.

49. Fais S (2007) Cannibalism: a way to feed on metastatic tumors. Cancer Lett 258: 155-164.

50. Peng Y, Jia XC, Liaofu L, Molnar J, Spengler G, et al. (2005) A theoretical model of cancerous and normal cells growth affected by entropy flow. In: Proceedings of International Seminar on Drug Resistance in cancer, Szeged, December 5: 10-14.

51. Fogg VC, Lanning NJ, Mackeigan JP (2011) Mitochondria in cancer: at the crossroads of life and death. Chin J Cancer 30: 526-539.

52. Weinberg F, Chandel NS (2009) Reactive oxygen species-dependent signaling regulates cancer. Cell Mol Life Sci 66: 3663-3673.

53. Vafa O, Wade M, Kern S, Beeche M, Pandita TK, et al. (2002) c-Myc can induce DNA damage, increase reactive oxygen species, and mitigate p53 function: a mechanism for oncogene-induced genetic instability. Mol Cell 9: 1031-1044.

54. Mansfield KD, Guzy RD, Pan Y, Young RM, Cash TP, et al. (2005) Mitochondrial dysfunction resulting from loss of cytochrome c impairs cellular oxygen sensing and hypoxic HIF-alpha activation. Cell Metab 1: 393-399.

55. Gogvadze V, Orrenius S, Zhivotovsky B (2009) Mitochondria as targets for cancer chemotherapy. Semin Cancer Biol 19: 57-66.

56. Fulda S, Galluzzi L, Kroemer G (2010) Targeting mitochondria for cancer therapy. Nat Rev Drug Discov 9: 447-464.

57. Wenger JB, Chun SY, Dang DT, Luesch H, Dang LH (2011) Combination therapy targeting cancer metabolism. Med Hypoth 76: 169-172.

58. Acharya A, Das I, Chandhok D, Saha T (2010) Redox regulation in cancer: a double-edged sword with therapeutic potential. Oxid Med Cell Longev 3: 23-34.

59. Guzman ML, Li X, Corbett CA, Rossi RM, Bushnell T, et al. (2007) Rapid and selective death of leukemia stem and progenitor cells induced by the compound 4-benzyl, 2-methyl, 1,2,4-thiadiazolidine, 3,5 dione (TDZD-8). Blood 110: 4436-4444.

60. Molnar J, Thornton BS, Molnar A, Gaal D, Luo L, et al. (2005) Thermodynamic aspects of cancer: possible role of negative entropy in tumor growth, its relation to kinetic and genetic resistence. Letters in Drug Design and Discovery 2: 429-438.

61. Keisari Y, Korenstein R (2013) *In situ* ablation of solid tumors by electric forces and its effect on the tumor microenvironment and anti-tumor immunity. Tumor Ablation The Tumor Microenvironment 5: 133-153.

29

Anti-Hyperglycemic Potency of *Jatropha Gossypiifolia* in Alloxan Induced Diabetes

Adetuyi BO*, Dairo JO and Didunyemi OM

Department of Biochemistry, College of Natural Sciences, Joseph Ayo Babalola University, Ikeji-Arakeji, Ilesa, Osun State, Nigeria

Abstract

The aqueous extract of *Jatropha Gossypiifolia* were studied for their anti-hyperglycemic activity, fifteen animals were taken and they were divided into five groups. First group act as the control, while the remaining four groups were induced diabetics by administering alloxan (120 mg/kg). Second group induced with diabetes with insulin treatment , third group induced with diabetes without treatment, fourth was infected with diabetes treated with 12 hours intervals oral dose of ethanolic extract of leaves (120 mg/kgbody weight) and fifth group was infected with diabetes treated with 12 hours intervals oral dose of ethanolic extract of leaves (240 mg/kg body weight/day). From the experiments, It was discovered that the aqueous extract of *Jatropha Gossypiifolia* at dose of 120 mg/kg and 240 mg/kg for 7 days has effects in reducing hyperglycemia, it was discovered that the body weight increased, in line with one of the symptoms of diabetes; obesity. The test carried out on three different types of microbes shows that the aqueous extract inhibit the growth of the micro-organisms at different concentration. Staphylococcus aureus is a gram +ve bacteria, this can be seen in the low zone of inhibition seen in *Klebsiella pneumonia* (gram -ve) and also Escherichia coli is a gram – ve. It was also discovered that the ethanolic extracts of *Jatropha Gossypiifolia* have a phytotoxic effect; that is, they inhibit the growth of plants as compared to the control. This could be trace to the difference in the phytochemical components of the ethanolic extract, alkaloids, tannins, saponins and glucosides are discovered to be present in the ethanolic extract.

Keywords: Diabetes; *Jatropha Gossypiifolia*; Anti-hyperglycemic; Alloxan

Introduction

The incidence of each type of diabetes varies widely throughout the world. The vast majority of diabetes patients have type 2 DM. About 90% of all diabetic patients have type 2 DM. There are more than 125 million persons with diabetic in the world today. There is increase in current interest and demand for herbs as worldwide phenomenon, WHO currently encourages, contains curcin, a toxalbumin which is highly irritant and produces deleterious effects on blood. The latex is acrid and irritable to the skin. Curcain, a protease has been isolated from the latex of *Jatropha curcas* [1]. Some of the ethnomedical uses of *Jatropha curcas* have received support from the results of scientific investigations in recent times. For example, some compounds with antitumor activities were reportedly found in this plant.

Furthermore various solvent extracts of *Jatropha curcas* have an abortive effect [2]. Traditionally it is taken internally with ripe banana to treat dysentery in adults. The sap from twigs is considered styptic and is used for dressing wounds and ulcer. The bark rubbed with asafetida and buttermilk is reportedly taken internally in Konkan to relieve dyspepsia and diarrhea. A decoction of bark is used externally for treating rheumatism and leprosy. The decoction of root bark is used to rinse the mouth to relieve toothache and sore throat among the tribal inhabitants of

Southern Andhra Pradesh [3]. Some anecdotal reports are there, which reveals plant has been used in the indigenous system of medicine and literature in the treatment of various ailments. Its leaves have acrid taste, which is considered as an excretory product or secondary metabolites, may be of therapeutic use and have action on metabolism [4-6]. Since diabetes is considered as metabolic disorder so action on liver or pancreas can be postulated hence an attempt has been focused for its anti-diabetic activity.

In the present work, we investigated the anti-hyperglycemic potency of *jatropha gossypiifolia* in alloxan induced diabetes. Phytochemical screening was carried out on the plant extract, antimicrobial Sensitivity Assay was carried out. Also, the activities of serum and liver GGT, the activities of serum and liver BILIRUBIN, the activities of serum and liver ALP were evaluated in the treated rats. To the best of our knowledge, no data have been reported on the effects of these naturally occurring compounds on alloxan-induced diabetes., and, thus, the study was undertaken to fill the lacuna in this regard.

Animals

The albino rats (Rattus norvegicus) of both sexes, weighing from 120-180g were purchased from Ayo Ola Farms, Kwara State, Ilorin, Nigeria. They were kept under usual management conditions in conventional animal house of Biochemistry, Department of Chemical science, Joseph Ayo Babalola University, Ikeji-Arakeji, Ilesa, Nigeria. Rats were given standard laboratory diet and free access to water *ad libitum*.

Chemicals

Alloxan was purchased from Sigma Aldrich Chemicals Pvt , Ltd, Bangalore. All other chemicals and reagents used were of analytical grade.

*Corresponding author: Adetuyi BO, Department of Biochemistry, College of Natural Sciences, Joseph Ayo Babalola University, Ikeji-Arakeji, Ilesa, Osun State, Nigeria, E-mail: krebcycle4u@yahoo.com

Reagent kits for biochemical analysis (Infopia and Randox)

Glucose levels were measured using Fine Test strips and Fine Test Glucometer manufactured by Infopia Co. Ltd in Korea. Alkaline phosphates, were determined using commercially available reagent kits (Randox Laboratories Limited, UK). All other chemicals used were of analytical grade and obtained from BDH (London).

Plants Material

The plant *Jastropha Gossypiifolia* was selected for my study. The leaves of plant *Jastropha Gossypiifolia* (Family- Euphorbiaceae) was collected in the month of March, 2011 from Ikeji-Arakeji in Osun-State, Nigeria. The plant was taken to the Department of plant science Joseph Ayo Babalola University, Ikeji- Arakeji, Ilesa for identification.

Bacterial isolates

The microorganism for antimicrobial are *Escherichia coli*, *Klebsiella pneumonia* and *Staphylococcous aureus*

Extract preparation

The freshly collected leaves of *Jatropha Gossypiifolia* were first air dried for four days. It was blended into powder using an industrial blender. 50 g of crude fibre was extracted with ethanol by soaking in 500 ml of 98% ethanol for 72 hours. The sample was then filtered using whatman filter paper. The filtrate was evaporated into a syrup using a water bath at 70°C. The extract was stored in a refrigerator for use in subsequent experiment.

Phytochemical screening of *Jatropha Gossypiifolia*

Basic phytochemical screening analysis of ethanolic extract were carried out for the detection of Saponins, Alkaloids, Tannins, Anthraquinone, Ardenolides and phylobatannins.

Test for alkaloids: About 0.2 g of each extract was stirred in 5 ml of 1% hydrochloric acid in a steam bath. 1 ml of the filtrate was treated with few drops of drigen droff reagent. Turbidity or precipitation was taken as the preliminary evidence for the preliminary presence of alkaloids in the extract being evaluated Horbane, 1973.

Test for saponin: Saponin was detected by vigorously shaking 0.5 g of extract in 5 ml of distilled water in a test tube to observe a stable froth persistent on warming.

Test for tannins: About 0.2 g of each portion of plant extract was stirred with 5 ml of distilled water, filtered and ferric chloride (0.1%) reagent was added to the filtrate. A blue black green or blue green precipitate was taken as evidence for the presence of tannin Trease and Evan, 1978.

Test for phlobatannins: Deposition of red precipitate when an aqueous extract of the plant part boiled with 1% aqueous Hcl was taken as evidence for the presence of phylobatannins Trease and Evans, 1978.

Test for anthraquinone: About 0.2 g of the extract was shaken with 5 ml concentration benzene and 5 ml of 1% NH3 solution was added to the filtrate. The mixture was shaken and the presence of pink, red or violet colour in ammoniacal (lower) phase indicate the presence of free anthraquinones.

Test for cardiac glucosides: The extract was dissolved in pyridine and few drops of 20% NaOH were added. A deep red colour, which faded to brownish yellow, indicate the presence of cardenlider.

Antimicrobial Sensitivity Assay

Media preparation

Nutrient Agar was prepared according to specification (Appendix 1) and then sterilized in autoclave at 121°C for 15 minutes. Agar plates were seeded with 0.5 ml of an overnight culture of each bacterial isolates: *E.coli, S. aureus, K. pneumonia*.

Extract were tested for inhibitory activity (invitro) against *Escherichia coli, Klebsiella pneumonia* and *Staphylococcous aureus* at different concentration of extract using the agar well diffusion (pop late technique method).

About 1 ml of 18 hours broth culture of the test organisms were introduced into a separated sterile petridish. Exactly 20 ml of sterile molten nutrient agar was poured into the petridish containing the test organisms. The agar was to set and holes were bored into the plates using sterile cork borer of 7 mm in diameter each. The wells bored on the plates were filled with the crude extract at different concentration of 25 mg/ml, 50 mg/ml, 75 mg/ml and 100 mg/ml respectively. A control experiment was set up the same way, however instead of the extract, sterile water was introduced into the holes bored in each plate. The petri dishes were incubated upright at 37°C for 24 hours. The relative sensitivity of the organisms to the extract were indicated by clear zones of inhibition around the well which were observed, measured and recorded in millimeters.

Preparation of citrate buffer (0.1M at pH 4.5)

1.4705 g of sodium citrate was dissolve in the 50 ml of distilled water and was poured into a 100 ml volumetric flask on a magnetic stirrer, 1.125 g of citric acid is used to maintain the pH of the solution to 4.5.

Experimental design

Fifteen albino rats weighing between 50 – 160 g each were used for the experiment. They were divided into five groups with three rats per group. As shown in the (Table 1).

Experimental induction of diabetes

All animals were allowed to adapt to cages for 15 days, after which they were fasted overnight and 65 mg/kg of alloxan monohydrate freshly dissolved in normal citrate buffer was injected with intra-peritoneally. After alloxan treatment, all animals were given free access to food and water. Blood glucose levels were measured 5 days after alloxan injection. All treatments started 5 days after alloxan injection.

Serum and tissue preparation

At the end of the treatment period, rats in each group were starved overnight but had access to water *ad libitum,* weighed and sacrificed by cervical dislocation while under anesthesia, 2 ml blood was collected from each rat by cardiac puncture into plain tube [7,8]. The blood was allowed to stand for 5 minutes and then centrifuged at 3500 rpm (Beckman GS-6R, Germany) for 10 minutes at 4°C. Serum was obtained at the supernatant for measuring fasting blood sugar level and enzyme (ALP and GGT) levels [9,10]. Liver and kidney were quickly excised, rinsed in Isotonic Sterile Saline (ISS), bottled dry on a filter paper and weighed. Each tissue was then placed in a separate plastic vial containing ice-cold ISS and stored at -4°C until required for further analysis.

Groups of rats	No of rats	Description
A	3	Uninduced rats that were given 1 ml distitilled water daily.
B	3	Rats infected with diabetes with insulin treatment.
C	3	Rats infected with diabetes without treatment.
D	3	Rats infected with diabetes treated with 12 hours intervals oral dose of 120mg/kg b.w. aqueous extract of Jatropha Gossypiifolia.
E	3	Rats infected with diabetes treated with 12 hours intervals oral dose of 240 mg/kg b.w. aqueous extract of Jatropha Gossypiifolia.

Table 1: Rats grouping.

Preparation of tissue homogenate

1 g of each of liver and kidney was cut out chopped into small pieces and then homogenized using pre-cooled pestle and mortar in a bowl of ice cubes. The tissue homogenate 5 ml of Isotonic Sterile Saline and centrifuge at 3500 rpm for 10 minutes and stored at -4°C until further analysis was carried out.

Biochemical assays

Serum glucose concentration was determined by means of Bayer Elite. Alkaline Phosphatase (ALP), Total Billirubin and GGT activities were determined using commercially available enzymatic test kits (Randox Laboratories Ltd, San Francisco, USA) method following the manufacturer's instructions.

Results

Phytochemical screening

The table below shows the result obtained for the phytochemical screening of the ethanolic extract Jatropha Gossypiifolia. The ethanolic extract revealed the presence of alkaloids, saponins, tannins and glycosides (Table 2).

Antimicrobial sensitivity assay

The table below shows the inhibition zone (mm) for the antimicrobial activity of ethanolic extract Jatropha Gossypiifolia at different concentration against bacterial isolates (Table 3) (Figures 1-3).

Result of body weight and blood glucose level

The Result of body weight and blood glucose level are shown in (Table 4).

Biochemical Assay

This shows the result of effect of ethanolic extract of Jatropha Gossypiifolia leaf on the activities of serum and organs in GGT, Bilirubin and ALP of serum and organ damage in rats. Each value is a mean of '3 determination ± S.D (Figure 4-6) Graph of ALP activity against Treatment Groups (Figure 5).

Discussions

In light of the result, our study indicate that ethanolic extract of Jatropha Gossypiifolia have good antidiabetic activity but there was a paralysis in one leg and lesion on the side of the paralysed legs, and some behavioural sign like loss of appetite and tiredness was observed.

Diabetes mellitus arises from the irreversible destruction of the pancreatic beta cells causing degranulation and reduction of insulin

secretion. The renewal of beta cells in diabetes have been studied in several animals model [11]. The present study demonstrated that the 50% ethanolic extract of *Jatropha Gossypiifolia* had an antihyperglycemic effect in the alloxan induced diabetic rats when

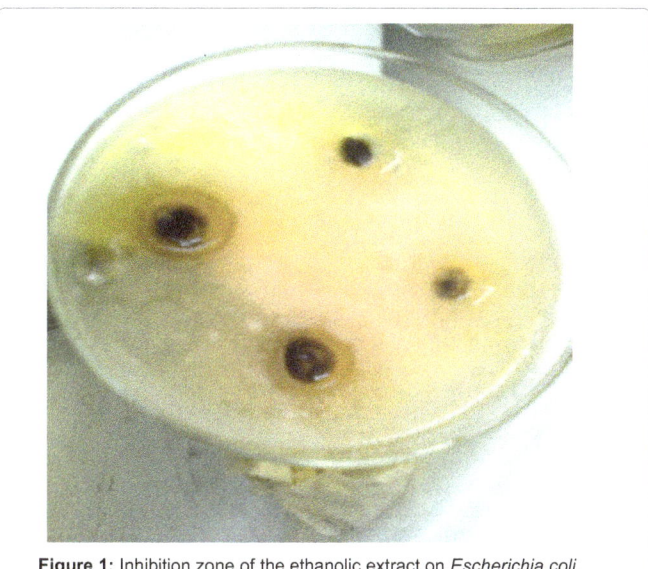

Figure 1: Inhibition zone of the ethanolic extract on *Escherichia coli.*

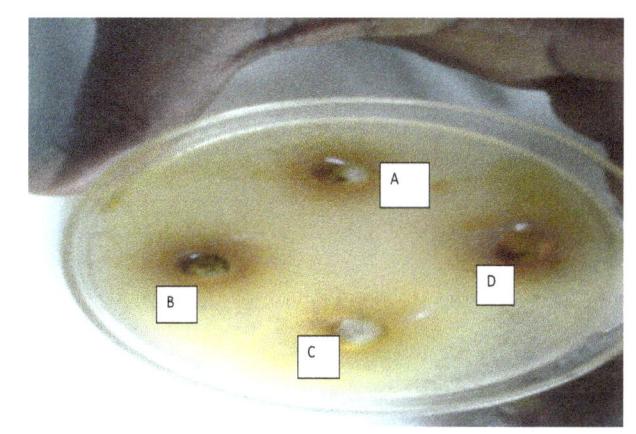

Figure 2: Inhibition zone of the ethanolic extract on *Klebsiella pneumonia.*

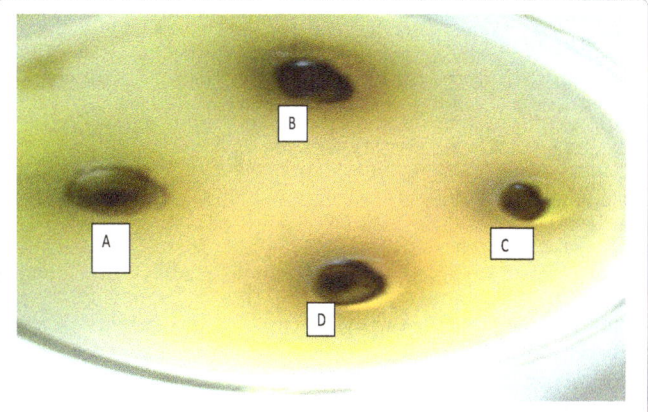

Figure 3: Inhibition zone of the ethanolic extract on *Staphylococcus aureus.*

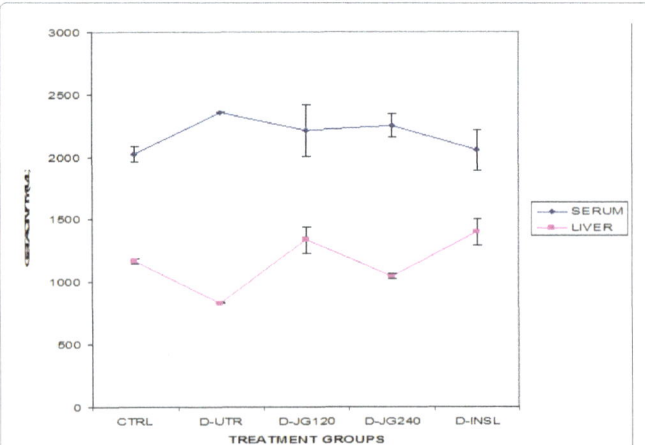

Note: CTRL - CONTROL RATS
D-UTR – DIABETES RATS WITHOUT TREATMENT
D-JG120- DIABETES RATS TREATED WITH *JATROPHA GOSSYPIIFOLIA* CONCENTRATION OF 12O mg/kg
D-JG240- DIABETES RATS REATED WITH *JATROPHA GOSSYPIIFOLIA* CONCENTRATION OF 240 mg/kg
D-INSL – DIABETES RATS TREATED WITH INSULIN

Figure 4: Effect of ethanolic extract of *Jatropha Gossypiifolia* leaf on the activities of serum and liver GGT of serum and liver damage in rats. Each value is a mean of '3 determination ±S.D.

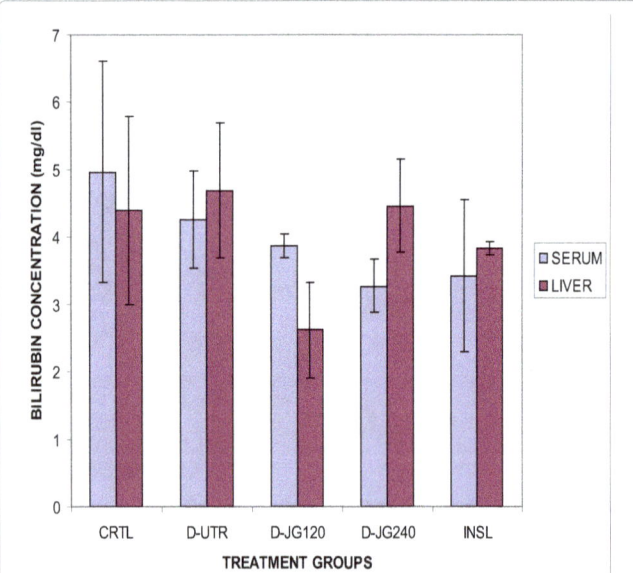

Note : CTRL - CONTROL RATS
D-UTR – DIABETES RATS WITHOUT TREATMENT
D-JG120- DIABETES RATS TREATED WITH *JATROPHA GOSSYPIIFOLIA* CONCENTRATION OF 12O mg/kg
D-JG240- DIABETES RATS TREATED WITH *JATROPHA GOSSYPIIFOLIA* CONCENTRATION OF 240 mg/kg
D-INSL – DIABETES RATS TREATED WITH INSULIN

Figure 5: Effect of ethanolic extract of *Jatropha Gossypiifolia* leaf on the activities of serum and liver BILIRUBIN of serum and liver damage in rats. Each value is a mean of '3 determination ±S.D.

administered orally. It has been demonstrated that insulin deficiency in diabetes mellitus leads to a variety of derangements in metabolic and regulatory process, which in turns leads to accumulation of lipids such as cholesterol and triglyceride in diabetic patients. The abnormal high concentration of serum lipids in the diabetic subject is mainly due to

increase in the mobilization of free fatty acids from the peripheral fat depots [12]. In present study, the 50% ethanolic extract of leaves of *J. curcas* decrease the cholesterol and triglyceride levels in the significant manner.

From the experiments conducted in the albino rats. It was found that the aqueous extract of *Jatropha Gossypiifolia* at dose of 120 mg/kg and 240 mg/kg for 7 days has effects in reducing hyperglycemia, it was seen that the body weight increased, in line with one of the symptoms of diabetes; obesity [13].

The test carried out on three different types of microbes shows that the aqueous extract inhibit the growth of the micro-organisms at different concentration. *Staphylococcus aureus* is a gram +ve bacteria, this can be seen in the low zone of inhibition seen in *Klebsiella pneumonia* (gram -ve) and also *Escherichia coli* is a gram – ve.

From (Table 2), it was discovered that the ethanolic extracts of *Jatropha Gossypiifolia* have a phytotoxic effect; that is, they inhibit the growth of plants as compared to the control. This could be trace to the difference in the phytochemical components of the ethanolic extract, as observed in this research project, alkaloids, tannins, saponins and glucosides are discovered to be present in the ethanolic extract.

Conclusion

The ethanolic extract of *Jatropha Gossypifolia* effectively reduced the alloxan-induced changes in blood glucose level. The current study provides some useful insight into the antihyperglycemic potency of *Jatropha curcas* leaves in alloxan induced diabetes. However, we

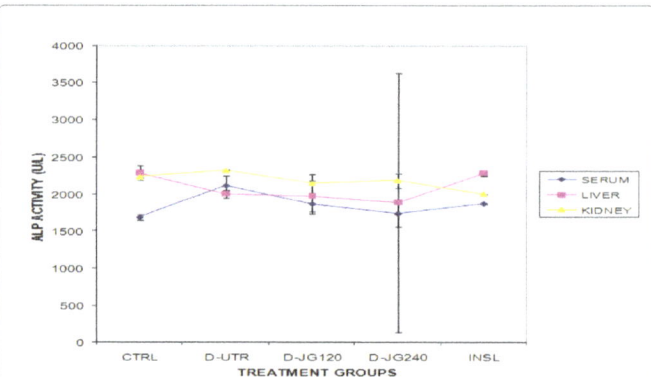

Note:
CTRL - CONTROL RATS
D-UTR – DIABETES RATS WITHOUT TREATMENT
D-JG120- DIABETES RATS TREATED WITH *JATROPHA GOSSYPIIFOLIA* CONCENTRATION OF 12O mg/kg
D-JG240- DIABETES RATS TREATED WITH *JATROPHA GOSSYPIIFOLIA* CONCENTRATION OF 240 mg/kg
D-INSL – DIABETES RATS TREATED WITH INSULIN

Figure 6: Effect of ethanolic extract of *Jatropha Gossypiifolia* leaf on the activities of serum, kidney and liver ALP of serum and liver and kidney damage in rats. Each value is a mean of '3 determination ± S.D.

s/no	Phytochemical component	Jatropha Gossypiifolia ethanolic extract
1	Alkaloids	Positive
2	Saponins	Positive
3	Tannins	Positive
4	phlobatannins	Negative
5	Anthraquinone	Negative
6	Glycosides	Positive

Table 2: Result of phytochemical screening.

Test organism	Different concentration			
	25 mg/ml (mm)	50 mg/ml (mm)	75 mg/ml (mm)	100mg/ml (mm)
Escherichia coli	12	8	13	11
Klebsiella pneumonia	14	10	12	15
Staphylicoccous aureus	10	12	13	14

Table 3: Result for Inhibition zone of antimicrobial sensitivity assay.

GROUP	Body weight (g)			Blood Glucose (mg/dl)		
Groups	Final	Initial	% Change	Final	Initial	% Change
Group A(Control)	95.27 ± 16	93.13 ± 9.2	2.14	100.2 ± 0.5	92.1 ± 7.5	8.79
Group B(UTR-D))	130.0 ± 4.6	154.8 ± 18	24.8	193.12 ± 4.2	158.32 ± 4.9	21.98
Group C(DJG120)	87.167 ± 2.9	95.53 ± 1.2	8.36	111.5 ± 20	288.5 ± 6.9	61.35
Group D(DJG240)	124.167 ± 5.0	137.3 ± 19	13.33	178 ± 3.3	248 ± 32	28.22
Group E(Insulin)	196.4 ± 5.3	146.17 ± 2.5	50.23	118 ± 14	121.67 ± 22	3.02

The results are the mean of 3 determinations ± S.D

Table 4: Weight and blood glucose in experimental and control rats before and after treatment with aqueous extract of ethanolic *Jatropha gossypifolia leaves.*

suggest that further work should be carried out at molecular level to find out the absolute mechanism of action of plant *Jatropha Gossypifoli* in experimental diabetes.

References

1. Nath LK , Dutta SK (1991) Extraction and purification of curcain, a protease from the latex of Jatropha curcas Linn. J Pharm Pharmacol 43: 111-114.

2. Goonasekera MM , Gunawardana VK, Jayasena K, Mohammed SG, Balasubramaniam S (1995) Pregnancy terminating effect of Jatropha curcas in rats. J Ethnopharmacol 47: 117-123.

3. Parotta JA (2001) Healing plants of peninsular india. CAB international. Wallingford U.K 299-300.

4. Lambert P, Polly J Bingley (2002) "What is Type 1 Diabetes?". Medicine 30: 1-5.

5. Dubois HFW, Bankauskaite V (2005) "Type 2 diabetes programmes in Europe" (PDF). Euro Observer 7: 5-6.

6. Lawrence JM, Contreras R, Chen W, Sacks DA (2008) Trends in the prevalence of preexisting diabetes and gestational diabetes mellitus among a racially/ ethnically diverse population of pregnant women, 1999-2005. Diabetes Care 31: 899-904.

7. Cooke DW , Plotnick L (2008) Type 1 diabetes mellitus in pediatrics. Pediatr Rev 29: 374-384.

8. Saydah SH , Miret M, Sung J, Varas C, Gause D, et al. (2001) Postchallenge hyperglycemia and mortality in a national sample of U.S. adults. Diabetes Care 24: 1397-1402.

9. Adler AI, Stratton IM, Neil HA, Yudkin JS, Matthews DR, et al. (2000) Association of systolic blood pressure with macrovascular and microvascular complications of type 2 diabetes (UKPDS 36): prospective observational study. BMJ 321: 412-419.

10. Narayan KM , Boyle JP, Thompson TJ, Sorensen SW, Williamson DF (2003) Lifetime risk for diabetes mellitus in the United States. JAMA 290: 1884-1890.

11. Junod A, Lambert AE, Stauffacher W, Renold AE (1969) Diabetogenic action of streptozotocin: relationship of dose to metabolic response. J Clin Invest 48: 2129-2139.

12. Selvin E , Steffes MW, Zhu H, Matsushita K, Wagenknecht L, et al. (2010) Glycated hemoglobin, diabetes, and cardiovascular risk in nondiabetic adults. N Engl J Med 362: 800-811.

13. Risérus U, Willett WC, Hu FB (2009) Dietary fats and prevention of type 2 diabetes. Prog Lipid Res 48: 44-51.

30

A Novel Application of Wutou (*Aconitum carmichaeli*) and Banxia (*Pinellia ternat*) Aqueous Extract on Wound Healing of Rats

Xia Xichao[1], Liu Hongyang[2], Wang Weina[1], Liu Fei[3], Hu Qingfu[1], Liang Guina[1], Zhang Dong[1] and Liu Rongzhi[1]*

[1]*Department of Basic Medicine, Nanyang Medical College, Nanyang, 473041, Henan Province, China*
[2]*Department of Plant Pathology, Nanyang Agriculture School, Nanyang, 473002, Henan Province, China*
[3]*Department of Clinical Medicine, Nanyang Medical College, Nanyang, 473041, Henan Province, China*

Abstract

Objective: The purpose of current study was to investigate effects of application of Wutou and Banxia aqueous extract in the wound rats.

Methods: Rats were fulfilled a surgical lesion with a 2.0 cm resecting tissue in the dorsal fascia. Following, animals were divided into 3 groups, including model group, control group treated with 1 mg/mL of Yunnan Baiyao, and Wutoubanxia group administrated 1 mg/mL of Wutou and Banxia extract. Wound contractions in day 0, 3, 7, 11 were calculated by an image analyzer. The histological analysis was detected using hematoxilin and eosin. The levels of tumor necrosis factor α (TNF-α), interleukin-2 (IL-2), transforming growth factor-β1 (TGF-β1), and basic Fibroblast Growth Factor (bFGF) transcripts in the wound tissue were determined by real-time quantitative PCR.

Results: Compared with the control group, rats in the model group showed poor re-modeling and re-epithelization characterized by a significant decrease of neovascularization, epithelialization and fibroblast. Furthermore, the expression levels of TNF-α, IL-2 were significantly increased, and TGF-β1 and bFGF significantly decreased in the model group in contrasted with that in the control group. By contrast, the treatment of Wutoubanxia extract reversed the above-mentioned conditions caused by wound.

Conclusion: The results suggest that administration of Wutou and Banxia extract has a promoting role in wound healing of rats possibly through enhancing anti-inflammatory ability and inducing fibroblast formation.

Keywords: Wutou and Banxia aqueous extract; Wound healing; Rat; Anti-inflammatory ability; Fibroblast formation

Introduction

In the resent years, wounds showed a gradually elevating-trend, and perhaps last for this status in the future with respect of unpredictable of natural disasters, increasing traffic accidents, abruptly physical injuries and so on [1,2]. Therefore, great efforts have been required to explore the candidates for wound healing and elucidate their mechanism in wound healing [3-5]. Process of wound healing is divided into three overlapping phases: inflammation (0-3 days), cellular proliferation (3-12 days), and remodeling (3-6 months) [6-8]. During the inflammatory stage, the pro-inflammatory cytokines are considered as key mediators to promote cutaneous inflammatory events [6]. In the second stage, the fibroblasts facilitate the formation of granulation tissue, proliferation moves into the wound, causing extracellular matrix production, connective tissue fibers and neovessels [8]. Accordingly, a new therapeutic candidate with more efficiency applied in the two stages should have a direct impact on the wound healing [9-11]. Meanwhile, it is exciting that great progresses have achieved along application of herbs in the wound healing [12-15].

Wutou, the axial root of *Aconitum carmichaeli*, has been extensively used to treat colds, polyarthralgia, diarrhea, heart failure, beriberi, and edema for thousands of years [16,17]. Banxia, the rootstock of *Pinellia ternate*, has a therapeutic effect on treatment of cough, infection and inflammation [18]. In Traditional Chinese Medicine (TCM), if several herbs are prescribed for treat a well-defined disease they should comply with formulas in which some herbs can't be used together *in vivo*, such as 18-against and 19-fear recorded in a classical TCM book [19]. Wutou against Banxia is an example of 18-against, but their use together in vitro remains large unknown [16,17,20,21]. Considering here, the current study was performed to investigate effects of Wutou and Banxia aqueous extract on the wound rats by analysis of the expressions of pro-inflammatory cytokines and fibroblast growth factors.

Methods

Preparation of aqueous extract

Wutou and Banxia were kindly provided by Hospital of Traditional Chinese Medicine of Nanyang Medical University. 350 g Wutou and 50 g Banxia were weighted, chopped and dried in shade, and powered mechanically. Power was immersed in water at room temperature for 4 h with constant stirring, boiled distilled water for 2 h, filtered through a filter paper, concentrated by rotary evaporator R52002K (Changyu Biochemical Instrument Factory, Shanghai, China). Residual was collected and dissolved in sterilized water to form Wutou and Banxia aqueous extract with a concentrate at 1 mg/mL.

Animals and treatment

Adult male Sprague-Dawley rats (150-200 g) were obtained at Henan Animals Center for Medical Science and Research, housed under standard conditions of temperature (22 ± 2°C), relative humidity (55 ± 5%) and light (12 h light/dark cycles). The animals care and use in

*Corresponding author: Rongzhi Liu, Department of Basic Medicine, Nanyang Medical College, Nanyang, China, E-mail: liurongzhi@sina.com

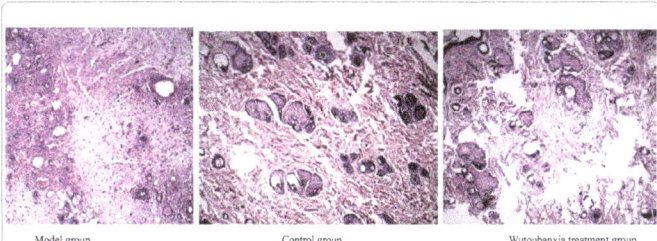

Figure 1: Histopathological view of epidermal/dermal in wound healing rats on day 11. Haematoxylin–eosin stain × 400. Control animals showing poor collagenization, fibroblasts and poor neovascularization. Control animals and Wutoubanxia treatment animal showing better healing and higher collagen deposition.

the experiment were approved by Nanyang Medical University Animal Care and Use Committee.

Wound healing activity was evaluated using excisional wound model. On the day 0, animals were anesthetized with 80 mg/kg ketamine and 10 mg/kg xylazine intramuscularly, and placed on operation table in its natural position. An impression was performed on area of 5 cm long × 4 cm wide, located in the thoracolumbar region. In the center trichotomized area was treated antisepsis with alcoholic clorexedine and fulfilled a surgical lesion with metallic punch with 2.0 cm in diameter resecting all tissue in the dorsal fascia. The rats were divided into 3 groups 30 animals per group, including model group, control group treated with 1 mg/mL of Yunnan Baiyao, and Wutoubanxia group administrated 1 mg/mL of Wutou and Banxia extract. All drugs were sprayed on wound by injector for twice daily in a volume of 100 ul.

Wound assessment and sample collection

Wound assessment starting from day 0, digital photograph was taken at day 0, day 3, day 7, and day 11. Wound size was measured by an image analyzer (image measurement standard v4.01, Bersoft, Puerto Plata, Dominican Republic) to assess the size changes during healing process. At corresponding days, 6 animals per group were deeply anaesthetized with chiloralhydrate at a concentration of 350 mg/kg, the full-thickness biopsy specimens of dorsal skin including periwound margin were dissected either for histological analysis or immediately frozen in liquid nitrogen, and then stored at -80°C for real-time PCR analysis.

Wound contraction % = (original wound area – specific day wound area)/ original wound area × 100.

Histological analysis

The specimen sample were fixed in fixative (60% of absolute alcohol, 30% of formaldehyde, 10% of glacial acetic acid) and embedded with paraffin. The specimens were cut in 4 um thick sections, and then stained by routine Hematoxilin and Eosin (H&E) for histological analysis. Briefly, the slides were deparaffinized in xylene, and rehydrated in descending order of ethanol. Following, the slides were dipped in hematoxylin, washed in tap water and dehydrated in ascending order of ethanol. Finally, the slides were stained with eosin and washed with absolute ethanol and xylene. The sections were analyzed under a light microscope (Olympus BX50, Barcelona, Spain) at 400 × magnifications.

Quantitative real-time PCR

Total RNA was isolated from the wound tissue using TRIzol (Invitrogen Life Technologies, Shanghai, China) according to the protocol set by manufacturer. The quality of RNA was confirmed by

1.2% agarose gel electrophoresis. The first-strand cDNA was synthesized using RTase M-MLV reverse transcriptase (Takara, Dalian, China). The cDNA was used as the template for real-time PCR reaction.

To determine the gene transcription levels of tumor necrosis factor α (TNF-α), interleukin-2 (IL-2), transforming growth factor-β1 (TGF-β1) and basic Fibroblast Growth Factor (bFGF) transcripts in the wound tissue, real-time quantitative PCR was performed using SYBR Premix Ex Taq™ (Takara, Dalian, China) according to the manufacture's instruction with the primers that were synthesized by Sangon (Shanhai, China). PCR was performed using an ABI 7500 Real-Time Detection System (ABI, Foster City, CA, USA). The expression levels of TNF-α, IL-2, TGF-β1 and bFGF were calculated using $2^{-\Delta C_T}$.

Statistical analysis

The data were expressed as the mean ± S.E.M. The results of the study were analyzed by one-way analysis of variance (ANOVA) with the aid of Statistical Package for Social Sciences (SPSS) software. P Values with $P<0.05$ were considered as statistically significant.

Results

Effects of Wutou and Banxia extract on wound healing in excisional rat

Animals contractions in the Wutoubanxia treated groups were significantly increase from day 3 to 7 at a level 98.61%, day 7 to day 11 at 47.73%, and the complete wound healing occurred at day 11 compared with that of the model group. Similar results were also observed in the control group animal those s were received Yunnan Baiyao. Poor re-modeling and re-epithelization were detected in the model group. Faster keratinization characterized with minor intraepithelial cornification was occurred in the control group and the Wutoubanxia treatment group. Histopathological sections from Wutoubanxia treated group showed significant increase of neovascularization, epithelialization and fibroblast in which showed matured epidermis with keratinization and mature hair follicles, fibroblasts in dermis that are the proof of completion of healing in contrasted with the model group (Figure 1).

Effects of Wutou and Banxia extract on mRNA levels of TNF-α and IL-2 in excisional rats

TNF-α and IL-2 expression levels in rats of the model group, the control group and the Wutoubanxia treatment group were within the significant increase throughout the experiment compared with that of day 0. The mRNA levels of TNF-α and IL-2 was significantly increase in the model group (Figures 2 and 3) compared with that of the control group. After administration of Wutou and Banxia extract, the TNF-α expression decrease by 34.9% (P<0.05) during whole experiment (Figure 2). Moreover, the IL-2 expression reduced 28.9% (P<0.05) and 41.46% (P<0.01) at day 3 and day 7, respectively (Figure 3).

Effects of Wutou and Banxia extract on mRNA level of TGF-β1 in the excisional rats

TGF-β1mRNA levels in rats of the model group, the control group and the Wutoubanxia treatment group showed a fluctuation throughout the experiment. Compared with the model group, TGF-β1 expressions in rats of the Wutoubanxia treatment group were increased 114.3% (P<0.01) in the day 3, 72.3% (P<0.01) in the day 7, but decreased 55.4% (P<0.01) in the day 11 (Figure 4). The change tread in animals of the Wutoubanxia treatment group was also detected in those of the control group at corresponding time.

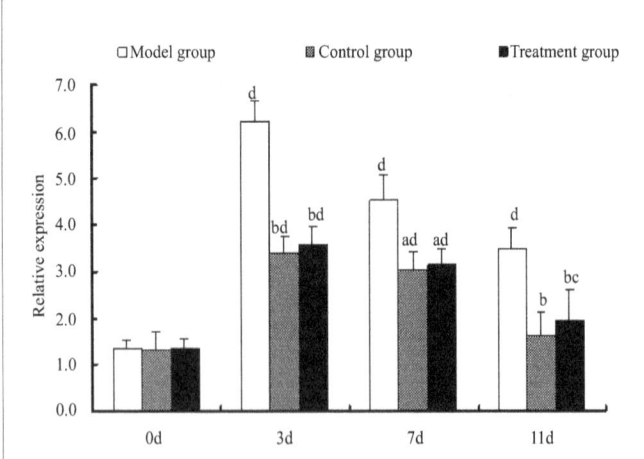

Figure 2: Effects of Wutou and Banxiag aqueous extract on the TNF-α mRNA levels in wound healing rats
N=6, [a]P<0.05, [b]P<0.01 vs model group, [c]P<0.05, [d]P<0.01 vs 0 day.

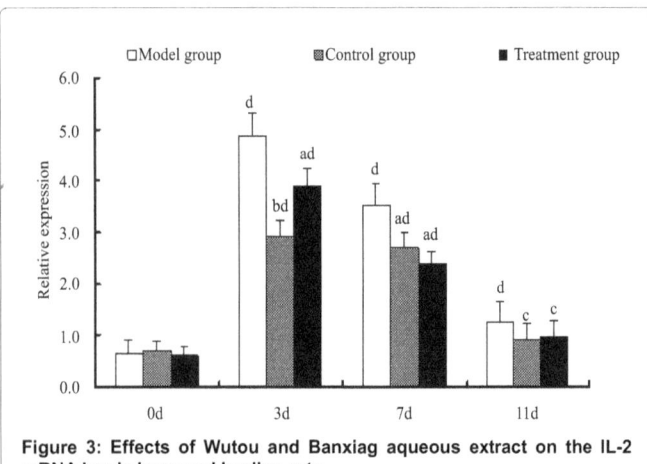

Figure 3: Effects of Wutou and Banxiag aqueous extract on the IL-2 mRNA levels in wound healing rats
N=6, [a]P<0.05, [b]P<0.01 vs model group, [c]P<0.05, [d]P<0.01 vs 0 day.

Effects of Wutou and Banxia extract on mRNA level bFGF in the excisional rats

Like the TGF-β1 mRNA levels change trend, the bFGF mRNA levels of rats in the three groups were also showed a fluctuation. Compared with that of the model group, the bFGF expression level in rats of the Wutoubanxia treatment group increased 74.7% (P<0.01) on day 3. On day 7, the bFGF mRNA level has not significant difference in contrasted with that of the model group, but was still significantly increase than that of day 0. Finally, it decreased 36.7% (P<0.05) in contrasted with that of the model group (Figure 5). Similar change tread was also detected in the control group.

Discussion

Tissue repair in the wound healing is a complex cascade of biological events regulated by numerous cytokines and growth factors that provide local signals to mediate cellular migration, angiogenesis, matrix synthesis, collagen deposition, formation of granulation and tissue remodeling [22,23]. In the CTM, many herbs play a positive role in the wound healing through acting on cytokines and growth factors [24,25].

Our results show that the administration of Wutou and Banxia aqueous extract contribute to wound healing in the incisions rats: an elevation of contraction, an acceleration of neovascularization, epithelialization and fibroblast, a down-regulation of TNF-α and IL-2 expression were observed. These results suggest that the application of Wutou and Banxia extract in wound rats has a promoting-role on wound healing. Inflammation cascade, occurring in the original stage of wound healing, is initiated by the innate immune system that pro-inflammatory cytokines, such as TNF-α, IL-2, IL-6 and IL-8, have a key role in the inflammatory response [26,27]. Inflammatory response is taken as a direct pathogenic-signal in the traumatized tissues [28]. Previous studies demonstrated that over-expression of these pro-inflammatory mediators may lead to wound condition deterioration [29]. Meanwhile, inflammatory response of wound tissue is coordinated by the interplay of anti-inflammatory cytokine and pro-inflammation cytokines, where a low level of pro-inflammation cytokines and/or a high level of anti-inflammatory cytokines should be helpful to tissue repair [30]. So, one key factor of wound healing acceleration from Wutou and Banxiag treatment is attribute to suppress of TNF-α and IL-2 expression.

In addition, remarkable gene up-regulation of TGF-β1 and bFGF in response to Wutou and Banxia extract treatment that reveals administration of Wutou and Banxia results in an acceleration of fibroblast formation in the wound healing through regulating certain

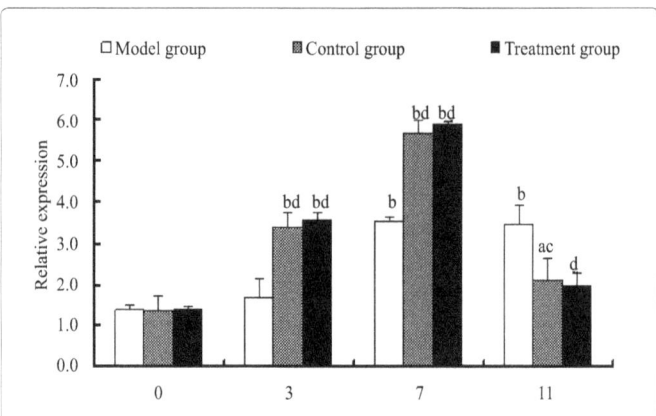

Figure 4: Effects of Wutou and Banxiag aqueous extract on the TGF-β1 levels in wound healing rats
N=6, [a]P<0.05, [b]P<0.01 vs model group, [c]P<0.05, [d]P<0.01 vs 0 day.

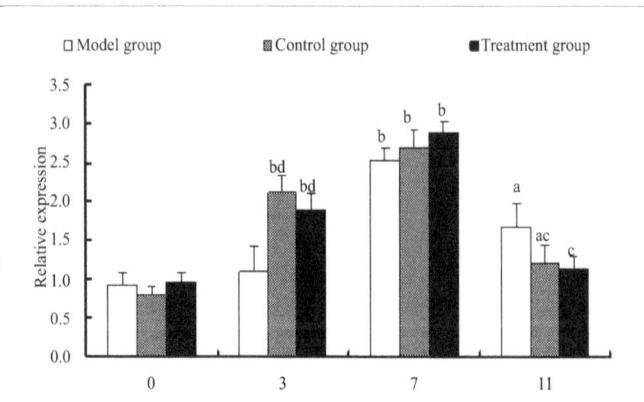

Figure 5: Effects of Wutou and Banxiag aqueous extract on the bFGF mRNA levels in wound healing rats
N=6, [a]P<0.05, [b]P<0.01 vs model group, [c]P<0.05, [d]P<0.01 vs 0 day.

genes expression. Literature has indicated that induction of TGF-β1 expression contributes to wound healing because TGF-β1 may initiate fibroblast, collagen synthesis and extracellular matrix formation [31,32]. In addition, TGF-β1 also has an ability to stimulate the expressions of other cytokines, such as matrix metalloproteinase 9 vascular endothelial growth factor-A and monocyte/macrophage chemotactic protein-1 [33]. bFGF, an important Fibroblast Growth Factor, can stimulate re-epithelialization and mediates in mesenchymal-epithelial interactions to promote epithelial proliferation and migration within the wounded area, which facilitates differentiation of new epidermis once combination with its receptor through [34-36]. Based on mentions, administration of Wutou and Banxia extract causes the induction of TGF-β1 and bFGF that may lead to fibrosis in the cellular proliferation stage of wound rat [23,37,38].

Wutou and Banxia are considered as an instance of 18-against in the classical TCM book [39,40]. In the present study, Wutou co-administration with Banxia plays a positive role in wound healing by application in vitro that is paradoxical with the traditional view. In the earliest pharmacopeia of China, Wutou possesses an evil reputation in duce it is consider as an extremely toxic plant in which toxic aconite alkaloids are contained which serve as highly toxic to myocardium, nerves, stomach and intestine through hyperpolarization and activation effect on the voltage-dependent sodium channels of the [41,42] Banxia also has few side effects and can leads to tongue numbing and swelling, salivation, slurred speech, and hoarsenes [42]. For a long time, the exact reasons of that Wutou and Banxia can't be used together in vivo remain large unknown [39,40,43]. But, the medical affect of Wutou combination with other herbs in vitro are constantly explored in resent years. The combinational use of *A. carmichaeli* and *Paeonia lactiflora* was showed to produce better efficacy in preventing and curing secondary adjuvant arthritis in rats [44,45]. Modern clinical studies have evidenced that the application of Fuzi, the lateral root of *A. carmichaeli*, in combination with other herbs have anti- arthritis property in the therapy of patients, indicating its promising therapeutic potential against arthritis [46,47]. These studies reveal the application of Wutou co-administration with Banxia in vitro should has potential scenario and is deserved to shed light of mechanism. So, there is still a long and exciting road ahead to fully understand and explain the mechanism of Wutou and Banxiag aqueous extract in the wound healing.

Nevertheless, the features of TNF-α, IL-2, TGF-β1, and bFGF acted by Wutou and Banxiag extract is not similar, for example the disparity of these genes expression in different time of sampling, imply that is likely related with order of these elements involved in cascade reaction in wound healing. On another hand, it is likely that many components existed in the Wutou and Banxiag have different regulatory pathways on these growth factors.

The current study demonstrated that treatment of Wutou and Banxia aqueous extract promote wound healing activity in rat incision. Further study shows the down-regulation of TNF-α and IL-2 expressions, and up-regulation TGF-β1 and bFGF expressions from Wutou and Banxia extract treatment is one value pathway to promote the wound healing.

Acknowledgement

We gratefully acknowledge the contribution of Pro Liu Rongzhi to this research program. This research was funded by the National Natural Science Foundation of Henan (No. 12B35002).

References

1. Brand HS, Veerman EC (2013) Saliva and wound healing. Chin J Dent Res 16: 7-12.

2. Kosins AM, Scholz T, Cetinkaya M, Evans GR (2013) Evidence-based value of subcutaneous surgical wound drainage: the largest systematic review and meta-analysis. Plast Reconstr Surg 132: 443-450.

3. Bae SH, Bae YC, Nam SB, Choi SJ (2012) A skin fixation method for decreasing the influence of wound contraction on wound healing in a rat model. Arch Plast Surg 39: 457-462.

4. Sharifi R, Rastegar H, Kamalinejad M, Dehpour AR, Tavangar SM, et al. (2012) Effect of topical application of silymarin (*Silybum marianum*) on excision wound healing in albino rats. Acta Med Iran 50: 583-588.

5. Tarameshloo M, Norouzian M, Zarein-Dolab S, Dadpay M, Mohsenifar J, et al. (2012) Aloe vera gel and thyroid hormone cream may improve wound healing in Wistar rats. Anat Cell Biol 45: 170-177.

6. Hajhashemi V, Ghannadi A, Heidari AH (2012) Anti-inflammatory and wound healing activities of Aloe littoralis in rats. Res Pharm Sci 7: 73-78.

7. Ryu HM, Oh EJ, Park SH, Kim CD, Choi JY, et al. (2012) Aquaporin 3 expression is up-regulated by TGF-β1 in rat peritoneal mesothelial cells and plays a role in wound healing. Am J Pathol 181: 2047-2057.

8. Lin YH, Lin JH, Wang SH, Ko TH, Tseng GC (2012) Evaluation of silver-containing activated carbon fiber for wound healing study: In vitro and in vivo. J Biomed Mater Res B Appl Biomater 100: 2288-2296.

9. Bhaskar A, Nithya V (2012) Evaluation of the wound-healing activity of *Hibiscus rosa sinensis* L (Malvaceae) in Wistar albino rats. Indian J Pharmacol 44: 694-698.

10. Simonetti O, Lucarini G, Cirioni O, Zizzi A, Orlando F, et al. (2013) Delayed wound healing in aged skin rat models after thermal injury is associated with an increased MMP-9, K6 and CD44 expression. Burns 39: 776-787.

11. Peplow PV, Baxter GD (2012) Gene expression and release of growth factors during delayed wound healing: a review of studies in diabetic animals and possible combined laser phototherapy and growth factor treatment to enhance healing. Photomed Laser Surg 30: 617-636.

12. Jain AK, Dixit A, Mehta SC (2012) Wound healing activity of aqueous extracts of leaves and roots of Coleus aromaticus in rats. Acta Pol Pharm 69: 1119-1123.

13. Mekonnen A, Sidamo T, Asres K, Engidawork E (2013) In vivo wound healing activity and phytochemical screening of the crude extract and various fractions of Kalanchoe petitiana A. Rich (Crassulaceae) leaves in mice. J Ethnopharmacol 145: 638-646.

14. Koca U, Süntar I, Akkol EK, Yilmazer D, Alper M (2011) Wound repair potential of Olea europaea L. leaf extracts revealed by in vivo experimental models and comparative evaluation of the extracts' antioxidant activity. J Med Food 14: 140-146.

15. Adetutu A, Morgan WA, Corcoran O (2011) Antibacterial, antioxidant and fibroblast growth stimulation activity of crude extracts of Bridelia ferruginea leaf, a wound-healing plant of Nigeria. J Ethnopharmacol 133: 116-119.

16. Fan YF, Xie Y, Liu L, Ho HM, Wong YF, et al. (2012) Paeoniflorin reduced acute toxicity of aconitine in rats is associated with the pharmacokinetic alteration of aconitine. J Ethnopharmacol 141: 701-708.

17. Tong P, Wu C, Wang X, Hu H, Jin H, et al. (2013) Development and assessment of a complete-detoxication strategy for Fuzi (lateral root of *Aconitum carmichaeli*) and its application in rheumatoid arthritis therapy. J Ethnopharmacol 146: 562-571.

18. Zhang ZH, Zhao YY, Cheng XL, Dai Z, Zhou C, et al. (2013) General toxity of *Pinellia ternata* (Thunb.) Berit. in rat: a metabonomic method for profiling of serum metabolic changes. J Ethnopharmacol 149: 303-310.

19. Chen C, Li SX, Wang SM, Liang SW (2011) A support vector machine based pharmacodynamic prediction model for searching active fraction and ingredients of herbal medicine: Naodesheng prescription as an example. J Pharm Biomed Anal 56: 443-447.

20. Peter K, Schinnerl J, Felsinger S, Brecker L, Bauer R, et al. (2013) A novel concept for detoxification: complexation between aconitine and liquiritin in a Chinese herbal formula ('Sini Tang'). J Ethnopharmacol 149: 562-569.

21. Lu G, Dong Z, Wang Q, Qian G, Huang W, et al. (2010) Toxicity assessment of nine types of decoction pieces from the daughter root of *Aconitum carmichaeli* (Fuzi) based on the chemical analysis of their diester diterpenoid alkaloids. Planta Med 76: 825-830.

22. Gu XY, Shen SE, Huang CF, Liu YN, Chen YC, et al. (2013) Effect of activated autologous monocytes/macrophages on wound healing in a rodent model of experimental diabetes. Diabetes Res Clin Pract 102: 53-59.

23. Esposito D, Rathinasabapathy T, Schmidt B, Shakarjian MP, Komarnytsky S, et al. (2013) Acceleration of cutaneous wound healing by brassinosteroids. Wound Repair Regen 21: 688-696.

24. Mukherjee H, Ojha D, Bharitkar YP, Ghosh S, Mondal S, et al. (2013) Evaluation of the wound healing activity of Shorea robusta, an Indian ethnomedicine, and its isolated constituent(s) in topical formulation. J Ethnopharmacol 149: 335-343.

25. Majtan J, Bohova J, Garcia-Villalba R, Tomas-Barberan FA, Madakova Z, et al. (2013) Fir honeydew honey flavonoids inhibit TNF-α-induced MMP-9 expression in human keratinocytes: a new action of honey in wound healing. Arch Dermatol Res 305: 619-627.

26. Kang R, Tang D, Lotze MT, Zeh Iii HJ (2013) Autophagy is required for IL-2-mediated fibroblast growth. Exp Cell Res 319: 556-565.

27. Spits H, Di Santo JP (2011) The expanding family of innate lymphoid cells: regulators and effectors of immunity and tissue remodeling. Nat Immunol 12: 21-27.

28. Cakmak GK, Tascilar O, Tekin IO, Ucan BH, Emre AU, et al. (2008) Experimental obstructive jaundice results in oxidized low-density-lipoprotein accumulation in surgical wound of rats. Acta Chir Belg 108: 725-731.

29. Kumar N, Mishra J, Narang VS, Waters CM (2007) Janus kinase 3 regulates interleukin 2-induced mucosal wound repair through tyrosine phosphorylation of villin. J Biol Chem 282: 30341-30345.

30. Kimura T, Sugaya M, Blauvelt A, Okochi H, Sato S (2013) Delayed wound healing due to increased interleukin-10 expression in mice with lymphatic dysfunction. J Leukoc Biol 94: 137-145.

31. Ponugoti B, Xu F, Zhang C, Tian C, Pacios S, et al. (2013) FOXO1 promotes wound healing through the up-regulation of TGF-β1 and prevention of oxidative stress. J Cell Biol 203: 327-343.

32. Fang F, Shangguan AJ, Kelly K, Wei J, Gruner K, et al. (2013) Early growth response 3 (Egr-3) is induced by transforming growth factor-β and regulates fibrogenic responses. Am J Pathol 183: 1197-1208.

33. Robinson PM, Chuang TD, Sriram S, Pi L, Luo XP, et al. (2013) MicroRNA signature in wound healing following excimer laser ablation: role of miR-133b on TGFβ1, CTGF, SMA, and COL1A1 expression levels in rabbit corneal fibroblasts. Invest Ophthalmol Vis Sci 54: 6944-6951.

34. Anitua E, Muruzabal F, Alcalde I, Merayo-Lloves J, Orive G (2013) Plasma rich in growth factors (PRGF-Endoret) stimulates corneal wound healing and reduces haze formation after PRK surgery. Exp Eye Res 115: 153-161.

35. Andres C, Hasenauer J, Ahn HS, Joseph EK, Isensee J, et al. (2013) Wound-healing growth factor, basic FGF, induces Erk1/2-dependent mechanical hyperalgesia. Pain 154: 2216-2226.

36. Shi HX, Lin C, Lin BB, Wang ZG, Zhang HY, et al. (2013) The anti-scar effects of basic fibroblast growth factor on the wound repair in vitro and in vivo. PLoS One 8: e59966.

37. Yan L, Wu W, Wang Z, Li C, Lu X, et al. (2013) Comparative study of the effects of recombinant human epidermal growth factor and basic fibroblast growth factor on corneal epithelial wound healing and neovascularization in vivo and in vitro. Ophthalmic Res 49: 150-160.

38. Hamuy R, Kinoshita N, Yoshimoto H, Hayashida K, Houbara S, et al. (2013) One-stage, simultaneous skin grafting with artificial dermis and basic fibroblast growth factor successfully improves elasticity with maturation of scar formation. Wound Repair Regen 21: 141-154.

39. Hikino H, Konno C, Takata H, Yamada Y, Yamada C, et al. (1980) Antiinflammatory principles of Aconitum roots. J Pharmacobiodyn 3: 514-525.

40. Sato H, Yamada C, Konno C, Ohizumi Y, Endo K, et al. (1979) Pharmacological actions of aconitine alkaloids. Tohoku J Exp Med 128: 175-187.

41. Zhang FS, Wu JY, Jia ZH, Sun JN (2012) Dose-toxicity relationship study for cardiotonic effect of aconitine. Chinese Journal of Experimental Traditional Medical Formulae 13: 341-344.

42. Qin L, Peng X, Li XL, Zhang SH, Sun R (2000) Acute toxicity experiment of white peony root and Radix Aconiti using together or separately. J Shangdong University of TCM 24: 453-455.

43. Xie Y, Zhou H, Wong YF, Xu HX, Jiang ZH, et al. (2008) Study on the pharmacokinetics and metabolism of paeonol in rats treated with pure paeonol and an herbal preparation containing paeonol by using HPLC-DAD-MS method. J Pharm Biomed Anal 46: 748-756.

44. Liu ZQ, Zhou H, Liu L, Jiang ZH, Wong YF, et al. (2005) Influence of co-administrated sinomenine on pharmacokinetic fate of paeoniflorin in unrestrained conscious rats. J Ethnopharmacol 99: 61-67.

45. Liu ZQ, Jiang ZH, Liu L, Hu M (2006) Mechanisms responsible for poor oral bioavailability of paeoniflorin: Role of intestinal disposition and interactions with sinomenine. Pharm Res 23: 2768-2780.

46. Tang L, Gong Y, Lv C, Ye L, Liu L, et al. (2012) Pharmacokinetics of aconitine as the targeted marker of Fuzi (Aconitum carmichaeli) following single and multiple oral administrations of Fuzi extracts in rat by UPLC/MS/MS. J Ethnopharmacol 141: 736-741.

47. Peng WW, Li W, Li JS, Cui XB, Zhang YX, et al. (2013) The effects of Rhizoma Zingiberis on pharmacokinetics of six Aconitum alkaloids in herb couple of Radix Aconiti Lateralis-Rhizoma Zingiberis. J Ethnopharmacol 148: 579-586.

31

Alterations in the Expression of Transcription Factors PPARγ and NFκ B in the Brain of Models of Chronic Pain

Amy M Birch[1][#], Jonathan Cheung[1][#], Christianah Oluwadare[1], James Burton[1], Wenlong Huang[2], Amparo Novejarque[2], Julia Inglis[3] and Magdalena Sastre[1]*

[1]Division of Brain Sciences, Imperial College London, Hammersmith Hospital, W12 0NN, UK
[2]Department of Surgery and Cancer, Imperial College London, Chelsea and Westminster Hospital, SW10 9NH, UK
[3]School of Medicine and Pharmacology, University of Western Australia, Perth, WA 6009, Australia
[#]Equal contribution

Abstract

Recent evidence has highlighted the role of nuclear receptors Peroxisome Proliferator-Activated Receptor (PPAR) α and PPARγ in the neuroinflammatory state associated with acute inflammatory and neuropathic pain. Its relevance in the control and treatment of pain has been confirmed by the beneficial effects of treatment with Thiazolidinediones and fibrates. The aim of this study was to evaluate the expression of PPARα, PPARγ, and Nuclear Factor kappa B (NFκB) in the brains of rodent models of inflammatory pain, peripheral neuropathy and peripheral nerve injury, including the collagen induced arthritis (CIA), Spinal Nerve Transection (SNT) and Anti-Retroviral (ART) models. Our results reveal that PPARγ levels are generally reduced in models of persistent pain, while NFκB expression is upregulated, with no major changes in PPARα expression. These alterations seem to be linked with the inflammatory state associated with the CIA model, but are present in nerve damage models as well. This was further confirmed *in vitro*, using neuroblastoma cells incubated with pro-inflammatory cytokines, with similar changes in the expression of these transcription factors. Therefore, these results point to a common pathway in the aetiologies of these different models contributing to further exacerbation of pain symptomatology and suggest that this pathway may serve as a target for the development of analgesic drugs.

Keywords: Inflammation; Transcription factors; Neuropathic pain; Collagen induced arthritis; Stavudine

Introduction

Despite chronic pain being a widespread health issue, current management and treatments for the condition are far from satisfactory [1]. There are three key causes for chronic pain: tissue injury leading to inflammatory pain; nerve damage causing neuropathic pain; and tumour growth eliciting cancer pain [2].

Pain is one of the classic signals of the inflammatory process. Inflammatory conditions alone can lead to debilitating and persistent pain [3]. Inflammation can also be a consequence of conditions such as neuropathic pain, where inflammation is secondary to damage to the somatosensory nervous system [4]. Inflammatory mediators, such as prostaglandins, nerve growth factor, nitric oxide, cytokines, and chemokines are released from injury sites and can activate or modify nociceptor activities. This directly elicits various forms of pain, resulting in peripheral and central sensitisation and ultimately, a chronic pain state [5-7]. In fact, inflammatory reactions increase nociceptor responsiveness, allowing low-intensity stimuli access to the nociceptive pathway and produce pain [8]. In line with this, a widely used approach to treat chronic pain is by non-steroidal anti-inflammatory drugs (NSAIDs), which prevent nociceptor sensitization. NSAIDs inhibit the synthesis of prostaglandins, hence diminishing peripheral and central sensitization. However, it is not fully understood whether the inflammatory mediators cause and or maintain neuropathic pain.

Several studies suggest that the transcription factor Nuclear Factor kappa B (NFκB) could be involved in pain [9]. A significant increase in the percentages of activated NFκB immunoreactive neurons and GFAP-positive cells under inflamed conditions was reported in the dorsal root ganglia of rats [10].

In addition, recent evidence suggests the involvement of Peroxisome proliferator-activated receptors (PPARs) in pain regulation [4,11,12]. These nuclear receptors are primarily known for their roles in metabolic processes and have garnered recent interest in mediating inflammatory responses [13-15]. Pioglitazone, a PPARγ synthetic ligand, has been shown to present anti-nociceptive and anti-edematogenic effects to various animal models [16]. In animal models of neuropathic pain, the endogenous PPARγ agonist, 15-deoxy-Δ12,14-PGJ2 (15d-PGJ2, a cyclopentanone prostaglandin), decreased mechanical and cold hypersensitivity in a dose-dependent manner [17]. Similar findings were reported using rosiglitazone, a synthetic PPARγ agonist [17]. The 15d-PGJ2 was also effective in alleviating inflammatory pain [6]. In addition, LoVerme et al. [18] investigated the effects of the PPARα agonists GW7647 and Palmitoyl Ethanilamide (PEA), and both reduced hyperalgesia in acute and inflammatory pain models.

Hence, we hypothesize that alterations in the expression of these transcription factors in the CNS may contribute to exacerbate allodynia and hyperalgesia. Therefore, it is relevant to investigate whether these transcription factors are changed during chronic pain. The aim of this study was to investigate whether the expression of NFκB and PPAR subtypes, γ and α, is affected by different models of chronic pain, including a model of inflammatory and two different models of neuropathic pain, a nerve injury model and the Anti-Retroviral (ART) model of peripheral neuropathy.

*Corresponding author: Magdalena Sastre, Division of Brain Sciences, Imperial College London, Hammersmith Hospital, Du Cane Road, London W12 0NN, UK, E-mail: m.sastre@imperial.ac

Materials and Methods

Materials and antibodies

Antibodies used were PPARγ H-100: sc-7196 (Santa Cruz), PPARα P0369 (Sigma), anti-p65 (Cell signalling), β-actin (Abcam). TNFα was obtained from Roche. All other reagents were obtained from Sigma and Invitrogen.

Ethical standards

All animal experiments conformed to the British Home Office Regulations (Animal Scientific Procedures, Act 1986) and International Association for the Study of Pain guidelines [19] for the care and use of animals. We followed the ARRIVE guidelines for reporting the behavioral studies in preparing this report [20].

Animals

In this study, three different models of pain were investigated: Collagen Induced Arthritis (CIA) mice as model of inflammatory pain [21,22]; and Spinal Nerve Transection (SNT) and Anti-Retroviral Neuropathy (ART) rats as models for neuropathic pain. Animals were housed and maintained at a temperature of 21 ± 2°C. Sample size estimation was not conducted, as the group number was according to the need of the current study, which is mainly a molecular biology, based study. Animals were fed with normal chow food (RM1 pelleted form; Special Diet Services, Essex, UK) and tap water ad libitum, and allowed to acclimatize in their housing environment for at least 48 h after arrival.

Brain tissue from 11 mice (5 Controls; 6 CIA) was provided by Julia Inglis (Kennedy Institute). Adult male DBA/1 mice (Charles River) ages 10–12 weeks were used. Mice were immunized by subcutaneous injection at the base of the tail with 2 50-μl injections of bovine type II collagen (2 mg/mL) in CFA (Becton Dickinson, Twickenham, UK), as described previously [22]. Fourteen to 28 days following immunization the mice developed arthritis and were sacrificed [22]. The rationale for choice of route of administration and drug dose were based on your previous publication.

For the ART and the SNT models, male adult Wistar rats (180–200 g; Charles River, UK) were used. Only rats that developed hind paw mechanical hypersensitivity of at least 25% change from the baseline were included. The experimenter was blinded to the treatments received and had no knowledge of the experimental group to which an animal was randomized. The rationale for choice of a brief general anesthetic, route of administration, and drug dose were based on your previous publication.

The ART model was obtained by injecting the HIV antiretroviral drug stavudine (d4T) in Wistar rats (n=4 per group) [23]. After 2 intravenous injections, i.e. via a tail vein under a brief general anaesthesia (1–2% isoflurane [Abbott, UK] in O_2 and N_2O at a 1:1 ratio), of d4T (a gift from Pfizer Ltd., UK; 50 mg/kg, 4 days apart), rats developed hind paw mechanical hypersensitivity, which plateaued at 21 days after initial d4T injection, as described previously [23]. Vehicle control animals received equivalent volumes of sterile saline using the same administration protocol for d4T (n=4).

For the spinal nerve transection (SNT: 4 controls; 4 treated) Wistar rats and their controls were produced at Chelsea & Westminster Hospital as described in previous publications [24]. Surgery was performed under general isofluorane anaesthesia and aseptic surgical conditions. Perioperative analgesia (0.05 ml bupivacaine, AstraZeneca,

UK) and antibiotic treatment (Enrofloxacin ("Baytril"): 0.2 ml/kg, Bayer Ltd, Dublin, Ireland) were injected subcutaneously at the start of the spinal nerve transection surgery. A 1-2 cm midline skin incision was made level with the iliac crests. The left paraspinal muscles were separated from spinous processes of L4 to S2 vertebrae using blunt dissection. Using anatomical landmarks, the L6 transverse process was identified and a small laminectomy performed, exposing L4 and L5 spinal nerve roots. The left L5 was tightly ligated (4-0 Mersilk, Ethicon) and transected 1-2 mm distal to the ligation. Transection of the L5 nerve root was confirmed post-mortem in all SNT animals. The wound was sutured and animals received intraperitoneal post-operative analgesia (20% carprofen ("Rimadyl"), 0.5 ml/kg; Pfizer, UK) 4 h post-surgery. Naive animals did not undergo any surgical procedure but were transported and housed in their cages in the surgical room for an equivalent period.

Behavioural testing

For the CIA model, animals were scored for clinical signs of inflammation, as follows: 0: Normal; 1: Slight swelling and/or erythema; 2: Pronounced edematous swelling; and 3: Joint rigidity. Each limb was graded, thus allowing a maximum score of 12 per mouse. This experiment was repeated on 3 separate occasions [22]. Thermal hyperalgesia was assessed using the Hargreaves plantar apparatus (Ugo Basile, Varese, Italy), as described previously [22]. The mice were placed in the equipment used to assess hyperalgesia on at least 2 occasions prior to pain evaluation, in order to reduce stress-induced behavioral changes. Thermal hyperalgesia was assessed using the Hargreaves plantar apparatus (Ugo Basile, Varese, Italy). Briefly, mice were placed in a Perspex box, and an increasing thermal stimulus was delivered to the plantar surface of the hind paw. The amount of time until lifting of the paw was recorded.

Behavioural data using the hind paw mechanical hyper-sensitivity are provided to confirm the validity of the models (Supplementary information, Figures S1A-S1B) [25]. Animals were tested in individual Plexiglas observation chambers ($23 \times 18 \times 14$ cm) by a single observer, 'blinded' to group allocation. The hind paw withdrawal threshold (PWT) in response to punctate static mechanical stimulation was assessed 14 days post-injury or 18 days following the first d4T injection using an electronic 'von Frey' device (Somedic AB, Hörby, Sweden). The calibrated force transducer (0.5 mm² diameter tip) was manually applied to the mid-plantar surface of both left and right hind paw alternately (8-15 g/s) until an active limb withdrawal response was observed. The threshold value was calculated as the mean of five measurements. Two sessions of habituation (40-50 min each) to the testing area were conducted. Then, two baseline values were obtained for all rats prior to surgery. Mechanical hypersensitivity was defined as a post-operative change in the hind paw withdrawal of at least -30% from baseline for the SNT model and -25% from baseline for the ART model.

Brains from all experiments were sub-dissected into frontal cortex, midbrain, brainstem, cerebellum, and spinal cord. All tissue was snap-frozen and kept at -80°C for further analysis.

Cell culture

Mouse neuroblastoma of the N2a cell line were cultured in Dulbecco's Modified Eagle's Medium (DMEM) supplemented with 10% fetal bovine serum and penicillin/streptomycin on a 35 mm diameter plates. Cells were grown in a 5% CO_2 incubator at 37°C and were incubated overnight with TNFα (30 ng ml⁻¹).

Western blot

Brain regions and cells were homogenized in radio-immunoprecipitation assay buffer (RIPA; 1% Triton X-100, 1% sodium deoxycholate, 0.1% SDS, 150 mM NaCl, 50 mM Tris-HCl, pH 7.2) supplemented with Roche Complete protease® inhibitor cocktail. Proteins were separated on 10% sodium dodecyl sulphate-polyacrylamide (SDS-PAGE) gels and transferred to Immobilon-P polyvinylidene fluoride (PVDF). Following appropriate blocking, membranes were incubated with a primary antibody (all at 1:1000 dilution) overnight at 4°C and then incubated with secondary antibodies. Membranes were developed using ECL˜ (GE Amersham, UK) reagents and Hyperfilm ECL˜ audioradiography film in an automated developer (Konica, SRX 101A). The intensity of the bands was quantified by densitometry using Image J software (NIH) and normalized to β-actin.

Statistical analyses

The sample number was based on biostatistical advice and previous experience, indicating that group sizes of 4-5 animals are sufficient to detect even subtle changes for protein expression analysis. Data analysis was performed with GraphPad Prism version 5.01. Unpaired t-tests were used to compare the expression of transcription factors and pro-inflammatory mediators in control *versus* CIA, ART, and SNT models. In all cases, $p < 0.05$ was considered statistically significant.

Results

The expression of PPARs and NFκB is altered in animal models of chronic pain

To allow better understanding towards the underlying mechanisms involved in the generation of chronic pain in the CNS, we investigated the potential changes in the expression of transcription factors NFkB and PPARs in the brain of CIA, SNT, and ART models of chronic pain. Because multiple areas all over brain are involved in pain, including those involved in sensory-discriminative, cognitive/affective responses and endogenous pain control, from cortex to brainstem, we decided to test the expression of transcription factors in frontal cortex, midbrain, brainstem and cerebellum.

Western blot analysis for PPARγ in different brain regions revealed a general reduction in the levels of these receptors in the frontal cortex, brainstem cerebellum of all the pain models (Figures 1A-1D). In contrast, we observed the opposite tendency in NFκB levels, with marked increases in p65 fragment in most brain regions of SNT model of neuropathic pain, and midbrain and brainstem of the CIA and ART models (Figure 2). On the other hand, no major changes were detected in PPARα expression in brains of the SNT and CIA models, although PPARα levels were reduced in certain brain areas of the ART model of pain (Figure 3).

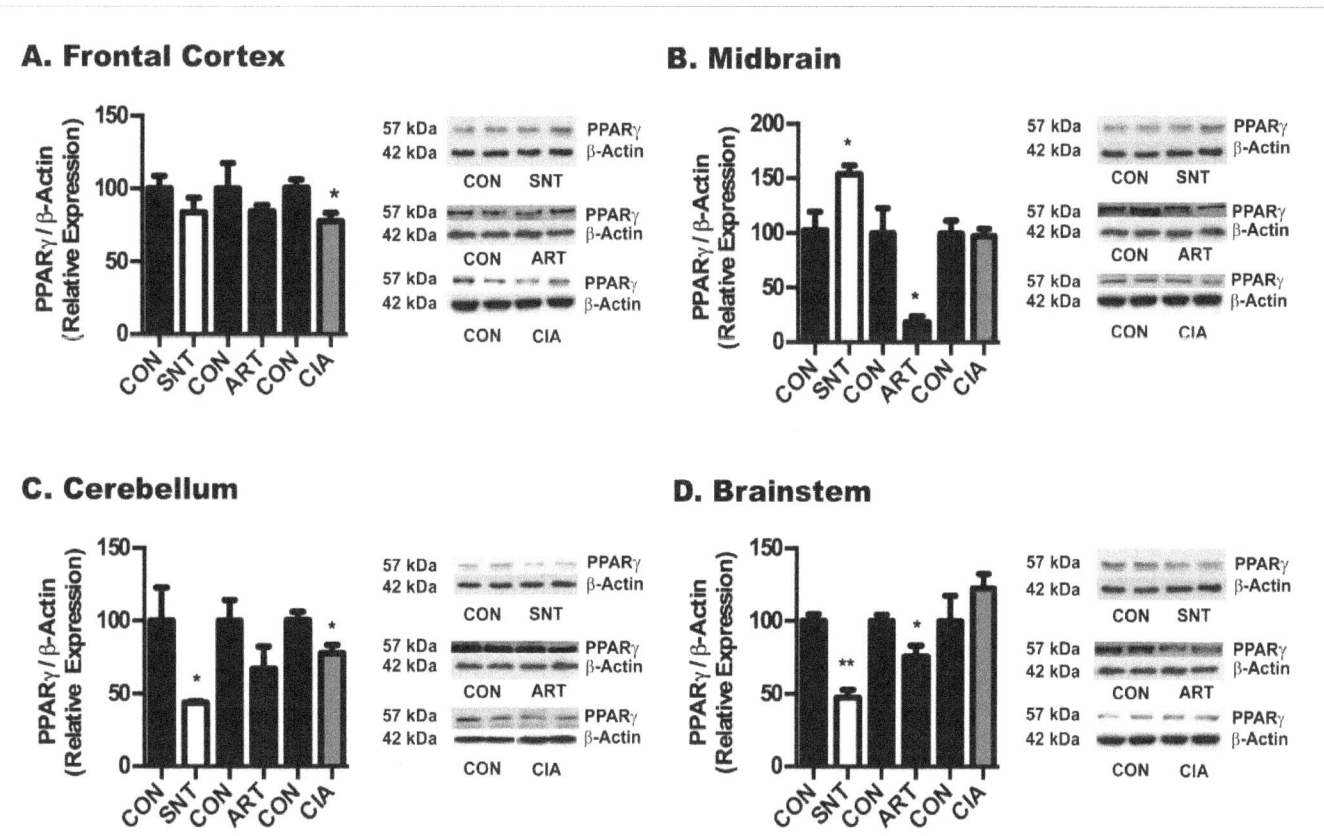

Figure 1: PPARγ expression in models of chronic pain. A) Representative western blots and quantification of PPARγ expression in the frontal cortex of spinal nerve spinal nerve transection (SNT), the anti-retroviral model (ART) associated neuropathy model and the collagen induced arthritis (CIA) models of chronic pain (n=3-5 per group). B) Representative western blots and quantification of PPARγ expression in in the midbrain of the SNT, the ART associated neuropathy model and the CIA models of chronic pain (n=2-5 per group). C) Representative western blots and quantification of PPARγ expression in the cerebellum of the SNT, the ART associated neuropathy model and the CIA models of chronic pain (n=3-5 per group). D) Representative western blots and quantification of of PPARγ expression in the brainstem of the SNT, the ART associated neuropathy are represented by *$p < 0.05$ and **$p < 0.01$.

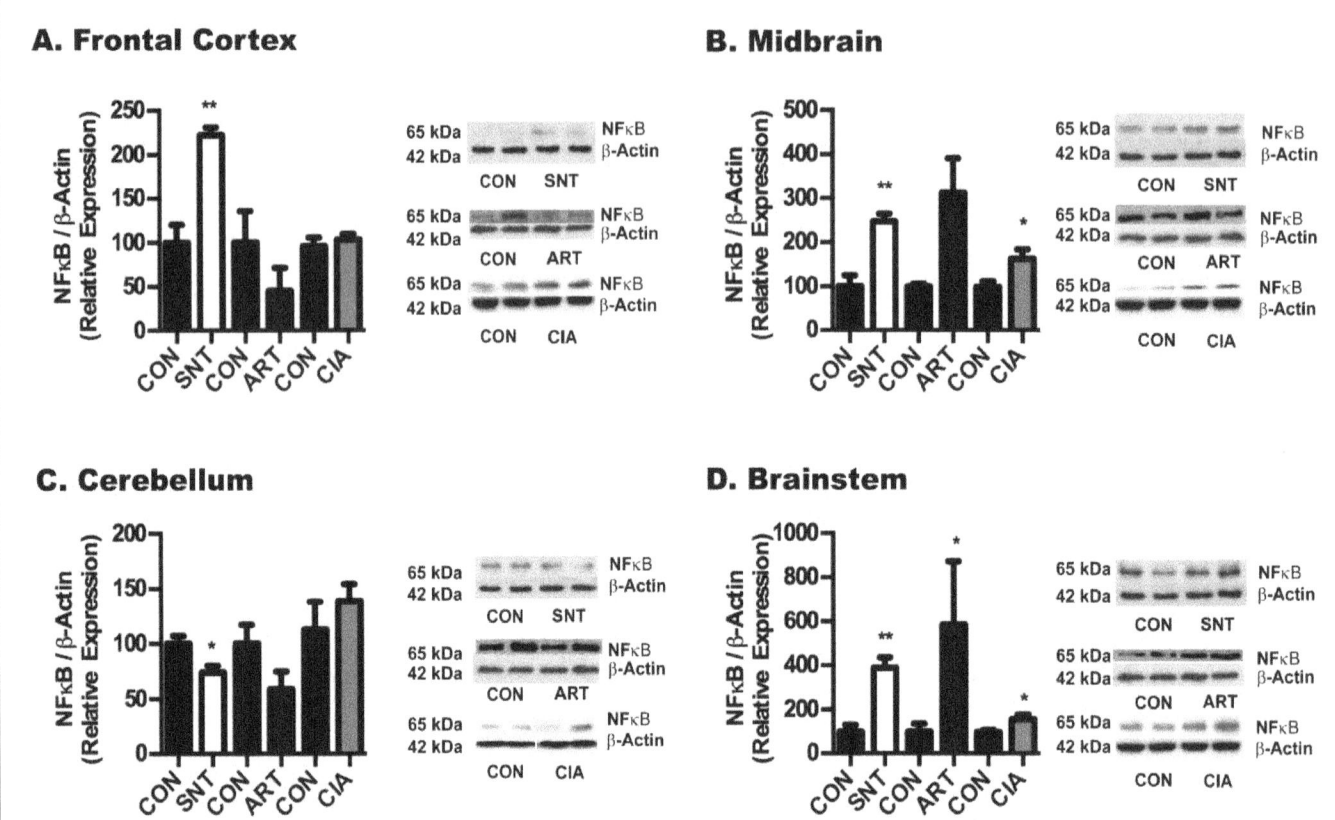

Figure 2: NFκB expression in models of chronic pain. A) Representative western blots and quantification of NFκB expression in the frontal cortex of spinal nerve spinal nerve transection (SNT), the ART associated neuropathy model and the collagen induced arthritis (CIA) models of chronic pain (n=3-5 per group). B) Representative western blots and quantification of NFκB in the midbrain of the SNT, the ART associated neuropathy model and the CIA models of chronic pain (n=2-5 per group). C) Representative western blots and quantification of NFκB expression in the cerebellum of the SNT, the ART associated neuropathy model and the CIA models of chronic pain (n=3-5 per group). D) Representative western blots and quantification of NFκB expression in the brainstem of the SNT, the ART associated neuropathy model and the CIA models of chronic pain (n = 4-5 per group). Columns represent mean ± SEM. Statistical differences are represented by *$p < 0.05$ and **$p < 0.01$.

Effect of pro-inflammatory cytokines on the expression of PPARs and NFκB

In order to confirm whether the changes in PPARs and NFκB expression in the animal models were consequence of the inflammatory component of the model, we repeated the same measurements in N2a cells, which were treated with either vehicle or with 30 ng ml^{-1} of TNFα, because this cytokine has been found increased in CIA models [26]. When treated with TNFα, N2a cells shown a significant decrease in PPARα (c.24%, $p < 0.05$) and PPARγ expression (c.19%, $p < 0.05$) (Figures 4A and 4B respectively). On the other hand, a significant increase (c.65%, $p < 0.005$) in p65 was detected under inflammatory conditions (Figure 4C), suggesting that changes in inflammatory mediators may affect the transcription of PPARs and NFκB, thus explaining the changes detected in animal models of chronic pain.

Discussion

Our results identified substantial changes in the expression of PPARγ and NFκB across various brain regions in different models of persistent pain, in particular those associated with inflammatory pain, such as the CIA model. This was further confirmed *in vitro*, showing that changes in PPARα, PPARγ, and NFκB expression in cultured N2a cells under inflammatory conditions suggested that the inflammatory component of CIA models were likely to be involved in the changes of transcription factors.

So far, there are no publications reporting changes in the expression of PPARs in animal models of pain. However, it has been previously suggested that PPARs might play a role in modulating thermal and pain sensations due to their prominent expression in the thalamus, particularly in the posterior part of the ventral medial nucleus, a site responsive to pain and cold stress and on spinal cord [27,28].

Recent publications have suggested PPARγ as a new target for treating chronic pain [17,29]. Treatment with PPARγ ligands, such as pioglitazone, in the SNT model indicates that pioglitazone alleviates neuropathic pain through the attenuation of the up-regulation in proinflammatory cytokines [30]. The effect of pioglitazone in reducing pain may be mediated by a decrease in glial activation and through neuropathic non-genomic and genomic activity [31]. It has been shown that inflammatory cytokines and oxidative stress decrease the expression of PPARγ mRNA in adipocytes [32] and thiazolidinediones reverse this effect [33]. Similarly, we have previously demonstrated that certain combinations of inflammatory cytokines can decrease PPARγ gene transcription and PPRE activity in neuronal cells [34], and this effect is suppressed by incubation with NSAIDs. In line with this, it has been reported that TNFα suppresses PPARγ2 transcription by inhibiting the binding of C/EBPδ to the PPARγ2 promoter in adipocytes [35]. However, we did not observe changes in the levels of pro-inflammatory cytokines in brain areas of the SNT model and in the ART model (data do not shown). This result is in agreement with previous publications reporting neither peripheral nor central

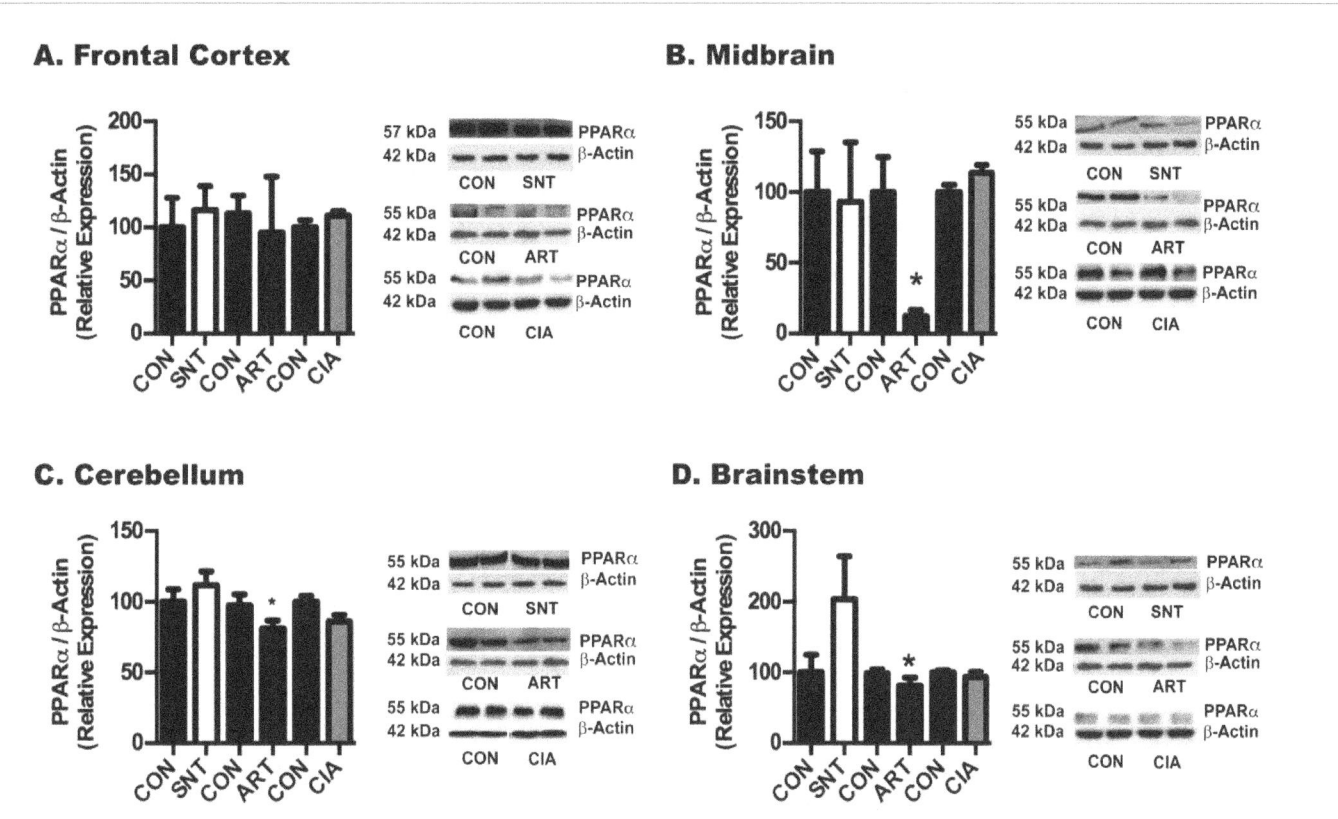

Figure 3: PPARα expression in models of chronic pain. A) Representative western blots and quantification of PPARα expression in the frontal cortex of spinal nerve spinal nerve transection (SNT), the ART associated neuropathy model and the collagen induced arthritis (CIA) models of chronic pain (n=3-5 per group). B) Representative western blots and quantification of PPARα expression in the midbrain of the SNT, the ART associated neuropathy model and the CIA models of chronic pain (n=2-5 per group). C) Representative western blots and quantification of PPARα expression in the Cerebellum (n=3-5 per group). D) Representative western blots and quantification of PPARα expression in the brainstem of the SNT, the ART associated neuropathy model and the CIA models of chronic pain (n = 4-5 per group). Columns represent mean ± SEM. Statistical differences are represented by $*p < 0.05$.

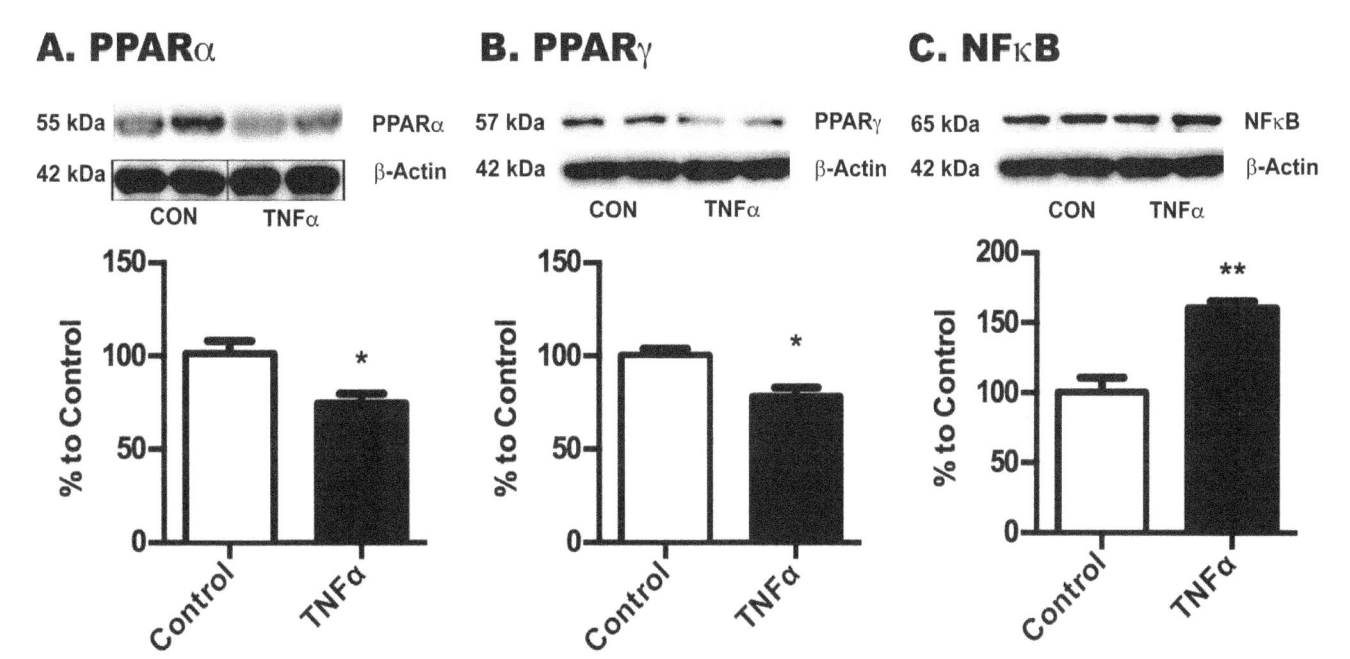

Figure 4: Effect of inflammation in the levels of PPARγ, PPARα and NFκB. Representative western blots and quantification of PPARα (A), PPARγ (B) and NFκB (C) in N2a cells incubated with 30 ng/mL of TNFα (n=3). Columns represent mean ± SEM. Statistical differences are represented by $*p < 0.05$ and $**p < 0.01$.

inflammatory cytokine secretion, or neuronal death, or metabolic dysregulation contributing to the development of hyperalgesia in the model of stavudine orally-induced hyperalgesia (the ART model) in rats [36]; however, results in HIV patients taking this medication seem to indicate alterations in the levels of adiponectin, which is modulated by TNFα [37]. Interestingly, PPARγ agonists have been involved in the regulation of this adipose-specific plasma protein that possesses anti-atherogenic properties [38]. Performing further analysis including other inflammatory mediators such as chemokines in the brain of SNT and ART models would be necessary to address this point [39].

Both *in vitro* and *in vivo* studies have demonstrated that neuronal PPARγ prevents COX-2 increase, which in turn may reduce prostaglandin synthesis [40]. Hence, the reduction of PPARγ in pain models might contribute towards the loss of control of COX-2 upregulation, ultimately causing pain. Alternatively, the analgesic effect of PPARγ agonists could rely upon endogenous opioid activity [6]; PPARγ may modulate the transcription of pain receptors, such as opioid receptors, and consequently affect nociception. Interestingly, both natural and synthetic PPARγ agonists show rapid effects, within 5 minutes of injection, suggesting a transcription-independent pathway of action [11] and mechanism of action. The anti-allodynia effects of PPARγ agonists are PPARγ-dependent, which confirms its involvement in pain regulation [17].

Although PPARα synthetic agonists, such as fenofibrates, have shown beneficial effects in acute and chronic models of inflammatory and neuropathic pain [16,18,41,42], no major changes were observed in their expression in the CIA and SNT models of chronic pain in the present study. However, in diet-induce obese rats the levels of PPARα were found down-regulated in spinal cord, and facilitated the susceptibility to peripheral inflammatory challenge by increasing inflammatory response, contributing to augmented peripheral inflammation and inflammatory hyperalgesia [43]. This is in agreement with the reduced levels of PPARα found in the ART model and in cells incubated with TNFα. Similar to the PPARγ, it has been hypothesised that PPARα agonists decrease pain via a non-transcriptional mediated mechanism, most likely regulating the activity of ion channels [4]. PPARα has been demonstrated to affect NFkB expression [41], as the PPARα agonist Fenofibrate upregulates IκBα expression, leading to the repression of the p50 subunit of NFkB and C/EBP [44].

The increased NFκB expression in the models of chronic pain observed in the present study is in agreement with existing publications that suggest that NFκB is regulated by inflammation and could be a mediator of pain [9,45]. In rat models of paw inflammation, R-flurbiprofen has both antinociceptive and anti-inflammatory effects [46]. Other studies demonstrate that R-flurbiprofen potently inhibits NFκB activation and its target genes [45], suggesting the involvement of NFκB in both the hyperalgesic and inflammatory component of the CIA model. On the other hand, activated p50 would seem to be a very interesting target to investigate in pain since p50 knockouts mice demonstrated reduced acute and inflammatory nociceptive responses [47].

In summary, PPARγ and NFκB seem to be oppositely regulated in models of chronic pain. In fact, PPARγ has been shown to be able to block NFkB actions by several mechanisms, including I-κBα induction [48] or by transcriptional transrepression, also known as squelching, receptor mutual antagonism, or cross-coupling, therefore interfering with NFκB transcriptional activity [49,50].

Conclusion

In conclusion, the results of this study identify alterations in a common signalling pathway in different models of persistent pain

and suggest that changes in PPARs and NFκB seem to be secondary to neuroinflammation, therefore contributing to further exacerbation of pain symptomatology. The result of interferences with the PPAR signalling pathway that has become evident in pain has far reaching consequences that extend beyond the pain scenario, affecting other conditions where PPARs have a role, including neurological pathologies such as Alzheimers disease [34]. Further research needs to be highlighted in these areas, as there is the potential that modification of this signalling pathway can ameliorate or even reverse these pathologies.

Acknowledgement

This project was partly funded by a grant from the Fundacio Marato TV3, ref 072610 (Catalonia, Spain). We thank Prof. Andrew S. Rice for his collaboration in the ART and SNT models.

References

1. Rice AS, Smith BH, Blyth FM (2016) Pain and the global burden of disease. Pain 157: 791-796.

2. Gao YJ, Ji RR (2008) Activation of JNK pathway in persistent pain. Neurosci Lett 437: 180-183.

3. Svensson CI, Zattoni M, Serhan CN (2007) Lipoxins and aspirin-triggered lipoxin inhibit inflammatory pain processing. J Exp Med 204: 245-252.

4. Maeda T, Kishioka S (2009) PPAR and Pain. In G.C.M.T.S.T. Bagetta and S. Sakurada, (eds). International Review of Neurobiology, Academic Press pp: 165-177.

5. Abbadie C (2005) Chemokines, chemokine receptors and pain. Trends Immunol 26: 529-534.

6. Napimoga MH, Souza GR, Cunha TM, Ferrari LF, Clemente-Napimoga JT (2008) 15d-Prostaglandin J2 Inhibits Inflammatory Hypernociception: Involvement of Peripheral Opioid Receptor. J Pharmacol Exp Ther 324: 313-321.

7. Scholz J, Woolf CJ (2002) Can we conquer pain? Nat Neurosci 5: 1062-1067.

8. Woolf CJ, Ma Q (2007) Nociceptors--noxious stimulus detectors. Neuron 55: 353-364.

9. Niederberger E, Geisslinger G (2008) The IKK-NF-kappaB pathway: a source for novel molecular drug targets in pain therapy? FASEB J 22: 3432-3442.

10. Ma W, Bisby MA (1998) Increased activation of nuclear factor kappa B in rat lumbar dorsal root ganglion neurons following partial sciatic nerve injuries. Brain Res 797: 243-254.

11. Fehrenbacher JC, Loverme J, Clarke W, Hargreaves KM, Piomelli D, et al. (2009) Rapid pain modulation with nuclear receptor ligands. Brain Res Rev 60: 114-124.

12. Quintanilla RA, Utreras E, Cabezas-Opazo FA (2014) Role of PPARγ in the Differentiation and Function of Neurons. PPAR Res 2014: 768594.

13. Berger J, Moller DE (2002) The mechanisms of action of PPARs. Annu Rev Med 53: 409-435.

14. Tan NS, Michalik L, Desvergne B, Wahli W (2005) Multiple expression control mechanisms of peroxisome proliferator-activated receptors and their target genes. J Steroid Biochem Mol Biol 93: 99-105.

15. Desvergne B, Wahli W (1999) Peroxisome proliferator-activated receptors: nuclear control of metabolism. Endocr Rev 20: 649-688.

16. Oliveira ACP, Bertollo CM, Rocha LT, Nascimento EB, Costa KA, et al. (2007) Antinociceptive and antiedematogenic activities of fenofibrate, an agonist of PPAR alpha, and pioglitazone, an agonist of PPAR gamma. European Journal of Pharmacology 561: 194-201.

17. Churi SB, Abdel-Aleem OS, Tumber KK, Scuderi-Porter H, Taylor BK (2008) Intrathecal rosiglitazone acts at peroxisome proliferator-activated receptor-gamma to rapidly inhibit neuropathic pain in rats. J Pain 9: 639-649.

18. LoVerme J, Russo R, La Rana G, Fu J, Farthing J, et al. (2006) Rapid broad-spectrum analgesia through activation of peroxisome proliferator-activated receptor-alpha. J Pharmacol Exp Ther 319: 1051-1061.

19. Zimmermann M (1983) Ethical guidelines for investigations of experimental pain in conscious animals. Pain 16: 109-110.

20. Kilkenny C, Browne W, Cuthill IC, Emerson M, Altman DG (2011) Animal research: reporting in vivo experiments-the ARRIVE guidelines. J Cereb Blood Flow Metab 31: 991-993.

21. Holmdahl R, Bockermann R, Bäcklund J, Yamada H (2002) The molecular pathogenesis of collagen-induced arthritis in mice-a model for rheumatoid arthritis. Ageing Res Rev 1: 135-147.

22. Inglis JJ, Notley CA, Essex D, Wilson AW, Feldmann M, et al. (2007) Collagen-induced arthritis as a model of hyperalgesia: functional and cellular analysis of the analgesic actions of tumor necrosis factor blockade. Arthritis & Rheumatism 56: 4015-4023.

23. Huang W, Calvo M, Karu K, Olausen HR, Bathgate G, et al. (2013) A clinically relevant rodent model of the HIV antiretroviral drug stavudine induced painful peripheral neuropathy. Pain 154: 560-575.

24. Wallace VC, Segerdahl AR, Lambert DM, Vandevoorde S, Blackbeard J, et al. (2007) The effect of the palmitoylethanolamide analogue, palmitoylallylamide (L-29) on pain behaviour in rodent models of neuropathy. Br J Pharmacol 151: 1117-1128.

25. Wallace VC, Blackbeard J, Pheby T, Segerdahl AR, Davies M, et al. (2007) Pharmacological, behavioural and mechanistic analysis of HIV-1 gp120 induced painful neuropathy. Pain 133: 47-63.

26. Rioja I, Bush KA, Buckton JB, Dickson MC, Life PF (2004) Joint cytokine quantification in two rodent arthritis models: kinetics of expression, correlation of mRNA and protein levels and response to prednisolone treatment. Clin Exp Immunol 137: 65-73.

27. Xing G, Zhang L, Heynen T (1995) Rat PPAR? contains a CGG triplet repeat and is prominently expressed in the thalamic nuclei. Biochemical and Biophysical Research Communications 217: 1015-1025.

28. Hathway GJ, Koch S, Low L, Fitzgerald M (2009) The changing balance of brainstem-spinal cord modulation of pain processing over the first weeks of rat postnatal life. J Physiol 587: 2927-2935.

29. Morgenweck J, Griggs RB, Donahue RR, Zadina JE, Taylor BK (2013) PPARγ activation blocks development and reduces established neuropathic pain in rats. Neuropharmacology 70: 236-246.

30. Maeda T, Kiguchi N, Kobayashi Y, Ozaki M, Kishioka S (2008) Pioglitazone attenuates tactile allodynia and thermal hyperalgesia in mice subjected to peripheral nerve injury. J Pharmacol Sci 108: 341-347.

31. Griggs RB, Donahue RR, Adkins BG, Anderson KL, Thibault O, et al. (2016) Pioglitazone Inhibits the Development of Hyperalgesia and Sensitization of Spinal Nociresponsive Neurons in Type 2 Diabetes. J Pain 17: 359-373.

32. Xing H, Northrop JP, Grove JR, Kilpatrick KE, Su JL, Ringold GM (1997) TNF alpha-mediated inhibition and reversal of adipocyte differentiation is accompanied by suppressed expression of PPARgamma without effects on Pref-1 expression. Endocrinology 138: 2776-2783.

33. Gimble JM, Robinson CE, Wu X, Kelly KA, Rodriguez BR, et al. (1996) Peroxisome proliferator-activated receptor-gamma activation by thiazolidinediones induces adipogenesis in bone marrow stromal cells. Mol Pharmacol 50: 1087-94.

34. Sastre M, Dewachter I, Rossner S, Bogdanovic N, Rosen E, et al. (2006) Nonsteroidal anti-inflammatory drugs repress beta-secretase gene promoter activity by the activation of PPARγ. Proc Natl Acad Sci USA 103: 443-448.

35. Kudo M, Sugawara A, Uruno A, Takeuchi K, Ito S (2004) Transcription suppression of peroxisome proliferator-activated receptor gamma2 gene expression by tumor necrosis factor alpha via an inhibition of CCAAT/ enhancer-binding protein delta during the early stage of adipocyte differentiation. Endocrinology 145: 4948-4956.

36. Weber J, Mitchell D, Veliotes D, Mitchell B, Kamerman PR (2009) Hyperalgesia induced by oral stavudine administration to rats does not depend on spinal neuronal cell death, or on spinal or systemic inflammatory cytokine secretion, or metabolic dysregulation. Neurotoxicology 30: 423-429.

37. Lindegaard B, Keller P, Bruunsgaard H, Gerstoft J, Pedersen BK (2004) Low plasma level of adiponectin is associated with stavudine treatment and lipodystrophy in HIV-infected patients. Clin Exp Immunol 135: 273-279.

38. Maeda N, Takahashi M, Funahashi T, Kihara S, Nishizawa H, et al. (2001) PPARγ ligands increase expression and plasma concentrations of adiponectin, an adipose-derived protein. Diabetes 50: 2094-2099.

39. Freitag CM, Miller RJ (2014) Peroxisome proliferator-activated receptor agonists modulate neuropathic pain: a link to chemokines? Front Cell Neurosci 8: 238.

40. Zhao Y, Patzer A, Herdegen T, Gohlke P, Culman J (2006) Activation of cerebral peroxisome proliferator-activated receptors gamma promotes neuroprotection by attenuation of neuronal cyclooxygenase-2 overexpression after focal cerebral ischemia in rats. FASEB J 20: 1162-75.

41. Genolet R, Wahli W, Michalik L (2004) PPARs as drug targets to modulate inflammatory responses? Curr Drug Targets Inflamm Allergy 3: 361-375.

42. Taylor BK, Dadia N, Yang CB, Krishnan S, Badr M (2002) Peroxisome proliferator-activated receptor agonists inhibit inflammatory edema and hyperalgesia. Inflammation 26: 121-127.

43. Wang J, Zhang Q, Zhao L, Li D, Fu Z, et al. (2014) Down-regulation of PPARa in the spinal cord contributes to augmented peripheral inflammation and inflammatory hyperalgesia in diet-induced obese rats. Neuroscience 278: 165-178.

44. Kleemann R, Gervois PP, Verschuren L, Staels B, Princen HM, et al. (2003) Fibrates down-regulate IL-1-stimulated C-reactive protein gene expression in hepatocytes by reducing nuclear p50-NFkappa B-C/EBP-beta complex formation. Blood 101: 545-551.

45. Tegeder I, Niederberger E, Israr E, Gühring H, Brune K, et al. (2001) Inhibition of NF-kappaB and AP-1 activation by R- and S-flurbiprofen. FASEB J 15: 595-597.

46. Geisslinger G, Ferreira SH, Menzel S, Schlott D, Brune K (1994) Antinociceptive actions of R(-)-flurbiprofen-a non-cyclooxygenase inhibiting 2-arylpropionic acid-in rats. Life Sci 54: PL173-PL 177.

47. Niederberger E, Schmidtko A, Gao W, Kahlein H, Ehnert C, et al. (2007) Impaired acute and inflammatory nociception in mice lacking the p50 subunit of NF-κB. Eur J Pharmacol 559: 55-60.

48. Dehmer T, Heneka MT, Sastre M, Dichgans J, Schulz JB (2004) Protection by pioglitazone in the MPTP model of Parkinson's disease correlates with I kappa B alpha induction and block of NF kappa B and iNOS activation. J Neurochem 88: 494-501.

49. Ghisletti S, Huang W, Ogawa S, Pascual G, Lin ME, et al. (2007) Parallel SUMOylation-dependent pathways mediate gene- and signal-specific transrepression by LXRs and PPARgamma. Mol Cell 25: 57-70.

50. Grommes G, Landreth GE, Heneka MT (2004) Antineoplastic effects of peroxisome proliferator-activated receptor gamma agonists. Lancet Oncol 5: 419-429.

32

Alpha-Tocopherol Counteracts Cognitive and Motor Deficits Induced by Repeated Treatment with Reserpine

Aldair José Sarmento-Silva[1], Ramón Hypolito Lima[1], Alicia Cabral[1], Ywlliane Meurer[1], Alessandra Mussi Ribeiro[1,2] and Regina Helena Silva[1,3*]

[1]Memory Studies Laboratory, Physiology Department, Federal University of Rio Grande do Norte, Natal, Brazil
[2]Department of Biosciences, Federal University of São Paulo, Santos, Brazil
[3]Department of Pharmacology, Federal University of São Paulo, São Paulo, Brazil

Abstract

Previous studies showed that chronic administration of the monoamine depleting agent reserpine in low doses promotes progressive cognitive and motor impairments in rats, and this protocol has been used as a pharmacological progressive model of Parkinson's disease. These behavioral alterations are accompanied by increased brain oxidative stress. We aimed to verify the effects of the concomitant treatment with the antioxidant agent alpha-tocopherol on the motor and cognitive deficits induced by chronic reserpine in rats. Rats were repeatedly treated with 0.1 mg/kg reserpine with or without a concomitant treatment with 40 mg/kg alpha-tocopherol. Across the treatment, motor and cognitive performances were evaluated by the catalepsy and novel object recognition tests, respectively. As expected, reserpine-treated rats showed progressively increased duration of catalepsy together with short-term memory deficits in the object recognition test. Importantly, these detrimental outcomes due to reserpine treatment were prevented by concomitant daily administration of the antioxidant agent alpha-tocopherol. The results show a preventive role of alpha-tocopherol on behavioral alterations induced by repeated reserpine treatment. This is relevant to the investigation of possible neuroprotective interventions in Parkinson's disease.

Keywords: Reserpine; Parkinson's disease; α-tocopherol; Motor impairment; Short-term memory impairment

Abbreviations: NOR: Novel Object Recognition; PD: Parkinson's Disease; RES: Reserpine; ROS: Reactive Oxygen Species; TOC: Alpha-Tocopherol; VR: Vehicle For Reserpine; VT: Vehicle For Alpha-Tocopherol; PKC: Protein Kinase C

Introduction

Reserpine precludes the storage of monoamines through the blockage of the synaptic vesicles transporters [1]. Consequently, synaptic vesicles are still available but there is a reduction in the amount of dopamine in the synaptic cleft. Because an important loss of dopaminergic neurons is the core feature of Parkinson´s disease (PD) [2], reserpine administration to rodents is a valid approach to study this disease in animal models [3-5]. The acute administration of a high dose of reserpine (above 1.0 mg/kg) leads to severe motor impairment [4]. In addition, acute injection of reserpine in lower doses causes memory deficits in the absence of motor damage [6,7]. However, although both cognitive and motor impairments are symptoms of PD, their emergence shortly after an acute injection is not compatible with the gradual progression of symptoms found in the clinical situation. More recently, studies have shown that the chronic administration of reserpine in low doses can promote progressive cognitive and motor impairments, along with decreased tyrosine hydroxylase levels in the nigrostriatal pathway [8]. This protocol is suggested as a progressive pharmacological model of PD [8,9].

Besides its classical mechanism of action (i.e. blockage of the vesicular transport of monoamines), there is clear evidence that reserpine also causes an increase in cellular oxidative stress, possibly potentiated by the rise in the levels of dopamine in the cytoplasm, which undergoes oxidative metabolism [10]. In this respect, the central nervous system is quite vulnerable to reactive oxygen species (ROS), which play a very important function in the pathogenesis of neurodegenerative disorders, including PD [11]. For example, there is evidence that the inclusion of antioxidant agents in the pharmacological

treatment of PD has advantages over the treatment based only in dopamine replacement [11-13]. In addition, the repeated treatment with reserpine that induces progressive features compatible with PD also leads to increased brain oxidative stress [9]. However, it is unclear if a possible oxidative damage is responsible for the behavioral deficits presented by animals repeatedly treated with reserpine.

Antioxidant agents mainly act as a reinforcement of endogenous antioxidant defenses. An important antioxidant agent is vitamin E (alpha-tocopherol; TOC), which plays an essential role in protecting the body against the damaging effects of ROS. Specifically, TOC blocks the propagation step of lipid peroxidation of polyunsaturated fatty acids in membranes and lipoproteins [14], mainly by neutralizing the effects of peroxides and oxygen free radicals [15].

The aim of this study was to evaluate the effects of the antioxidant agent TOC on motor, cognitive and neuronal parameters in animals submitted to a progressive pharmacological animal model of PD, i.e., the repeated treatment with a low dose of reserpine.

Material and Methods

Animals

We used 75 five-month-old male Wistar rats (300-500 g). The

*Corresponding author: Regina Helena Silva, Departamento de Farmacologia – UNIFESP, Rua Botucatu, 862, Edificio Leal Prado, 1º.andar, CEP 04023062 - São Paulo, SP, Brasil, E-mail: reginahsilva@gmail.com

animals were obtained from the Physiology Department at the Federal University of Rio Grande do Norte, and were housed in groups of four, in plastic cages, under controlled conditions of ventilation, temperature (23 ± 1ºC), and light/dark cycle (12h/12h, lights on 6:30 a.m.), with free access to water and food. The rats were handled according to the Brazilian law for the use of animals in scientific research (Law Number 11.794) and all the procedures described were approved by the local ethical committee (CEUA/UFRN nº 051/2011).

Drugs

Reserpine (RES; Sigma Chemical Co., St. Louis, MO) was dissolved in acetic acid and further diluted in distilled water at the concentration of 0.1 mg/mL, pH ≈ 6.5. We used this vehicle (glacial acetic acid diluted in water) as a control for reserpine treatment (VR). RES and VR were given s.c. on alternate days. The antioxidant alpha-tocopherol (TOC; Sigma Chemical Co., St. Louis, MO) was diluted in distilled water with Tween-80 at the concentration of 40 mg/mL. We used the vehicle used to dilute TOC (VT) as a control for TOC treatment. These solutions were injected i.p. daily. The volume of injection was 1 mL/kg of body weight in all cases. We prepared all solutions every 48 hours and kept them at 4ºC between administrations.

Experimental design

The rats were randomly assigned to the following groups: VR + VT (n=18), RES + VT (n=19), RES + TOC (n=19) and VR + TOC (n=19). Drug treatment lasted 30 days. Animals received 15 s.c. injections of RES (0.1 mg/kg) or VR every 48 hours, concomitantly to daily i.p. administration of TOC (40 mg/kg) or VT.

Before the beginning of the experiments, all animals were submitted to a daily 5-minute handling session for five consecutive days. Throughout the treatment, all the animals were subjected to catalepsy tests (performed daily) and part of the animals (n=35, 7-11 per group) went through the novel object recognition (NOR) tasks (days 2, 12 and 18 of treatment). The experimental design is shown in Figure 1. Both behavioral tests were performed as described in our previous study [8] and were conducted before the injections of that day. Thus, all behavioral evaluations were performed 48h after the last injection of reserpine in order to avoid acute effects of the drug. NOR sessions were recorded with a digital camera fixed above the arena and the behavior was analyzed through video-tracking software (Anymaze, Stoelting Co, Wood Dale, Illinois, and USA). Before each experimental procedure, the apparatuses were cleaned with a 5% alcohol solution, and the experimental groups were alternated across testing.

Statistical analysis

We analyzed the performances in catalepsy test (total time spent in immobility until the animal removed both forepaws of the bar) by the two-way ANOVA with repeated measures followed by Tukey's multiple comparison post hoc test. In the NOR task we conducted one-way ANOVA followed by Bonferroni's multiple comparison post hoc test in order to compare old versus familiar object exploration. Analyses for the exploration ratio throughout test sessions and among experimental groups were conducted through two-way ANOVA followed by Tukey's Post Hoc test.

Results

Catalepsy

Figure 2 shows that from day 15 onwards there was an increase in catalepsy behavior of the group RES + VT compared to all other groups (RM two-way ANOVA; days of treatment [$F_{(29,2130)}$ = 16.72, P < 0.0001], treatment [$F_{(3,2130)}$ = 211.0, P < 0.0001] and days of treatment × treatment interaction effects [$F_{(87,2130)}$ = 4.876, P < 0.0001]). This increase was not detected for the group RES+TOC.

Novel object recognition

We found that all animals spent more time exploring the new object in the second day of protocol (first test; Figure 3A; one-way ANOVA [$F_{(7,62)}$ = 11.23; P < 0.0001]). Reserpine treatment impaired short-term memory after the 12th day of protocol (second and third tests). Conversely, treatment with α-tocopherol was able to prevent the short-term memory impairment (Figure 3B; one-way ANOVA [$F_{(7,74)}$ = 6.864; P < 0.0001] and Figure 3C; one-way ANOVA [$F_{(7,68)}$ = 10.00; P < 0.0001]). We also performed statistical analyses in order to evaluate the effect of drug administration in objects exploration ratio throughout test sessions and among experimental groups. We found that in the third test session animals' receiving RES differs on exploration rate of new (Table 1; two-way ANOVA [$F_{(6,89)}$ = 2.843; P < 0.05]) and old objects (Table 1; two-way ANOVA [$F_{(6,89)}$ = 2.843; P < 0.05]) when comparing to both VR + VT and RES + TOC. Yet, we found that only RES + VT group presented alterations in object discrimination across tests. More accurately, exploration of old and new objects increased and decreased, respectively, comparing first and second tests (Table 1; two-way ANOVA [$F_{(3,89)}$ = 2.760; P < 0.05]) and first and third tests (Table 1; two-way ANOVA [$F_{(3,89)}$ = 2.649; P < 0.05]).

Discussion

In this study, we investigated the effects of concomitant treatment with TOC on catalepsy behavior and NOR task in rats submitted to a

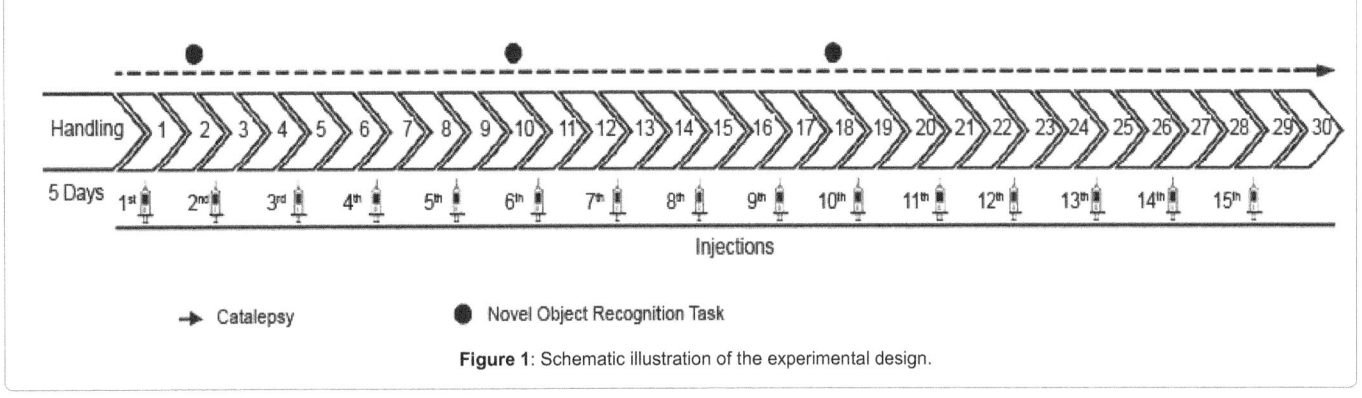

Figure 1: Schematic illustration of the experimental design.

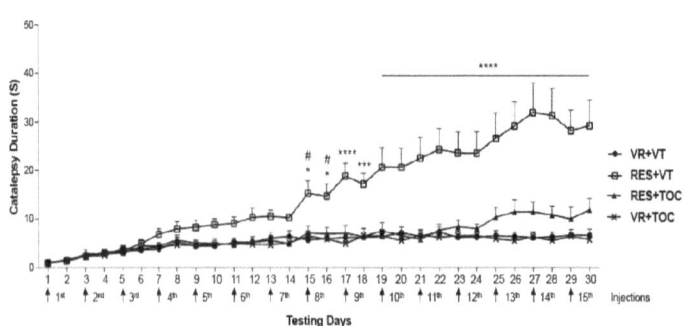

Figure 2: Repeated administration of reserpine increases catalepsy duration and this effect is prevented by α-tocopherol. Animals were placed daily in a catalepsy bar and the latency to step-down was registered. Arrows indicate reserpine (RES; 0.1 mg/kg) or vehicle (VR) s.c. injections, while α-tocopherol (TOC; 40 mg/kg) or its vehicle (VT) were administered through daily i.p. injections. Data are expressed as mean + SEM; (*) $P < 0.05$ for RES + VT vs. RES+TOC; (#) $P < 0.01$ for RES + VT vs. VR+VT; (***) $P < 0.001$ and (****) $P < 0.0001$ for RES + VT vs. all experimental groups in Tukey's multiple comparison post hoc test after RM two-way ANOVA.

chronic treatment with a low dosage of reserpine. We observed that the motor and cognitive impairments induced by chronic treatment with reserpine were prevented by treatment with TOC. These results can be seen in the evaluation of catalepsy behavior performed 48 h after each reserpine injection (Figure 2) as well as in the analysis of exploration time in the novel object recognition task (Figure 3 and Table 1).

As previously observed in studies by our group [8,9], repeated treatment with a low dose (0.1 mg/kg) of reserpine in rats induced the progressive appearance of motor impairment. This impairment is marked by a gradual increase in the duration of catalepsy behavior. Indeed, as one can see in Figure 2, reserpine-treated (RES + VT) animals start differing from control subjects after 7 reserpine s.c. injections. It is well documented that catalepsy in rodents indicates akinesia and rigidity that are important symptoms of PD [16-18]. Importantly, we did not observe this impairment in the group that was concomitantly treated with TOC. Indeed, the group RES + TOC (Figure 2) presented catalepsy duration similar to control across the treatment.

Besides motor assessment, the protocol used in the present study includes the cognitive evaluation. Cognitive deficits have been reported as symptoms of PD, and can even appear before the motor deficits. In a previous study, we have shown that the protocol of reserpine treatment used here induces short-term memory deficits before the appearance of increased catalepsy behavior and other motor signs [8]. The present study corroborates those findings. We used the NOR task, which involves recognition memory and executive functions, both functions that can be impaired in PD [19,20]. Our results corroborated the previous study showing that animals treated with reserpine failed to discriminate the objects in the test session (in the second and third tests, Figure 3). Further, similarly to that described for motor evaluations, the deficit was prevented by TOC administration. Indeed, animals treated with both reserpine and TOC presented increased novel object exploration in all tests, similarly to control subjects. In addition, comparisons among experimental groups showed that animals treated with RES had worse object discrimination compared to both control and RES + TOC groups in the third test. Finally, when performances across the three tests were analyzed, only the group treated with reserpine alone presented discrimination deficits in the second and third tests compared to the first test (Table 1). These additional analyses reinforce the prevention of the reserpine-induced object recognition impairment by co-treatment with TOC.

As mentioned, reserpine is a non-selective inhibitor of the vesicular monoamine transporter [1]. Thus, one could raise the possibility that the behavioral alterations induced by reserpine treatment are related exclusively to the dopamine depletion caused by this blockage. In other words, the alterations could be a consequence of an additive effect on dopaminergic function. However, there is evidence that favors the hypothesis that the progressive effect of the repeated treatment with reserpine is due to oxidative damage. First, a previous study has shown that the classical acute treatment (with a dose 10 times higher than the one we used) did not cause a reduction in tyrosine hydroxylase staining (an indicative of dopaminergic neuronal function), although causing an important motor impairment [21]. Conversely, the protocol used here (repeated treatment with a low dose) reduced tyrosine hydroxylase staining in the substantia nigra and striatum, and part of the alterations induced by the treatment were not recovered after 30 days of treatment withdrawal [8]. Second, it has been shown that reserpine treatment increases brain oxidative stress and this alteration is accompanied by behavioral deficits [10,22,23]. In addition, in a previous study [9] the repeated treatment with a low dose of reserpine induced an increase in striatal level of lipid peroxidation, which occurred concomitantly to the motor impairment. These results lead us to question if co-treatment with TOC would prevent the progressive motor and cognitive alterations induced by the repeated treatment with a low dose of reserpine. As discussed above, treatment with TOC was able to prevent these deficits. This preventive effect might be explained by a neuroprotection mechanism, probably by a reduction the in neurotoxic dopamine oxidation bioproducts [24].

Despite the well-known antioxidant properties of vitamin E, it is important to mention that tocopherol and other antioxidant agents can have pro-oxidant effects as well. Indeed, the ability of these compounds to accept and donate electrons enables them to cause oxidative damage under certain conditions [25]. However, this pro-oxidant action is mainly found in vitro, and under high concentrations [26,27]. Some in vivo studies have also shown pro-oxidant effects of classical antioxidants, but they are variable depending on substance, concentration, age of the subject and target molecules [25,28-30]. Further, it seems that their preferential action is antioxidant when an oxidant insult from another source is present [31]. In the case of the present results, there was no evidence of a pro-oxidant action regarding possible behavioral alterations.

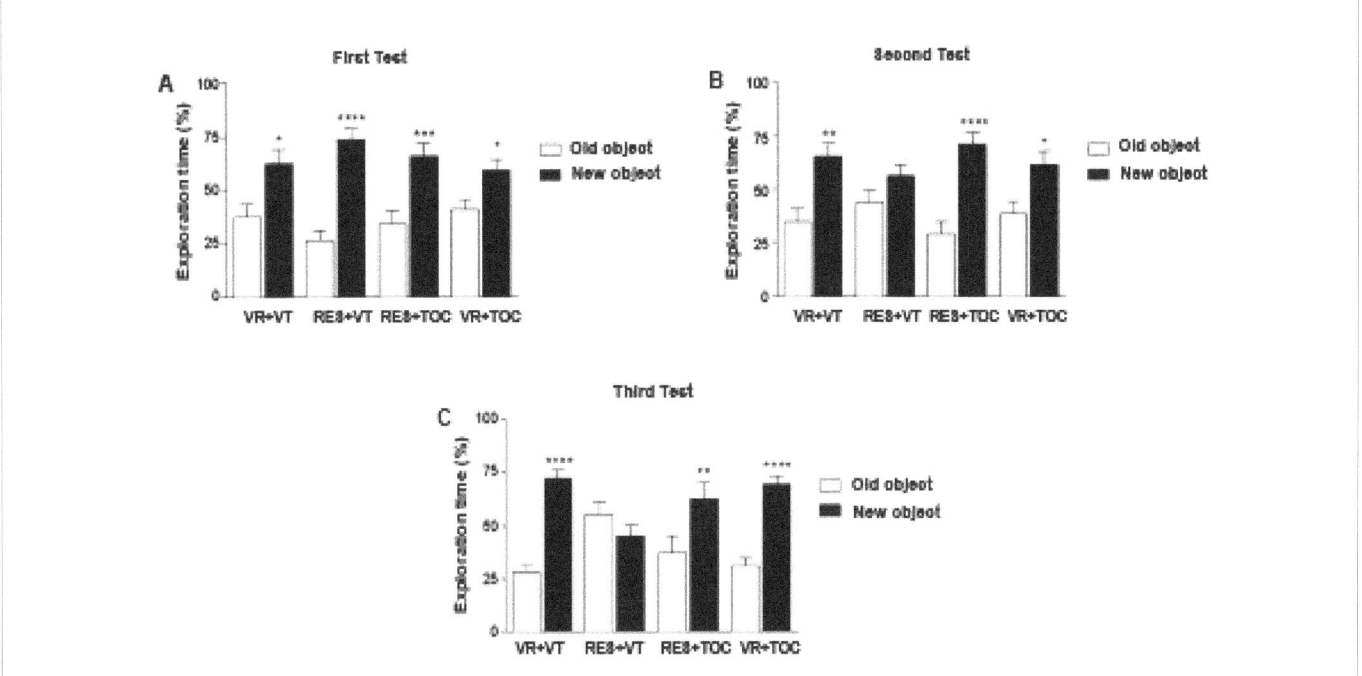

Figure 3: Animals were treated with reserpine (RES; 1.0 mg/kg) or vehicle (VR) through s.c. injections, and α-tocopherol (TOC; 40 mg/kg) or its vehicle (VT) with daily i.p. injections. Animals were tested on the following days of experiment: (A) 2nd, (B) 12th and (C) 18th. In each day, training (with two identical objects, data not shown) and test (with one familiar and one novel object) were performed with a one-hour interval in an open field arena. Data are expressed as mean ± SEM. (') P < 0.05; ('') P < 0.01; (''') P < 0.001 and ('''') P < 0.0001 when comparing old vs. new object exploration ratio in one-way ANOVA followed by Bonferroni's multiple comparison post hoc test.

Tests	Objects	Groups			
		VR + VT	RES + VT	RES + TOC	TOC
First Test	Old	36.94 ± 6.61	26.06 ± 5.01	34.11 ± 5.84	40.6 ± 4.91
Post 1st injection	New	63.06 ± 6.61	73.94 ± 5.01	65.89 ± 5.84	59.4 ± 4.91
Second Test	Old	34.69 ± 5.92	43.97 ± 5.31*	26.85 ± 5.87	39.17 ± 6.32
Post 6th injection	New	65.31 ± 5.92	56.03 ± 5.31*	73.15 ± 5.87	60.83 ± 6.32
Third Test	Old	27.71 ± 4.97	59.99 ± 6.95$^{\epsilon\#}$	31.99 ± 6.43'	37.07 ± 3.25
Post 9th injection	New	72.28 ± 4.97	40.01 ± 6.95$^{\epsilon\#}$	68.01 ± 6.43'	62.93 ± 3.25

Table 1: Exploration rate in the NOR task throughout the test sessions. Data are expressed as mean ± SEM. (') P < 0.05 and ($^{\epsilon}$) P < 0.01 when comparing RES + VT vs. RES + TOC and VR + VT vs. RES + VT respectively. (*) P < 0.05 and (#) P < 0.001 when comparing the first vs. second test and first vs. third test respectively. All statistical analyses were conducted through two-way ANOVA followed by Tukey's Post Hoc test.

Nevertheless, an antioxidant role of vitamin E in ameliorating neurodegeneration in PD has been consistently proposed by in vitro and animal studies [32-37]. On the other hand, despite strong evidence favoring an antioxidant effect, the exact mechanism of action of vitamin E in Parkinson's disease is still under investigation [32]. There is evidence that vitamin E, particularly alpha-tocopherol, can act through other mechanisms not related to modulation of oxidative stress. For example, studies showed that alpha-tocopherol regulates the expression of several genes [38,39] and inhibits protein kinase C (PKC) activity [40,41]. The later could be related to the neuroprotective action of this compound, because PKC activation has been implicated in cell death signaling pathways related to PD [42]. This relationship was found in studies with animal models of PD induced by the toxins 1-methyl-4-phenylpyridinium [43] and paraquat [44]. If PKC activation is also relevant for reserpine-induced Parkinsonism it is still unknown.

Regardless of the specific mechanism related to the prevention of behavioral alterations found in the present study, there is evidence that increased oxidative stress underlies the physiopathology of neurodegenerative diseases such as PD [45-48]. Further, clinical data suggest that neuroprotective treatments based on increasing antioxidant defenses are able to delay the progression of the pathology [49-56]. Thus, a neuroprotective intervention could be a relevant line of investigation in animal models of this disease. However, the usual acute pharmacological models include severe motor impairment upon a single injection of reserpine or specific neurotoxins [4,57-60]. This approach is not suitable for the investigation for testing neuroprotective interventions because they usually present a preventive and/or a neurodegeneration delaying profile. Further, most of the previous studies investigating the effects of vitamin E treatments on PD models did not investigate progressive behavioral deficits related to the clinical symptoms of the disease [33,35-37]. In this sense, the need for animal models of PD more compatible with clinical outcomes when investigating neuroprotective therapies has been pointed out. Thus, the present findings reinforce the idea that the protocol of progressive Parkinsonism induction with reserpine is suitable for investigating possible neuroprotective interventions in animal models of PD.

In conclusion, concomitant treatment with alpha-tocopherol prevents behavioral alterations induced by repeated reserpine. Although the antioxidant action of vitamin E is probably related, the exact mechanism underlying this preventive effect remains to be investigated. Finally, the progressive behavioral motor and cognitive alterations induced by repeated reserpine treatment seems an adequate protocol to investigate possible neuroprotective interventions for PD.

Acknowledgments

The authors would like to thank Antonio Carlos Queiroz de Aquino for capable technical assistance. This study was supported by grants from Conselho Nacional de Desenvolvimento Científico e Tecnológico (CNPq, Brazil), Fundação de Amparo a Pesquisa do Estado do Rio Grande do Norte (FAPERN, Brazil), and Coordenação de Aperfeiçoamento de Pessoal de Nível Superior (CAPES, Brazil).

References

1. Henry JP, Sagné C, Botton D, Isambert MF, Gasnier B (1998) Molecular pharmacology of the vesicular monoamine transporter. Adv Pharmacol 42: 236-239.

2. Dauer W, Przedborski S (2003) Parkinson's disease: mechanisms and models. Neuron 39: 889-909.

3. Alves CS, Andreatini R, da Cunha C, Tufik S, Vital MA (2000) Phosphatidylserine reverses reserpine-induced amnesia. Eur J Pharmacol 404: 161-167.

4. Colpaert FC (1987) Pharmacological characteristics of tremor, rigidity and hypokinesia induced by reserpine in rat. Neuropharmacology 26: 1431-1440.

5. Skalisz LL, Beijamini V, Joca SL, Vital MA, Da Cunha C, et al. (2002) Evaluation of the face validity of reserpine administration as an animal model of depression--Parkinson's disease association. Prog Neuropsychopharmacol Biol Psychiatry 26: 879-883.

6. Carvalho RC, Patti CC, Takatsu-Coleman AL, Kameda SR, Souza CF, et al. (2006) Effects of reserpine on the plus-maze discriminative avoidance task: dissociation between memory and motor impairments. Brain Res 1122: 179-183.

7. Fernandes VS, Ribeiro AM, Melo TG, Godinho M, Barbosa FF, et al. (2008) Memory impairment induced by low doses of reserpine in rats: possible relationship with emotional processing deficits in Parkinson disease. Prog Neuropsychopharmacol Biol Psychiatry 32: 1479-1483.

8. Santos JR, Cunha JA, Dierschnabel AL, Campêlo CL, Leão AH, et al. (2013) Cognitive, motor and tyrosine hydroxylase temporal impairment in a model of parkinsonism induced by reserpine. Behav Brain Res 253: 68-77.

9. Fernandes VS, Santos JR, Leão AH, Medeiros AM, Melo TG, et al. (2012) Repeated treatment with a low dose of reserpine as a progressive model of Parkinson's disease. Behav Brain Res 231: 154-163.

10. Abílio VC, Araujo CC, Bergamo M, Calvente PR, D'Almeida V, et al. (2003) Vitamin E attenuates reserpine-induced oral dyskinesia and striatal oxidized glutathione/reduced glutathione ratio (GSSG/GSH) enhancement in rats. Prog Neuro-Psychopharmacol Biological Psychiatry 27:109–114.

11. Ebadi M, Srinivasan SK, Baxi MD (1996) Oxidative stress and antioxidant therapy in Parkinson's disease. Prog Neurobiol 48: 1-19.

12. Bavarsad Shahripour R, Harrigan MR, Alexandrov AV (2014) N-acetylcysteine (NAC) in neurological disorders: mechanisms of action and therapeutic opportunities. Brain Behav 4: 108-122.

13. Pérez-H J, Carrillo-S C, García E, Ruiz-Mar G, Pérez-Tamayo R, et al. (2014) Neuroprotective effect of silymarin in a MPTP mouse model of Parkinson's disease. Toxicology 319: 38-43.

14. Halliwell B, Gutteridge JM (2007) Free Radicals in Biology and Medicine. Oxford University Press.

15. Jiang Q (2014) Natural forms of vitamin E: metabolism, antioxidant, and anti-inflammatory activities and their role in disease prevention and therapy. Free Radic Biol Med 72: 76-90.

16. Sanberg PR, Bunsey MD, Giordano M, Norman AB (1988) The catalepsy test: its ups and downs. Behav Neurosci 102: 748-759.

17. de Lau LM, Breteler MM (2006) Epidemiology of Parkinson's disease. Lancet Neurol 5: 525-535.

18. Duty S, Jenner P (2011) Animal models of Parkinson's disease: a source of novel treatments and clues to the cause of the disease. Br J Pharmacol 164: 1357-1391.

19. Higginson CI, Wheelock VL, Carroll KE, Sigvardt KA (2005) Recognition memory in Parkinson's disease with and without dementia: evidence inconsistent with the retrieval deficit hypothesis. J Clin Exp Neuropsychol 27: 516-528.

20. Lewis SJ, Dove A, Robbins TW, Barker RA, Owen AM (2003) Cognitive impairments in early Parkinson's disease are accompanied by reductions in activity in frontostriatal neural circuitry. J Neurosci 23: 6351-6356.

21. Caudle WM, Colebrooke RE, Emson PC, Miller GW (2008) Altered vesicular dopamine storage in Parkinson's disease: a premature demise. Trends Neurosci 31: 303-308.

22. Bergström T, Ersson C, Bergman J, Möller L (2012) Vitamins at physiological levels cause oxidation to the DNA nucleoside deoxyguanosine and to DNA--alone or in synergism with metals. Mutagenesis 27: 511-517.

23. Osiecki M, Ghanavi P, Atkinson K, Nielsen LK, Doran MR (2010) The ascorbic acid paradox. Biochem Biophys Res Commun 400: 466-470.

24. Palozza P, Calviello G, Serini S, Maggiano N, Lanza P, et al. (2001) Beta-carotene at high concentrations induces apoptosis by enhancing oxy-radical production in human adenocarcinoma cells. Free Radic Biol Med 30: 1000-1007.

25. de Oliveira BF, Veloso CA, Nogueira-Machado JA, Martins Chaves M (2012) High doses of in vitro beta-carotene, alpha-tocopherol and ascorbic acid induce oxidative stress and secretion of IL-6 in peripheral blood mononuclear cells from healthy donors. Curr Aging Sci 5: 148-156.

26. Winterbone MS, Sampson MJ, Saha S, Hughes JC, Hughes DA (2007) Pro-oxidant effect of alpha-tocopherol in patients with type 2 diabetes after an oral glucose tolerance test--a randomised controlled trial. Cardiovasc Diabetol 22: 6-8.

27. Nadeem N, Woodside JV, Kelly S, Allister R, Young IS, et al. (2012) The two faces of α- and γ-tocopherols: an in vitro and ex vivo investigation into VLDL, LDL and HDL oxidation. J Nutr Biochem 23: 845-851.

28. Reich EE, Montine KS, Gross MD, Roberts LJ 2nd, Swift LL, et al. (2001) Interactions between apolipoprotein E gene and dietary alpha-tocopherol influence cerebral oxidative damage in aged mice. J Neurosci 21: 5993-5999.

29. Vatassery GT (1992) Vitamin E. Neurochemistry and implications for neurodegeneration in Parkinson's disease. Ann N Y Acad Sci 669: 97-109.

30. Casani S, Gómez-Pastor R, Matallana E, Paricio N (2013) Antioxidant compound supplementation prevents oxidative damage in a Drosophila model of Parkinson's disease. Free Radic Biol Med 61: 151-160.

31. Fariss MW, Zhang JG (2003) Vitamin E therapy in Parkinson's disease. Toxicology 189: 129-146.

32. Miklya I, Knoll B, Knoll J (2003) A pharmacological analysis elucidating why, in contrast to (-)-deprenyl (selegiline), alpha-tocopherol was ineffective in the DATATOP study. Life Sci 72: 2641-2648.

33. Butterfield DA, Castegna A, Drake J, Scapagnini G, Calabrese V (2002) Vitamin E and neurodegenerative disorders associated with oxidative stress. Nutr Neurosci 5: 229-239.

34. Roghani M, Behzadi G (2001) Neuroprotective effect of vitamin E on the early model of Parkinson's disease in rat: behavioral and histochemical evidence. Brain Res 892: 211-217.

35. Azzi A (2007) Molecular mechanism of alpha-tocopherol action. Free Radic Biol Med 43: 16-21.

36. Azzi A, Gysin R, Kempná P, Munteanu A, Negis Y, et al. (2004) Vitamin E mediates cell signaling and regulation of gene expression. Ann N Y Acad Sci 1031: 86-95.

37. Ferri P, Cecchini T, Ambrogini P, Betti M, Cuppini R, et al. (2006) alpha-Tocopherol affects neuronal plasticity in adult rat dentate gyrus: the possible role of PKCdelta. J Neurobiol 66: 793-810.

38. Azzi A, Ricciarelli R, Zingg JM (2002) Non-antioxidant molecular functions of alpha-tocopherol (vitamin E). FEBS Lett 519: 8-10.

39. Kanthasamy A, Jin H, Mehrotra S, Mishra R, Kanthasamy A, et al. (2010) Novel cell death signaling pathways in neurotoxicity models of dopaminergic degeneration: relevance to oxidative stress and neuroinflammation in Parkinson's disease. Neurotoxicology 31: 555-561.

40. Chalimoniuk M, Stolecka A, Zieminska E, Stepien A, Langfort J, Strosznajder JB (2009) Involvement of multiple protein kinases in cPLA2 phosphorylation,

arachidonic acid release, and cell death in in vivo and in vitro models of 1-methyl-4-phenylpyridinium-induced parkinsonism--the possible key role of PKG. J Neurochem 110: 307-317.

41. Cristóvão AC, Barata J, Je G, Kim YS (2013) PKCδ́ mediates paraquat-induced Nox1 expression in dopaminergic neurons. Biochem Biophys Res Commun 437: 380-385.

42. Beal MF (2002) Oxidatively modified proteins in aging and disease. Free Radic Biol Med 32: 797-803.

43. Beal MF (2003) Mitochondria, oxidative damage, and inflammation in Parkinson's disease. Ann N Y Acad Sci 991: 120-131.

44. Cadenas E, Davies KJ (2000) Mitochondrial free radical generation, oxidative stress, and aging. Free Radic Biol Med 29: 222-230.

45. Younes-Mhenni S, Frih-Ayed M, Kerkeni A, Bost M, Chazot G (2007) Peripheral blood markers of oxidative stress in Parkinson's disease. Eur Neurol 58: 78-83.

46. Abdel-Salam OM (2008) Drugs used to treat Parkinson's disease, present status and future directions. CNS Neurol Disord Drug Targets 7: 321-342.

47. Beal MF (2009) Therapeutic approaches to mitochondrial dysfunction in Parkinson's disease. Parkinsonism Relat Disord 15 Suppl 3: S189-194.

48. Chen JJ, Ly AV (2006) Rasagiline: A second-generation monoamine oxidase type-B inhibitor for the treatment of Parkinson's disease. Am J Health Syst Pharm 63: 915-928.

49. De Araújo DP, Lobato Rde F, Cavalcanti JR, Sampaio LR, Araújo PV, et al. (2011) The contributions of antioxidant activity of lipoic acid in reducing neurogenerative progression of Parkinson's disease: a review. Int J Neurosci 121: 51-57.

50. Magyar K, Pálfi M, Tábi T, Kalász H, Szende B, et al. (2004) Pharmacological aspects of (-)-deprenyl. Curr Med Chem 11: 2017-2031.

51. Mayo JC, Sainz RM, Tan DX, Antolín I, Rodríguez C, et al. (2005) Melatonin and Parkinson's disease. Endocrine 27: 169-178.

52. Weber CA, Ernst ME (2006) Antioxidants, supplements, and Parkinson's disease. Ann Pharmacother 40: 935-938.

53. Weinreb O, Amit T, Bar-Am O, Youdim MB (2010) Rasagiline: a novel anti-Parkinsonian monoamine oxidase-B inhibitor with neuroprotective activity. Prog Neurobiol 92: 330-344.

54. Hsieh MH, Gu SL, Ho SC, Pawlak CR, Lin CL, et al. (2012) Effects of MK-801 on recognition and neurodegeneration in an MPTP-induced Parkinson's rat model. Behav Brain Res 229: 41-47.

55. Marin C, Aguilar E (2011) In vivo 6-OHDA-induced neurodegeneration and nigral autophagic markers expression. Neurochem Int 58: 521-526.

56. Salamone J, Baskin P (1996) Vacuous jaw movements induced by acute reserpine and low-dose apomorphine: possible model of parkinsonian tremor. Pharmacol Biochem Behav 53: 179-183.

57. Salamone JD, Ishiwari K, Betz AJ, Farrar AM, Mingote SM et al. (2008) Dopamine/adenosine interactions related to locomotion and tremor in animal models: possible relevance to parkinsonism. Parkinsonism Relat Disord 14: S130-134.

58. Tetrud JW, Langston JW (1989) MPTP-induced parkinsonism as a model for Parkinson's disease. Acta Neurol Scand Suppl 126: 35-40.

59. Itoh N, Masuo Y, Yoshida Y, Cynshi O, Jishage K, et al. (2006) gamma-Tocopherol attenuates MPTP-induced dopamine loss more efficiently than alpha-tocopherol in mouse brain. Neurosci Lett 403: 136-140.

60. Kamat CD, Gadal S, Mhatre M, Williamson KS, Pye QN, et al. (2008) Antioxidants in central nervous system diseases: preclinical promise and translational challenges. J Alzheimers Dis 15: 473-493.

Permissions

All chapters in this book were first published in BP, by OMICS International; hereby published with permission under the Creative Commons Attribution License or equivalent. Every chapter published in this book has been scrutinized by our experts. Their significance has been extensively debated. The topics covered herein carry significant findings which will fuel the growth of the discipline. They may even be implemented as practical applications or may be referred to as a beginning point for another development.

The contributors of this book come from diverse backgrounds, making this book a truly international effort. This book will bring forth new frontiers with its revolutionizing research information and detailed analysis of the nascent developments around the world.

We would like to thank all the contributing authors for lending their expertise to make the book truly unique. They have played a crucial role in the development of this book. Without their invaluable contributions this book wouldn't have been possible. They have made vital efforts to compile up to date information on the varied aspects of this subject to make this book a valuable addition to the collection of many professionals and students.

This book was conceptualized with the vision of imparting up-to-date information and advanced data in this field. To ensure the same, a matchless editorial board was set up. Every individual on the board went through rigorous rounds of assessment to prove their worth. After which they invested a large part of their time researching and compiling the most relevant data for our readers.

The editorial board has been involved in producing this book since its inception. They have spent rigorous hours researching and exploring the diverse topics which have resulted in the successful publishing of this book. They have passed on their knowledge of decades through this book. To expedite this challenging task, the publisher supported the team at every step. A small team of assistant editors was also appointed to further simplify the editing procedure and attain best results for the readers.

Apart from the editorial board, the designing team has also invested a significant amount of their time in understanding the subject and creating the most relevant covers. They scrutinized every image to scout for the most suitable representation of the subject and create an appropriate cover for the book.

The publishing team has been an ardent support to the editorial, designing and production team. Their endless efforts to recruit the best for this project, has resulted in the accomplishment of this book. They are a veteran in the field of academics and their pool of knowledge is as vast as their experience in printing. Their expertise and guidance has proved useful at every step. Their uncompromising quality standards have made this book an exceptional effort. Their encouragement from time to time has been an inspiration for everyone.

The publisher and the editorial board hope that this book will prove to be a valuable piece of knowledge for researchers, students, practitioners and scholars across the globe.

List of Contributors

Schulz S, Gundelach J, Hayn L and Koch M
Brain Research Institute, Department of Neuropharmacology, University of Bremen, 28359 Bremen, Germany

Svärd HK
University of Oulu, Department of Biology, FIN-90140 University of Oulu, Finland

Christian Agyare, Yaw Duah Boakye, John Susana Oteng Dapaah, Theresa Appiah and Adobea Adow
Department of Pharmaceutics, Kwame Nkrumah University of Science and Technology, Kumasi, Ghana

Antwi Apenteng
Department of Pharmaceutical Science, Central University College, Accra, Ghana

Baraka AM and Guemei A
Department of Clinical Pharmacology, Faculty of Medicine, Alexandria University, Egypt

Yogesh Chand Yadav
Department of Pharmacology, Pharmacy College Saifai, Uttar Pradesh University of Medical Sciences, UP, India

Muthu K
Department of Zoology, Raja Serfoji College, Thanjavur-622 404, Tamil Nadu, India

Krishnamoorthy P
Department of Biotechnology, J. J.College of Arts and Science, Pudukottai-622 404, Tamil Nadu, India

Okpala JC
Department of Biochemistry, Ahmadu Bello University, Zaria, Kaduna State, Nigeria

Igwe JC
Department of Pharmaceutical Microbiology, Ahmadu Bello University, Zaria, Kaduna State, Nigeria

Ifedilichukwu HN
Department of Medical Biotechnology, National Biotechnology Development Agency, Abuja, Nigeria

Zhang Guanglei
Engineering Research Center for Feed Safety and Efficient Utilization of Ministry of Education, Institute of Animal Nutrition, Hunan Agricultural University, Hunan, 410128, China

Fan Zhiyong
Engineering Research Center for Feed Safety and Efficient Utilization of Ministry of Education, Institute of Animal Nutrition, Hunan Agricultural University, Hunan, 410128, China
State Key Laboratory of Animal Nutrition, Beijing 100081, China

Wang Fenglai
State Key Laboratory of Animal Nutrition, Beijing 100081, China

Zhou Dinggang and Liang Zhe
College of Animal Science and Technology, Sichuan Agricultural University, Yaan, 625014, China

Wu Xin
Hunan Provincial Engineering Research Center of Healthy Livestock, Key Laboratory of Agro-ecological Processes in Subtropical Region, Institute of Subtropical Agriculture, Chinese Academy of Sciences, Changsha, Hunan 410125, China

Muhammad Tahir Haidry and Arif Malik
Institute of Molecular Biology and Biotechnology, The University of Lahore-Pakistan, Pakistan

Qiong Luo, Yang Sun, Biao Jin, Wei Zheng, Fenli Shao, Nan Hang and Qiang Xu
State Key Laboratory of Pharmaceutical Biotechnology, School of Life Sciences, Nanjing University, 22 Hankou Road, Nanjing 210093, China

Yongqian Shu and Yanhong Gu
Department of Oncology, The First Affiliated Hospital with Nanjing Medical University, 300 Guangzhou Road, Nanjing 210029, China

Xiaomin Li
Department of Emergency, The First People's Hospital of Lianyungang, Lianyungang, Jiangsu 222002, China

Tabarak Malik
Department of Biochemistry, Lovely Professional University-144402, India

Pandey DK
Department of Biotechnology, Lovely Professional University-144402, India

Gupta GSD
Division of Petroleum Toxicology, Indian Institute of Toxicology Research- 226 001, India

Eun Jung Park
Korean Medicine Convergence Research Division, Korea Institute of Oriental Medicine (KIOM), 1672 Yuseongdae-ro, Yuseong-gu, Daejeon, South Korea

Young Sook Kim, Nu Ri Kang and Jin Sook Kim
Korean Medicine Convergence Research Division, Korea Institute of Oriental Medicine (KIOM), 1672 Yuseongdae-ro, Yuseong-gu, Daejeon, South Korea
Korean Medicine Life Science, University of Science Technology (UST), 217 Gajeong-ro, Yuseong-gu, Daejeon, South Korea

Qin JD
Department of Pediatrics, The University of Chicago, Chicago, USA
Department of Biochemistry, Hebrew University School of Medicine, Jerusalem, Israel

Gatt S
Department of Biochemistry, Hebrew University School of Medicine, Jerusalem, Israel

Dagan A
Department of Biochemistry, Hebrew University School of Medicine, Jerusalem, Israel
Department of Biochemistry and Molecular Biology, Institute for Medical Research Israel-Canada, Hebrew-University-Hadassah School of Medicine, Jerusalem, Israel

Weiss L, Zeira M and Yekhtin Z
Department of Bone-Marrow Transplantation, Hadassah–Hebrew University of Medical Center, Jerusalem, Israel

Slavin S
Department of Bone-Marrow Transplantation, Hadassah–Hebrew University of Medical Center, Jerusalem, Israel
The International Center for Cell Therapy & Cancer Immunotherapy, Tel Aviv, Israel

Youping Yang
The first People's Hospital of Wenling, Wenling, Zhejiang, 317500, China

Hongxia Lin, Yangli Zhu, Hongwei Wu, Ruoyan Wang, Jianmin Zhang and Rongbiao Ying
Taizhou Cancer Hospital, Wenling, Zhejiang, 317500, China

Linghui Zeng and Ximei Wu
Zhejiang University, Hangzhou, Zhejiang, 310058, China

Pushparani DS
Department of Biochemistry, SRM Dental College, SRM University, Ramapuram, Chennai-600089, Tamil Nadu, India

Oliveira AG and Gomes-Marcondes MCC
Department of Structural and Functional Biology, Institute of Biology, State University of Campinas – UNICAMP Campinas, Brazil

Ashu Michael Agbor
Universite des Montagnes, Dental surgery, Bangangte, Cameroon

Barrow K, Jiang C and Lü J
Department of Biomedical Sciences, School of Pharmacy, Texas Tech University Health Sciences Center, 1300 South Coulter Street, Amarillo, TX79106, USA

Saimei Yan, Ting Wang and Cui Yang
Key Laboratory of Ethnic Medicine Resource Chemistry, State Ethnic Affairs Commission & Ministry of Education, Yunnan Minzu University, Kunming 650500, P.R. China

Changhong Zhang, Peng Wang and Xiangting Xu
School of Pharmaceutical Science & Yunnan Key Laboratory of Pharmacology for Natural Products, Kunming Medical University, Kunming 650500, P.R. China

Jihong Yang
School of Pharmaceutical Science & Yunnan Key Laboratory of Pharmacology for Natural Products, Kunming Medical University, Kunming 650500, P.R. China
Guangxi Weimei Biotechnology Co., Ltd., Nanning 530100, P.R. China

Umoren EB and Osim EE
Department of Physiology, College of Medical Sciences, University of Calabar, Calabar, Nigeria

Xin-shang Wang, Zhen Tian, Xu-bo Li, Le Yang, Ming-gao Zhao and Shui-bing Liu
Department of Pharmacology, School of Pharmacy, Fourth Military Medical University, Xi'an, Shaanxi 710032, China

Hong-liang Guo
Department of Pharmacology, School of Pharmacy, Fourth Military Medical University, Xi'an, Shaanxi 710032, China
Department of Pharmacy, Fifth Hospital of PLA, Yin chuan, Ning xia 750004, China

Jiao Tian
Department of Pediatrics, Tangdu Hospital, Fourth Military Medical University, Xi'an, Shaanxi 710038, China

Rui-hua Xu
Department of Medical Oncology, Sun Yat-Sen University Cancer Center, State Key Laboratory of Oncology in Southern China, Guangzhou 510060, People's Republic of China

Hui-yan Luo
Department of Medical Oncology, Sun Yat-Sen University Cancer Center, State Key Laboratory of Oncology in Southern China, Guangzhou 510060, People's Republic of China
Department of Biomedical Engineering, School of Engineering, Sun Yat-sen University, Guangzhou, Guangdong 510006, People's Republic of China

Heba MI Abdallah, Rehab F Abdel-Rahman, Gehad A Abdel Jaleel, Salma A El-Marasy, Samir AE Bashandy and Mahmoud S Arbid
Department of Pharmacology, National Research Centre, Cairo, Egypt

Heba AM Abd El-Kader
Department of Cell Biology, National Research Centre, Cairo, Egypt

Eman R Zaki
Department of Molecular Biology, National Research Centre, Cairo, Egypt

Abdel Razik H Farrag
Department of Pathology, National Research Centre, Cairo, Egypt

Muñoz O
Chemistry Department, Faculty of Science, University of Chile, Santiago, Chile
Chilean Society of Phytotherapy (SOCHIFITO), Chile

Bustamante S
Chilean Society of Phytotherapy (SOCHIFITO), Chile
Program of Molecular and Clinical Pharmacology, Faculty of Medicine, University of Chile, Avda, Independencia 1027, Santiago, Chile

Muñoz R
School of Medicine, University of Chile, Avda, Independencia 1027, Santiago, Chile

Adegbegi J Ademuyiwa and Jose R Adeolu
Department of Science Laboratory Technology, Rufus Giwa Polytechnic, Owo, Ondo State, Nigeria

Adefegha S Adeniyi
Department of Biochemistry, Federal University of Technology, Akure, Ondo State, Nigeria

Boucherit Hanane, Chikhi Abdelouahab, Bensegueni Abderrahmane, Merzoug Amina, Hioual Khadidja Soulef and Mokrani El Hassen
Laboratory of Applied Biology and Health, Department of Biochemistry-Microbiology, Faculty of Natural And Life Sciences, Mentouri University, Constantine, Algeria

Hyunshun Shin and Heather Whitehead
Department of Chemistry and Biochemistry, McMurry University, McM station Box 158, Abilene, TX 79697, USA

Xian Zhou
Department of Chemistry, University of Iowa, Iowa City, IA 52242-1294, USA

Karl L Banta and Juliet V Spencer
Department of Biology, University of San Francisco, 2130 Fulton Street, San Francisco, CA 94117, USA

Myung K Cho and Sung-Kun Kim
Department of Chemistry and Biochemistry, Baylor University, Waco, TX 76798-7348, USA

Omale James, Abbah Okpachi Christopher, Ojogbane Eleojo Berikisu, David Ede Patience and Adah Gabriel Onuche
Faculty of Natural Sciences, Department of Biochemistry, Kogi State University, P.M.B. 1008, Anyigba, Kogi State, Nigeria

Joseph Molnár, Ilona Mucsi, Helga Engi and Gabriela Spengler
Institute of Medical Microbiology and Immunobiology, University of Szeged, Szeged, Hungary

Leonard Amaral
Institute of Medical Microbiology and Immunobiology, University of Szeged, Szeged, Hungary
Travel Medicine, Center for Malaria and other Tropical Diseases (CMDT), Institute of Hygiene and Tropical Medicine of Lisbon, Universidade Nove de Lisboa, Lisbon, Portugal

Attila Zalatnai
Department of Pathology, University of Semmelweis, Budapest, Hungary

Qi Wang
Department of Respiratory Medicine, the Second Affiliated Hospital of Dalian Medical University, Dalian, China

Ben Efraim Shlomo
Department of Human Microbiology Sackler, Faculty of Medicine, Tel-Aviv –University, Tel Aviv, 62155, Israel

Adetuyi BO, Dairo JO and Didunyemi OM
Department of Biochemistry, College of Natural Sciences, Joseph Ayo Babalola University, Ikeji-Arakeji, Ilesa, Osun State, Nigeria

Xia Xichao, Wang Weina, Hu Qingfu, Liang Guina, Zhang Dong and Liu Rongzhi
Department of Basic Medicine, Nanyang Medical College, Nanyang, 473041, Henan Province, China

Liu Hongyang
Department of Plant Pathology, Nanyang Agriculture School, Nanyang, 473002, Henan Province, China

Liu Fei
Department of Clinical Medicine, Nanyang Medical College, Nanyang, 473041, Henan Province, China

Amy M Birch, Jonathan Cheung, Christianah Oluwadare, James Burton and Magdalena Sastre
Division of Brain Sciences, Imperial College London, Hammersmith Hospital, W12 0NN, UK

Wenlong Huang and Amparo Novejarque
Department of Surgery and Cancer, Imperial College London, Chelsea and Westminster Hospital, SW10 9NH, UK

Julia Inglis
School of Medicine and Pharmacology, University of Western Australia, Perth, WA 6009, Australia

Aldair José Sarmento-Silva, Ramón Hypolito Lima, Alicia Cabral and Ywlliane Meurer
Memory Studies Laboratory, Physiology Department, Federal University of Rio Grande do Norte, Natal, Brazil

Alessandra Mussi Ribeiro
Memory Studies Laboratory, Physiology Department, Federal University of Rio Grande do Norte, Natal, Brazil
Department of Biosciences, Federal University of São Paulo, Santos, Brazil

Regina Helena Silva
Memory Studies Laboratory, Physiology Department, Federal University of Rio Grande do Norte, Natal, Brazil
Department of Pharmacology, Federal University of São Paulo, São Paulo, Brazil

Index